Clinical Forensic Psychology and Law

The International Library of Psychology
Series Editor: David Canter

Titles in the Series:

Human Perception
Marco Bertamini and Michael Kubovy

Environmental Psychology
David Canter, Terry Hartig and Mirilia Bonnes

Hypnosis
Michael Heap and Irving Kirsch

Interpersonal Development
Brett Laursen and Rita Žukauskienė

Counseling Psychology
Frederick Leong

Psychology of Aging
Martin Orrell and Aimee Spector

Psychology and Law
Ronald Roesch and Nathalie Gagnon

Clinical Forensic Psychology and Law
Ronald Roesch and Kaitlyn McLachlan

Parapsychology I
Richard Wiseman and Caroline Watt

History of Psychology Revisited
William Woodward

Clinical Forensic Psychology and Law

Edited by

Ronald Roesch and Kaitlyn McLachlan

Simon Fraser University, Canada

ASHGATE

Published by
Ashgate Publishing Limited
Gower House
Croft Road
Aldershot
Hampshire GU11 3HR
England

Ashgate Publishing Company
Suite 420
101 Cherry Street
Burlington, VT 05401-4405
USA

Ashgate website: http://www.ashgate.com

British Library Cataloguing in Publication Data
Clinical forensic psychology and law. – (International library of psychology)
1. Law – Psychological aspects 2. Forensic psychology
I. Roesch, Ronald, 1947 –II. Mclachlan, Kaitlyn
340. 1′ 9

Library of Congress Cataloging-in-Publication Data
Clinical forensic psychology and law / edited by Ronald Roesch and Kaitlyn McLachlan
p. ; cm. – (International library of psychology)
Includes bibliographical references and index.
ISBN: 978-0-7546-2619-0 (Hardback: alk paper)
1. Forensic psychology. I. Roesch, Ronald, 1947– II. McLachlan, Kaitlyn. III. Series
[DNLM: 1. Forensic Psychiatry – Collected Works. 2. Psychology –legislation & jurisprudence – Collected Works. W 740 C6405 2007]

RA1148.C57 2007
614'.15–dc22

2007002018

ISBN: 978-0-7546-2619-0

Printed in Great Britain by TJ International Ltd, Padstow, Cornwall

Contents

PART III FORENSIC TREATMENT

PART IV YOUTH ASSESSMENT AND INTERVENTION

Acknowledgements

The editors and publishers wish to thank the following for permission to use copyright material.

American Medical Association for the essay: Linda A. Teplin, Karen M. Abram, Gary M. McClelland, Mina K. Dulcan and Amy A. Mericle (2002), 'Psychiatric Disorders in Youth in Juvenile Detention', *Archives of General Psychiatry*, **59**, pp. 1133–43. Copyright © 2002 American Medical Association.

American Psychological Association for the essay: Donald N. Bersoff, Jane Goodman-Delahunty, J. Thomas Grisso, Valerie P. Hans, Norman G. Poythress Jr and Ronald G. Roesch (1997), 'Training in Law and Psychology: Models from the Villanova Conference', *American Psychologist*, **52**, pp. 1301–10. Copyright © 1997 American Psychological Association; R. Karl Hanson and Kelly E. Morton-Bourgon (2005), 'The Characteristics of Persistent Sexual Offenders: A Meta-Analysis of Recidivism Studies', *Journal of Consulting and Clinical Psychology*, **73**, pp. 1154–63. Copyright © 2005 American Psychological Association; Randy K. Otto and Kirk Heilbrun (2002), 'The Practice of Forensic Psychology: A Look Toward the Future in Light of the Past', *American Psychologist*, **57**, pp. 5–18. Copyright © 2002 American Psychological Association; Stuart A. Greenberg and Daniel W. Shuman (1997), 'Irreconcilable Conflict Between Therapeutic and Forensic Roles', *Professional Psychology Research and Practice*, **28**, pp. 50–57. Copyright © 1997 American Psychological Association; Edward P. Mulvey and Elizabeth Cauffman (2001), 'The Inherent Limits of Predicting School Violence', *American Psychologist*, **50**, pp. 797–802. Copyright © 1997 American Psychological Association.

Blackwell Publishing Limited for the essay: Robert E. Emery, Randy K. Otto and William T. O'Donohue, (2005), 'A Critical Assessment of Child Custody Evaluations: Limited Science and a Flawed System', *Psychological Science in the Public Interest*, **6**, pp. 1–29. Copyright © 2005 American Psychological Association, Inc.

British Psychological Society for the essay: Kevin S. Douglas, David N. Cox and Christopher D. Webster (1999), 'Violence Risk Assessment: Science and Practice', *Legal and Criminological Psychology*, **4**, pp. 149–84. Copyright © 1999 British Psychological Society.

Cambridge University Press for the essay: Rolf Loeber and David P. Farrington (2000), 'Young Children Who Commit Crime: Epidemiology, Developmental Origins, Risk Factors, Early Interventions, and Policy Implications', *Development and Psychopathology*, **12**, pp. 737–62. Copyright © 2000 Cambridge University Press.

Elsevier Ltd for the essays: Randall T. Salekin (2002), 'Psychopathy and Therapeutic Pessimism: Clinical Lore or Clinical Reality?', *Clinical Psychology Review*, **22**, pp. 79–112. Copyright © 2002 Clinical Psychology Review; David J. Cooke, Christine Michie, Stephen D. Hart and Danny Clark (2005), 'Searching for the Pan-Cultural Core of Psychopathic Personality Disorder', *Personality and Individual Differences*, **39**, pp. 283–95. Copyright © 2005 Elsevier Ltd.

International Journal of Forensic Mental Health for the essay: Henrik Belfrage and Kevin S. Douglas (2002), 'Treatment Effects on Forensic Psychiatric Patients Measured with the HCR-20 Violence Risk Assessment Scheme', *International Journal of Forensic Mental Health*, **1**, pp. 25–36. Copyright © 2002 International Association of Forensic Mental Health.

John Wiley and Sons Ltd for the essay: Richard J. Bonnie (1992), 'The Competence of Criminal Defendants: A Theoretical Reformulation', *Behavioral Sciences and the Law*, **10**, pp. 291–316. Copyright © 1992 John Wiley and Sons Ltd; Merith Cosden, Jeffrey K. Ellens, Jeffrey L. Schnell, Yasmeen Yamini-Diouf and Maren M. Wolfe (2003), 'Evaluation of a Mental Health Treatment Court with Assertive Community Treatment', *Behavioral Sciences and the Law*, **21**, pp. 415–27. Copyright © 2003 John Wiley and Sons Ltd.

Lippincott Williams and Wilkins for the essay: Charles M. Borduin (1999), 'Multisystemic Treatment of Criminality and Violence in Adolescents', *Journal of the American Academy of Child and Adolescent Psychiatry*, **38**, pp. 242–49. Copyright © 1999 American Academy of Child and Adolescent Psychiatry.

Sage Publications Inc for the essays: Caroline Friendship, Ruth E. Mann and Anthony R. Beech (2003), 'Evaluation of a National Prison-Based Treatment Program for Sexual Offenders in England and Wales', *Journal of Interpersonal Violence*, **18**, pp. 744–59. Copyright © 2003 Sage Publications; Francis T. Cullen and Paul Gendreau (2001), 'From Nothing Works to What Works: Changing Professional Ideology in the 21st Century', *Prison Journal*, **81**, pp. 313–38. Copyright © 2001 Sage Publications; Randy Borum (2003), 'Managing At-Risk Juvenile Offenders in the Community: Putting Evidence-Based Principles into Practice', *Journal of Contemporary Criminal Justice*, **19**, pp. 114–37. Copyright © 2003 Sage Publications.

Springer for the essays: Kirk Heilbrun (1997), 'Prediction Versus Management Models Relevant to Risk Assessment: The Importance of Legal Decision-Making Context', *Law and Human Behavior*, **21**, pp. 347–59. Copyright © 1997 American Psychology - Law Society; Patricia A. Zapf and Ronald Roesch (2005), 'An Investigation of the Construct of Competence: A Comparison of the FIT, the MacCAT-CA, and the MacCAT-T', *Law and Human Behavior*, **29**, pp. 229–52. Copyright © 2005 Springer Science; Paul S. Appelbaum and Thomas Grisso (1995), 'The MacArthur Treatment Competence Study I: Mental Illness and Competence to Consent to Treatment', *Law and Human Behavior*, **19**, pp. 105–26. Copyright © 1995 Plenum Publishing Corporation; Pamela Clark Robbins, John Monahan and Eric Silver (2003), 'Mental Disorder, Violence, and Gender', *Law and Human Behavior*, **27**, pp. 561–71. Copyright © 2003 American Psychology - Law Society; William J. Koch, Melanie O'Neill and Kevin S. Douglas (2005), 'Empirical Limits for the Forensic Assessment of PTSD Litigants', *Law and Human Behavior*, **29**, pp. 121–49. Copyright © 2005 Springer Science and Business Media Inc.; Thomas Grisso, Laurence Steinberg, Jennifer Woolard, Elizabeth Cauffman, Elizabeth Scott, Sandra Graham, Fran Lexcen, N. Dickon Reppucci and Robert Schwartz (2003), 'Juveniles' Competence to Stand Trial: A Comparison of Adolescents' and Adults' Capacities as Trial Defendants', *Law and Human Behavior*, **27**, pp. 333–63. Copyright © 2003 American Psychology; Robert A. Nicholson and Steve Norwood (2000), 'The Quality of Forensic Psychological Assessments, Reports, and Testimony: Acknowledging the Gap Between Promise and Practice', *Law and Human Behavior*, **24**, pp. 9–44. Copyright © 2000 American Psychology - Law Society; John Petrila (2004), 'Emerging Issues in Forensic Mental Health', *Psychiatric Quarterly*, **75**, pp. 3–19. Copyright © 2004 Human Science Press, Inc; Candice L. Odgers, Marlene Moretti and N. Dickon Reppucci (2005), 'Examining the Science and Practice of Violence Risk Assessment with Female Adolescents', *Law and Human Behavior*, **29**, pp. 7–27. Copyright © 2005 American Psychology - Law Society.

Every effort has been made to trace all the copyright holders, but if any have been inadvertently overlooked the publishers will be pleased to make the necessary arrangement at the first opportunity.

Series Preface

Psychology now touches every corner of our lives. No serious consideration of any newsworthy topic, from eating disorders to crime, from terrorism to new age beliefs, from trauma to happiness, is complete without some examination of what systematic, scientific psychology has to say on these matters. This means that psychology now runs the gamut from neuroscience to sociology, by way of medicine and anthropology, geography and molecular biology, connecting to virtually every area of scientific and professional life. This diversity produces a vibrant and rich discipline in which every area of activity finds outlets across a broad spectrum of publications.

Those who wish to gain an understanding of any area of psychology therefore either have to rely on secondary sources or, if they want to connect with the original contributions that define any domain of the discipline, must hunt through many areas of the library, often under diverse headings.

The volumes in this series obviate those difficulties by bringing together under one set of covers, carefully selected existing publications that are the definitive papers that characterize a specific topic in psychology.

The editors for each volume have been chosen because they are internationally recognized authorities. Therefore the selection of each editor, and the way in which it is organized into discrete sections, is an important statement about the field.

Each volume of the International Library of Psychology thus collects in one place the seminal and definitive journal articles that are creating current understanding of a specific aspect of present-day psychology. As a resource for study and research the volumes ensure that scholars and other professionals can gain ready access to original source material. As a statement of the essence of the topic covered they provide a benchmark for understanding and evaluating that aspect of psychology.

As this International Library emerges over the coming years it will help to specify what the nature of 21st century psychology is and what its contribution is to the future of humanity.

DAVID CANTER
Series Editor
Professor of Psychology
University of Liverpool, UK

Introduction

Many trace the beginning of psychology and law to the early part of the twentieth century. In 1908 Hugo Munsterberg published *On the Witness Stand*, a book in which he presented a case for increased roles for psychologists in the legal system on issues such as eyewitness testimony, false confessions and even hypnotism. Munsterberg's book was promptly met with criticism, notably by John Henry Wigmore (1909), who put Munsterberg 'on trial' for making false claims about the value of psychology's contributions to the law. At about the same time, psychology and law was gaining a foothold in Europe. Pozzulo, Bennell and Forth (2006) note that the first witness to provide expert testimony (on the topic of the effect of pre-trial publicity on memory) in Europe took place in Germany in 1896, and later, in 1911, a Belgian psychologist testified in a murder case about the reliability of child witnesses.

Although these early activities are important from an historical perspective, it was some time before psychology began to develop a major role in the legal arena. Indeed, no substantive growth of psychology and law took place until the latter part of the twentieth century when an increasing number of psychologists became attracted to the field, professional associations were formed, and journals devoted solely to psychology and law topics were initiated. In this Introduction we will provide a brief overview of the field and a discussion of the sub-areas of psychology and law that are reflected in this volume.

Psychology and Law Defined

Psychology and law is a broad field that encompasses a range of roles that psychologists may play in providing psychological knowledge, expertise or services to the legal system. The field is sometimes referred to as forensic psychology, but others refer to it as legal psychology or simply as psychology and law. 'The Specialty Guidelines for Forensic Psychologists' define forensic psychology as referring to:

> … all forms of professional psychological conduct when acting, with definable foreknowledge, as a psychological expert on explicitly psycholegal issues, in direct assistance to courts, parties to legal proceedings, correctional and forensic mental health facilities, and administrative, judicial, and legislative agencies acting in an adjudicative capacity. (Committee on Ethical Guidelines for Forensic Psychologists, 1991, p. 657)[1]

For convenience, in this Introduction we will use the terms 'forensic psychology' and 'psychology and law' to refer to the involvement of psychologists in the legal system in a broad range of roles. This includes psychologists with backgrounds and training in clinical, social,

[1] We had originally intended to include the 'Specialty Guidelines' in this volume, but they are currently undergoing a major revision so we instead refer the interested reader to the update on the American Psychology-Law Society webpage (http://www.ap-ls.org/links/professionalsgfp.html).

developmental, neuropsychological or other subdisciplines of psychology. One prominent area for forensic psychologists is court-ordered assessments. This includes assessments of risk for violence, competence to stand trial, criminal responsibility (the insanity defence), treatment amenability, child custody, child sexual abuse and many others. Other clinical forensic contributions include the treatment of offenders.

Forensic psychologists are also involved in many other activities that are not clinical in nature. Research is, of course, one area that encompasses forensic psychologists from different subdisciplines. Other applied activities include trial consultancy, in which psychologists help legal teams select trial jurors or conduct surveys to examine effects of pre-trial publicity on a given case. Another area is research and expert testimony on eyewitness reliability. Thus, there are many roles for psychologists as clinicians, researchers and legal scholars. The complexity and differing roles that psychology can play in the legal arena is captured in an encompassing model provided by Craig Haney (1980).

Haney's Taxonomy

Haney (1980) has developed a threefold taxonomy for understanding the multiple relationships of psychology and law: psychology *in* the law, psychology *and* law, and psychology *of* law. Psychology *in* the law refers to the 'explicit and conventional use of psychology by lawyers in the legal process' (Haney, 1980, p. 153). Examples include psychological testimony on legal issues such as the insanity defence or competency to stand trial, but also expert consultation in jury trials, including jury selection. Psychology *and* law involves the use of 'psychological principles to analyse and examine the legal system' (ibid., p. 154). Examples include research on eyewitness accuracy, false confessions and judicial decision-making. Psychology *of* law, in which psychologists study issues such as why people need the law and why people obey the law, is the third relationship.

Haney notes that the roles and expectations of psychologists are different for each of these three relationships. In the first relationship, psychologists have a more passive role, since the law defines the legal concepts that psychologists are asked to address. The second and third relationships provide more autonomous roles for psychologists in that they can define the legal issues which they address. Haney comments that while the majority of psychologists are involved *in* the law, it is the other two relationships in which psychologists might have the most impact on legal change through research that examines how the law actually works or studies of changes that might improve legal procedures. An example of this is the research on police line-ups, which formed the basis for recommendations by an APLS subcommittee for changes in line-up and photospread procedures, many of which have been adopted by police throughout the United States (see Wells *et al.*, 1998).

Training in Psychology and Law

When the field of psychology and law began to expand in the 1970s, the majority of psychologists who conducted research or engaged in practice were not specifically trained in psychology and law. This began to change with the creation of the first psychology and law graduate programme by the University of Nebraska in 1973 (Krauss and Sales, 2006).

Since then, programmes have been established in many other universities in the United States, Canada, Europe, Australia and elsewhere in the world. Some of them adopt the scientist–practitioner model of clinical training, offering basic training in clinical psychology but with an emphasis on forensic applications. Other programmes are non-clinical in nature, focusing on training in more traditional fields of psychology, such as social, developmental or other experimental areas of psychology. A few universities offer joint degrees, with students obtaining a PhD and a law degree (see Bersoff *et al.*, Chapter 25, this volume, for a discussion of training models). In addition to graduate programmes, forensic psychologists participate in workshops and other continuing education programmes in order to keep up to date with the latest advances in psychology and law.

Professional Associations

There are a number of professional groups that represent forensic psychology. In North America, the primary group is the American Psychology - Law Society (APLS), which is an interdisciplinary organization devoted to scholarship, practice and public service in psychology and law (see Grisso, 1991 for a history of the APLS). The APLS is a free-standing organization as well as a division (Division 41) of the American Psychological Association. In Europe, the European Association of Psychology and Law (EAPL) is the representative association, and in Australia and New Zealand, it is the Australian and New Zealand Association for Psychiatry, Psychology and the Law (ANZAPPL). The three associations hold a joint scholarly conference every four years, in order to promote international collaborations and presentation of the latest research findings. Law and Human Behavior, which began publication in 1977, was the first journal devoted entirely to law and psychology. Since then, many new journals have entered the field, reflecting the substantial increases in research and practice that psychology and law has enjoyed over the past 40 years. The list is extensive but includes *Criminal Behavior and Mental Health, Behavioral Sciences and the Law and Legal and Criminological Psychology.*

Volume Overview

This book is one of two volumes in the International Library of Psychology series published by Ashgate. The other volume (Roesch and Gagnon, 2007) includes essays on five major areas within psychology and law: eyewitnesses, memory, and the law; police investigations, lie detection and false confessions; jury research; civil forensic issues; and social science and the law.

The essays selected for this volume were limited to papers published in journals and they reflect five primary sub-areas of clinical forensic psychology: criminal forensic assessment; civil forensic assessment; forensic treatment; youth assessment and intervention; and forensic practice: professional and ethical issues. A brief overview of each of these sections is offered below.

Criminal Forensic Assessment

The criminal forensic assessment literature spans a broad range of theoretical and practice issues across a number of assessment areas. For Part I of this volume we have chosen to include essays that address the two major practice areas within criminal forensic assessment – risk prediction and the assessment of criminal competency. There are many other forensic assessment topics, but limitations of space precludes their inclusion (the interested reader is referred to Heilbrun, 2001; Heilbrun, Marczyk and DeMatteo, 2002; Roesch, Viljoen and Hui, 2004).

Within the last 20 years, the forensic risk assessment literature has witnessed a boom in research on risk factors and the development of risk assessment instruments. During the 1960s and 1970s the primary conclusion from the small amount of research on predicting risk was that there was an excessively high number of false positives (those predicted to be violent but who were not), supporting the view that mental health professionals were not accurate predictors of violence (Litwack and Schlesinger, 1999; Monahan, 1981). In the early 1980s the amount of research and subsequent improvements in risk assessment began to change, stimulated in large part by John Monahan's *Predicting Violent Behavior* (1981). In this book Monahan acknowledged the poor record of clinicians, but also identified a number of promising approaches that could help advance the field. This second generation of research led to more sophisticated and empirically-based risk assessment instruments. Research using these instruments showed that accuracy rates improved substantially (Borum, 1996; Douglas and Webster, 1999; Monahan and Steadman, 1994). However, despite these advances, prediction errors, while fewer, remain an important consideration in judging the utility of risk assessments. As Otto has commented, 'mental health professionals still make a considerable number of incorrect predictions, with false positives being the most common type of error' (1992, p. 128).

These and other risk assessment issues are discussed Chapter 1. Here, Kevin Douglas, David Cox and Christopher Webster outline a scientifically informed conceptual framework for violence risk assessment guided by the scientist–practitioner model of training in clinical psychology, which explicitly bases clinical practice on research findings when possible. In the area of risk assessment this has resulted in substantial improvements in the ability to make predictions about future risk and, perhaps more importantly, about how to manage risk (Borum, 1996; Heilbrun, 2001; Litwack, Zapf, Groscup and Hart, 2006). Douglas and his colleagues review key conceptual issues for clinicians, including definitions of violence and violence risk assessment, clinical versus actuarial prediction, and the validity of violence risk prediction. They also present a series of robust risk factors for the prediction of violence and discuss the importance of empirically-validated structured clinical decision-making.

In Chapter 2 Kirk Heilbrun describes two models of risk assessment relevant to various legal decisions, including both risk prediction and risk management. In contrast to the focus on risk prediction in much of the theoretical and historical literature, Heilbrun makes the case for an increased emphasis on risk reduction. His essay includes an informative discussion regarding the appropriateness of these models within a variety of different legal decision-making contexts and also describes the relevance of management/treatment-oriented risk decisions. As a result of this rich clinical–legal review, Heilbrun concludes that careful consideration of the legal context in which forensic mental health professionals are working will help to increase the relevance and accuracy of the information that they provide to legal decision-makers.

Turning from broader to more narrow considerations within the field of criminal forensic assessment and the risk prediction literature, the next two chapters in Part I have been selected as informative examples of specific issues encountered by forensic mental health practitioners. In Chapter 3 David Cooke, Christine Michie, Stephen Hart and Danny Clark generally introduce personality disorder and psychopathy and provide an instructive discussion of cross-cultural issues. In their study the authors investigate the cross-cultural validity of the construct of psychopathy, as measured by the Psychopathy Checklist-Revised (PCL-R), by comparing the psychopathy ratings of offenders from Canada, the United States and a number of European countries, and their results provide evidence for significant cultural bias in PCL-R ratings. This study also employs a sophisticated statistical evaluation of the psychometric properties of the PCL-R across cultural samples, which will be useful as a model for students and practitioners interested in conducting this type of research. Chapter 4 moves from the assessment of violence risk towards the specific risk factors associated with sexual recidivism. Karl Hanson and Kelly Morton-Bourgnon present the results from their meta-analysis of 82 recidivism studies and identify several major predictors of sexual recidivism for adult and adolescent sexual offenders. The authors suggest that their findings, in addition to informing forensic clinicians involved in applied risk assessments with sexual offenders, may also be useful for professionals and researchers who wish to develop new, or improve existing, treatment programmes for sexual offenders.

The final two chapters in Part I focus on the second major area within criminal forensic assessment, and review issues relevant to the assessment of criminal competence. The legal concept of competence to stand trial has its foundation in English common law and is designed to protect the rights of defendants to a fair trial (Roesch, Zapf, Golding and Skeem, 1999). A defendant can be found incompetent to stand trial if he or she is unable to understand or participate adequately in his or her defence. If found incompetent, trial proceedings are suspended and the defendant is treated until competence is restored, at which time the trial may then resume. Psychologists have developed a number of forensic assessment instruments to assess trial competence (see Poythress *et al.*, 1999; Roesch, Zapf and Eaves, 2006).

Chapter 5, by Richard Bonnie, was selected because it constitutes a major theoretical turning point for the conceptualization of the construct of criminal competence. Bonnie's reformulation of competency continues to inform forensic mental health professionals and researchers working in this field today. In this essay he proposes two primary types of competence. The first, competence to assist counsel, refers to the minimum conditions required to participate in one's own defence, such as understanding the charges and ability to communicate with counsel. The second is decisional competence, which focuses on a defendant's decision-making ability regarding legal options. He argues that the standards for evaluating each type of competence should be fundamentally different. He notes that defendants unable to assist counsel would need to be found incompetent and proceedings suspended until competence is restored. However, defendants who have diminished decision-making ability could proceed with a defence if a lawyer is able to present a defence and make decisions on behalf of the client. Bonnie also reviews important legal principles informing criminal competence.

The final chapter in Part I is a research essay, by Patricia Zapf and Ronald Roesch, examining the issue of criminal competence. They investigate the construct of competence in two different domains and the specific abilities required of different competencies. They question the appropriateness of a North American legal position that there is to be one standard or level for evaluating all types of criminal competence and suggest that decisions about competence should be influenced by the type and complexity of the expected legal proceedings. Their factor analysis, which uses three forensic instruments designed to assess various forms of competence, finds that a single common construct does appear to underlie different types of competence. While much of the work in conceptualizing competence has been theoretical in nature, this study represents a good first step in examining competence through empirical methods.

Civil Forensic Assessment

Forensic mental health practitioners are also heavily involved in civil cases, conducting assessments in cases involving child custody, personal injury, civil competency and informed consent to treatment and research. In Part II we have included essays that represent these key civil issues.

The deinstitutionalization movement in North America and Europe resulted in many changes to the manner in which individuals could be detained involuntarily (Bennett and Morris, 1983; Mosher, 1983; Roesch and Golding, 1985). It also led to the release of many mental patients into the community, although mental health services were unable to meet patients' needs as most communities failed to provide the resources necessary to meet the new demands. The result was an increasing number of mentally ill homeless individuals as well as an increase in the number of mentally ill in prison (Roesch, 1995). The downsizing of mental hospitals has also led to sometimes controversial alternatives, such as outpatient civil commitment (Petrila, 2007), which allows for involuntary mental health treatement in the community. Another controversial area, at least in the United States, is the use of civil commitment to involuntarily detain sexual offenders who have completed prison sentences (Petrila, 2007).

Given the changes to civil commitment laws in the US and many other countries, the legal position of a civilly committed patient is a precarious one, and the field of psychology and law has seen significant attention devoted to the civil rights of these individuals over the past four decades. The opening chapter in Part II, by J. Legemaate, gives an informative overview of the legal position of psychiatric patients and the major developments that have occurred in the area of mental health law in several countries.

The essay by Paul Appelbaum and Thomas Grisso (Chapter 8) deals with issues surrounding the abilities and rights of persons with a mental illness to make decisions about psychiatric treatment. This essay is the first in a three-part series introducing the MacArthur Treatment Competence Study – a large-scale project that aimed to develop reliable and valid information with which to address clinical and policy questions in this area. In this introductory essay, the authors present a brief history of legal principles, an overview of research on decision-making capacities and mental illness, and review the various design considerations involved in the conceptualization of this study.

As mental health and legal professionals have begun to reconsider assumptions concerning individuals with mental illness hospitalized in the civil system, the relationship between mental illness and violence has increasingly come into question (Monahan *et al.*, 2001; Mulvey, 1994). In Chapter 9 Pamela Robbins, John Monahan and Eric Silver present data from their study investigating the relationship between gender and violence in a group of acute psychiatric patients. They find similar rates of violence between men and women one year following their release from hospital, but discuss interesting differences in the situational context of the violence committed. For example, men were more likely to have been using substances or alcohol and less likely to have been adhering to prescription medications prior to committing violence, and, when violent, were more likely to cause serious injury than women. By contrast, women were more likely to be violent towards family members and in the home, and were less likely than men to be arrested after committing a violent act.

As we noted, forensic mental health professionals are called on with increasing frequency to conduct evaluations in cases involving the psychological impact of trauma in tort litigation and child custody (Committee on Professional Practice and Standards, 1994; Condie, 2003; Simon, 1995). The final two chapters in Part II review a number of clinical and legal issues that mental health professionals should take into consideration when making these decisions. In Chapter 10 William Koch, Melanie O'Neill and Kevin Douglas review the limits of expert opinion on post-traumatic stress disorder in personal injury claims and offer suggestions for improving forensic practice. In Chapter 11 Robert Emery, Randy Otto and William O'Donohue review the theoretical, psychological and legal issues that complicate child custody evaluations. Both essays provide a thorough review of relevant legal principles, psychological research, and assessment instruments and methods with the aim of improving the state of practice in these areas.

Forensic Treatment

As noted earlier, research on forensic assessment has dramatically increased in the last few decades. By comparison, research on effective forensic treatment has been far less common. Over the same period there has been a substantial increase in the number of adolescents and adults with mental problems in both the juvenile and criminal justice systems (see Teplin, Abram, McClelland, Dulcan, and Mericle, Chapter 18, this volume; and Roesch, 1995). At times, the view has prevailed that treatment is not effective in these circumstances, but a careful review of the research supports the conclusion reached by Gendreau, Coggin, French and Smith that 'it is clear that correctional treatments founded on sound empirical principles do work in reducing antisocial behavior' (2006, p. 743). In Part III of this volume we present five essays dealing with aspects of the forensic treatment of adults.

In Chapter 12 Francis Cullen and Paul Gendreau provide a historical overview of the treatment philosophies and approaches geared towards offenders over the past four decades. Although their essay considers these issues from within the field of criminology, we chose to include it in this volume because it closely parallels similar developments and changing ideologies within the field of clinical forensic psychology. Cullen and Gendreau trace a recent trend that has moved away from the pessimistic belief that 'nothing works' towards the development of a professional ideology that asks 'what works' in the treatment of offenders. Importantly, Cullen and Gendreau remind readers of a within-discipline tendency to become locked in particular paradigms of understanding the world – a problem that crosses disciplinary boundaries.

Historically, clinicians and researchers have taken an attitude of significant pessimism when conceptualizing the therapeutic effectiveness of clinical intervention with psychopaths.

Clinical lore regarding the intractability of psychopathic traits can have far-reaching consequences for individuals who are assigned this label in the real world. In Chapter 13 Randall Salekin challenges this assumption and reviews the lack of scientifically-based evidence for these conclusions in the literature. After reviewing the important limitations with regard to the research on psychopathy and treatment, he makes suggestions for both clinicians and researchers interested in these issues.

When searching the clinical forensic treatment literature, we were struck by the absence of published studies examining treatment outcomes for sexual offenders, and the lack of well-designed outcome studies in this area. The study by Caroline Friendship, Ruth Mann and Anthony Beech (Chapter 14) is one example of a control group design that sheds some light on sex offender treatment. They describe the findings from a treatment efficacy study examining the outcomes of a sexual offender treatment programme implemented in UK prisons. Overall, they find that the treatment group had somewhat lower two-year sexual and/or violent reconviction rates than the comparison group. However, this study is not without its limitations, and the authors acknowledge several methodological problems inherent in their study. Nevertheless, they make helpful recommendations for future research directions and describe effective methodological approaches that readers may find informative.

In Chapter 15 Henrik Belfrage and Kevin Douglas report their findings from a study making innovative use of a structured, clinical judgement risk assessment instrument – the HCR-20. In the study they compared time of admission risk scores with scores spanning an 18-month period of institutionalization in a sample of forensic psychiatric patients in Sweden and found that patients with longer treatment times had lower scores on two of the three HCR-20 scales. The authors discuss the implications of their results in terms of confirming the underlying dynamic nature of violence risk factors and also suggest that clinicians and administrators can use the HCR-20 and similar tools when considering treatment plans and intervention.

The final essay in Part III concerns the advent of mental health treatment courts. Authors Merith Cosden, Jeffrey Ellens, Jeffrey Schnell, Yasmeen Yamini-Diouf and Maren Wolfe discuss the implementation of a mental health treatment court and assertive community treatment programme in California. They provide a thorough review of the special needs of offenders with mental health and substance abuse problems and describe the revolving-door phenomenon in which individuals are bounced between the courts, jails, community mental health services and psychiatric hospitals without ever having their treatment needs met. This study is unique in that it was able to compare the experiences of offenders randomly assigned to either a traditional adversarial court and the accompanying traditional mental health referral routes or to a newly developed non-adversarial criminal processing and intensive court-supervision programme adapted from the drug court model. The essay reviews the findings from this study and its implications for community outcomes.

Youth Assessment and Intervention

We have included a separate section on 'Youth Assessment and Intervention' because issues of assessment and treatment are substantially different for youth, compared to adults. For example, with regard to risk assessment, the prevailing view is that long-term predictions of recidivism or violence should be avoided. It is also likely that youth are more amenable to treatment. The reasons for these differences are many, but they primarily centre on developmental issues. The importance of considering developmental issues in adolescent assessment and intervention was emphasized in a decision by the US Supreme Court. In *Roper* v. *Simmons* (2005), the Court considered whether it was permissible, under the US Constitution, to execute a juvenile offender (older than 15 but younger than 18) when a capital crime was committed. The *Simmons* case is important for both the decision and the reasoning that lay behind it. The Court considered briefs by a number of groups that presented evidence on the capacities of adolescents. Notable among these briefs to the Court was one submitted by the American Psychological Association (APA). The APA brief reviewed the developmental research that shows that adolescents have considerably less capacity than adults in terms of judgement and decision-making. Adolescence is marked by an increase in risk-taking (Arnett, 1992), including engaging in criminal behaviour. As Moffitt (1993) notes, this involvement in criminal activity, particularly when initiated in adolescence rather than in childhood, typically does not persist into adulthood, and may reflect the fact that adolescents are immature and are more heavily influenced by peers. Adolescents are also less future-oriented and are less likely to weigh the consequences of their decisions (Cauffman and Steinberg, 2000). One compelling explanation for these differences between adolescents and adults is that the cognitive capacities of adolescents are simply underdeveloped. Recent research on brain development shows that adolescent brains have not reached adult maturity, particularly in the frontal lobes which control executive functions of the brain related to decision-making (Giedd *et al.*, 1999). This area of the brain is typically not fully developed until the early twenties.

The first essay in Part IV by Rolf Loeber and David Farrington (Chapter 17) has been included because it provides a broad overview of the developmental background of young offenders: the developmental pathway to delinquency; the rates and course of adolescent delinquency; risk and protective factors pertaining to individual youths, their peers, families, schools and neighbourhoods as they affect development; and preventive and responsive intervention programmes as they impact on delinquency. This thorough review represents an excellent introduction to the multitude of factors that require special consideration when dealing with youths in the criminal justice system.

Until recently, little was known about the prevalence of mental health symptomatology in the juvenile offender population and even less about the characteristics of young offenders with mental illness. Moving from broad youth delinquency to the consideration of mental illness and youth criminality, in Chapter 18 Linda Teplin and her colleagues present a preliminary prevalence estimate for several mental health problems based on a sample of adolescent offenders from Chicago, Illinois. They find that a substantial number of adolescent offenders meet one or more diagnostic criteria and discuss the implications of their findings in terms of their impact on both the juvenile justice system and community mental health system.

Violence risk assessment has also become an important issue for clinicians working with adolescent offenders. However, researchers have questioned the appropriateness of directly extending downwards forensic risk assessment approaches used with adults to the assessment of adolescents. Candice Odgers, Marlene Moretti and Dickon Reppucci (Chapter 19) consider the empirical evidence for the assessment, prediction and management of violence in adolescent girls and review many associated limitations. They also introduce a series of practice recommendations aimed towards informing clinicians who currently undertake risk assessments of adolescent girls.

The next essay was included in an effort to address the recent rise in attention devoted to school violence – a type of violence that is unique to early developmental periods. In Chapter 20 Edward Mulvey and Elizabeth Cauffman put recent media attention to school violence into perspective and provide recommendations for appropriately improving the safety of schools.

Over the past few decades criminal courts have begun to acknowledge the importance of ensuring that adolescents are competent to participate in criminal trials and make other types of important legal decisions. In Chapter 21 Thomas Grisso and his colleagues describe the results from a large-scale study in which they compared the adjudicative competence of adults and adolescents in juvenile detention facilities across the United States. They found that youths under the age of 15 performed more poorly than adults, and discuss a variety of important developmental differences in the manner in which adolescents think about and process information relevant to criminal justice system in comparison with adults. Implications for policy and practice are also presented.

Finally, clinicians and researchers have proposed a variety of unique intervention approaches that focus on the specific, developmentally informed treatment needs of adolescent offenders. In Chapter 22 Charles Borduin describes a family-based therapeutic approach – multisystemic therapy – that has increasingly been seen as a promising form of treatment for delinquent adolescents. Borduin introduces and reviews this approach in terms of its theoretical, empirical and clinical features and reviews a series of effectiveness studies. He also considers a number of possible reasons why this form of therapy has demonstrated preliminary success. Randy Borum (Chapter 23) also discusses treatment approaches for adolescent offenders, focusing on community management strategies. His essay not only provides a thorough distillation of the literature in this area but also makes several recommendations for intervention planning in practice.

Forensic Practice: Professional and Ethical Issues

The essays presented in Part V address a number of important professional and ethical issues confronted by those working in the field of clinical forensic psychology today. We begin with an essay by Randy Otto and Kirk Heilbrun (Chapter 24) that provides a broad overview of the field of forensic psychology as a professional discipline. Otto and Heilbrun review the attainment of various landmarks within the development of the field, including publication sources, professional memberships, practice standards, credentialing and training programmes. They also assess the state of forensic assessment procedures and instruments and make a number of important recommendations with regard to future directions for the discipline.

Over the past few decades forensic psychology has become significantly more popular as a field of study. Yet, despite the impressive growth within the profession, until recently little had been done in the way of working towards creating effective training programmes and streamlining the practice of forensic psychology. In 1995 a number of invited professionals gathered at a national conference held at Villanova's law school and formed working groups to formulate education and training models appropriate for undergraduate and graduate students interested in pursuing careers in psychology and law. The essay by Donald Bersoff *et al.* (Chapter 25) describes the product of this conference and outlines a variety of education and training programmes available to students and scholars interested in joining this exciting discipline.

The very nature of the discipline means that forensic mental health professionals encounter difficult professional and ethical issues. Indeed, the intersection of psychology and law gives rise to a number of unique challenges beyond those encountered in daily standard clinical practice. All forensic mental health professionals must familiarize themselves with these special problems, and Chapter 26 provides a comprehensive introduction to these issues. Here, Stuart Greenberg and Daniel Shuman describe the challenge of role conflicts and outline key differences between therapeutic and forensic relationships. Readers will also appreciate the manner in which they situate these issues within the body of existing professional guidelines.

The next essay focuses on practice challenges related to the content, nature and quality of assessments carried out by forensic mental health professionals. Robert Nicholson and Steve Norwood (Chapter 27) review the transformation that has taken place within the last ten years in the practice and standards set by the field with respect to psychological evaluations within legal contexts. They compare the current state of practice against aspirational standards and guidelines, and identify several significant areas of weakness.

Chapter 28 by John Petrila nicely integrates much of the work presented in this volume and directs readers towards a number of emerging issues in forensic mental health. Petrila applauds the field for overcoming a number of challenging milestones over the past few decades, but also highlights a need for continued improvement in a number of areas. He describes the need for better integration of treatment and risk, the implications associated with the emergence of special jurisdiction courts, the problematic 'criminalization' of adolescent offenders, and a need for better understanding of the use of coercion in community treatment.

References

Arnett, J. (1992), 'Reckless Behavior in Adolescence: A Developmental Perspective', *Developmental Review*, **12**, pp. 339–73.

Bennett, D. and Morris, I. (1983), 'Deinstitutionalization in the United Kingdom', *International Journal of Mental Health*, **11**, pp. 5–23.

Borum, R. (1996), 'Improving the Clinical Practice of Violence Risk Assessment: Technology, Guidelines, and Training', *American Psychologist*, **51**, pp. 945–56.

Cauffman, E. and Steinberg, L. (2000), '(Im)maturity of Judgment in Adolescence: Why Adolescents May Be Less Culpable Than Adults', *Behavioral Sciences and the Law*, **18**, pp. 741–60.

Committee on Ethical Guidelines for Forensic Psychologists (1991), 'Specialty Guidelines for Forensic Psychologists', *Law and Human Behavior*, **6**, pp. 655–65.

Committee on Professional Practice and Standards (1994), 'Guidelines for Child Custody Evaluations in Divorce Proceedings', *American Psychologist*, **49**, pp. 677–80.

Condie, L.O. (2003), *Parenting Evaluations for the Court: Care and Protection Matters*, New York: Kluwer Academic/Plenum.

Douglas, K.S. and Webster, C.D. (1999), 'Predicting Violence in Mentally and Personality Disordered People', in R. Roesch, S.D. Hart and J.R. Ogloff (eds), *Psychology and Law: The State of the Discipline*, New York: Plenum.

Gendreau, P., Coggin, C., French, S. and Smith, P. (2006), 'Practicing Psychology in Correctional Settings', in I.B. Weiner and A.K. Hess (eds), *Handbook of Forensic Psychology* (3rd edn), New York: Wiley, pp. 722–50.

Giedd, J., Blumenthal, J., Jeffries, N., Castellanos, F., Liu, H., Ijdenbos, A., Paus, T., Evans, A. and Rapoport, J. (1999), 'Brain Development During Childhood and Adolescence: A Longitudinal MRI Study', *Nature Neuroscience*, **2**, pp. 861–63.

Grisso, T. (1991), 'A Developmental History of the American Psychology-Law Society', *Law and Human Behavior*, **15**, pp. 213–31.

Haney, C. (1980), 'Psychology and Legal Change: On the Limits of a Factual Jurisprudence', *Law and Human Behavior*, **4**, pp. 147–99.

Heilbrun, K. (2001), *Principles of Forensic Mental Health Assessment*, New York: Plenum.

Heilbrun, K., Marczyk, G.R. and DeMatteo, D.S. (2002), *Principles of Forensic Health Assessment: A Casebook*, New York: Oxford University Press

Krauss, D.A. and Sales, B.D. (2006), 'Training in Forensic Psychology: Training for What Goal?', in I.B. Weiner and A.K. Hess (eds), *Handbook of Forensic Psychology* (3rd edn), New York: Wiley, pp. 851–71.

Litwack, T.R. and Schlesinger, L. (1999), 'Dangerousness Risk Assessments: Research, Legal, and Clinical Considerations', in A.K. Hess and I.B. Weiner (eds), *The Handbook of Forensic Psychology* (2nd edn), Hoboken, NJ: Wiley, pp. 171–217.

Litwack, T.R., Zapf, P.A., Groscup, J.L. and Hart, S.D. (2006), 'Violence Risk Assessment: Research, Legal, and Clinical Considerations', in I.B. Weiner and A. K. Hess (eds), *Handbook of Forensic Psychology* (3rd edn), New York: Wiley, pp. 487–533.

Moffitt, T.E. (1993), 'Adolescence-Limited and Life-Course-Persistent Antisocial Behavior: A Developmental Taxonomy', *Psychological Review*, **100**, pp. 674–701.

Monahan, J. (1981), *Predicting Violent Behavior*, Beverly Hills, CA: Sage.

Monahan, J. and Steadman, H.J. (1994), *Violence and Mental Disorder: Developments in Risk Assessment*, Chicago, IL: Univesity of Chicago Press.

Monahan, J., Steadman, H.J., Silver, E., Appelbaum, A., Robbins, P., Mulvey, E., Roth, L., Grisso, T. and Banks, S. (2001), *Rethinking Risk Assessment: The MacArthur Study of Mental Disorder and Violence*, New York: Oxford University Press.

Mosher, L.R. (1983), 'Radical Deinstitutionalization: The Italian Experience', *International Journal of Mental Health*, **11**, pp. 129–36.

Mulvey, E.P. (1994), 'Assessing the Evidence of a Link Between Mental Illness and Violence', *Hospital and Community Psychiatry*, **45**, pp. 663–68.

Munsterberg, H. (1908), *On the Witness Stand*, New York: Doubleday Page.

Otto, R. (1992), 'The Prediction of Dangerous Behavior: A Review and Analysis of "Second Generation" Research', *Forensic Reports*, **5**, pp. 103–33.

Petrila, J. (2007), 'Recent Civil Decisions: Implications for Forensic Mental Health Experts', in A.M. Goldstein (ed.), *Forensic Psychology: Emerging Topics and Expanding Roles*, Hoboken, NJ: Wiley, pp. 209–31.

Poythress, N., Nicholson, R., Otto, R.K., Edens, J.F., Bonnie, R.J., Monahan, J. and Hoge, S.K. (1999), *The MacArthur Competence Assessment Tool – Criminal Adjudication: Professional Manual*, Odessa, FL: Psychological Assessment Resources.

Pozzulo, J., Bennell, C. and Forth, A. (2006), *Forensic Psychology*, Toronto: Pearson.

Roesch, R. (1995), 'Creating Change in the Legal System: Contributions from Community Psychology', *Law and Human Behavior*, **19**, pp. 325–43.

Roesch, R., and Gagnon, N. (eds) (2007), *Psychology and Law: Criminal and Civil Perspectives*, Aldershot: Ashgate.

Roesch, R. and Golding, S.L. (1985), 'The Impact of Deinstitutionalization', in D.P. Farrington and J. Gunn (eds), *Current Research in Forensic Psychiatry and Psychology: Aggression and Dangerousness*, New York: Wiley, pp. 209–39.

Roesch, R., Viljoen, J.L. and Hui, I. (2004), 'Assessing Intent and Criminal Responsibility', in W. O'Donohue and E. Levensky (eds), *Handbook of Forensic Psychology: Resource for Mental Health and Legal Professionals*, New York: Academic Press, pp. 157–74.

Roesch, R., Zapf, P.A. and Eaves, D. (2006), *Fitness Interview Test—Revised: A Structured Interview for Assessing Competency to Stand Trial*, Sarasota, FL: Professional Resource Press.

Roesch, R., Zapf, P.A., Golding, S.L. and Skeem, J. L. (1999), 'Defining and Assessing Competency to Stand Trial', in I.B. Weiner and A.K. Hess (eds), *Handbook of Forensic Psychology* (2nd edn) New York: Wiley, pp. 327–49).

Simon, R.I. (1995), *Posttraumatic Stress Disorder in Litigation: Guidelines for Forensic Assessment*, Washington, DC: American Psychiatric Press.

Wells, G.L., Small, M., Penrod, S., Malpass, R.S., Fulero, S.M. and Brimacombe, C.A.E. (1998), 'Eyewitness Identification Procedures: Recommendations for Lineups and Photospreads', *Law and Human Behavior*, **22**, pp. 603–47.

Wigmore, J.H. (1909), 'Professor Munsterberg and the Psychology of Evidence', *Illinois Law Review*, **3**, pp. 399–445.

Case Cited

Roper v. *Simmons*, 543 US 551 (2005).

Part I
Criminal Forensic Assessment

[1]

Violence risk assessment: Science and practice

Kevin S. Douglas* and **David N. Cox**

Simon Fraser University, Canada

Christopher D. Webster

Simon Fraser University, University of Toronto (Psychiatry and Criminology) and Earlscourt Child and Family Centre, Toronto, Canada

Within the conceptual framework of the scientist–practitioner model, this paper describes how the science of risk assessment has progressed to a point where it can be of definite assistance to clinicians. Similarly, clinicians can be of marked help to researchers as they play a role in concept definition and as they design and carry out studies to determine the accuracy of their predictions. Risk assessments ought to be carried out in accord with state-of-the-discipline knowledge. Until fairly recently, it may have been argued that the state of knowledge did not provide any sort of reliable or trustworthy direction on violence risk assessment. This position seems no longer tenable. Topic areas discussed include violence and risk assessment generally, the actuarial–clinical prediction debate, the validity of violence risk assessments, predictors of violence, violence risk assessment schemes (empirically validated structured clinical decision-making), communication of risk assessment findings, and implications for training.

In recent years, there has been an encouraging number of well conceived and executed research studies showing that, contrary to earlier opinion, there is every justification for trying to improve the accuracy of predictions of violence and the quality of assessments of violence risk (for a review, see Douglas & Webster, 1999*a*). The authors wish to describe a *process* through which violence risk assessments can be carried out. This process, involving the use of violence risk assessment schemes, calls for collaboration among researchers and clinicians and can, it is to be hoped, benefit some patients, convicted persons, and even young children inclined toward early aggression and violence.

The authors believe that the gap between scientists and practitioners is wide, and is narrowing only slowly, if at all. Routine practice is little influenced by strong scientific findings, and frequently research has minimal links to the actualities of everyday clinical life. The authors' position, however, is that each sphere must

*Requests for reprints should be addressed to Kevin S. Douglas, Simon Fraser University, 8888 University Drive, Burnaby, British Columbia, V5A 1S6, Canada (e-mail: kdouglas@arts.sfu.ca).

inform the other in order to attain a level of sophistication in both the science and practice of violence risk assessment that is commensurate with its importance.

This paper is based on the scientist–practitioner model of training in clinical psychology. In such a model, clinical work is guided as much as possible by research findings. Violence risk assessment entails making clinical decisions that, more often than not, can have important consequences. The well-known dilemma is that persons who would not be violent if they were released may end up being detained, and violent individuals, who really ought to be confined to an institution, are released. Both types of errors are serious, and it is highly desirable to reduce them. The authors' position is that the goal of minimizing errors can be forwarded by adopting violence risk assessment strategies that are based in research—'empirically validated' violence risk assessments. This paper first lays a conceptual foundation based on the scientist–practitioner model of clinical psychology, and then discusses how it may apply to the contemporary science and practice of violence risk assessment.

Science and practice

The 1949 Boulder Conference established a model for training clinical psychologists which has endured since that time. Simply put, clinical psychologists would be trained both as researchers and as practitioners. It has been described as a 'grand aspiration that rarely has been achieved in individual psychologists' (Stricker & Trierweiler, 1995, p. 995). Goldfried & Wolfe (1996) state that since this conference 'the field has struggled to foster the synergy between therapy, research and practice' (p. 104). They go on to suggest that the differences between practice and research need to be examined very closely, as it is a dysfunctional relationship in which both sides view the other with disdain. Kanfer (1990) acknowledges that some individuals have demonstrated how effective practice is based on a knowledge of science; however, his concern is that there is only minimal support for those who are systematically involved in building the relationship between the two. He states: 'A failure to resolve the "scientist–practitioner crisis" not only would lessen the potential impact of advances in psychological science on practice but would also endanger the credibility of a psychological profession by dismantling its most substantial foundation' (p. 269). Nezu (1996) concludes, like Kanfer, that the debate which exists between practitioners and researchers in psychology could have major negative consequences if it continues, as ultimately both sides will lose. He comments that 'despite the definition of psychology as being the *science* of human and animal behavior, those individuals engaged in the *attainment* of psychological knowledge continue to be at odds with those engaged in the *application* of such knowledge' (p. 161; emphasis in original).

While practitioners criticize researchers for being out of touch with the realities of clinical work, researchers suggest that clinicians who are out of touch with the research literature cannot provide effective treatment. What is of greatest concern is the apparent lack of any willingness to reconcile differences. Hayes (1996), while acknowledging that psychology is still a very young field, describes the 'virtual disconnection' that still exists between science and practice. Beutler, Williams, Wakefield & Entwistle (1995) believe that it is the body of knowledge behind these two positions which is the basis for conflict. Researchers feel that empirical findings are a necessity for correct clinical practice, and clinicians argue that researchers are insensitive to the practicalities of their needs and fail to demonstrate relevance in the context of clinical concerns. They point out that the scientist–practitioner duality pervades disciplines where the scientific method is the primary source of knowledge. Following a national survey of psychologists, they concluded that clinicians use research findings in their work more than academics give them credit for, while academics are less likely to acknowledge the usefulness of clinical work. They take the further position that 'it should be remembered that scientists are more dependent on the practitioner community for the survival of their findings than practitioners are on scientists' (p. 991).

An extreme position is that taken by Fensterheim & Raw (1996), who believe that integration of research and practice is not possible. They feel that it is a model which does not work, as these are two distinct fields. Their plea is for deintegration, as they feel that integration impedes progress. They argue that the two areas should interact on the basis of mutual respect while remaining independent. Somewhat in contrast to this position is Meehl's (1954) concept of the 'honest clinician', an individual who constantly questions success and seeks to know through maintaining a research-scholarly attitude, if it is possible to do better. As Stricker (1992) points out, the honest clinician derives certainty from empirical evidence and recognizes the responsibility to maintain a scholarly attitude that is intended to provide clients with the best treatment possible on the basis of current knowledge. This position is perhaps most strongly stated by Singer (1990), who believes that a central ethic of clinical practice is that it is based on a current knowledge of the research literature.

This concern is crucial to the present discussion of risk assessment as it raises the issue of ethical practice. In summarizing Singer's concerns, Stricker (1992) states: 'Thus, the position that research drives practice is endorsed, and it is also elevated to a principle of ethics. Not only are practitioners who are not informed by research offering an inferior brand of treatment, not only are they less than honest clinicians, but they are unethical in their practice' (p. 546). Stricker pursues his concerns in a convincing manner while attempting to determine the ethical issues involved. He concludes initially that it is not unethical to practice in the absence of specific evidence, as such certainty is not possible within the limits of the existing body of knowledge. However, he states that 'although it may not be unethical to practice in the absence of knowledge it is unethical to practice in the face of knowledge. We all must labor with the absence of affirmative data, but there is no excuse for ignoring contradictory data. An insistence on relying on overlearned, favored, but invalid approaches is not justifiable' (p. 546). He cautions against rigid adherence to a particular approach, while recognizing that no clinician, no matter how well experienced or educated, can be competent in all approaches. Out of this recognition comes the ethical obligation to refer clients to other practitioners who possess the necessary competence to deal with a specific problem. This concern over the ethical implications of ignoring the scientific method is perhaps stated most strongly by Meehl (1997) who, in condemning a reliance on clinical experience rather than empirical findings, concludes that: 'As for our many prescientific practices, I believe that if we do not take strong steps to clean up our act, some smart lawyers and sophisticated judges will either discipline or discredit us' (p. 98).

It is in this context that the authors' concern about the current 'state-of-the-discipline' knowledge with respect to violence risk assessment becomes relevant. Borum (1996), in his article on how risk assessment in clinical practice might be improved, cites the statement made by Webster, Douglas, Eaves & Hart (1997*b*) that 'the greatest challenge in what remains of the 1990s is to integrate the almost separate worlds of research on the prediction of violence and the clinical practice of assessment. At present the two domains scarcely intersect' (p. 1). It is a balance in the scientist–practitioner model that is sought, and yet, as the preceding paragraphs have suggested, it is not clear how this balance is to be attained. Within the area of risk assessment the authors have commented that it is this balance that is in urgent need of being achieved (Webster & Cox, 1997). The indications are, as discussed in this article, that the science of risk assessment has progressed to the point where it is important, and perhaps ethically necessary, that this information be made available to, and be used by, clinicians in assisting them make what has been described as one of the most complex predictions in behavioural science and law (Grisso & Appelbaum, 1992).

A worthwhile by-product of this process is that an example may be provided of how a truly workable scientist–practitioner model can be achieved. Clearly it is possible to focus on the failings of the model. This may give rise to a sense of the differences between research and practice as being insurmountable. Yet the present authors' position inclines toward optimism. Research and practice should benefit one another. The synergy described earlier is a real possibility. As Stricker (1992) has pointed out, there are different levels of research use in which a practitioner can engage. The first occurs simply through an awareness of research. The second involves the active consideration of the implications that research has for practice. The third possibility, which is identified as the highest order of use, involves the active integration of research and practice. Recently Sobell (1996), in a discussion of strategies for bridging the gap between science and practice, suggests that real integration has yet to occur. She describes this as an elusive alliance that requires more than mere recognition as an issue. The rest of this article demonstrates the workability of combining the goals of research and practice in the context of risk assessment. The authors have chosen to call this 'empirically validated violence risk assessment'.

Empirically validated violence risk assessment

Definition of violence

Given that violence is at the core of risk assessment, it is perhaps surprising that its definition has received little attention in risk assessment research compared to other facets of this research. The present authors adopt a definition that can be found in recent literature on violence risk assessment (i.e. Boer, Hart, Kropp &

Webster, 1998; Hart, 1998; Lyon, Hart & Webster, in press; Webster *et al.* 1997*b*). Webster *et al.* (1997*b*) define violence as 'actual, attempted, or threatened harm to a person or persons' (p. 24). Included under this statement are acts that can reasonably be considered to harm another person. Threats of harm ought to be non-ambiguous to be counted as violent. Boer *et al.* (1998) define sexual violence as 'actual, attempted, or threatened sexual contact with a person who is nonconsenting or unable to give consent' (p. 9).

Lyon *et al.* (in press) point out that definitions that focus on consequences of actions may be too narrow, and exclude such patently violent acts as firing a gun into a group of people but hitting no one. However, these autors also point out that definitions that include non-physical acts such as threatening may be considered too broad. In the large-scale MacArthur risk assessment project in the United States, researchers created categories of violence depending on seriousness (Steadman *et al.*, 1998). For instance, Steadman *et al.* (1998) define violence as 'battery that resulted in physical injury, sexual assaults, assaultive acts that involved the use of a weapon, or threats made with a weapon in hand' (p. 395). They then define 'other aggressive acts' as 'battery that did not result in physical injury' (p. 395). Other researchers have made a distinction between physical and non-physical violence (Douglas, Ogloff, Nicholls & Grant, in press; McNiel & Binder, 1989, 1994*a,b*).

The present authors think that there is merit to the fairly flexible definition of violence used by Boer *et al.* (1998) or Webster *et al.* (1997*b*). It is capable of being divided along relevant dimensions such as seriousness (i.e. Steadman *et al.*, 1998), physical/non-physical (i.e. Douglas *et al.*, in press; McNiel & Binder, 1989, 1994*a,b*), sexual/non-sexual (i.e. Boer *et al.*, 1998), or instrumentality (Cornell, Warren, Hawk, Stafford, Oram & Pine, 1996). This approach allows researchers to capture the broad spectrum of violent acts as well as to pare down conceptualizations into meaningful categories, which can themselves be subjected to study. This approach also facilitates the identification of predictors that may be most important for different types or categories of violence.

The authors are mindful of the fact that there are many other important considerations regarding violence, such as its measurement (official records vs. self-report vs. observation; Convit, Isay, Gadioma & Volavka, 1988; Douglas & Hart, 1999; Mulvey, Shaw & Lidz, 1994; Steadman *et al.*, 1998); its setting (institutional vs. community; Douglas & Hart, 1999; McNiel & Binder, 1989); its targets (family vs. strangers vs. professionals; Estroff & Zimmer, 1994; Mulvey & Lidz, 1995); its density (number of acts in a specified time period); and its breadth (number of different types of violent acts). These sorts of concerns can and should be integrated into research projects and into clinicians' considerations, and can be fitted within the flexible definition outlined above.

Definition of violence risk assessment

Hart (1998) has provided a useful definition of violence risk assessment as '*the process of evaluating individuals to (1) characterize the likelihood they will commit acts of violence and (2) develop interventions to manage or reduce that likelihood*' (p. 122; emphasis in original). There are several important parts to this definition. First, the fact that risk assessment is described as a process denotes a continuing assessment procedure. Reed (1997) makes this point clearly when, in writing of the English Care Programme Approach (CPA; Department of Health, 1990), he states that 'risk assessment is not a one-off event but part of an ongoing process of assessment, review and re-assessment' (p. 5). Secondly, risk assessment requires a characterization of the likelihood of future violence, or a prediction of violence. Thirdly, the process of risk assessment invites consideration of what can or cannot be done to avert further similar violence in the future. This leads to the concept of violence risk management, which is vitally important, though perhaps has not been recognized as such until fairly recently (Heilbrun, 1997; Heilbrun, Philipson, O'Neill, Paninopolous, Strohman & Bowman, 1998; Monahan & Steadman, 1994*b*; Reed, 1997; Snowden, 1997; Webster *et al.*, 1997*b*).

This description of violence risk assessment implies that the task is much broader than the mere prediction of violence. Prediction surely is required, but so too is action that stems from the prediction. Prediction requires that the most accurate estimate of future violence probability is forwarded. Management requires that steps are taken to provide treatment, programming, release plans and other mitigating strategies to reduce the likelihood of violence. As Hart (1998) describes, a prediction of 'high' likelihood of violence must be coupled with efforts to disprove the prediction. That is, to suggest or provide interventions or management strategies that will reduce or prevent violence risk is a necessary component of the risk assessment process. Similarly, Reed (1997) discusses the ethical obligation or responsibility of clinicians to act in their professional capacity to reduce and effectively manage violence risk. Just as risk assessment is conceived of as a process rather than a static event, so too should risk management be considered such a process. Snowden (1997) defines risk management as 'the process of systematically focusing on methods of reducing both the severity and frequency of recognized adverse clinical risks for each individual patient' (p. 33). Several commentators have written about the usefulness of having *a priori* risk management strategies that flow from risk assessments (Boer *et al.*, 1998; Heilbrun *et al.*, 1998; Monahan & Steadman, 1996; Webster *et al.*, 1997*b*).

Clinical vs. actuarial prediction

One of the persisting controversies in the risk assessment field is the clinical vs. actuarial prediction debate. This debate requires some explanation and also some comment regarding how it may fit into the risk assessment approach described in this article (or, conversely, how the risk assessment approach may fit within the clinical–actuarial debate). The clinical–actuarial distinction and debate has close parallels to the larger framework of this article, the scientist–practitioner model. Traditionally, actuarial prediction may be considered to be aligned with the scientist side of the debate, and clinical prediction with the practitioner side.

Meehl (1954) is often credited with bringing the statistical–clinical prediction debate or controversy to light in the field of psychology. Generally, statistical (or actuarial, or mechanical) prediction 'involves a formal, algorithmic, objective procedure (e.g. equation) to reach the decision' (Grove & Meehl, 1996, p. 293). Clinical prediction 'relies on an informal, "in the head," impressionistic, subjective conclusion, reached (somehow) by a human clinical judge' (Grove & Meehl, 1996, p. 294). It is important to emphasize that clinical and actuarial prediction refers to the *process* of offering predictions, and not to the types of variables used. Clinical variables, as defined herein, refer to dynamic factors that can change. They could as easily be subjected to clinical prediction methods as they could to actuarial ones. Similarly, it actually makes little sense to speak of 'actuarial variables', as the term 'actuarial' refers to process, not content. Often when variables are referred to as actuarial, what is meant is that they are static or historical. However, static variables, again, may be subjected to either clinical or actuarial prediction methods.

As Hart (1998) points out, perhaps the most important advantage of actuarial prediction is that it improves the validity (accuracy) and consistency of predictions. Grove & Meehl (1996) report the results of a meta-analysis of studies that compared clinical vs. actuarial prediction. Of 136 such studies, 8 resulted in greater predictive accuracy for the clinical method, 64 showed more accurate prediction for the actuarial method, and 64 showed no difference.

What seems clear is that actuarial prediction methods, which typically lack the biases, idiosyncrasies and imperfections of human clinical judgment, are superior to clinical prediction methods in terms of accuracy. Nevertheless, many clinicians are reticent to accept this superiority. In fact, some make the argument that the actuarial method is 'of little use' (Grubin, 1997, p. 17). It is argued here, conversely, that the actuarial method, while useful, is not a panacea, and that it has limitations in the risk assessment field. The function of actuarial prediction methods is simply that—prediction. Risk assessment as conceived here is broader than prediction. Prediction is a necessary first step. Yet risk management and prevention are equally necessary steps. Once a person is defined as high risk, it is in everyone's best interest to suggest means by which such risk can be attenuated.

Hart (1998) notes several other potential problems. One of these is that actuarial methods tend to involve a small number of variables that are assumed to have equally useful predictive value across different groups of people in different settings. This point is also made by Grubin (1997), who claims that actuarial methods may miss the individual and rare variables that may be of most interest to the case at hand. For instance, if an actuarial risk assessment tool places a person at low risk, but that person has just issued a serious threat to kill some person, should that person in fact not be considered high risk, despite the actuarial forecast?

Grove & Meehl (1996) anticipate this (and other) criticisms of actuarial prediction, and in fact refer to this particular objection as the 'broken leg case' (p. 307).[1] Grubin (1997) argues that one cannot realistically apply actuarial predictive models, derived on aggregate data, to individual cases. Grove & Meehl

[1]The authors give the example of knowing, through an actuarial prediction, that the probability of a certain professor going to a movie on Friday night is .84. However, the professor has a broken leg, making the trip to a movie very unlikely, and broken limbs were not taken into account in the actuarial prediction model. What should the decision be?

(1996) put forth that, though such cases give rise to an important dilemma for the actuary, such cases are also relatively infrequent. In the hypothetical example, the broken leg is a clear objective fact with equally clear implications. As such, countervailing the actuarial equation may be warranted. The danger of ascribing 'broken leg' status to large numbers of predictions is the application of non-optimal weights to the 'broken leg' events or factors, and doing so inconsistently over cases (Grove & Meehl, 1996).

Hart (1998) also argues that an actuarial prediction method, calibrated and even validated on a certain sample, may not possess the same psychometric and predictive characteristics in other samples and settings. As such, wholesale adoption of an actuarial model into a setting that has distinct differences from the validation sample may be untenable. Again, Grove & Meehl (1996) counter this point. They assert that there is little evidence to support the notion that an actuarial instrument will not generalize to other settings. Using their example, they are probably right. They argue that if an instrument has been shown to work in several psychiatric clinics, there is little reason to suspect that it will not generalize to another psychiatric clinic. Even if accuracy decreases by 10%, they assert, the actuarial approach will still be superior to clinical judgment.

What if, however, settings are substantially different? Can a risk assessment tool that is validated on forensic psychiatric patients be applied with confidence to medium security prisoners? This is a researchable question, the answer to which cannot be taken for granted or assumed. In some cases, it may seem quite reasonable to decide on the basis of careful and logical thought, attention to demographics of samples, the nature of predictions being made, the consequences of those decisions, and so forth, that a certain actuarial tool can be applied at least tentatively. However, in certain cases, there may be convincing evidence that it might very well not apply, and should not be used. In response to this point, Grove and Meehl argue: either revalidate the prediction model, or develop your own.

Clearly, this debate is complex and has not subsided. The present authors' view is that, generally, actuarial prediction has been demonstrated to be superior to clinical prediction purely in terms of predictive validity. However, this statement has qualifications. Their argument is not so much that global clinical judgment would be superior to actuarial judgment when, say, the actuarial method is deemed inapplicable to a certain setting. This is not a useful comparison (i.e. global clinical impression vs. an inapplicable algorithm). Rather, it is argued here that *empirically validated, structured decisions* can be used to avoid some of the problems described above with actuarial prediction: concern over generalization to a certain setting; failure to account for salient idiosyncratic risk markers; and tendency to focus only on prediction to the exclusion of management, prevention and amelioration issues. By the term 'empirically validated structured decisions' the authors mean assessments that are guided by factors that have received empirical support in the literature. This approach is described fully below. Empirically validated, structured clinical assessment (as opposed to unstructured 'in the head', impressionistic, global clinical judgment) brings in the notion of 'conditional prediction' (Mulvey & Lidz, 1995). That is, a person may be considered to be at high risk given certain other conditions (lack of community supervision; medication noncompliance), but at lower risk under certain conditions (access to appropriate treatment; supportive family). Reed (1997) discusses the importance of specifying which future circumstances may aggravate or mitigate risk, and whether proposed interventions can reasonably be expected to reduce risk. Further, this approach recognizes that violence risk is not static, but rather is dynamic and fluctuates with changing conditions. As such, as pointed out above, and as others have noted (Reed, 1997; Snowden, 1997), risk assessment, ideally, is a process that continues over time. Actuarial prediction typically involves the offering of a prediction index of some sort at time *A*, and then passive observation to confirm or refute the prediction at some time, *B*. Conversely, the view here is that risk assessments should reach into the future, specifying level of risk as functions of possible conditions. Treatment and management planning can then be organized specifically to disconfirm the decision of high risk.

The present authors' view, then, is that something more than mere prediction is normally needed. The use of actuarial devices, once it is decided that they are appropriate for the sample and setting, may be important *as part of the overall assessment procedure* to help inform risk level decisions. Use of such actuarial instruments, however, does not abrogate clinicians' responsibilities for their assessments and opinions. A broad approach is called for, one that goes beyond passive prediction and involves risk management, risk re-evaluation, recognition of 'critical items',[2] and statements about future events that may aggravate or mitigate risk. This approach, however, ought also to be grounded in scientifically validated knowledge. As Snowden (1997) states: '[i]f one makes important treatment or management decisions without adequate information, this is a clinical *gamble*' (p. 32; emphasis in original). The approach ought to be structured to promote systematic assessment of violence factors. These features are what separate scientifically validated structured clinical assessments from mere global clinical impressions. It is systematic, data-based, yet not so inflexible that it cannot find practical application.

Although the process of empirically validated, structured clinical assessment is discussed more fully below, the authors' general meaning is that the broad assessment approach described here ought to be rooted in knowledge that, for the most part, has been subjected to and validated by research. They do not advocate simple adoption of algorithmic prediction. As explained, their conception of risk assessment includes but goes beyond prediction. What they do insist upon, however, is the use of an assessment model that is grounded in well-substantiated research. Risk assessment schemes or guides that have been developed from a consideration of the research may improve both the clinical practice of risk assessment as well as risk assessment technology (Borum, 1996). These ideas are introduced here to provide a context for the remainder of the article. Two important questions are now discussed: (1) how accurate is risk assessment?, and (2) what predicts violence?

[2]These, as explained by Kropp, Hart, Webster & Eaves (1998), are items that are of such immediate salience so as to warrant, on their own, decisions of high risk. An example may be homicidal ideation.

Validity of violence prediction

Having outlined conceptual and theoretical issues in risk assessment in some detail, the validity (accuracy) of violence prediction is summarized here. The authors do not wish to suggest that this is an easy task. As Hart (1998) adeptly describes, there are many complex decisions that go into planning a single risk assessment study. To provide a 'simple' summary of validity data is not so simple. Perhaps the best starting point is where others often start—with the few studies that existed in the 1960s and 1970s.

As Cocozza & Steadman (1976) put it, in the 1960s and 1970s there was 'clear and convincing evidence' (p. 1084) for the inability of mental health professionals to predict violence accurately. In fact, Monahan's (1981) review of the topic revealed that only one in three positive predictions of violence were accurate. Since that time, given the pressure placed on mental health professionals by courts and statutes to predict violence (Douglas, Macfarlane & Webster, 1996), a good deal of research on the topic has been carried out. Conclusions from recent reviews of the subject are decidedly more positive. The increase in predictive accuracy is due at least in part to the use of improved methodologies and statistical analyses.

Studies appearing over the last few years have used better methodology than their forerunners. They have obtained correspondingly larger effect sizes. One of the important methodological advances was comprehensive follow-up procedures aimed at detecting more of the community violence that was actually occurring (see e.g. Mulvey *et al.*, 1994; Steadman *et al.*, 1998). Lines of study were published in the 1980s that showed that predictions of violence could reach at least moderate levels of accuracy.[3]

McNiel, Binder and colleagues have published numerous studies starting in the 1980s which have investigated various correlates of psychiatric inpatient violence (Binder & McNiel, 1988, 1990; McNiel & Binder, 1989, 1994*a*), and the accuracy of predictions of violence (McNiel & Binder, 1991, 1994*b*, 1995; McNiel, Binder & Greenfield, 1988). Some of these studies investigated clinical (as opposed to actuarial) prediction (McNiel & Binder, 1991, 1995; McNiel *et al.*, 1988). These studies have shown consistently that certain diagnoses, symptoms, and previous aggressive behaviours are related to inpatient violence. Also, McNiel & Binder (1994*b*) developed a screening instrument, guided by their numerous investigations, for assessing inpatient violence. It improved over chance by 25% (i.e. relative improvement over chance = 25%). Klassen & O'Connor (1988*a*,*b*,*c*, 1989) conducted several studies on the risk of community violence. They identified several domains of variables[4] which related prospectively to violence. Using this measure, 75.8% of patients were correctly classified as violent or non-violent. A moderate size multiple regression coefficient (.32) was obtained. Menzies, Webster & Sepejak (1985) developed the Dangerous Behaviour Rating Scheme (DBRS), consisting of 22 items such as anger, rage, hostility and environmental support. This instrument correlated at .34 with later violence.

[3]According to Cohen (1988), a moderate effect size in correlation terms is ± .30, and a large effect size is ± .50.

[4]These are: (1) early family quality; (2) current intimate relationships; (3) arrest history; (4) admissions history; (5) assault in the presenting problem (Klassen & O'Connor, 1989).

Studies appearing in the 1990s have shown sustained and even enhanced levels of predictive accuracy. The large-scale MacArthur risk assessment project (Steadman *et al.*, 1994) has produced a clinically-relevant actuarial violence prediction tool that relies upon a 'regression tree' approach to classify civil psychiatric patients into various risk categories (Monahan *et al.*, in press; Steadman *et al.*, in press). This approach requires the clinician to ask certain questions and consider certain risk markers depending on the answer to previous questions. A large number of variables (18) entered into logistic regression-based classification trees. This approach was able to obtain a strong relationship with violence.

Harris, Rice & Quinsey (1993; see also Quinsey, Harris, Rice & Cormier, 1998; Rice, 1997; Rice & Harris, 1995) found that a set of 12 variables, selected statistically from a much larger set, produced a multiple correlation with violence of .44. Coefficients in some groups were as high as .53. Lidz, Mulvey & Gardner (1993), in a well-designed study, showed that clinicians could actually offer predictions of violence that exceed chance. This group (Gardner, Lidz, Mulvey & Shaw, 1996) also developed a screening instrument for use with psychiatric patients. Using four variables (young age, multiple [3 +] previous violent acts, heavy drug use, and hostility) in a 'regression tree' design akin to that used by the MacArthur group, the researchers were able to demonstrate excellent specificity[5] (true negative rate was 99%), but poor sensitivity[6] (true positive rate was 7%). Douglas *et al.* (in press) found that the HCR-20 violence risk assessment scheme, discussed in greater detail below, was consistently and strongly associated with violence in a sample of 193 civil psychiatric patients. One promising and robust finding is the relationship between psychopathy as measured by the Hare Psychopathy Checklist—Revised (PCL–R; Hare, 1991) or Screening Version (PCL:SV; Hart, Cox & Hare, 1995). Two recent meta-analyses have shown that the link between psychopathy and violence is at least moderate (Hemphill, Hare & Wong, 1998) to large (Salekin, Rogers & Sewell, 1996).

In the 1990s, there has been a recognition of the value of statistical techniques apart from correlation, regression and classification models. For instance, Mossman (1994) has recommended the relative advantage of receiver operating characteristic (ROC) analyses over other techniques because they are much less dependent on base-rates of violence. ROC analyses produce a statistical index called the 'Area under the Curve' or AUC which is derived from plotting sensitivity against specificity for various cut-offs on a predictive measure. The AUC can range from 0 (perfect negative prediction) to .50 (chance prediction) to 1.0 (perfect positive prediction). The AUC represents the probability that a randomly chosen, actually violent person will score greater than a randomly chosen, actually non-violent person. AUC values in the mid-.70s and up may be considered large effects. Researchers have used these advantageously (Douglas *et al.*, in press; Grann, Belfrage & Tengström, in press; Rice & Harris, 1995; Strand, Belfrage, Fransson & Levander, 1999). Other techniques, such as Item Response Theory (IRT) analyses

[5]Specificity or true negative rate is the proportion of persons who are not violent who were not predicted to be violent.

[6]Sensitivity or true positive rate is the proportion of persons who are violent who were predicted to be so.

are useful for identifying which items in a scale carry the most information about the underlying characteristic in question (Cooke & Michie, 1997).

In his quantitative review of some violence risk assessment studies, Mossman (1994) determined that predictive accuracy was improved in more recent studies over older studies, that actuarial prediction outperformed clinical prediction, and that, overall, predictive accuracy across 58 data sets was appreciable. Current reviews, then, along with some recent risk assessment studies, suggest that violence can be predicted with moderate to large effect sizes. This statement is possible largely owing to the improved methodology used in the 1980s and 1990s. Researchers have been able to identify higher base rates of violence than in the past because of more sensitive data detection methodology (e.g. see Convit *et al.*, 1988; Mulvey & Lidz, 1994; Steadman *et al.*, 1998). Also, statistical techniques such as ROC analyses, survival curves and hierarchical regression are well-suited to identifying relationships that exist in the data.

What does 'large effect size' translate into in 'real terms', however? Some examples will help. Correlation (or regression coefficients) in the area of .50 are considered large effect sizes (Cohen, 1992). A correlation of .50 translates roughly into an odds ratio of 9.0. This would mean that a person who is predicted to be violent is nine times more likely to be violent than a person not so predicted. Douglas *et al.* (in press) found an AUC of .80 for the HCR-20 violence risk assessment scheme for predicting violent crime (Webster *et al.*, 1997*b*). This means that the probability is .80 (80%) that a randomly chosen, actually violent person will score above a given cut-off of the HCR-20, and a non-violent person will score below it. The base rate of violence in this case (violent criminal recidivism) was only 9.8%. This indicates that the prediction was improved vastly over chance. In fact, persons scoring above the median of the HCR-20 were 13 times more likely to incur violent criminal charges than those scoring below the median. Similarly, Rice (1997) reports that the AUC for the Violence Risk Appraisal Guide (VRAG) was .76, which was equivalent to a Cohen's *d* of 1.0. The MacArthur risk assessment studies (Monahan *et al.*, in press; Steadman *et al.*, in press) have found AUC values of up to .80 and .82. Again, these represent large effect sizes, and considerable accuracy in prediction. Mossman's (1994) quantitative review, which does not include the most recent and promising research, found a median AUC of .73.

To take a convincing example from outside the risk assessment arena, Cohen (1988) describes that large effect sizes are clearly discernible from observation of the data. He cites as one objective example of a large effect size the difference in height between 13- and 18-year-old women. When compared to other disciplines, how do the effects obtained in risk assessment research 'measure up'? Lipsey & Wilson (1993) carried out a meta-analysis of over 300 meta-analyses—a meta-meta-analysis. Some of the effects that they found are shown in Table 1. What seems clear is that some of the effects seem surprisingly low. For instance, chemotherapy for breast cancer produces a small effect size, as does the use of cyclosporine for organ transplants. Should, therefore, patients be dissuaded from accepting such treatments? The answer is clearly 'No' since when these effects are translated into real-life terms, they are in fact quite substantial. For instance, a correlation between treatment and recidivism of − .20 equates to a 20% drop in the chance

Table 1. Comparison of effect sizes across disciplines

Type of study	Effect (d)
Medical	
Effect of by-pass surgery on angina	.80
Use of AZT for AIDS	.47
Cyclosporine for organ transplants	.30
Chemotherapy for breast cancer	.08–.11
Drug treatment for arthritis; various outcomes	.45–.77
Psychological	
Psychotherapy, general[a]	.76
Psychotherapy, cognitive behavioural/behaviour modification[a]	.64
Treatment programmes for offenders[a]	.36
Effect of ECT on depression	.80
Drug treatment for behavioural disorders . . .	.28–.74
Drug treatment for hyperactivity; cognitive . . .	.47–.96
Neuroleptic drugs for dementia; effects on agitation	.37
Hypertensive drug therapy; effects on quality of life	.11–.28
Risk Assessment[b]	
Douglas *et al.* (in press)[c]	.91–1.07
Kropp *et al.* (1999)[d]	1.70
Rice (1997)	1.0
Strand *et al.* (1999)	1.19

Note. Adapted from Table 6 of Lipsey & Wilson (1993).
[a]Mean effect sizes calculated by the present authors from the data presented in Lipsey & Wilson (1993).
[b]Effects not from the Lipsey & Wilson (1993) meta-analysis.
[c]Calculation, though based on data by Douglas *et al.* (1998), not presented in their manuscript.
[d]Effect was calculated by the present authors from data presented in Kropp *et al.* (1998), and indicates difference in Total Scores on the SARA between groups of inmates who had or did not have spousal assault histories.

of reoffending. Over data pooled across thousands of persons, the overall benefit of treatment cannot be doubled. When the effect sizes listed in the upper parts of Table 1 are compared to the recent effect sizes being obtained in risk assessment research, it appears that this field is faring well relative to others. This is not an endorsement for complacency. Rather, it serves to demonstrate that risk assessments can indeed be made with respectable accuracy. The old question—can violence be predicted?—is not a good one. More interesting and practical is the somewhat more convoluted question: Which groups of subjects, with which particular characteristics, followed over what periods of time, are likely to exhibit precisely defined kinds of violent behaviour (see Jackson, 1997)?

Substance of risk assessment

What predicts violence? Several major factors have been shown to predict violence. Most of these have been found to cut across types of samples and settings, and are discussed globally. Although literally hundreds of specific variables have been demonstrated to associate with violence, the following focuses on several higher-order constructs that have been shown in various studies to relate to violence with some robustness. In focusing on these groupings of risk factors, the authors are aware that others could be included, and that this discussion is not exhaustive. Readers are referred to more comprehensive accounts (Borum, 1996; Douglas & Webster, 1999*a*; Lyon *et al.*, in press; Monahan & Steadman, 1994*a*; Webster *et al.*, 1997*a,b*).

Historical and static factors. Under the broad category of historical and static items are included diverse risk factors. Some historical factors are simply indices of past behaviour. For instance, current young age (Harris *et al.*, 1993; Swanson, 1994), young age at time of first violence (Harris, Rice & Cormier, 1991; Harris *et al.*, 1993; Hodgins, 1983), and a history of violent behaviour (Binder & McNiel, 1990; Klassen & O'Connor, 1989; McNiel & Binder, 1994*a,b*) all have been shown in numerous studies, primarily of personality and mentally disordered persons, to predict violence. Maladjustment at an early age in various contexts has been shown to predict violence (Convit *et al.*, 1988; Harris *et al.*, 1993; Klassen & O'Connor, 1989).

Other historical or static risk markers may be rooted in adult past, but, like the childhood factors already mentioned, cannot be changed. A history of substance abuse is clearly a very strong marker for violence (Swanson, 1994; Steadman *et al.*, 1998). Similarly, though not without controversy and negative findings (Bonta, Law & Hanson, 1998; Harris *et al.*, 1993; Steadman *et al.*, 1998), major mental illness, generally, elevates the odds for violence (Douglas & Hart, 1999; Lindqvist & Allebeck, 1990; Swanson, 1994; Wessely, Castle, Douglas & Taylor, 1994). So too does a diagnosis of personality disorder (Douglas, Ogloff & Nicholls, 1997; Harris *et al.*, 1993) and, in particular, personality disorders characterized by anger, impulsivity and hostility (Kropp *et al.*, 1999). Examples of adult maladjustment that predict violence are relationship instability (Harris *et al.*, 1993; Klassen & O'Connor, 1988*b*; Saunders, 1992) and employment problems (Menzies & Webster, 1995; Shaffer, Waters & Adams, 1994). For people who already have been processed by the mental health or criminal justice systems, having attempted or completed an escape from custody, or more generally violating the terms of a conditional release, predicts violence (Harris *et al.*, 1993; Hoffman & Beck, 1985).

An important risk factor that, in theory, is relatively stable over the life-span, is psychopathy. First discussed in its modern conception by psychiatrist Hervey Cleckley (1941), the clinical construct of psychopathy has been refined, developed, and set to reliable and valid measurement by Hare (1991, 1993, 1996). Hare (1991) developed the PCL–R as a measure of psychopathy. There have been dozens of studies carried out in support of its relationship with violence and other antisocial acts. Two recent meta-analyses summarize the literature well, and, as previously noted, place the effect size between psychopathy and violence between moderate (Hemphill *et al.*, 1998) and large (Salekin *et al.*, 1996).

Dynamic and clinical factors. Although historical factors have more substantiated support behind them than dynamic, changeable aspects of persons, various clinical constructs have also been found to predict violence. For instance, lack of impulse control and behavioural inhibition, or impulsivity—one of the items on the PCL–R, and the HCR-20—is often thought to be a strong correlate of violence (Barratt, 1994; Hollander & Stein, 1995; Webster & Jackson, 1997). In a related way, antisocial attitudes and beliefs (Andrews & Bonta, 1995), anger (Novaco, 1994) and hostility (Menzies & Webster, 1995) are states that, if currently afflicting a person, will probably elevate violence risk. Whether a person is amenable to treatment, or rather is resistant to remediation attempts, also has relevance for violence (Bartels, Drake, Wallach & Freeman, 1991).

Although, as discussed earlier, some researchers have found that mental illness, on a global level, does not relate to violence, or in fact relates negatively, numerous studies have found that persons with major mental disorders are actually at an increased risk for violence. Some have suggested that it is the active, florid states of mental illness that are the key ingredient in the relationship between violence and mental illness (Buchanan, 1997; Douglas & Hart, 1999; Monahan, 1992). For instance, certain aspects of delusions, such as being able to identify evidence or support for the belief, and being made afraid because of the belief, have been shown to elevate the chances that a person will act on a delusion (Buchanan, 1997). A concept known as threat-control override (TCO) psychotic symptoms, which involves the perceived loss of control over decisional functions (e.g. thought insertion) in concert with perceived threats to personal safety (e.g. beliefs that others are following and out to cause one harm), has been shown to be related to violence (Link & Stueve, 1994; Swanson, Borum, Swartz & Monahan, 1996). In a meta-analysis of over 100 studies on the topic of psychosis and violence, Douglas & Hart (1999) found that not only was there an association between major mental disorders and violence generally, but that this relationship was stronger when analyses used symptoms as the level of measurement, rather than the more gross categorization of diagnosis of disorder. Other dynamic markers for violence risk include suicidal or self-harm intent (Hillbrand, 1995), sadistic fantasies (MacCulloch, Snowden, Wood & Mills, 1983) and homicidal ideation.

Risk management factors. This category of violence risk markers has substantial importance to the violence risk assessment task in that these variables, if targeted, can help to ameliorate risk. Since they are, in fact, changeable, these markers could be included under the previous section. However, their distinguishing qualities are that they tend not to relate to characteristics of persons themselves, but rather to aspects of the situation or environment in which a person will be living upon release (or at least at some future time, or to the person–situation interaction).

For instance, whether a release plan is feasible (i.e. developed to suit a person's particular requirements) may have a bearing on violence risk (Andrews, Zinger, Hoge, Bonta, Gendreau & Cullen, 1990). Unfeasible, poorly thought out or weak plans are likely to increase violence risk. Further, people who have access to the appropriate amount and type of professional help are at reduced risk to act violently (Estroff & Zimmer, 1994). In a parallel manner, personal support from family and friends is an important part of ameliorating violence risk (Estroff &

Zimmer, 1994; Klassen & O'Connor, 1989), so long as family and friends are understanding of relevant mental health and violence issues. Obviously, such support must act as buffers to violence relapse, rather than as triggers to ignite it. Concerning triggers in a different light, it is important that assessors evaluate whatever destabilizers are likely to aggravate violence risk. Such factors are idiosyncratic and personalized depending on a person's criminogenic propensities. For example, a paedophile who is released to live beside a school will encounter, on a daily basis, children playing and coming to and from school. This circumstance is apt to be destabilizing, and surely increases violence risk. Finally, salient stressors may make coping with the demands of everyday life less manageable than otherwise, and hence increase the probability of poorly judged or thought out reactions, including possibly violent ones (Felson, 1992; Klassen & O'Connor, 1994).

Process of risk assessment: empirically validated structured clinical decision-making

Much of the above discussion of risk assessment focuses on the science of the task. How does this translate into clinical action? As should be clear by this stage, an ordered, systematic approach to structured clinical decision-making is endorsed. This may involve first deciding if any or all of a number of actuarial schemes are suited to the task. Such an analysis requires thoughtful comparison between the characteristics of the individual under assessment and the features of the population for which the actuarial scale was developed. It may even be necessary, locally, to array data from comparable individuals and determine the extent to which the individual under consideration does or does not fit group-based characteristics. If an actuarial scheme is considered applicable, it should be used *as part of the overall assessment procedure*. It may be an important data point for a clinician to consider as he or she forms an opinion about violence risk.

Use of actuarial schemes does not remove the necessity of clinical decision-making. There most likely will remain the legal and ethical obligation to ameliorate violence risk after making predictions of 'high' violence risk (Hart, 1998). That is, decisions regarding risk management and prevention are required, and are as crucial as the first step of making a violence prediction. The use of actuarial tools also does not remove the necessity of clinical skill and judgment. For instance, the VRAG (Harris *et al.*, 1993), an actuarial scare that has been shown to relate strongly to violence, requires ratings for psychopathy, schizophrenia and personality disorder. Diagnosis of these conditions is an inherently clinical task. Clinicians also have to decide when an actuarial process is not indicated. The VRAG was calibrated on a sample of male forensic psychiatric patients. Whether its predictive properties generalize to, say, female prisoners or to other settings is a researchable but as yet unanswered question. Its use in certain settings is ruled out by its own construction, in that it contains several items that presume the existence of an index offence (e.g. offence severity, gender of victim). In some settings where violence is a clinical and legal concern though is not inherent to the setting (e.g. civil psychiatric), these variables may not apply, as persons may be civilly committed without having perpetrated actual violence against others.

The use of an empirically based guide or *aide-mémoire* to structure the clinical assessment is forwarded as an appropriate and comprehensive violence risk assessment model. Several of these that have, of late, been developed rationally from consideration of the scientific and professional literatures are reviewed here. These instruments, though capable of being used as actuarial predictors, are better conceptualized as assessment protocols. These clinical guides embody what is meant by 'empirically validated structured clinical decision-making'.

The rationale underlying such instruments is to integrate the tasks of prediction, assessment, management, prevention and communication. Four schemes are highlighted that may be described as guides for structured clinical decision-making: the HCR-20; the Spousal Assault Risk Assessment (SARA) guide; the Sexual Violence Risk-20 (SVR-20); and the Early Assessment Risk List for Boys (EARL-20B; Augimeri, Webster, Koegl & Levene, 1998). The first of these, the HCR-20, is meant to apply to assessments for violence generally. The SARA was designed for the assessment of spousal violence risk. The SVR-20 was created for assessing risk for sexual violence. The EARL-20B, as its name implies, is intended to assist clinicians to assess violence risk in childhood.

These schemes have commonalities. At a conceptual level, they are manifestations of the scientist–practitioner philosophy, in that each possesses risk factors that were selected through review of the scientific and professional literatures, and through consultation with clinicians in respective fields. They were conceived rationally, or analytically. Each was designed to be used by clinicians, as well as to be testable according to conventional research standards. Items can be scored by clinicians in an applied setting, and may also be coded reliably by researchers (or researcher-clinicians) in research applications. Making these schemes 'user friendly' was a driving concern in their development. Complex scoring procedures and cumbersome assessment protocols cannot feasibly be integrated into routine clinical practices. The four risk assessment guides discussed here were created to be easily adopted into day-to-day clinical regimes. Some adaptation to suit local circumstances was anticipated. Although all were devised as guides or *aide-mémoires*, each also is capable of being treated as an actuarial device, in that numbers can be aggregated in some fashion and linked to subsequent violence. However, these risk assessment schemes are intended to include, but be broader than, instruments designed principally to offer a numerical index of risk.

Each instrument recommends a certain method of use. Generally, persons are rated on the presence of the relevant risk factors. Then, a 'summary risk rating' of high, moderate or low risk is given, based on the clinician's overall appraisal. This approach clearly does call for clinical judgment—but it is structured. Advocates of pure actuarial approaches would probably label this approach as 'clinical judgment'. The present authors agree. Yet they assert that there may be defining differences between clinical opinion, as conceptualized by Meehl (1954) and Grove & Meehl (1996) and the present approach to structuring assessment procedures. Grove and Meehl call clinical prediction impressionistic and subjective. The present authors think that the approach propounded in this paper need be neither impressionistic nor subjective. It also is not necessarily algorithmic or mechanical, as actuarial prediction is defined to be. Recent research supports the utility of this approach.

Using the SARA, Kropp *et al.* (1999) showed that the 'summary risk ratings' made by clinicians (which would fall into the 'clinical' camp in the traditional debate) actually outperformed the relationship between the sum of the instrument's individual items and violence (actuarial prediction). As Kropp *et al.* note, this was the first time, to their knowledge, in the violence risk assessment field, that 'clinical' judgment outperformed actuarial methods. Dempster (1998) also found that structured clinical ratings of risk using the SVR-20 added incremental validity to actuarial predictions. While these findings do not, of course, overturn the many findings that have found actuarial prediction to out-predict clinical impressions, they do provide some support for the structured clinical decision-making approach.

In this family of violence risk assessment schemes that follow, clinicians are called upon systematically to assess violence risk markers, indicate their presence, and then assign an overall risk rating based on the importance of these factors for the person being assessed. These tools also feature the option of 'critical items', which are variables that are of such salient importance for the current assessee that, alone, they warrant ratings of high risk. Clinicians are encouraged to base risk ratings on the items, but there is no specific concrete recommendation for cut-offs. Part of the reason for this stems from the fact that a person can be at high risk with the presence of a single (critical) risk marker. However, clinicians may devise their own procedures for rating people as high, moderate and low risk that are guided by score ranges, number of items present, and types of items present. One of the schemes, the SARA (Kropp *et al.*, 1999), provides guidance through the display of percentile tables and by placing certain scores into 'zones' of risk.

It is the present authors' contention that the flexibility afforded by this approach to risk assessment is an advantage when it comes to dealing with treatment and rehabilitation issues. Though flexible, the assessment method also is structured, guided and empirically based. As discussed earlier, this approach recognizes that the clinician is ultimately responsible for decisions, that (existing) actuarial tools may not be entirely appropriate and completely relevant in some settings, and that actuarial tools may fail to allow clinicians to 'flag' important markers in individual cases. If an individual issues definite and serious threats to kill some other person, but 'homicidal ideation or intent' did not make it into the regression equation, then the individual could probably erroneously be rated as low risk.

Violence risk assessment schemes

HCR-20. The HCR-20 applies to the assessment of violence risk generally (i.e. it does not target but includes sexual violence and spousal violence). Its three scales, as shown in Table 2, capture past (Historical), present (Clinical) and future (Risk Management) aspects of violence risk. Each of the 20 items are scored 0, 1, 2. A score of 0 indicates that the item is definitely absent; a score of 1 indicates that the item is possibly present or present in less serious form; a score of 2 indicates that the item is definitely present or present in more serious form. This scoring procedure was adopted from the PCL–R (Hare, 1991) because it appears to promote reliability, and it is easily understandable by clinicians and researchers

Table 2. Items in the HCR-20 risk assessment scheme

Subscales	Items
Historical scale	
H1	Previous violence
H2	Young age at first violent incident
H3	Relationship instability
H4	Employment problems
H5	Substance use problems
H6	Major mental illness
H7	Psychopathy
H8	Early maladjustment
H9	Personality disorder
H10	Prior supervision failure
Clinical scale	
C1	Lack of insight
C2	Negative attitudes
C3	Active symptoms of major mental illness
C4	Impulsivity
C5	Unresponsive to treatment
Risk management scale	
R1	Plans lack feasibility
R2	Exposure to destabilizers
R3	Lack of personal support
R4	Noncompliance with remediation attempts
R5	Stress

Note. Adapted from Webster, Douglas, Eaves & Hart (1997*b*).

alike. Each of the 20 items enjoys at least some backing from current published research. Support for the validity of the HCR-20 has been found in samples of civil psychiatric patients, forensic psychiatric patients, and correctional inmates. Much of this research is unpublished, given the HCR-20's relative youth.

There have been two civil psychiatric samples that have yielded several manuscripts and presentations. Douglas *et al.* (in press) completed the HCR-20 on 193 psychiatric patients who were released into the community. Using ROC analyses, AUCs ranged from .76 (for any violent act and for physical violence) to .77 (for fear-inducing or threatening behaviour), to .80 (for arrest for violent offences). These effects are large in size. In fact, persons who scored above the median of the HCR-20 were 13 times more likely to be arrested for violent offences than those who scored below the median. The PCL:SV (Hart *et al.*, 1995) also was coded in this study, and it too produced respectable AUCs (range from .68 to .79), as well as an odds ratio of approximately 13 for violent offences. A direct comparison of the two instruments revealed that the HCR-20 produced a statistically significantly greater AUC for the prediction of any violence and for fear-inducing/threatening behaviour. Regression analyses revealed that the HCR-20 and its scales were more consistently related to violence than the PCL:SV. Nicholls, Ogloff & Douglas (1997) found that, generally, the HCR-20 performed well for women in addition to men, although it was not as strongly related to the physical violence of women (AUC = .63) as it was for men.

In another civil psychiatric setting, Ross, Hart & Webster (1998) found, in their sample of 131 acute psychiatric inpatients, that AUCs ranged from .68 to .75 for the prediction of community violence. For inpatient violence in this sample, AUCs were smaller (.63 to .68), although still of moderate size and significantly greater than chance. The PCL:SV also was coded for this study, and its AUCs were somewhat smaller than those for the HCR-20, ranging from .65 to .70 for community violence, and averaging .61 for inpatient violence (although the statistical significance of differences was not reported).

Reliability in these civil psychiatric settings is acceptable. Douglas *et al.* (in press) report an overall intraclass correlation coefficient (ICC_1) between raters of .80. Ross *et al.* (1999) also found inter-rater reliability to be .82. In terms of internal reliability or consistency, Cronbach's alpha was reported by Ross *et al.* to be .74 for the Historical scale, .64 for the Clinical scale, and .69 for the Risk Management scale.

In forensic psychiatric samples, seven data sets have provided various disseminations on reliability and validity. Five of these samples have offered some validity data—for instance, Strand, Belfrage, Fransson & Levander (1999), in a Swedish sample of 40 male forensic psychiatric patients,[7] 22 of whom were recidivists, and 18 of whom were non-recidivist, matched controls. This research also used the PCL:SV. The AUC for the HCR-20 was .80, and for the PCL:SV, .70. The mean HCR-20 score for the recidivist group was 30.8, and for the non-recidivist group 22.4. This eight-point difference translates into a Cohen's d of 1.19, which is clearly a large effect size.[8] Every person who scored above 34/40 on the HCR-20 (N = 11/40) recidivated. Surprisingly, items from the Clinical and Risk Management scales were most powerful in terms of discriminating the two groups. This may stem from the fact that, as Strand *et al.* report, the two groups were quite homogeneous on the Historical items.

In another Swedish sample, Grann, Belfrage & Tengström (in press) compared the Historical scale of the HCR-20 to the VRAG (Harris *et al.*, 1993) in 404 forensic patients and mentally disordered offenders. They carried out analyses on the entire sample, as well as on subgroups of schizophrenic patients (N = 293) and personality disordered patients (N = 111). The Historical scale AUC for the entire sample was .71, and for the VRAG it was .68. Similarly, in the personality disordered group, the AUC for the Historical scale was .71, and for the VRAG it was .68. In the schizophrenic cohort, the AUC was lower for the Historical scale, at .66. The AUC for the VRAG was not greater than chance.

[7]This research project, in addition to all others carried out in Sweden, used the Swedish translation of the HCR-20 (Belfrage & Fransson, 1997). This is a literal translation of Version 2 of the HCR-20 (Webster *et al.*, 1997*b*), and hence findings based upon it ought to be interpretable as support for the HCR-20 generally.

[8]This d was calculated by the present authors. According to Cohen (1988, 1992), a d score (which is $[M_1 - M_2]$/pooled SD) of .80 + is considered large in magnitude. A d of 1.19, as in Strand *et al.*'s study, means that the difference between the groups' means is 1.19 times their average standard deviation.

In a Canadian sample of 80 male forensic psychiatric patients, Wintrup (1996; see also Douglas, Webster & Wintrup, 1996) found that both the HCR-20 and PCL–R correlated at approximately .30 with several measures of later community violence. The HCR-20 was quite strongly related to subsequent re-admissions to the forensic facility ($r = .38$) and to civil psychiatric hospitalization ($r = .45$).[9]

Finally, in another Canadian sample of 175 consecutively assessed forensic psychiatric patients, Douglas, Klassen, Ross, Hart & Webster (1998) studied the concurrent validity of the HCR-20 through its relationship with the PCL–R, the Brief Psychiatric Rating Scale (BPRS; Overall & Klett, 1962), and indices of violent and other antisocial behaviour. The HCR-20 total score correlated strongly with both the PCL–R ($r = .61$) and BPRS ($r = .54$). However, the relationship between particular HCR-20 scales and these other instruments differed importantly from the overall correlation. For instance, the Historical scale was very strongly related to the PCL–R ($r = .75$) whereas the Clinical and Risk Management scales were related with small/moderate effects (*rs* = .21 and .18, respectively). Conversely, the latter two scales were strongly related to most of the factors on the BPRS (*rs* = .63 and .59), whereas the former was not. This pattern of findings makes conceptual sense, given the content of the various scales. With respect to the HCR-20's relationship with criminal record, people scoring above the median of the HCR-20 were approximately two to four times more likely to have criminal histories of violence offences, past assault charges, and juvenile criminal histories than those scoring below the median. For these analyses, Item H1 (Previous violence) was removed from analyses to prevent artificial inflation of the effects.

Concerning the reliability of the HCR-20 within forensic samples, Belfrage (1998), in another Swedish sample, had six clinicians rate the same 43 patients. Using multivariate inter-relater reliability analyses, Kendall's $W = .81$ for the total scale. In this same study, internal consistency for the total scale, using Cronbach's alpha, was .95. In the Douglas *et al.* (1998) sample, inter-rater reliability was determined using the ICC, both single measure (ICC_1) and average measure (ICC_2). Here, $ICC_1 = .80$ and $ICC_2 = .89$. Also in this study, Cronbach's alpha for the total scale was .79. In a sample of 100 forensic patients in Germany, Müller-Isberner & Jöckel (1997)[10] found that the mean Kappa for the Historic scale was .89, with 91% of cases being rated by two clinicians within 1 point. For the Clinical scale, mean Kappa was lower, at .49, with 71% of cases being within 1 point.

Lastly, there have been three completed studies of the HCR-20 in correctional or prison samples. Belfrage, Fransson & Strand (1999) carried out a prospective study of violence within two maximum security prisons in Sweden, using the HCR-20. Eight of the 41 (19.5%) inmates were violent in the prison. The Clinical scale, Risk Management scale, and HCR-20 Total Score differentiated between the violent and non-violent groups. The HCR-20 Total Score was 33.4 in the violent group, and 24.6 in the non-violent group. All HCR-20 Risk Management scale items were

[9] According to Cohen (1988, 1992) a Pearson correlation coefficient of ± .30 is considered moderate in magnitude, and ± .50 is considered large.

[10] The German version of the HCR-20 contains three items not in the original HCR-20, and is based on Version 1 (Webster *et al.*, 1995), not Version 2 (Webster *et al.*, 1997*b*) of the HCR-20. It was not possible to rate the Risk Management scale.

significantly greater among the violent group than the non-violent group. The Historical scale was not predictive of violence, except for Item H10. In a sub-group of 30 psychopaths, defined with the PCL:SV, the Risk Management scale and HCR-20 Total Score were significantly higher in the violent inmates. Four of the five Risk Management scale items were higher in the violent psychopaths compared to the non-violent psychopaths. The authors comment that the Historical scale was not predictive in this sample because inmates (being maximum security violent inmates) were homogeneous with respect to most historical factors. The Clinical and Risk Management factors did, however, provide for a means of separating violent from non-violent inmates. These results are consistent with those of Strand *et al.* reported above. The results of the study, though limited by a small sample, provide support for the importance of risk management concerns for high-risk violent offenders.

In a second study, Douglas & Webster (1999*b*) evaluated the concurrent validity of the HCR-20 in 72 male prisoners who had been referred to a regional health centre of the federal Canadian prison system. They were rated on the Historical and Clinical scales of the HCR-20,[11] the PCL–R and the VRAG. Correlations between these scales and past violence, again with Item H1 (Previous violence) removed from analyses, were, respectively, .50 and .30 (for the HC composite, $r = .44$). The VRAG correlated at .20 and the PCL–R at .41, with past violence. Scores above the median of the HC composite increased the odds of various types of past violent and other antisocial behaviour by an average of four times. Hierarchical regression analyses showed that the HCR-20 (particularly the Historical scale) added incremental validity to the relationship between the PCL–R and violence, and the VRAG and violence. The converse was not true—that is, neither the VRAG nor the PCL–R added appreciably to the relationship between the HCR-20 and violence. This was particularly so for the VRAG. In this study, inter-rater reliability between two raters, using Pearson *r*, was .80. In another postdictive study, Dunbar (1999) observed correlations of .33 to .63 between the HCR-20 and violence in a sample of American hate crime perpetrators.

In summary, across civil psychiatric, forensic psychiatric and correctional samples, the HCR-20 has demonstrated effect sizes with violence that typically are either large or moderate in size by conventional definitions. In the few studies that have compared its validity to other measures (PCL:SV; PCL–R; VRAG) it has performed well. Reliability has ranged from acceptable to good, with most inter-rater indices being in the .80s. Internal consistency has been rated in the high .70s to the .90s.

SARA. The SARA possesses conceptual underpinnings similar to the HCR-20, but is intended to be applied in cases where there is a known or suspected background or concern about violence against spouses or partners. The SARA also possesses 20 items that are scored 0, 1, 2. These items are grouped differently from the HCR-20 items. As shown in Table 3, the SARA is divided into four types of risk factors: Criminal History; Psychosocial Adjustment; Spousal Assault History; and Alleged

[11]It was not possible to complete the Risk Management scale because most prisoners had not yet been considered for release from prison.

Table 3. Items in the SARA risk assessment scheme

Subscales	Items
Criminal History	
1	Past assault of family members
2	Past assault of strangers or acquaintances
3	Past violation of conditional release of community supervision
Psychosocial Adjustment	
4	Recent relationship problems
5	Recent employment problems
6	Victim of and/or witness to family violence as a child or adolescent
7	Recent substance use/dependence
8	Recent suicidal or homicidal ideation/intent
9	Recent psychotic and/or manic symptoms
10	Personality disorder with anger, impulsivity, or behavioural instability
Spousal Assault History	
11	Past physical assault
12	Past sexual assault/sexual jealousy
13	Past use of weapons and/or credible threats of death
14	Recent escalation in frequency or severity of assault
15	Past violation of 'no-contact' orders
16	Extreme minimization or denial of spousal assault history
17	Attitudes that support or condone spousal assault
Alleged (Current) Offence	
18	Severe and/or sexual assault
19	Use of weapons and/or credible threats of death
20	Violation of 'no-contact' orders

Note. Adapted from Kropp, Hart, Webster & Eaves (1999).

(Current) Offence. The Criminal History section deals with past crimes generally. Psychosocial Adjustment contains risk markers that span various areas from relationships to psychosis. The Spousal Assault History section contains items that are related specifically to previous spouse assault. Finally, the section dealing with the Alleged (Current) Offence has raters consider three items that are similar to the previous spouse assault items but apply only to the present index offence.

The SARA manual (Kropp *et al.*, 1999) provides appreciable validity and reliability data. These analyses were carried out on samples totalling more than 2300 probationers and inmates. Validity was estimated according to known-groups and concurrent validity strategies. Impressively, every item, scale score and summary score had higher scores for participants with known histories of spousal assault than for those without.

In terms of concurrent validity, the PCL:SV, VRAG, and the General Statistical Information on Recidivism (GSIR; Nuffield, 1982) were correlated with the SARA. All SARA ratings (summary risk ratings, total scores, scale scores, and number of items present) were moderately to highly correlated with the PCL:SV. The GSIR and VRAG, on the other hand, were moderately to highly correlated with only the general violence items of the SARA, but were not related to the spousal violence section scores or to summary risk ratings. Kropp *et al.* interpret this pattern of findings as support for the convergent validity of the general violence part of the SARA and for the discriminant validity of the spousal assault part of the SARA.

Finally, in a post-diction analysis of a subset of known recidivist and non-recidivist spouse assaulters, various SARA indices discriminated between recidivists and non-recidivists. For instance, recidivists had higher scores on the number of critical items present, number of items present, and summary risk ratings. Generally, differences were larger for the spousal assault section rather than the general violence section. It is important to point out that these groups did not differ on important demographic variables (e.g. age, education, employment, marital status, ethnicity), history of assault or on treatment variables (except one).

A very important finding was that summary risk ratings ('clinical' prediction) outperformed total scores ('actuarial' prediction) in terms of their relationship to spousal assault recidivism. The type of clinical prediction facilitated by the SARA is, of course, empirically guided structured decision-making, rather than the unstructured, global, impressionistic, clinical decision-making that is typically considered in debates over clinical vs. actuarial prediction.

In terms of reliability, internal consistency for the total scale, as measured by Cronbach's alpha, was .78. Item homogeneity, as estimated by mean inter-item correlations (MIC), was .15 for the total scale. Inter-rater reliability indices were very good—$ICC_1 = .84$ and $ICC_2 = .91$. Inter-rater reliability was (expectedly) somewhat lower for summary risk ratings, though still good—$ICC_1 = .77$ and $ICC_2 = .77$.

The SVR-20. As with the HCR-20 and SARA, the SVR-20 was constructed rationally from a consideration of the scientific and professional literatures on sexual violence. The obvious difference is that its purpose is the assessment of sexual violence risk. It, too, has 20 items that are scored on the 0, 1, 2 basis. A slight deviation from the HCR-20 and SARA item coding is that SVR-20 items are rated Present (Y), Absent (N) or Unsure (?). In practice and in research, however, the scoring system is the same as the PCL-R, HCR-20 and SARA. One useful addition to the scoring of the SVR-20 is the allotment of a 'recent change' score for each item. Assessors can indicate whether each risk factor has become more or less salient in some recent specified period of time. As with the other guides, the SVR-20 provides assessment guidelines, recommendations for the communication of assessment findings, and management strategies based on ratings of high, moderate or low risk. Table 4 shows that the 20 items are divided into three categories: Psychosocial Adjustment; Sexual Offences; and Future Plans.

The one completed study on the SVR-20 was carried out by Dempster (1998), who coded the SVR-20, along with other sexual violence and forensic assessment instruments, on 95 sexual offenders who had been incarcerated in federal Canadian institutions. Both the 'actuarial' (summed total of items) and 'structured clinical' (ratings of high, medium and low risk) forms of completing the SVR-20 had moderate-sized univariate correlations with sexual violence (the former correlating

Table 4. Items in the SVR-20 risk assessment scheme

Subscales	Items
Psychosocial Adjustment	
1	Sexual deviation
2	Victim of child abuse
3	Psychopathy
4	Major mental illness
5	Substance use problems
6	Suicidal/homicidal ideation
7	Relationship problems
8	Employment problems
9	Past nonsexual violent offences
10	Past nonviolent offences
11	Past supervision failure
Sexual Offences	
12	High density sex offences
13	Multiple sex offence types
14	Physical harm to victim(s) in sex offences
15	Uses weapons or threats of death in sex offences
16	Escalation in frequency or severity of sex offences
17	Extreme minimization or denial of sex offences
18	Attitudes that support or condone sex offences
Future Plans	
19	Lacks realistic plans
20	Negative attitudes toward intervention

Note. Adapted from Boer, Hart, Kropp & Webster (1998).

at .31 and the latter at .34, with sexual violence). The SVR-20 clinical ratings produced an AUC of .77 with sexual recidivism, which was equal to or greater than concurrent measures of sexual violence risk. The SVR-20 clinical ratings were one of two measures (of a total of six) that were able to distinguish between sexual recidivism vs. non-sexual but otherwise violent recidivism. A powerful finding by Dempster was that, for the prediction of sexual recidivism, the SVR-20 structured clinical ratings had incremental validity above and beyond that of various actuarial predictive scales of sexual violence risk. That is to say, using a hierarchical Cox regression model, the SVR-20 clinical ratings produced significant model improvements above the sole inclusion of the actuarial predictors. For some of these analyses, both the actuarial and clinical predictions remained significant once both predictors were entered, and for one analysis only the clinical ratings retained significance.

EARL-20B. This device evolved from the Earlscourt Child and Family Centre (ECFC) in Toronto, Canada. The agency assists children under age 12 and their families. Most of the children are referred by the police because of conduct problems. Although theft and fire-setting are often referral issues, the most

Table 5. Items in the Early Risk List for Boys (EARL-20B)

Subscales	Items
Family	
F1	Household circumstances
F2	Caregiver continuity
F3	Supports
F4	Stressors
F5	Parenting style
F6	Antisocial values and conduct
Child	
C1	Developmental problems
C2	Onset of behavioural difficulties
C3	Trauma
C4	Impulsivity
C5	Likeability
C6	Peer socialization
C7	School functioning
C8	Structured community attitudes
C9	Police contact
C10	Antisocial attitudes
C11	Antisocial behaviour
C12	Coping ability
Amenability	
A1	Family responsivity
A2	Child treatability

Note. Adapted from Augimeri, Webster, Koegl & Levene (1998).

pressing concerns usually centre around aggression and violence. The EARL-20B was developed from a longer 56-item checklist (Augimeri & Levene, 1997) and, using some of the ideas derived from the HCR-20, the SARA and SVR-20 noted above, was reduced to an assessment manual with 20 items. As with the other devices, much time was devoted to both scouring the literature and consulting with clinicians. Some colleagues will ask, perfectly reasonably, whether such a focus on the assessment of aggression in boys might be wise in persons so young, that there can be dangers in 'labelling' children so early. Issues such as these do, of course, require thoughtful and respectful consideration. But in the end it is necessary to decide whether the benefits to clients are likely to outweigh the costs and, if so, to move forward cautiously.

As can be seen in Table 5, the EARL-20B is comprised of three sections: Family Factors; Child Factors; and Amenability Factors. Family factors attempt to tap whether there is nurturance, support and supervision in the home. Child factors expand upon core constructs of sociability and spontaneity. Amenability factors are concerned with the resilience and competence of the child and family. Many of these items are similar to those found in the HCR-20 (e.g. stressors, antisocial values and attitudes, supports). Of course, there is strong focus on issues of childhood. Many of these risk factors are considered under a single HCR-20 risk factor (H8: Early maladjustment). In childhood, however, these factors are not necessarily historical, as in the HCR-20, but may be currently affecting a child.

As with the other devices, the EARL-20B is intended to inform treatment and management decisions. The identification of critical items (as in other of the devices) does a great deal to galvanize prompt and effective interventions. It helps to sort out not just how many factors are important, but assists in settling the order in which problems might best be tackled. There is also the chance that the EARL-20B will help in determining, perhaps from total scores or numbers of critical items, which children and families must receive immediate intensive service. It may even be helpful to complete the EARL-20B with the child's parent as a way of reaching agreement with parents over the exact nature of the problem and the best way of tackling it. It should be pointed out that similar scheme for use with girls is being developed. It is likely that the sorts of issues that are important for aggression in boys and girls warrant separate attention.

Communicating the results of risk assessments

Above it was explained that violence risk assessment may be able to be carried out with some respectable degree of accuracy, and that there are schemes available to promote this. When this is so, how should a clinician communicate the findings of his or her risk assessment? What degree of precision is warranted by the empirical research? This is a major issue in the risk assessment field (see Monahan & Steadman, 1996; Schropp, 1996). In the past, predictions were often given in Yes/No terms. An individual was deemed 'dangerous' or 'not dangerous'. Such an approach is probably too simple and begs for errors. Some researchers advocate communicating violence risk estimates in terms of precise probability levels, such as .82 over 10 years (Quinsey *et al.*, 1998). Others prefer more general statements that speak of such terms as 'low', 'moderate' and 'high' risk (Monahan & Steadman, 1996; Webster *et al.*, 1997*b*).

The authors favour the latter approach—use of broad categories such as 'low', 'moderate', 'high', and 'imminent', somewhat along the lines suggested by Monahan & Steadman (1996). The present authors' argument is that the specification of precise probabilities probably conveys a level of exactitude that can be misleading. Consider the idea of 'conditional prediction' offered by Mulvey & Lidz (1995). These commentators argued that risk for violence is conditional upon a great many factors that may occur post-release, after an initial risk assessment has been completed. Risk assessment, as the present authors consider it, is by no means solely a static process. The dynamic and conditional nature of risk assessment as a continuous, changing construct belies the possibility of giving precise, static estimates of violence risk. For instance, does the probability remain precisely fixed for every person with a given score on an instrument? If Person A returns to substance abuse (a known risk factor) while Person B receives appropriate treatment by diligent and trained professionals and is reunited with a supportive and strong family, the probabilities may not remain the same. When this idea is coupled with another concept—that of relative risk—the form of violence risk communication that is considered appropriate includes categories of *low*, *moderate*, *high* and *imminent* risk for violence (see Monahan & Steadman, 1996), that are *conditional upon* (may be aggravated or mitigated by) X and Y factors, and are *relative to* other inmates/patients/insanity acquittees with similar demographic characteristics from similar institutions.

The idea of risk management discussed at points throughout this article integrates some of these ideas. For instance, a person may be considered to be at moderate risk for violence relative to, say, other persons released from the same institution, based on an assessment of historical, clinical and risk management factors. This risk may be conditional upon the risk management factors remaining the same. If, for instance, the person fails to comply with medication, absconds from treatment, and begins abusing substances, then risk may be considered to be high. The advantages of such an approach are the implications for management that flow from the assessment (Boer *et al.*, 1998; Monahan & Steadman, 1996; Webster *et al.*, 1997*b*) and the flexibility to change violence risk communications should conditions change.

It should be evident from the above that the authors do not disagree with calculating the percentage of people who act violently as a function of being in one or other of various risk categories. In fact, this exercise would be useful in order to validate the risk communication approach; it also yields descriptive information to users about risk assessment models that employ such communication statements. But, as well as this, the authors favour explicating the violence risk factors that are relevant to the case at hand, and specifying those that are changeable.

Risk assessment training

Much of what has been said above has strong implications for training. Programmes that provide clinical training ought surely to include a component on violence risk, and should offer training on validated assessment methods. There is also a need to guide education about research on violence risk assessment. An example of a training module that could be found as part of a graduate, medical or other professional programme that included emphasis on forensic issues is outlined in Table 6. Introduction to both the science and practice of risk assessment proceeds from very introductory-level activities such as reading and clinical case or video review to carrying out independent research studies and handling a clinical caseload. Borum (1996) has suggested as well that violence risk assessment be declared a proficiency area within the mental health professions. It is, as he reminds us, disconcerting that training students and professionals in violence risk assessment is not more entrenched, given that many, if not most, professionals will come across a situation where risk assessment is called for in some manner.

Implications for clinical practice and research

What lessons for clinical practice and research follow from the ideas forwarded in this paper? In terms of practice, the implications seem relatively straightforward.

Table 6. Violence risk assessment training curriculum

Research	Practice
Level 1	Level 1
Lectures; reading	Observation, reading
Level 2	Level 2
Literature reviews	Videotape case reviews
Research proposals	Mock risk assessments/reports
Level 3	Level 3
Research assistantship	Clinical assistantship
Run pre-planned studies	Assist case preparation/file review
Assist in data processing/analyses	Assist in risk determination
Assist in write-up and dissemination	Assist in case write-up
Level 4	Level 4
Supervised minor research project	Supervised clinical risk assessment
Plan; conduct; write; disseminate	Assess; interview; write; opine
Mock/actual research presentation	Case conference/grand rounds
Level 5	Level 5
Major research project/thesis	Clinical caseload/practicum

Clinicians should base decisions on substantiated assessment procedures. This also means that they should contribute to the development and testing of such devices. Researchers should be at pains to help consolidate the scientific literature in ways that have practical use to clinicians. This means that they should have, where possible, familiarity with actual individual assessment cases and be challenged to deal with them in the light of prediction and assessment schemes.

The general framework for this article is the scientist–practitioner model. This approach, generally, holds that the practice of psychology (and by extension the other mental health professions) should be informed by scientific research. It is argued that this model has an apt fit in the risk assessment field. Despite the fact that much research knowledge is of recent origin, the authors agree with Borum (1996) that there has been enough advance of late to allow general consensus about key areas of risk assessment. Guidelines can, it would seem, be written responsibly. The authors assert further that science *ought* to inform practice. As indicated above, it may be ethically questionable for practitioners to fail to avail themselves of easily available research and technology. In tort law, professionals may be held to be negligent if they do not perform as a reasonable professional would, and injury ensues as a result. It certainly is reasonable for practitioners to be expected to be familiar with the state of their discipline in terms of practice *and* research. Ethical guidelines of professional associations require as much (APA, 1992). Failure to be so familiar could result in professional negligence. The authors do not advocate blind adoption of any research findings, but critical evaluation of research and adoption of reliable and valid findings that could be reasonably expected to generalize to the setting at hand.

The approach outlined above with the HCR-20, SARA, SVR-20 and EARL-20B does seem to be a slightly new addition to that aspect of forensic mental health practice which is concerned with assessing and managing risk for violence. This is not to say that others have not been at pains to produce guides in the past. Monahan's (1981) text was turning in that direction, and certainly the MacArthur Risk Assessment Project in the United States (Monahan & Steadman, 1994*b*; Monahan *et al.*, in press; Steadman *et al.*, 1994, 1998, in press) offers much in this regard. As a result of the present authors' experience to date, they think that this kind of conceptualization opens the way for different kinds of scientific and professional literatures to be connected to the literature on risk assessment. What they are mainly discussing here is the very large body of literature which deals with the scientist vs. practitioner debate, discussed earlier.

In advancing this alternative, somewhat more flexible and clinically collaborative line, the authors do not for a moment argue against the continuing effort to establish in more 'linear' fashion the exact links between clearly defined predictions and clearly defined outcomes. Once the basis for the four scales described here reaches a sufficient level of firmness, it seems that colleagues begin to use standard methodology to confirm the guides' reliability and validity. The authors have observed that colleagues tend to go over these instruments with painstaking care. Well in advance of wanting to test them formally in their own settings, they wish to be sure that they understand the terms and the method of scoring. The authors have found it necessary to be somewhat flexible about the coding of some items. A good example of this occurs in the German version of the HCR-20 (Müller-Isberner, Jöckel & Cabeza 1998). They call their version the 'HCR-20 + 2' to indicate that they collect somewhat more information, in a slightly different way, than is captured in the original. At a more general level, one seems to be trying as a first step to find a level of professional comfort with these devices. Always assuming that this process does not invite departure from what the scientific literature is informing one about various risk factors, there seems much to be gained from a plan of action that draws clinicians and researchers together in the common intent of making decisions that affect so vitally the lives and freedoms of persons suffering from mental and personality disorders who are in trouble with the law.

Concluding comment

This paper attempts to illustrate how the clinical practice of violence risk assessment ought to be informed by research, and how research also should be responsive to the realities of clinical practice. On the clinical side of the issue, practitioners need to be in touch with state-of-the-discipline research, demonstrate their competence in the clinical domain of risk assessment, and consider employing assessment guides. On the research side of the matter, scientists ought at least to consult with clinical colleagues, develop their research in clinically meaningful and helpful ways, and communicate this information to practitioners through clear channels.

Borum (1996) argued that '[d]espite substantive advances in knowledge about the risk for violent behavior among people with mental disorder, there have been virtually no systematic efforts to incorporate this information into a useful, empirically based framework for clinical assessment' (p. 947). He suggests that risk assessment schemes of the sort discussed in this article represent such integration and may facilitate the improvement of the clinical practice of risk assessment as well as risk assessment technology. What the present authors wish to show is that clinical practice may be flawed when it comes to risk assessment. At the same time, they wish to stress that research comes with its own limitations and liabilities. There needs to be some housecleaning on both sides of the semi-detached mansion and some thought about how best to tear down the walls which separate clinicians and researchers. This, of course, is no new issue, for it links directly to the debates around the scientist–practitioner model, and the actuarial–clinical prediction distinction, discussed earlier. It is suggested that clinical risk assessments could be better effected than at present, and that normative research could be designed so as to improve both the practice and science of violence risk assessment.

References

American Psychological Association (1992). Ethical principles of psychologists and code of conduct. *American Psychologist*, **47**, 1597–1611.

Andrews, D. A. & Bonta, J. (1995). *The psychology of criminal conduct.* Cincinnati, OH: Anderson Publishing.

Andrews, D. A., Zinger, I., Hoge, R. D., Bonta, J., Gendreau, P. & Cullen, F. T. (1990). Does correctional treatment work: A clinically relevant and psychologically informed meta-analysis. *Criminology*, **28**, 369–404.

Augimeri, L. K. & Levene, K. S. (1997). Outreach programme: Risk factors associated with possible conduct disorders and non-responders. Unpublished manuscript. Toronto, Ontario: Earlscourt Child and Family Centre.

Augimeri, L. K., Webster, C. D., Koegl, C. J. & Levene, K. S. (1998). *Early Assessment Risk List for Boys (Version 1): Consultation Edition.* Toronto, Ontario: Earlscourt Child and Family Centre.

Barratt, E. S. (1994). Impulsiveness and aggression. In J. Monahan & H. J. Steadman (Eds), *Violence and mental disorder: Developments in risk assessment*, pp. 61–79. Chicago, IL: University of Chicago Press.

Bartels, S. J., Drake, R. E., Wallach, M. A. & Freeman, D. H. (1991). Characteristic hostility in schizophrenic outpatients. *Schizophrenia Bulletin*, **17**, 163–171.

Belfrage, H. (1998). Implementing the HCR-20 scheme for risk assessment in a forensic psychiatric hospital: Integrating research and clinical practice. *Journal of Forensic Psychiatry*, **9**, 328–338.

Belfrage, H. & Fransson, G. (1997). *HCR-20: Bedömning av risk för framtida våld: Manual med instruktioner och kommentarer.* Forskningsenheten: Psykiatrist Regionvårdscentrum.

Belfrage, H., Fransson, G. & Strand, S. (1999). Prediction of violence within the correctional system using the HCR-20 risk assessment scheme. Manuscript under review.

Beutler, L. R., Williams, R. E., Wakefield, P. J. & Entwistle, S. R. (1995). Bridging scientist and practitioner perspectives in clinical psychology. *American Psychologist*, **50**, 984–994.

Binder, R. L. & McNiel, D. E. (1988). Effects of diagnosis and context on dangerousness. *American Journal of Psychiatry*, **145**, 728–732.

Binder, R. L. & McNiel, D. E. (1990). The relationship of gender to violent behavior in acutely disturbed psychiatric patients. *Journal of Clinical Psychiatry*, **51**, 110–114.

Boer, D. P., Hart, S. D., Kropp, P. R. & Webster, C. D. (1998). *Manual for the Sexual Violence Risk – 20: Professional guidelines for assessing risk of sexual violence.* Vancouver: British Columbia Institute Against Family Violence.

Bonta, J., Law, M. & Hanson, R. K. (1998). The prediction of criminal and violent recidivism among mentally disordered offenders: A meta-analysis. *Psychological Bulletin*, **123**, 123–142.

Borum, R. (1996). Improving the clinical practice of violence risk assessment. *American Psychologist*, **51**, 945–956.

Buchanan, A. (1997). The investigation of acting on delusions as a tool for risk assessment in the mentally disordered. *British Journal of Psychiatry*, **170** (s32), 12–16.

Buchanan, A., Reed, A., Wessely, S., Garety, P., Taylor, P., Grubin, D. & Dunn, G. (1993). Acting on delusions. II: The phenomenological correlates of acting on delusions. *British Journal of Psychiatry*, **163**, 77–81.

Cleckley, H. (1941). *The mask of sanity*. St Louis, MO: Mosby.

Cocozza, J. J. & Steadman, H. J. (1976). The failure of psychiatric predictions of dangerousness: Clear and convincing evidence. *Rutgers Law Review*, **29**, 1084–1101.

Cohen, J. (1988). *Statistical power analysis for the behavioral sciences*, 2nd ed. Hillsdale, NJ: Lawrence Erlbaum.

Cohen, J. (1992). A power primer. *Psychological Bulletin*, **112**, 155–159.

Convit, A., Isay, D., Gadioma, R. & Volavka, J. (1988). Underreporting of physical assaults in schizophrenic inpatients. *Journal of Nervous and Mental Disease*, **176**, 507–509.

Cooke, D. J. & Michie, C. (1997). An item response theory analysis of the Hare Psychopathy Checklist—Revised. *Psychological Assessment*, **9**, 3–14.

Cornell, D., Warren, J., Hawk, G., Stafford, E., Oram, G. & Pine, D. (1996). Psychopathy in instrumental and reactive violent offenders. *Journal of Consulting and Clinical Psychology*, **64**, 783–790.

Dempster, R. J. (1998). Prediction of sexually violent recidivism: A comparison of risk assessment instruments. Unpublished master's thesis. Simon Fraser University, Burnaby, British Columbia, Canada.

Department of Health (UK) (1990). *The care programme approach for people with a mental illness referred to the specialist psychiatry service*. London: Department of Health.

Douglas, K. S. & Hart, S. D. (1999). Psychosis as a risk factor for violence: A quantitative review of the research. Manuscript under review.

Douglas, K. S., Klassen, C., Ross, C., Hart, S. D. & Webster, C. D. (1998). *Psychometric properties of HCR-20 violence risk assessment scheme in insanity acquittees*. Poster presented at the Annual meeting of the American Psychological Association, August, San Francisco.

Douglas, K. S., Macfarlane, E. & Webster, C. D. (1996). Predicting dangerousness in the contemporary Canadian mental health and criminal justice systems. *Canada's Mental Health*, **43**, 4–11.

Douglas, K. S., Ogloff, J. R. P. & Nicholls, T. L. (1997). *The role of personality disorders in community violence among civil psychiatric patients*. Paper presented at the Fifth International Congress of the Disorders of Personality, June, Vancouver, Canada.

Douglas, K. S., Ogloff, J. R. P., Nicholls, T. L. & Grant, I. (in press). Assessing risk for violence among psychiatric patients: The HCR-20 risk assessment scheme and the Psychopathy Checklist: Screening Version. *Journal of Consulting and Clinical Psychology*.

Douglas, K. S. & Webster, C. D. (1999*a*). Predicting violence in mentally and personality disordered individuals. In R. Roesch, S. D. Hart & J. R. P. Ogloff (Eds), *Psychology and law: The state of the discipline*, pp. 175–239. New York: Plenum.

Douglas, K. S. & Webster, C. D. (1999*b*). The HCR-20 violence risk assessment scheme: Concurrent validity in a sample of incarcerated offenders. *Criminal Justice and Behavior*, **26**, 3–19.

Douglas, K. S., Webster, C. D. & Wintrup, A. (1996). *The HCR-20 Risk Assessment Scheme: Psychometric properties in two samples*. Poster presented at the annual convention of the American Psychological Association, August, Toronto, Ontario.

Dunbar, E. (1999). A psychographic analysis of violent hate crime perpetrators: Aggressive, situational and ideological characteristics of bias motivated offenders. Manuscript under review.

Estroff, S. E. & Zimmer, C. (1994). Social networks, social support, and violence among persons with severe, persistent mental illness. In J. Monahan & H. J. Steadman (Eds), *Violence and mental disorder: Developents in risk assessment*, pp. 259–295. Chicago, IL: University of Chicago Press.

Felson, R. B. (1992). 'Kick 'em when they're down': Explanations of the relationship between stress and interpersonal aggression and violence. *Sociological Quarterly*, **33**, 1–16.

Fensterheim, H. & Raw, S. D. (1996). Psychotherapy research is not psychotherapy practice. *Clinical Psychology: Science and Practice*, **3**, 168–171.

Gardner, W., Lidz, C. W., Mulvey, E. P. & Shaw, E. C. (1996*a*). A comparison of actuarial methods for identifying repetitively violent patients with mental illnesses. *Law and Human Behavior*, **20**, 35–48.

Gardner, W., Lidz, C. W., Mulvey, E. P. & Shaw, E. C. (1996*b*). Clinical versus actuarial predictions of violence in patients with mental illness. *Journal of Consulting and Clinical Psychology*, **64**, 602–609.

Goldfried, M. R. & Wolfe, B. E. (1996). Psychotherapy practice and research. *American Psychologist*, **51**, 1007–1016.

Grann, M., Belfrage, H. & Tengström, A. (in press). Actuarial assessment of risk for violence: Predictive validity of the VRAG and the historical part of the HCR-20. *Criminal Justice and Behavior.*

Grisso, T. & Appelbaum, P. S. (1992). Structuring the debate about ethical predictions of future violence. *Law and Human Behavior*, **17**, 482–485.

Grove, W. M. & Meehl, P. E. (1996). Comparative efficiency of informal (subjective, impressionistic) and formal (mechanical, algorithmic) prediction procedures: The clinical–statistical controversy. *Psychology, Public Policy, and Law*, **2**, 293–323.

Grubin, D. (1997). Predictors of risk in serious sex offenders. *British Journal of Psychiatry*, **170**, s17–s21.

Hare, R. D. (1991). *Manual for the Hare Psychopathy Checklist—Revised.* Toronto: Multi-Health Systems.

Hare, R. D. (1993). *Without conscience: The disturbing world of the psychopaths among us.* Toronto: Pocket Books.

Hare, R. D. (1996). Psychopathy: A clinical construct whose time has come. *Criminal Justice and Behavior*, **23**, 25–54.

Harris, G. T., Rice, M. E. & Cormier, C. A. (1991). Psychopathy and violent recidivism. *Law and Human Behavior*, **15**, 625–637.

Harris, G. T., Rice, M. E. & Quinsey, V. L. (1993). Violent recidivism of mentally disordered offenders: The development of a statistical prediction instrument. *Criminal Justice and Behavior*, **20**, 315–335.

Hart, S. D. (1998). The role of psychopathy in assessing risk for violence: Conceptual and methodological issues. *Legal and Criminological Psychology*, **3**, 121–137.

Hart, S. D., Cox, D. & Hare, R. D. (1995). *The Hare Psychopathy Checklist: Screening Version (PCL:SV).* Toronto, Ontario: Multi-Health Systems.

Hart, S. D., Webster, C. D. & Menzies, R. J. (1993). A note of portraying the accuracy of violence predictions. *Law and Human Behavior*, **17**, 695–700.

Hayes, S. C. (1996). Creating the empirical clinician. *Clinical Psychology: Science and Practice*, **3**, 179–181.

Heilbrun, K. (1997). Prediction versus management models relevant to risk assessment: The importance of legal decision-making context. *Law and Human Behavior*, **21**, 347–359.

Heilbrun, K., Philipson, J., O'Neill, M., Paninopolous, M., Strohman, L. & Bowman, Q. (1998). *Expert and practitioner approaches to communicating violence risks.* Paper presented at the annual convention of the American Psychological Association, August, San Francisco.

Hellman, D. & Blackman, J. (1966). Enuresis, firesetting and cruelty to animals: A triad predictive of adult crime. *American Journal of Psychiatry*, **122**, 1431–1435.

Hemphill, J. F., Hare, R. D. & Wong, S. (1998). Psychopathy and recidivism: A review. *Legal and Criminological Psychology*, **3**, 139–170.

Hillbrand, M. (1995). Aggression against self and aggression against others in violent psychiatric patients. *Journal of Consulting and Clinical Psychology*, **63**, 668–671.

Hodgins, S. (1983). A follow-up study of persons found incompetent to stand trial and/or not guilty by reason of insanity in Quebec. *International Journal of Law and Psychiatry*, **6**, 399–411.

Hoffman, P. B. & Beck, J. L. (1985). Recidivism among released federal prisoners: Salient factor score and five-year follow-up. *Criminal Justice and Behavior*, **12**, 501–507.

Hollander, E. & Stein, D. J. (Eds) (1995). *Impulsivity and aggression.* Toronto: Wiley.

Jackson, J. (1997). A conceptual model for the study of violence and aggression. In C. D. Webster & M. A. Jackson (Eds), *Impulsivity: Theory, assessment and treatment*, pp. 233–247. New York: Guilford.

Kanfer, F. H. (1990). The scientist–practitioner connection: A bridge in need of constant attention. *Professional Psychology: Research and Practice*, **21**, 264–270.

Klassen, D. & O'Connor, W. A. (1988*a*). Crime, inpatient admissions, and violence among male mental patients. *International Journal of Law and Psychiatry*, **11**, 305–312.

Klassen, D. & O'Connor, W. A. (1988*b*). Predicting violence in schizophrenic and non-schizophrenic patients: A prospective study. *Journal of Community Psychology*, **16**, 217–227.

Klassen, D. & O'Connor, W. A. (1988*c*). A prospective study of predictors of violence in adult male mental health admission. *Law and Human Behavior*, **12**, 143–158.

Klassen, D. & O'Connor, W. A. (1989). Assessing the risk of violence in released mental patients: A cross-validation study. *Psychological Assessment: A Journal of Consulting and Clinical Psychology*, **1**, 75–81.

Klassen, D. & O'Connor, W. A. (1994). Demographic and case history variables in risk assessment. In J. Monahan & H. J. Steadman (Eds), *Violence and mental disorder: Developments in risk assessment*, pp. 229–258. Chicago, IL: University of Illinois Press.

Kropp, P. R., Hart, S. D., Webster, C. D. & Eaves, D. (1999). *Manual for the Spousal Assault Risk Assessment Guide*, 3rd ed. Toronto: Multi-Health Systems.

Lidz, C. W., Mulvey, E. P. & Gardner, W. (1993). The accuracy of predictions of violence to others. *Journal of the American Medical Association*, **269**, 1007–1111.

Lindqvist, P. & Allebeck, P. (1990). Schizophrenia and crime: A longitudinal follow-up of 644 schizophrenics in Stockholm. *British Journal of Psychiatry*, **157**, 345–350.

Link, B. G. & Stueve, A. (1994). Psychotic symptoms and the violent/illegal behavior of mental patients compared to community controls. In J. Monahan & H. J. Steadman (Eds), *Violence and mental disorder: Developments in risk assessment*, pp. 137–159. Chicago, IL: University of Chicago Press.

Lipsey, M. W. & Wilson, D. B. (1993). The efficacy of psychological, educational, and behavioral treatment: Confirmation from meta-analyses. *American Psychologist*, **48**, 1181–1209.

Lyon, D. R., Hart, S. D. & Webster, C. D. (in press). Violence and risk assessment. In R. Schuller & J. R. P. Ogloff (Eds), *Law and psychology: Canadian perspectives*. Toronto: University of Toronto Press.

MacCulloch, M. J., Snowden, P. R., Wood, P. J. W. & Mills, H. E. (1983). Sadistic fantasy, sadistic behaviour, and offending. *British Journal of Psychiatry*, **143**, 20–29.

McNiel, D. E. & Binder, R. L. (1989). Relationship between preadmission threats and later violent behavior by acute psychiatric inpatients. *Hospital and Community Psychiatry*, **40**, 605–608.

McNiel, D. E. & Binder, R. L. (1991). Clinical assessment of the risk of violence among psychiatric inpatients. *American Journal of Psychiatry*, **148**, 1317–1321.

McNiel, D. E. & Binder, R. L. (1994*a*). The relationship between acute psychiatric symptoms, diagnosis, and short-term risk of violence. *Hospital and Community Psychiatry*, **45**, 133–137.

McNiel, D. E. & Binder, R. L. (1994*b*). Screening for risk of inpatient violence: Validation of an actuarial tool. *Law and Human Behavior*, **18**, 579–586.

McNiel, D. E. & Binder, R. L. (1995). Correlates of accuracy in the assessment of psychiatric inpatients' risk of violence. *American Journal of Psychiatry*, **152**, 901–906.

McNiel, D. E., Binder, R. L. & Greenfield, T. K. (1988). Predictors of violence in civilly committed acute psychiatric patients. *American Journal of Psychiatry*, **145**, 965–970.

Meehl, P. E. (1954). *Clinical versus statistical prediction*. Minneapolis, MN: University of Minnesota Press.

Meehl, P. (1997). Credentialed persons, credentialed knowledge. *Clinical Psychology: Science and Practice*, **4**, 91–98.

Menzies, R. & Webster, C. D. (1995). Construction and validation of risk assessments in a six-year follow-up of forensic patients: A tridimensional analysis. *Journal of Consulting and Clinical Psychology*, **63**, 766–778.

Menzies, R. J., Webster, C. D. & Sepejak, D. S. (1985). Hitting the forensic sound barrier: Predictions of dangerousness in a pre-trial psychiatric clinic. In C. D. Webster, M. H. Ben-Aron & S. J. Hucker (Eds), *Dangerousness: Probability and prediction, psychiatry and public policy*, pp. 115–143. New York: Cambridge University Press.

Monahan, J. (1981). *Predicting violent behavior: An assessment of clinical techniques*. Beverly Hills, CA: Sage.

Monahan, J. (1984). The prediction of violent behavior: Toward a second generation of theory and policy. *American Journal of Psychiatry*, **141**, 10–15.

Monahan, J. (1988). Risk assessment of violence among the mentally disordered: Generating useful knowledge. *International Journal of Law and Psychiatry*, **11**, 249–257.

Monahan, J. (1992). Mental disorder and violent behavior. *American Psychologist*, **47**, 511–521.

Monahan, J. (1996). Violence prediction: The last 20 and the next 20 years. *Criminal Justice and Behavior*, **23**, 107–120.

Monahan, J. & Steadman, H. J. (Eds) (1994*a*). *Violence and mental disorder: Developments in risk assessment.* Chicago, IL: University of Chicago Press.

Monahan, J. & Steadman, H. J. (1994*b*). Toward a rejuvenation of risk assessment research. In J. Monahan & H. J. Steadman (Eds), *Violence and mental disorder: Developments in risk assessment*, pp. 1–17. Chicago, IL: University of Chicago Press.

Monahan, J. & Steadman, H. J. (1996). Violent storms and violent people: How meteorology can inform risk communication in mental health law. *American Psychologist*, **51**, 931–938.

Monahan, J., Steadman, H. J., Appelbaum, P. S., Robbins, P. C., Mulvey, E. P., Silver, E., Roth, L. H. & Grisso, T. (in press). Developing a clinically useful actuarial tool for assessing violence risk. *British Journal of Psychiatry.*

Mossman, D. (1994). Assessing predictions of violence: Being accurate about accuracy. *Journal of Consulting and Clinical Psychology*, **62**, 783–792.

Müller-Isberner, J. R. & Jöckel, D. (1997). *The implementation of the HCR-20 in a German hospital order institution.* Paper presented at the Seventh European Conference on Psychology and Law, September, Solna, Sweden.

Müller-Isberner, R., Jöckel, D. & Cabeza, S. G. (1998). *Die Vorhersage von Gewalttaten mit dem HCR 20.* Haina: Institut für Forensische Psychiatrie Haina.

Mulvey, E. P. & Lidz, C. W. (1995). Conditional prediction: A model for research on dangerousness to others in a new era. *International Journal of Law and Psychiatry*, **18**, 129–143.

Mulvey, E. P., Shaw, E. & Lidz, C. W. (1994). Why use multiple sources in research on patient violence in the community? *Criminal Behaviour and Mental Health*, **4**, 253–258.

Nezu, A. M. (1996). What are we doing to our patients and should we care if anyone else knows? *Clinical Psychology: Science and Practice*, **3**, 160–163.

Nicholls, T. L., Ogloff, J. R. P. & Douglas, K. S. (1997). Comparing risk assessments with female and male psychiatric outpatients: Utility of the HCR-20 and Psychopathy Checklist: Screening Version. In J. R. P. Ogloff (Chair), *Involuntary civil commitment—patient characteristics, review panel decision making, and risk assessment.* Symposium conducted at the annual convention of the American Psychological Association, August, Chicago.

Novaco, R. W. (1994). Anger as a risk factor for violence among the mentally disordered. In J. Monahan & H. J. Steadman (Eds), *Violence and mental disorder: Developments in risk assessment*, pp. 21–59. Chicago, IL: University of Chicago Press.

Nuffield, J. (1982). *Parole decision-making in Canada: Research towards decision guidelines.* Ottawa: Ministry of Supply and Services Canada.

Overall, J. E. & Klett, C. J. (1962). The brief psychiatric rating scale. *Psychological Reports*, **10**, 799–812.

Pfohl, S. J. (1978). *Predicting dangerousness: The social construction of psychiatric reality.* Lexington, MA: Lexington Books.

Quinsey, V. L., Harris, G. T., Rice, G. T. & Cormier, C. A. (1998). *Violent offenders: Appraising and managing risk.* Washington, DC: American Psychological Association.

Reed, J. (1997). Risk assessment and clinical risk management: The lessons from recent inquiries. *British Journal of Psychiatry*, **170**, s4–s7.

Rice, M. E. (1997). Violent offender research and implications for the criminal justice system. *American Psychologist*, **52**, 414–423.

Rice, M. E. & Harris, G. T. (1995). Violent recidivism: Assessing predictive validity. *Journal of Consulting and Clinical Psychology*, **63**, 737–748.

Ross, D. J., Hart, S. D. & Webster, C. D. (1998). *Aggression in psychiatric patients: Using the HCR-20 to assess risk for violence in hospital and in the community.* Port Coquitlam, British Columbia: Riverview Hospital.

Salekin, R. T., Rogers, R. & Sewell, K. W. (1996). A review and meta-analysis of the Psychopathy Checklist and Psychopathy Checklist—Revised: Predictive validity of dangerousness. *Clinical Psychology: Science and Practice*, **3**, 203–215.

Saunders, D. G. (1992). Woman battering. In R. T. Ammerman & M. Hersen (Eds), *Assessment of family violence: A clinical and legal sourcebook*, pp. 208–235. New York: Wiley.

Schopp, R. F. (1996). Communicating risk assessments: Accuracy, efficacy, and responsibility. *American Psychologist*, **9**, 939–944.

Shaffer, C. E., Waters, W. F. & Adams, S. G. (1994). Dangerousness: Assessing the risk of violent behavior. *Journal of Consulting and Clinical Psychology*, **62**, 1064–1068.

Singer, J. L. (1990). The scientific basis of psychotherapy practice: A question of values and ethics. *Psychotherapy: Theory, Research, and Practice*, **17**, 372–383.

Snowden, P. (1997). Practical aspects of clinical risk assessment and management. *British Journal of Psychiatry*, **170**, s32–s34.

Sobell, L. C. (1996). Bridging the gap between scientists and practitioners: The challenge before us. *Behavior Therapy*, **27**, 297–320.

Steadman, H. J., Monahan, J., Appelbaum, P. S., Grisso, T., Mulvey, E. P., Roth, L. H., Robbins, P. C. & Klassen, D. (1994). Designing a new generation of risk assessment research. In J. Monahan & H. J. Steadman (Eds), *Violence and mental disorder: Developments in risk assessment*, pp. 297–318. Chicago, IL: University of Chicago Press.

Steadman, H. J., Mulvey, E., Monahan, J., Robbins, P. C., Appelbaum, P. S., Grisso, T., Roth, L. H. & Silver, E. (1998). Violence by people discharged from acute psychiatric inpatient facilities and by others in the same neighborhoods. *Archives of General Psychiatry*, **55**, 393–401.

Steadman, H. J., Silver, E., Monahan, J., Appelbaum, P. S., Robbins, P. C., Mulvey, E. P., Grisso, T., Roth, L. H. & Banks, S. (in press). *Law and Human Behavior.*

Strand, S., Belfrage, H., Fransson, G. & Levander, S. (1999). Clinical and risk management factors in risk prediction of mentally disordered offenders: More important than actuarial data? *Legal and Criminological Psychology*, **4**, 67–76.

Stricker, G. (1992). The relationship of research to clinical practice. *American Psychologist*, **47**, 543–549.

Stricker, G. & Trierweiler, S. J. (1995). The local clinical scientist: A bridge between science and practice. *American Psychologist*, **50**, 995–1002.

Swanson, J. W. (1994). Mental disorder, substance abuse, and community violence: An epidemiological approach. In J. Monahan & H. J. Steadman (Eds), *Violence and mental disorder: Developments in risk assessment*, pp. 101–136. Chicago, IL: University of Chicago Press.

Swanson, J. W., Borum, R., Swartz, M. & Monahan, J. (1996). Psychotic symptoms and disorders and the risk of violent behavior in the community. *Criminal Behaviour and Mental Health*, **6**, 317–338.

Webster, C. D. & Cox, D. N. (1997). Integration of nomothetic and ideographic positions in risk assessment: Implications for practice and the education of psychologists and other mental health professionals. *American Psychologist*, **52**, 1245–1246.

Webster, C. D., Dickens, B. M. & Addario, S. M. (1985). *Constructing dangerousness: Scientific legal and policy implications.* Toronto, Ontario: University of Toronto Centre of Criminology.

Webster, C. D., Douglas, K. S., Eaves, S. D. & Hart, S. D. (1997*a*). Assessing risk of violence to others. In C. D. Webster & M. A. Jackson (Eds), *Impulsivity: Theory, assessment, and treatment*, pp. 251–277. New York: Guilford.

Webster, C. D., Douglas, K. S., Eaves, D. & Hart, S. D. (1997*b*). *HCR-20: Assessing Risk for Violence (Version 2).* Vancouver: Mental Health, Law, and Policy Institute, Simon Fraser University.

Webster, C. D., Eaves, D., Douglas, K. S. & Wintrup, A. (1995). *The HCR-20 scheme: The assessment of dangerousness and risk.* Vancouver, B.C.: Mental Health Law and Policy Institute, and Forensic Psychiatric Services Commission of British Columbia.

Webster, C. D. & Jackson, M. A. (Eds) (1997). *Impulsivity: Theory, assessment, and treatment.* New York: Guildford.

Wessely, S. C., Castle, D., Douglas, A. J. & Taylor, P. T. (1994). The criminal careers of incident cases of schizophrenia. *Psychological Medicine*, **24**, 483–502.

Wintrup, A. (1996). Assessing risk of violence in mentally disordered offenders with the HCR-20. Unpublished master's thesis. Simon Fraser University, Burnaby, British Columbia, Canada.

[2]

Prediction Versus Management Models Relevant to Risk Assessment: The Importance of Legal Decision-Making Context

Kirk Heilbrun[1]

Most of the theoretical and empirical literature on violence risk to date has focused on the task of predicting who will behave violently. In the present article, it is argued that at least two models of risk assessment may be applied to the varying legal decisions in which violence risk is a consideration: prediction *(with an emphasis on overall accuracy) and* management *(with an emphasis on risk reduction). These two models are described, and discussed in the contexts of the literatures on forensic assessment and therapeutic jurisprudence. The implications for research, policy, and practice are considered.*

The use of science to inform legal decision-making has been one of the most important goals for the field of law and psychology. During the last two decades, this field has witnessed the emergence of formal interdisciplinary predoctoral and postdoctoral training programs, the establishment of an APA division, the development of a procedure for board certification in forensic psychology, and the initiation of several interdisciplinary journals. Through each runs the theme of "better-informed legal decision-making." Whether empirical data are obtained from laboratory studies, field studies with quasi-experimental designs, or simply formal efforts to obtain better base rates, we hope they can be used to assist courts in making better decisions. When scientific studies are applied to improving the measurement of the psychological constructs underlying legal issues, as with the Interdisciplinary Fitness Interview (Golding, Roesch, & Schreiber, 1984) or the more recent approach to the measurement of adjudicative competence taken by the MacArthur Research Network on Mental Health and Law (Hoge et al., 1997), the result should be a better quality of practice in forensic mental health assessment (FMHA), and better-informed decisions from the courts that are the "consumers" of FMHA.

[1]Law-Psychology Program, Department of Clinical and Health Psychology, Allegheny University of the Health Sciences, Mail Stop 626, Broad & Vine, Philadelphia, PA 19102-1192; e-mail: HEILBRUN@ALLEGHENY.EDU.

This article will focus on FMHA and the context of legal decision-making. "Context" will be considered broadly, to include the consequences of legal judgments. The goals, substance, and form of communication of FMHA may be substantially different when this "context" varies. In the course of this description, I will incorporate Grisso's (1986) model of legal competencies, Poythress's (1987, 1990) contributions in the areas of negligent release and risk management, Monahan and Steadman and the MacArthur Research Network's efforts (1994) in risk assessment, and Wexler and Winick's (1991, 1996) work in therapeutic jurisprudence.

I have chosen risk assessment as the example of forensic assessment to use in this analysis because of its importance to society and the significant research advances that have been observed in this area during the last decade. Risk assessment is not a legal issue in the conventionally-understood sense that competence to stand trial, child custody, or criminal responsibility (to name a few of many) are legal issues. Nevertheless, it is an important part of many legal decisions (e.g., civil commitment, end of sentence commitment as a "sexual predator," sentencing, juvenile transfer, NGRI release). Because violent behavior is of widespread concern within our legal system and our larger society, it is associated with a number of circumstances in which some form of "control" is exercised over those thought to be potentially violent, and risk-reduction management strategies implemented. Violence also has a significant history as an outcome that has been "predicted," both through research studies and the clinical activity of mental health professionals (Meehl, 1954; Monahan, 1981). In short, risk assessment is well-suited to an analysis that uses the concepts of "prediction" and "management"[2] as integral parts.

SCIENTIFIC GOALS RELEVANT TO LEGAL DECISION-MAKING

A brief historical note provides a helpful context for the respective roles of *understanding* and *prediction/control* in scientific research. In a recent *American Psychologist* article relating prediction and control to the work of B. F. Skinner, Smith (1992) observed that reigning Aristotelian philosophy at the turn of the seventeenth century drew a sharp distinction between theoretical (or contemplative) knowledge, and lower forms of knowledge which Aristotle called *practical* and *productive*. Yet during the time of Francis Bacon, a series of technological innovations, including the compass, gunpowder, and the printing press, made it clear that human works were not merely artifacts of nature. Bacon promoted technological innovation not only for the power of its products, but also as a model of the knowledge process. The influence of Bacon's work on Skinner was important, particularly in Skinner's preference for a "technology of behavior" that emphasized prediction and control far more than understanding (Smith, 1992).

It is beyond the scope of this article to discuss the relative importance to courts of *understanding* vs. *prediction/control* of individuals involved in litigation. Certainly

[2]In my presidential address, I used the terms prediction and control to characterize two approaches to decision-making that can arise in the course of litigation. The term management has subsequently been substituted for control, because of the potentially pejorative connotations that could result from the latter label.

each may be identifiable within the structure of mental health laws. The information provided to legal decision-makers may be used to increase the court's understanding of scientific methods or results (particularly under *Daubert*, 1993); it may also help the court address relevant questions concerning prediction/control. However, it is worth noting that prediction and control are, in some important respects, distinct goals. This will be seen when we discuss the example of risk assessment.

SCIENTIFIC COMPONENTS OF LEGAL DECISION-MAKING

In theory, at least, the quality of the information provided to a decision-maker should affect the quality of the decision. In practice, the translation of scientific data into a form in which it can demonstrably improve legal decision-making can be a daunting task. Consider the generalizability problem. Variables defining a subpopulation relevant for a given court may include (among others) age, severity of disorder, jurisdiction, stage in the legal process, and setting. For a juvenile judge in Virginia interested in the question of how a 16-year-old defendant, currently incarcerated in the local detention facility, having a measured IQ of 74, diagnosed disorders of Attention Deficit Hyperactivity Disorder and substance abuse, and two prior juvenile arrests compares with other juvenile defendants in his appreciation of his plea options and the rationality of his decision-making for pleading, there are currently no answers. In considering what would be needed to address this question, assume a *best-case scenario*: a multistate study had been conducted with 1000 juvenile defendants in three states (including Virginia). The court was interested in only the Virginia data, which subdivided the sample into thirds. Data collection was further divided according to subject age, into categories of ≤12, 13-14, and ≤15 (Grisso, 1995), leaving approximately 110 subjects in the relevant age category. Further subdivision according to level of intellectual functioning, nature of psychopathology, and incarceration status could quickly leave the court with a comparison group smaller than the juvenile defendant's family. To make meaningfully empirically-supported decisions at this level, then, the supporting studies would need to be very large and very expensive.[3]

Hopefully this is not the only way in which behavioral scientists can prove helpful to legal decision-makers. There are any number of areas in which this best-case scenario would not be met, and the quality and quantity of available data would be far more limited. However, in addition to empirical data obtained from large samples, behavioral science can offer the following to legal decision-makers: (1) scientific reasoning, (2) idiographic analysis, and (3) FMHA that is relevant to legal context. Since the present focus will be on the third area, I will note only briefly that questions relevant to *scientific reasoning*—whether the relevant underlying constructs have been operationalized, and whether falsifiable hypotheses have been formulated and tested—are also helpful to judges attempting to weigh evidence to decide issues such as child custody or criminal responsible. Likewise, while

[3] I am grateful to John Monahan for his comments on this particular aspect of data analysis and generalizability from large data sets.

it may be useful for a judge to consider a given juvenile's capacities in relation to those of other juvenile defendants, it is also helpful to assess that individual's functioning relative to his potential, and consider how the level of "actual" functioning might be improved and whether that improvement would be "enough" in the present situation.

It is on the topic of legal decisions and their contexts, however, that I want to focus most attention. The consideration of legal context has recently been incorporated into the analyses of several commentators. Legal context has been applied to the consideration of programmatic interventions for sexual offenders (Small, 1992). It has also been argued recently that an emphasis on "dangerousness" is overly narrow when it fails to include situational influences on violence potential, and that broadening the conceptualization of risk provides a better linkage with legal decision-making on many risk issues of legal concern (Carson, 1994).

Legal context has also been incorporated into the literature on forensic assessment. For example, Grisso's (1986) model of legal competencies delineates the following characteristics:

Functional Characteristic—that which an individual can do or accomplish, as well as...the specific knowledge, understanding, or beliefs that may be necessary for the accomplishment.

Contextual Characteristic—some class of external situations to which a person must respond...each context is presumed to require certain types of functional abilities in order to manage one's role within that context.

Causal Characteristic—legal competency constructs require causal inferences to explain an individual's functional abilities or deficits related to a legal competency...(including) ascription of the deficit's cause, future consequences, or other meanings.

Interactive Characteristic—a focus on person–context interactions...asks, "Does this person's level of ability meet the demands of the specific situation with which the person will be (was) faced?" Defined more formally, a decision about legal competency is in part a statement about congruency or incongruency between (1) the extent of a person's functional ability, and (2) the degree of performance demand that is made by the specific instance of the context in that case.

Judgmental Characteristic—legal competency constructs require a judgment that person–context incongruency is of a sufficient magnitude to warrant a finding of legal incompetency and its dispositional consequences...addresses the question, "How much incongruency is enough to warrant a finding of incompetency?"

Dispositional Characteristic—a finding of incompetency gives the state the authority to act in some way toward the individual, in a way that involves deprivation of fundamental rights (e.g., liberty) (Grisso, 1986, pp. 15–27).

This model is the literature's closest approximation to a description of legal decision-making on forensically relevant issues; even though it describes legal competencies rather than "included" constructs such as risk assessment, it seems reasonably applicable for present purposes. The model contains two particular characteristics—*context* and *disposition*—that are particularly important in this discussion. Under context, we might ask about the "external situations" to which a person undergoing forensic evaluation must respond. To some of the more obvious elements (e.g., nature of charges or litigation, characteristics of attorney, community sentiment/media exposure) we might add the "characteristics of the disposition": where is the litigant placed if a judgment is made, and what is the level of control retained by the court (or exercised by another source) as part of this placement?

RELEVANT CHARACTERISTICS OF RISK ASSESSMENT

Attempts to determine whether an individual will behave violently in the future should first be considered as part of the classic "clinical vs. statistical prediction" issue addressed by Paul Meehl in the 1950s (Meehl, 1954), when he demonstrated convincingly that attempts at prediction were more accurate when they were actuarial, assuming that there was some basis for using an actuarial approach (i.e., the predictor and outcome variables could be operationalized, and there were preexisting data defining their relationship). This superiority of actuarial over clinical approaches is even more demonstrable today (Dawes, Faust, & Meehl, 1989). When Monahan (1981) wrote his seminal work on the clinical prediction of violent behavior, he clearly conceptualized prediction as the task, and used civil commitment as an example of a context in which predictions of violence were frequently made.

The focus on prediction as the scientific task has shifted somewhat, however, in the work of the MacArthur Research Network on Mental Health and Law, which identified a large sample of civilly committed individuals across three sites and followed them after release from hospitalization, in the attempt to determine what risk factors are most strongly associated with outcomes of violent behavior in the community (Monahan & Steadman, 1994). In a theoretical reconceptualization of the task of assessing violence risk, this group envisioned a shift from a focus on a single prediction of risk potential to ongoing decisions, made at different times, about the management and treatment of mentally disordered persons (Steadman et al., 1993).

Another approach to risk assessment that is more consistent with this reconceptualized approach has been developed under more applied circumstances. The Violent Behavior Analysis, developed by Norman Poythress and others[4] at Alabama's Taylor Hardin Secure Medical Facility, is an attempt to determine current violence risk for Not Guilty by Reason of Insanity acquittees being considered for transfer to a less secure unit, or for release into the community. The VBA is a semistructured interview, supplemented by collateral information, that assesses patterns of thinking, emotion, and behavior that recur across violent acts. A modified VBA (the Analysis of Aggressive Behavior (AAB);[5] Heilbrun, 1991), used with NGRI acquittees in Virginia since 1991, involves multiple administrations in the attempt to assess change in risk status over time, particularly at crucial "decision points" (involving the determination of whether an individual should be granted a requested privilege involving a lessening of restrictions in their situation, such as

[4]The VBA has not been published. Relevant hospital policy is available upon request from the Taylor Hardin Secure Medical Facility in Tuscaloosa, Alabama.
[5]The AAB is available upon request from the author.

Table 1. Risk Management Plan in Management Context[a]

Risk factor	Intervention plan	Status
1	1	1
2	2	2
N	N	N

[a]Ratings for Status Column: 1=no longer active, 2=currently contained, 3=currently partly contained, 4=not currently contained, 5=intervention refused, 6=intervention not attempted, 7=unknown, 8=other.

grounds privileges, community visits, transfer from a higher to a lower security unit, or conditional release into the community). It also includes the development and periodic updating of a Risk Management plan, in which risk factors common to violent episodes are identified in one column, a plan for treatment/rehabilitation/management is described next to the its respective risk factor, and a "status" column—to determine how successfully the plan is being implemented—is offered in the third column (see Table 1).

Civil commitment and NGRI graduated release are examples of legal decision contexts that are either *prediction*- or *management*-oriented. Using these examples, we can see how *prediction*- and *management*-oriented approaches to risk assessment differ in some important respects. As may be seen in Table 2, there are at least six differences between these models. First, the primary *goal* of using the prediction model is to attempt to determine, as accurately as possible, the probability of a specified event's occurrence within a given time period in the future. By contrast, the primary goal in using a management model is to reduce the risk of this the risk of this specified event's occurrence. The *nature of the risk factors* used in each model varies accordingly. In the prediction model, the risk factors (called predictor variables in regression-based designs) should be those which maximize predictive accuracy. They may be either *static* (not changeable through interventions; examples include gender and history) or *dynamic* (potentially changeable through intervention and other influences).

One of the important differences between prediction and control contexts is the *nature of the post-assessment control*. For the management model to be operative, there must be ongoing authority for monitoring and compliance ensurance; most often this would involve continued court jurisdiction.[6] If such authority is present, then decision-making may be conceptualized as an ongoing process, with a series of decisions over multiple occasions and the capacity to modify a previous decision in light of new information. If postassessment control in some form is *not* available, however, then the decision is better conceptualized as a single event in which the most accurate predictors will be employed *and there will be no chance for modification in light of further information.*

[6]Other examples of monitoring bodies under which a management model could operate include departments of parole and probation, psychiatric security review boards, and departments of welfare. Depending upon the applicable laws of the particular jurisdiction, such bodies may provide monitoring and reporting services, with decisions made by the courts, or may have some degree of decision-making authority themselves.

Table 2. Prediction vs. Management Models: Relevant Contrasts

	Prediction	Management
Goal	Violence prediction	Risk reduction
Nature of risk factors	Static and dynamic Strongest empirically	Dynamic Risk-relevant; can be affected by intervention
Post-assessment control	Variable	High
Number of times administered	One	Multiple, at different times
Sensitivity to change in risk status	Low	High
Implications for intervention	Minimal	Strong
Research measures	TP, TN, FP, FN Sensitivity, specificity Overall accuracy (receiver operating characteristics) Relative improvement over chance Future violent behavior	Association of respective risk factors with prior violent behavior Delivery of respective risk interventions (RIs) Compliance/progress in RIs Future violent behavior
Validation designs	Regression-based	Random or matched assignment to experimental and control groups Between-groups comparisons Risk reducing effect of satisfactory relevant intervention

An individual's risk status may change, for a variety of reasons. *Sensitivity to this change* is relatively high under the management model, because (a) assessments are multiple across time, and (b) the focus is particularly on dynamic risk factors, which are most relevant to overall change in risk status. A predictive approach is less sensitive to risk status changes, not only because of its more typical single-administration implementation, but because it is driven by a powerful, utterly static risk factor: history.

The *implications for intervention* under the prediction model are not likely to be significant. To the extent that dynamic risk factors are important elements in a given prediction, and interventions may be designed to address these risk factors, then there may be some such implications. The focus of assessment under the management model is risk reduction, however, so it directly addresses those dynamic risk factors and is designed for amenability to planning interventions and monitoring their impact.

LEGAL DECISION-MAKING CONTEXTS RELEVANT TO PREDICTION AND MANAGEMENT MODELS

There are certain kinds of legal decisions for which *either* prediction *or* management would clearly be preferable. Two of the variables in Table 2—"post-assessment control" and "number of times administered"—are particularly relevant. Legal decisions in which a single decision must be informed by the most accurate available information, and after which there is no continued jurisdiction, are those addressed by the prediction model. Examples include civil commitment and related decisions (e.g., outpatient commitment, end of sentence commitment as "sexual predator"). By contrast, those legal decisions for which there is ongoing legal jurisdiction, and may be made (or modified) at different times, are better served by the management model. Examples include NGRI graduated release decisions (including conditional release, if available), adult and juvenile sentencing decisions resulting in probation, or release decisions leading to parole. Another example, consistent with the management model but not involving risk assessment, would be the decision about the restorability of competence to stand trial under *Jackson v. Indiana* (1972) following an adjudication of incompetent to stand trial.

However, it may be that there are few legal contexts in which *only* a prediction *or* a management approach to risk is indicated. It might be preferable to characterize the applicability of each along two separate continua, designed to address the applicability of each model in a given legal context. For example, in civil commitment proceedings, there are several points at which the applicability of a prediction approach seems better (e.g., the initial commitment decision, the hospital discharge decision). However, there are times in this process at which a management model may be useful to consider as well; inpatient treatment-planning relevant to violence risk reduction is one example. While discussing the applicability of prediction and management models as opposing ends of the same continuum may be useful to illustrate their differences, therefore, it may be more helpful to consider separately the applicability of each to a given legal context. Even further, it may be that a single legal context may be viewed as a larger process, in which each of the respective models is more applicable at different points.[7]

PROMOTING CONGRUENCE: MATCHING FORENSIC ASSESSMENT APPROACHES WITH LAW'S DEMANDS

The goal of providing legal decision-makers with mental health assessment that is relevant to the psychological constructs underlying various legal competencies has been an explicit part of the forensic assessment literature for nearly three decades. The further goal of "expressing person-situation congruency"—providing information about the person's capabilities that are particularly relevant in a given situation—was offered by Grisso (1986) as a quality that enhances the value of a given approach. This is one useful way to view the use of prediction and management models in legal decision-making. Since violence risk is an "indirect" legal issue, often relevant to ultimate decisions but rarely defining the ultimate issue specifically, it should not be surprising that there has been relatively little attention to the variability in legal circumstances under which risk assessment is relevant to decision-making. Clearly there are potential benefits to this kind of analysis, dem-

[7]The comments of Bruce Winick were particularly helpful on this point.

onstrated by Bonnie's (1992) theoretical reformulation of the trial competency construct and the reinvigorated research efforts that have appeared subsequently (Hoge et al., 1996, 1997).[8]

Recognizing the applicability of prediction and management approaches to risk in different legal contexts, and conforming our clinical and research efforts to the particular needs of each context, can increase the relevance and congruence of information provided to the courts in different situations. In particular, there are implications for *data selection* (the use of static and dynamic risk factors), *data analysis* (whether these factors are combined actuarially, or whether they are designed to demonstrate current behavior in risk-relevant areas), and *communication* (whether communicated in numerical fashion or emphasizing verbal descriptions of behavior). Before elaborating on implications for research, policy, and practice, however, I would like to consider another way of viewing the use of prediction and control models in legal decision-making: therapeutic jurisprudence.

REDUCING RISK: THERAPEUTIC JURISPRUDENCE AS A LENS FOR VIEWING MANAGEMENT-ORIENTED RISK ASSESSMENT

Therapeutic jurisprudence addresses the issue of how "knowledge, theories, and insights of the mental health disciplines can help *shape* the development of the law" (Wexler, 1992, p. 32). It may be applicable to prediction and management in two ways: (1) through further illuminating how predictive and management models can help legal decision-makers interpret existing law in making better decisions, and (2) through enhancing our appreciation that the law may be *shaped* to specify the use of the different models according to context.

Several examples of the applicability of therapeutic jurisprudence to prediction- or control-oriented legal decisions are available in this literature. For instance, Wexler (1992) addresses the issue of violence risk under *Tarasoff v. Regents of the University of California* (1976) circumstances in this way:

> What does the literature say about those who make homicidal threats, about those against whom they are made, about the role of the victim in contributing to the violence, and about the best therapeutic approaches to take when violence is threatened against a specified other? What do those findings tell us about whether the *Tarasoff* requirement of warning or protecting potential victims is a good or bad rule in its likely aggregate impact? (Wexler, 1992, p. 35)

Here, Wexler clearly views *Tarasoff* as creating a circumstance in which therapists have a responsibility to act to reduce the risk of violence by their patients—a management context—and asks about the most effective way to accomplish this.

Consider another example, in which prediction and management are identified even more explicitly in a therapeutic jurisprudence analysis:

> Can health care compliance principles, recently synthesized by Meichenbaum and Turk, be brought into play in the insanity acquittee conditional release process? One such

[8]It may be that the violence risk data collected by the MacArthur Research Network will be as applicable for management purposes as for prediction, and will be analyzed with both in mind (particularly in light of the Network's reconceptualization of risk assessment from having a primary emphasis on single, prediction-oriented applications to an ongoing focus on risk status).

> principle is that compliance is greater among those who enter into behavioral contracts; another is that compliance is greater among those who make a public commitment to comply. If the use of behavioral contracts and public commitments increase patient compliance, can the conditional release and furlough system incorporate these devices? If so, courts might be able to structure conditional release proceedings so as not simply to *predict* whether a patient will continue to take medication if released, but also to actually *influence* and *facilitate* that compliance. Here, therapeutic compliance and public safety may presumably be enhanced without any sacrifice to liberty/justice principles [italics added]. (Wexler, 1992, p. 37)

Finally, consider what therapeutic jurisprudence might suggest about a circumstance in which a patient is proposed for release from civil commitment, which is a prediction circumstance (assuming there is no continuing hospital or agency control over the individual following release):

> Does the fear of being judged by hindsight in the event a released patient commits an act of violence lead releasing authorities to *delay* release—and hence to provide unnecessary and inappropriate institutional treatment for—mental patients who have been violent in the past? (Wexler, 1992, p. 35)

In this case, this question illuminates what may be inadequate predictive capacity on the part of hospital staff; more likely, however, it points to the attempt to transform a predictive circumstance into a management context (by keeping the patient hospitalized), and justifying such a transformation using the rationale that "more treatment is needed."

Recent works on therapeutic jurisprudence (e.g., Wexler & Winick, 1996) reveal its application to a broad range of legal issues. It may be applied to the present question by asking how the use of a prediction or a management model of risk assessment might (1) enhance the quality of legal decision-making, and (2) help in the design and implementation of risk-reduction interventions which could be viewed as a "working partnership" between clinician and patient. The first of these two possibilities has been discussed; to the extent that congruence between legal demand and available information can be enhanced, then decision-making quality should improve.[9] When a management model is used (in contexts in which it applicable), it can also have clear benefits for the working relationship between clinician and patient. Consider the following possibilities:

- rather than being the object of a prediction, the patient is a fuller participant in a process which
- specifies the target behavior clearly and
- enlists the patient's participation in working toward a (risk reduction) goal,
- the achievement of which is more within the patient's control, and
- with progress more directly related to reward, and lack of progress to absence of reward, in a way that is
- easier for the patient to understand, relying more on achievement of goals and less on "clinical judgment."

As these features would suggest, there may be significant benefits to the risk-reduction intervention process that go beyond improved planning. These benefits may

[9]It is also possible to ask (as therapeutic jurisprudence would have us do) how the law might be reshaped to more explicitly request information best obtained from each model in contexts in which that model is most applicable.

also encompass the implementation of the interventions, including the willingness, cooperation, and degree of commitment of the participants.

IMPLICATIONS FOR RESEARCH, PRACTICE, AND POLICY

The consideration of two contrasting models for the applications of risk assessment has certain larger implications for research, practice, and policy. One important implication involves the need to consider the extent to which different legal contexts are *management-* and *prediction*-oriented, respectively. Research questions can then focus on both *normative practice* (Do courts consider information and make decisions any differently under these circumstances? Do forensic evaluators select and combine variables, and communicate results, any differently?), *expressed preference* (Do judges perceive that the respective "predictive" and "control" assessment approaches provide them with more relevant information in those respective contexts? Do forensic clinicians perceive that describing these approaches, and their associated legal decisions, sharpens their thinking about risk assessment? Is the quality of risk communication enhanced by matching approach to decisional context?), and *differences in outcome* (Do "prediction" strategies result in more accurate predictions? Do "control" yield decisions that reduce the risk of future violent behavior? Does considering this distinction result in better decisions made by courts?).

When shaped by the results of such research, the practice of risk assessment by forensic clinicians will become more contextually sensitive. Depending on whether the assessment is performed under prediction or management circumstances, there may be implications for how the task is defined, whether there are additional "updates" added to the original assessment, and how the results are communicated (relative emphasis on nomothetic vs. idiographic considerations, the use of probabilities vs. the emphasis on behavioral observations, the status of risk reduction interventions, and the role of "protective factors" as well as risk factors relevant to violence).

Legal and mental health policy considerations could also diverge according to whether the decision was being considered in a prediction or a management context. Particularly when management decisions are made, there are a number of policy implications regarding how ongoing assessment might best be made and tailored to fit with existing risk-relevant interventions (and with additional interventions that may not yet exist). Three distinct activities—assessment, intervention, and decision-making—can blend more harmoniously when linked through comprehensive policy. When promising elements of *assessment* (the use of risk-relevant criteria with an emphasis on dynamic risk factors), *intervention* (applying therapeutic and rehabilitation efforts, and explicit consideration of situational influences on risk), and *decision-making* (consideration of multiple assessments, addressing identified risk factors, and the progress in risk relevant interventions, at the level of both individual clinicians or treatment teams and a review panel) are thus linked, the potential for improvement should be clear.

Legal context is important to consider if we are to increase the relevance and accuracy of information provided by forensic clinicians. Violence risk lends itself particularly well to a contextual analysis, but there may be other legally-relevant constructs whose use in legal decisions may be improved in this way as well. As the field of forensic mental health assessment matures, this kind of contextual analysis may complement the development of empirically-based instruments in helping to improve the quality of legal decision-making.

ACKNOWLEDGMENTS

An earlier version of this article was presented as the Presidential Address of the American Psychology-Law Society/Division 41 at the Annual Convention of the American Psychological Association, 'Ioronto, Ontario, Canada, August 1996. Appreciation is expressed to Joel Dvoskin, John Monahan, Hank Steadman, and Bruce Winick for their helpful comments on some of the ideas described in this article.

REFERENCES

Bonnie, R. (1992). The competence of criminal defendants: A theoretical reformulation. *Behavioral Sciences & the Law, 10*, 291–316.

Carson, D. (1994). Dangerous people: Through a broader conception of "risk" and "danger" to better decisions. *Expert Evidence, 3*, 51–69.

Daubert v. Merrell Dow Pharmaceuticals, Inc., 113 S.Ct. 2786 (1993).

Dawes, R., Faust, D., & Meehl, P. (1989). Clinical versus actuarial judgment. *Science, 243*, 1668–1674.

Golding, S., Roesch, R., & Schreiber, J. (1984). Assessment and conceptualization of competency to stand trial: Preliminary data on the Interdisciplinary Fitness Interview. *Law and Human Behavior, 9*, 321–334.

Grisso, T. (1986). *Evaluating competencies*. New York: Plenum.

Grisso, T. (August, 1995). The Competence of Adolescents as Trial Defendants. Distinguished Contribution to Research in Public Policy Award Address presented at the Annual Convention of the American Psychological Association, New York, NY.

Heilbrun, K. (1991). *The analysis of aggressive behavior*. Richmond, VA: Department of Mental Health, Mental Retardation, and Substance Abuse Services.

Hoge, S., Poythress, N., Bonnie, R., Eisenberg, M., Monahan, J., Feucht-Haviar, T., & Oberlander, L. (1996). Mentally ill and non-mentally ill defendants' abilities to understand information relevant to adjudication: A preliminary study. *Bulletin of the American Academy of Psychiatry and the Law, 24*, 187–197.

Hoge, S., Bonnie, R., Poythress, N., Monahan, J., Eisenberg, M., & Feucht-Haviar, T. (1997). The MacArthur Adjudicative Competence Study I: Development of a research instrument. *Law and Human Behavior, 21*, 141–179.

Jackson v. Indiana, 406 U.S. 715 (1972).

Meehl, P. (1954). *Clinical versus statistical prediction: A theoretical analysis and a review of the evidence*. Minneapolis: University of Minnesota Press.

Monahan, J. (1981). *Predicting violent behavior: An assessment of clinical techniques*. Beverly Hills, CA: Sage.

Monahan, J., & Steadman, H. (Eds.) (1994). *Violence and mental disorder: Developments in risk assessment*. Chicago: University of Chicago Press.

Poythress, N. (1987). Avoiding negligent release: A risk-management strategy. *Hospital and Community Psychiatry, 38*, 1051–1052.

Poythress, N. (1990). Avoiding negligent release: Contemporary clinical and risk management strategies. *American Journal of Psychiatry, 147*, 994–997.

Small, M. (1992). The legal context of mentally disordered sex offender (MDSO) treatment programs. *Criminal Justice and Behavior, 19*, 127–142.

Smith, L. D. (1992). On prediction and control: B. F. Skinner and the technological ideal of science. *American Psychologist, 47*, 216–223.

Steadman, H., Monahan, J., Robbins, P. C., Appelbaum, P., Grisso, T., Klassen, D., Mulvey, E., & Roth, L. (1993). From dangerousness to risk assessment: Implications for appropriate research strategies. In S. Hodgins (Ed.), *Mental disorder and crime*. Newbury Park, CA: Sage.

Tarasoff v. Regents of the University of California, 551 P.2d 334 (Cal.Sup.Ct. 1976).

Wexler, D. (1991). Health care compliance principles and the insanity acquittee conditional release process. *Criminal Law Bulletin, 27*, 18–41.

Wexler, D. (1992). Putting mental health into mental health law. *Law and Human Behavior, 16*, 27–38.

Wexler, D. (1996). Applying the law therapeutically. *Applied and Preventive Psychology, 5*, 179–186.

Wexler, D., & Winick, B. (Eds.) (1991). *Essays in therapeutic jurisprudence*. Durham, NC: Carolina Academic Press.

Wexler, D., & Winick, B. (Eds.) (1996). *Law in a therapeutic key*. Durham, NC: Carolina Academic Press.

[3]

Searching for the pan-cultural core of psychopathic personality disorder

David J. Cooke [a,*], Christine Michie [b], Stephen D. Hart [c], Danny Clark [d]

[a] *Glasgow Caledonian University and Douglas Inch Centre, 2 Woodside Terrace, G3 7UY, Glasgow, Scotland, UK*
[b] *Glasgow Caledonian University, G4 OBA, UK*
[c] *Simon Fraser University, Canada*
[d] *National Probation Service, SWIP 2AW, UK*

Received 14 April 2004; received in revised form 24 May 2004; accepted 17 January 2005
Available online 9 March 2005

Abstract

Previous research has reported that psychopathy ratings of offenders in Canada and the United States made using the Psychopathy Checklist-Revised were metrically equivalent with each other, but not with ratings of Scottish offenders or with ratings of offenders from the rest of the UK. In this study, we further evaluated the cross-cultural validity of psychopathic personality disorder by comparing ratings from a number of different continental European countries to those from North America. Overall, the findings indicated the presence of a significant culture bias in PCL-R ratings. Cross-cultural stability was highest for symptoms related to deficient affective experience, suggesting that they may be the pan-cultural core of the disorder. The findings are consistent with cultural facilitation models of psychopathology. They have important implications for cross-national comparisons of research based on the PCL-R and implications for the clinical and forensic application of the PCL-R in Europe.

Keywords: Psychopathy; PCL-R; Cross-cultural; Factor structure; Measurement problems

* Corresponding author. Tel.: +44 141 211 8000; fax: +44 141 211 8005.
E-mail address: djcooke@rgardens.vianw.co.uk (D.J. Cooke).

1. Introduction

Personality disorders are mental abnormalities characterized by chronic disturbances in relating to self, others, and the environment. Because personality is inherently relational in nature, manifested largely in the interpersonal sphere, culture may have a greater impact on personality disorders than on most other forms of mental disorder (Cross & Markus, 1999). Because complex and manifold social processes encourage interpersonal behaviors consistent with important norms and values (Weisz, Suwanlert, Chaiyasit, & Walter, 1987), personality disorders may tend to be an exaggeration of prevalent patterns of adaptation within a society (Alarcon, Foulks, & Vakkur, 1998).

There has been considerable debate concerning the impact of culture on the expression of psychopathic personality disorder. Historical and anthropological evidence suggests that psychopathic personality disorder is found across time and across cultures (Cooke, 1996), however, it has been speculated that the disorder may be more prevalent in highly individualistic cultures (Lykken, 1995; Paris, 1998). Individualistic cultures promote the development of self-identity that is independent of relationships with others; factors that at their extreme characterize psychopathy are highly valued in individualistic cultures (Cross & Markus, 1999).

To date, there has been little quantitative research on the cross-cultural validity of psychopathic personality disorder (Cooke, 1996). Some studies have examined the distribution of test scores or prevalence of diagnoses across different cultural groups (e.g., Compton et al., 1991; Loranger, 1999; Robins, Tipp, & Przybeck, 1991). Research of this sort is sometimes referred to as the "transport-and-test" approach (Cross & Markus, 1999): researchers take an existing measure, translate it into different languages, and then compare the distribution or reliability of scores across cultures. There are several problems with this strategy (Cooke & Michie, 2002; Cross & Markus, 1999; Lopez & Gaurnaccia, 2000; Rogler, 1999). First, although it is relatively straight-forward to translate a test into another language, it is not at all easy to ensure the *cultural equivalence* of literal translations. Second, tests may lack *cultural relevance*, even when they have been translated adequately. It is always possible to administer an old test in a new culture and obtain scores, but it is not at all certain that the validity of test scores is the same across cultures. Third, even assuming cultural equivalence, and cultural relevance of a test, most commonly-used statistics do not provide an adequate means of evaluating potential *cultural bias*. Methods and indexes commonly used to describe the distribution and structure of scores—such as the mean and standard deviation of total scores and the internal consistency—do not provide a strong test of whether individual items and total scores operate equivalently across cultures. Specialized techniques including Confirmatory Factor Analysis (CFA) and Item Response Theory (IRT) methods are preferable (Cooke & Michie, 2002; Embretson & Reise, 2000; Lopez & Gaurnaccia, 2000).

The PCL-R (Hare, 2003) is a 20-item symptom rating scale of psychopathic personality disorder intended for use in forensic settings. The test manual provides a definition of each item, and evaluators rate the lifetime presence of symptoms on a three-point scale (0–2) on the basis of an interview with the subject and a review of case history information.

The PCL-R is North American by birth: it was developed originally in Canada, written in English, and validated primarily in Canada and the United States. Psychometric evaluations conducted within the framework of Classical Test Theory (CTT) indicate that the test has high interrater, internal consistency, and test–retest reliabilities in North America (Hare, 2003); similar evaluations within the framework of IRT indicate that many test items and the total score provide useful information across the full range of the latent trait (Cooke & Michie, 1997). There is also a large body of research supporting the test's validity in North America (Cooke, Forth, & Hare, 1998).

Although born and raised in North America, the PCL-R has since traveled overseas—mostly to Europe (e.g., Af Klinteberg, Humble, & Schalling, 1992; Pham, 1998; Tengstrom, Grann, Langstrom, & Kullgren, 2000; but also to Asia, Australasia, and South America (e.g., Darke, Kaye, Finlay-Jones, & Hall, 1998; Howard, Payamal, & Neo, 1997).

In cross-cultural research, interest must be focused not on manifest variables such as test scores, but rather on the latent variables that underlie them (Meredith & Millsap, 1992; Waller, Thompson, & Wenk, 2000). Cross-cultural equivalence requires that the structure of the latent trait and the metric used to measure the latent trait are both invariant across cultures. Thus, two broad questions have to be addressed. First, is the factor structure invariant across cultures? This can be addressed through the application of CFA (Tanzer, 1995). Second, is the association between PCL-R ratings and the latent trait of psychopathy the same across cultures? This question can be addressed through the application of IRT methods (Embretson & Reise, 2000; Lopez & Gaurnaccia, 2000). These techniques are complementary and provide different information about the structure of data. We have conducted a small number of studies using CFA and IRT methods to examine cross-cultural differences (Cooke & Michie, 1997, 1999, 2001; Cooke, Kosson, & Michie, 2001; Cooke, Michie, Hart, & Clark, 2004; Cooke, Michie, Hart, & Clark, submitted). Three broad conclusions can be reached.

First, the disorder has a clear factor structure. Cooke and Michie (2001) used CFA methods to analyze 13 of the 20 PCL-R items that were conceptually distinct and, according to previous IRT findings, psychometrically non-redundant. A hierarchical structure in which the superordinate trait, psychopathy, overarched three highly correlated symptom facets: Arrogant and Deceitful Interpersonal Style, Deficient Affective Experience, and Impulsive and Irresponsible Behavioral Style fitted the data best. This factor structure replicated well in data from Scotland, as well as in ratings based on the Screening Version of the PCL-R (Hart, Cox, & Hare, 1995) and the various criterion sets used in the DSM-IV Antisocial Personality Disorder Field Trial (Widiger et al., 1996). This structure has been replicated by independent investigators (e.g., Skeem, Mulvey, & Grisso, 2003). These finding suggest that the syndromal structure of psychopathic symptoms may be invariant across cultures and measures.

Second, within North America there is little evidence of cross-cultural variation across ethnocultural groups (Cooke et al., 2001; Cooke & Michie, 1997). Cooke et al. (2001) examined the differences between samples of African-American and White offenders in the United States. The three factor structure replicated and was completely invariant across groups. Differential item functioning across the groups on 5 of 20 PCL-R items was observed; however, the differences were small in magnitude and inconsistent in direction, so that they canceled out each other when items were summed to form total scores.

Third, there appears to be structural invariance between Europe and North America but not metric invariance (Cooke & Michie, 1999; Cooke et al., submitted). In both these studies there was evidence of metric inequivalence with participants in the UK, on average, obtaining lower total scores for the same level of the underlying trait compared with North American participants:

the interpersonal features of the disorder showed greatest differences and the affective features the least.

In this paper we examine the generalizability of the PCL-R from North America to continental Europe. We examine four issues. First, is the syndrome of psychopathy specified by the same symptoms in both settings? Second, do PCL-R scores have the same meaning in both settings? Third, where are any differences in the disorder located? And fourth, which symptoms are most diagnostic of psychopathy?

2. Method

2.1. Participants

2.1.1. Europe

Participants included 1,563 adult male offenders and forensic psychiatric patients from continental Europe. The participants came from eight different samples from six different countries: forensic psychiatric patients from Belgium ($N = 94$), Denmark ($N = 212$), Norway ($N = 87$), and Sweden ($N = 651$); and offenders from Belgium ($N = 103$), Germany ($N = 100$), Spain ($N = 117$), and Sweden ($N = 199$).

2.1.2. North America

Participants were 2067 adult male offenders and forensic psychiatric patients from ten different convenience samples in Canada and the United States. These samples are described in detail elsewhere and have been used in previous comparisons of Scottish and UK samples (Cooke & Michie, 1997; Cooke et al., submitted).

2.2. Procedure

PCL-R ratings were made according to instructions in the test manual (Hare, 2003).

2.3. Data analyses

2.3.1. CFA

CFA permits quantification of a factor structure's fit in a particular sample. We assessed quality of fit using multiple indexes; χ^2, NNFI, CFI, RMSEA. Following convention, the criterion for adequate fit was defined as CFI and NNFI > 0.90 and RMSEA < 0.08 (Byrne, 1994).

CFA was performed using EQS (Bentler & Wu, 1995). Cases with missing data were deleted listwise.

2.3.2. IRT

IRT models estimate the relationship between item or test scores and a latent trait (θ) that underlies them. Essentially, the trait level for each individual is estimated from the pattern of their item scores, taking into account the characteristics of the individual items. Item characteristic curves (ICCs) index the association between the probability of an item score and θ; test charac-

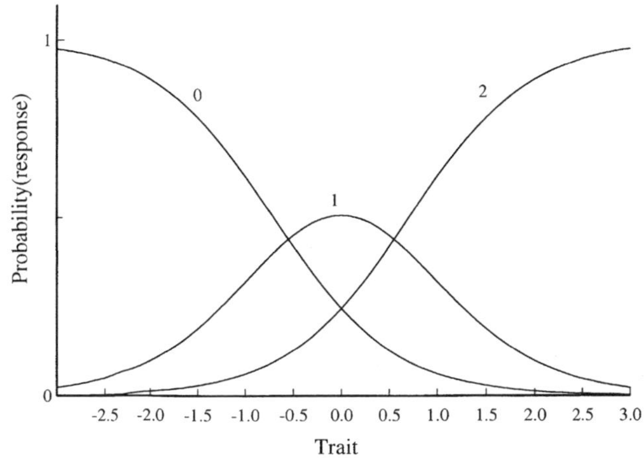

Fig. 1. Item characteristic curves.

teristic curves (TCCs) index the association between the probability of total scores and θ. The slopes of ICCs or TCCs reflect discriminating power, that is, the extent to which item or test scores are saturated with trait-relevant variance. The inflexion point of ICCs and TCCs reflect the extremity or difficulty of item or test scores. IRT methods also can be used to detect differential item functioning (DIF) or differential test functioning (DTF) across groups. DIF occurs when an item is more discriminating, or is more difficult or extreme, in one group as compared with another; DTF occurs when total scores on a test are more discriminating or more extreme in one group than another.

Samejima's Graded Model was used as the assumptions of the model are a good match to the structure of PCL-R ratings (e.g., Cooke & Michie, 1997). The probability of the three response options for a PCL-R item vis-à-vis the latent trait can be expressed by probability curves (Fig. 1). The curves for 0 and 2 ratings are symmetric logistic functions; the curve for the 1 response is found by subtraction. The shape and position of the curves can be summarized by the values of three parameters: a, b_1, and b_2 (Thissen, 1991). The a parameter is an index of slope; the b_i parameters are indexes of difficulty or extremity.

3. Results

First, we evaluated the extent to which the three-factor hierarchical model fits ratings from Europe. Following convention, adequate fit was determined by values of the NNFI and CFI greater than 0.90 and RMSEA less than 0.08: models that do not achieve these values can be regarded as mis-specified (Byrne, 1994). Using a combination of indices provides a more conservative and reliable evaluation of fit. The model was parameterized as outlined by Cooke and Michie (2001), using 13 of the 20 PCL-R items. The fit for this model for the European sample was good, χ^2

(56, $N = 729$) = 201.3, $p < 0.001$, NNFI = 0.94, CFI = 0.96, RMSEA = 0.06.[1] Also, neither the traditional two factor solution for the PCL-R nor the four factor model recently proposed in the PCL-R manual (see Hare, 2003, Fig. 7.3) fitted χ^2 (117, $N = 586$) = 874.8, $p < 0.001$, NNFI = 0.78, CFI = 0.81, RMSEA = 0.10 and χ^2 (131, $N = 585$) = 864.3, $p < 0.001$, NNFI = 0.80, CFI = 0.83, RMSEA = 0.10.

Second, as a more rigorous test of cross-sample structural invariance, we fitted the three-factor hierarchical model simultaneously to data from Europe versus Canada and the United States. The fit of the baseline (i.e., unconstrained) model was good, χ^2 (112, $N = 2723$) = 558.6, $p < 0.001$, NNFI = 0.95, CFI = 0.96, RMSEA = 0.04. The fit obtained when the loadings were constrained to be equal across cultures was good, χ^2 (125, $N = 2723$) = 662.4, $p < 0.001$, NNFI = 0.94, CFI = 0.96, RMSEA = 0.04, although significantly worse than the fit of the unconstrained model, $\Delta\chi^2$ (13, $N = 2723$) = 103.8, $p < 0.001$.

We conducted IRT analyses of the 13 PCL-R items incorporated in the three-factor hierarchical model. Initially, an unconstrained baseline model was generated in which the mean level of the latent trait and all item parameters were allowed to vary across the two groups (see Table 1). Constraining the *a* parameters (slopes) to be equal resulted in a significant increase in χ^2, $\Delta\chi^2(13) = 167.9, p < 0.001$, indicating that the discriminating power of items was significantly different across cultures.

The existence of DIF necessitated anchoring of the latent trait; to ensure continuity with other studies we chose one item from each of the three lower-order factors in the hierarchical model, consistent with previous analysis for the UK (Cooke et al., submitted). The anchors were Items 5 (*Conning/manipulative*), 6 (*Lack of Remorse or Guilt*), and 9 (*Parasitic lifestyle*).

Overall, the model fits the data well, with predicted responses for each item falling within 1% of the observed values. The IRT parameters for the constrained model are shown in Table 1. Given equivalent standing on the latent trait, participants from Europe had lower ratings on most of the 13 PCL-R items than did participants from North America.

Finally, we replicated the previous analysis for all 20 PCL-R items across cultures using the same three anchors, Items 5 (*Conning/manipulative*), 6 (*Lack of Remorse or Guilt*) and 9 (*Parasitic lifestyle*). The results were unchanged.

Bias at the item level (DIF) does not necessarily result in equivalent bias at the level of total scores (DTF), as summing items may either cancel out or amplify their bias. We plotted Test Characteristic Curves (TCCs) for ratings from Europe versus North America (Fig. 2). The TCCs indicated that the association between the latent trait and PCL-R scores varied across cultures. Participants from Europe obtained lower PCL-R total scores than did those from North America given the same level of θ, but only at lower levels of the trait (i.e., $\theta < 0.5$).

We calculated the root differential test function (rDTF; Raju, Linden, & Fleer, 1995); this indexes the average difference between TCCs in the metric of the test (i.e., raw score units). For the 13 items included in the three-factor hierarchical model, rDTF was 1.1 points ($p < 0.001$) mean score = 11.9 (SD = 6.8). For the 20-item PCL-R total scores, rDTF was 1.5 points ($p < 0.001$), mean score = 17.5 (SD = 9.8). Although statistically significant, the magnitude of the rDTF was relatively small in practical terms for individual scores.

[1] Additional information is available from the authors.

Table 1
IRT parameters for Europe versus Canada and the United States, 13 and 20 item models after anchoring

Item		13 items						20 items					
		Europe			Canada and the US			Europe			Canada and the US		
		a	b_1	b_2	a	b_1	b_2	a	b_1	b_2	a	b_1	b_2
1	Glibness/Superficial charm[a]	1.1	−0.3	1.5	1.5	−0.4	1.3	1.1	−0.4	1.4	1.4	−0.4	1.2
2	Grandiose sense of self–worth[a]	1.2	−0.5	1.1	1.7	−0.6	0.9	1.1	−0.6	1.1	1.6	−0.6	0.9
3	Need for stimulation[c]	1.3	−1.0	0.4	1.5	−1.6	−0.1	1.5	−1.0	0.2	1.7	−1.5	−0.1
4	Pathological lying[a]	2.0	−0.2	0.9	1.5	−0.9	0.8	2.0	−0.3	0.8	1.5	−0.9	0.8
5	Conning/Manipulative[a]	1.6	−0.7	0.7	1.6	−0.7	0.7	1.7	−0.7	0.6	1.7	−0.7	0.6
6	Lack of remorse or guilt[b]	2.0	−1.5	−0.3	2.0	−1.5	−0.3	1.9	−1.6	−0.3	1.9	−1.6	−0.3
7	Shallow affect[b]	1.8	−1.2	0.4	1.8	−1.1	0.4	1.6	−1.4	0.3	1.8	−1.1	0.4
8	Callous/lack of empathy[b]	1.5	−1.3	0.4	2.1	−1.3	0.3	1.5	−1.4	0.3	2.1	−1.3	0.2
9	Parasitic lifestyle[c]	1.1	−1.3	1.0	1.1	−1.3	1.0	1.2	−1.2	0.8	1.2	−1.2	0.8
10	Poor behavioral controls							1.5	−1.5	−0.2	1.1	−1.4	0.3
11	Promiscuous sexual behavior							0.9	−0.6	0.7	0.8	−1.1	0.4
12	Early behavioral problems							1.0	−0.7	0.3	1.0	−0.6	0.6
13	Lack of long term goals[c]	1.7	−1.1	0.1	1.2	−1.6	0.2	1.8	−1.1	0.0	1.3	−1.6	0.2
14	Impulsivity[c]	1.6	−1.5	−0.1	1.4	−2.2	−0.4	1.9	−1.5	−0.2	1.5	−2.0	−0.4
15	Irresponsibility[c]	1.8	−1.2	0.3	1.4	−2.1	−0.2	2.0	−1.2	0.2	1.5	−2.1	−0.2
16	Failure to accept responsibility[b]	1.8	−1.1	0.0	1.2	−1.5	0.2	1.7	−1.2	0.0	1.0	−1.6	0.2
17	Many short term marriages							0.6	0.8	2.5	0.7	0.5	1.9
18	Juvenile delinquency							1.1	−0.3	0.5	0.8	−1.0	0.2
19	Revocation of release							1.3	−0.5	−0.1	0.8	−1.7	−0.4
20	Criminal versatility							1.6	−0.3	0.8	0.9	−0.6	1.2

Note: PCL-R = Psychopathy Checklist-Revised (Hare, 2003).
[a] Items that load on Arrogant and Deceptive Interpersonal Style.
[b] Items that load on Deficient Affective Experience.
[c] Items that load on Impulsive and Irresponsible Behavioral Style.

To help identify the source of DTF observed, we conducted analyses comparing the test characteristic curves of the three lower-order factors of Cooke and Michie's hierarchical model. The TCCs for Factors 1, 2, and 3 are presented in Fig. 3. The TCC for Factor 2 (*Deficient Affective Experience*) indicates it was more discriminating than the other factors, with a steeper slope at the point of inflexion. It also discriminated over a wide range of scores around average values of the latent trait. In contrast, Factor 1 (*Arrogant and Deceitful Interpersonal Style*) discriminated well at high levels of the latent trait, but not at low levels; it also failed to reach its maximum score even at high levels of the trait (i.e., $\theta = 3.0$). By way of contrast, Factor 3 (*Impulsive and Irresponsible Behavioral Style*) discriminated best at low levels of the trait. It is noteworthy that DIF is present for high scores for Factor 1 but for low scores on Factor 3.

Next, we equated Factor scores across the samples using Items 5 (*Conning/manipulative*), 6 (*Lack of remorse or guilt*) and 9 (*Parasitic lifestyle*) as anchors, one anchor per factor. We then calculated rDTF with the following results: Factor 1, 0.29 ($p < 0.001$) mean = 2.6 (SD = 2.4); Factor 2, 0.07 ($p < 0.001$) mean = 4.2 (SD = 2.6); and Factor 3, 0.86 ($p < 0.001$) mean = 4.9 (SD = 3.1). Thus, cross-cultural bias was much smaller for Factor 2 than it was for Factors 1 and 3.

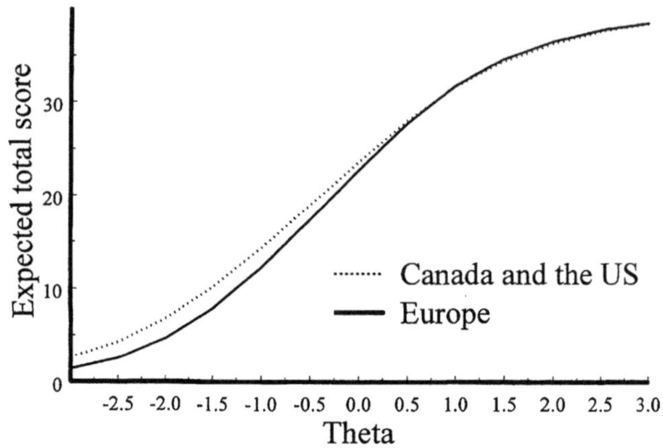

Fig. 2. Test characteristic curves for PCL-R total scores.

Finally, we estimated factor information functions, which provide an estimate of the precision of measurement. In contrast to traditional reliability indexes, information indicates measurement reliability, or precision, across the full range of the latent trait (Fig. 4). Factor 2 provided more information than the other factors across most of the range of the latent trait; only at high trait levels (i.e., $\theta > 1.0$) did Factor 1 provide more information. Factor 3 did not provide the most information at any point of the trait, despite the fact that it is made up of 5 items, versus 4 items for the other factors.

In summary, there was very little cross-cultural bias in ratings of affective symptoms of psychopathy, but distinct bias in ratings of the interpersonal and behavioral symptoms. In addition, the ratings of affective symptoms were, on average, more discriminating and more precisely measured than were ratings of the other symptoms. Taken together, these findings suggest that Deficient Affective Experience may be the pan-cultural core of psychopathy.

4. Discussion

We draw two major conclusions from our findings. First, there was no evidence of cross-cultural *structural* bias in PCL-R ratings. The comparability of factor structures across groups is a necessary but not sufficient condition for cross-cultural equivalence. CFA analyses indicated that the three-factor hierarchical model previously developed on samples from North America provided a good fit to data from continental Europe. The fit of the three-factor hierarchical model across cultures, together with the failure of the two- and four-factor models to provide an adequate fit, either within or across cultures, provides strong support for the generalizability of the model proposed by Cooke and Michie (2001), and thereby enhances its plausibility.

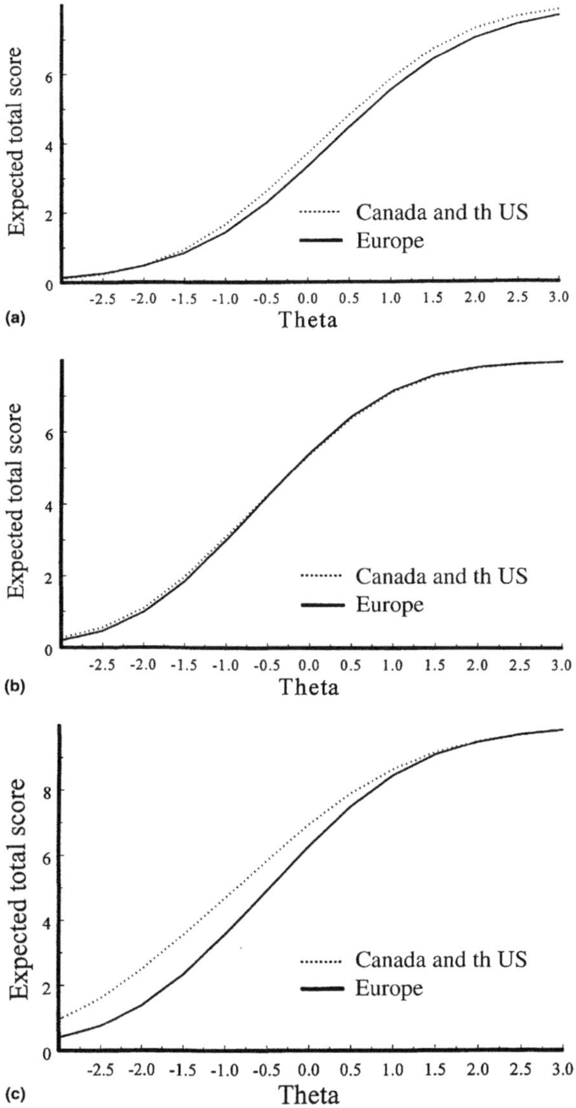

Fig. 3. (a) Test characteristic curves for Factor 1: Arrogant and Deceitful Interpersonal Style. (b) Test characteristic curves for Factor 2: Deficient Affective Experience. (c) Test characteristic curves for Factor 3: Impulsive and Irresponsible Behavioral Style.

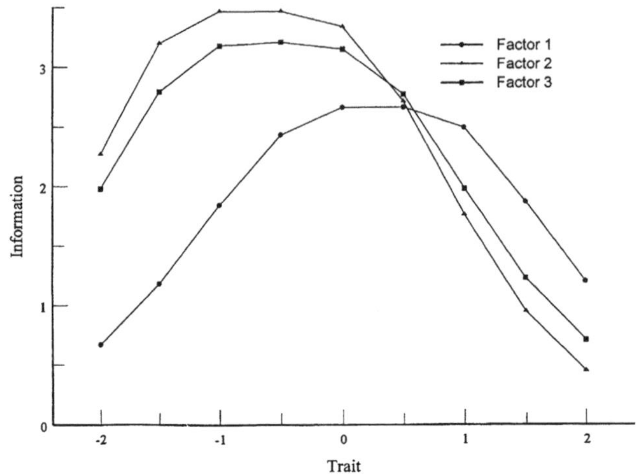

Fig. 4. Information functions for three-factor scores.

Second, there was some evidence of cross-cultural metric bias in ratings of psychopathic symptoms that was statistically significant and clinically meaningful. Specifically, IRT analyses indicated that some of the slopes of the ICCs and TCCs varied in magnitude across cultures. This suggests that some symptoms are more useful in North America as compared with Europe. Also, the intercepts of the ICCs and TCCs were significantly different across cultures. There was no clear pattern in these differences and it is impossible to tell whether they reflect differences in the relevance of the items in different contexts or problems in translating from (Canadian) English into a variety of European languages (Cooke & Michie, 2002). In general, PCL-R total, factor, and item scores were lower in European than North American samples, given equivalent standing on the latent trait of psychopathy. DTF was largest for Factors 1 and 3 of the hierarchical three-factor model, suggesting that symptoms reflecting deficient affective experience may comprise the pan-cultural core of psychopathy.

Our findings add further support to the cross-cultural validity of psychopathy, at least across cultures in industrialized Western nations. Importantly, the disorder appears to have a syndromal structure that is stable across cultures. The relative importance of individual symptoms in defining the syndrome also appears to be stable across cultures. In the absence of stability of this kind, it is impossible to conclude that a particular mental disorder even "exists" across cultures.

But our findings also suggest that culture had an important pathoplastic effect. These analyses replicate comparisons between North America and the United Kingdom (Cooke et al., submitted). The cultural effect differed across symptoms: It was strongest for interpersonal and behavioral symptoms, and weakest for affective symptoms. The presence of specificity of effect—certain facets of the disorder varied across cultures, whereas others did not—increases the plausibility of cultural facilitation (Susser, 1973).

This study did not allow us to determine the processes through which culture may influence the expression of psychopathic personality disorder. However, it is interesting to note that previous research also found the interpersonal features of the disorder to vary across the cultures (Cooke & Michie, 1999; Cooke et al., submitted). The *cultural facilitation model* suggests that complex social processes can shape the expression of interpersonal behaviors. Socialization and enculturation serves to suppress the development of certain aspects of behavioral and personality disorders and to facilitate others (Weisz et al., 1987).

When it comes to disorders of personality, socialization has been implicated in the development of antisocial personality: Lykken (1995) argues that the interplay between temperament and socialization is a key process in the ontogenesis of "sociopathy", with children who are temperamentally fearless and impulsive and who experience incompetent parenting being at greater risk of developing sociopathy. Studies of Antisocial Personality Disorder (ASPD) suggest that this disorder may be influenced by cultural processes. Compton et al. (1991) found substantial differences in the prevalence of ASPD when Taiwan and the USA were compared. Robins et al. (1991) predicted that the prevalence of ASPD would double across a generation within the USA; Paris (1998) argued that such changes were consequent on changes in socialization.

Future research on the cross-cultural validity of psychopathy should examine the generalizability of these findings across measures. There is a danger of over-reliance on the PCL-R: if researchers fail to use other measures the resulting mono-method bias will make it impossible to determine whether findings are a reflection of the test or of the latent trait. The development of a "culture-fair" measure of psychopathy is required. Only by comparing groups or populations on such an instrument can we be certain about the nature and extent of cross-cultural variation in the prevalence and presentation of this important disorder (Cooke & Michie, 2002).

The PCL-R has great potential for causing harm if misapplied. Because psychopathy is recognized as an important predictor of criminal behavior generally, and violent behavior in particular, it is a key variable in current risk assessment procedures (Quinsey, Harris, Rice, & Cormier, 1998; Steadman et al., 2000; Webster, Douglas, Eaves, & Hart, 1997). PCL-R scores influence important decisions about individuals, including granting of parole from prison, access to treatment, detention under dangerous offender legislation, and indeed, death sentence applications (Lyon & Ogloff, 2000). Thus, it is of paramount importance that the PCL-R is applied in an unbiased manner in settings and amongst populations on which it was not standardized.

The procedures adopted in this study allow a common metric of measurement to be used for the measurement of psychopathy in Europe and North America. We would recommend that a different diagnostic cut-off of 28 should be applied in Europe. However, adjusting the cut-off may not be enough for the valid use of the instrument. Bias in predictive validity can occur even in the absence of measurement bias (Millsap, 1997). Although the PCL-R has been shown to have predictive utility in Europe (e.g., Cooke, Michie, & Ryan, 2001; Tengstrom et al., 2000), it might be expected that cross-cultural differences, including differences in the performance of criminal-justice systems (e.g., detection rates, prosecution rates and sentencing policy) will have an impact on the predictive utility of the PCL-R. From a practical perspective, until a test's cross-cultural validity is firmly established, users must be cautious about the possibility of a bias in measurement that may render scores difficult or impossible to interpret accurately (Cooke, Michie, & Hart, in press).

Acknowledgements

We would like to thank all our colleagues who generously gave us access to their data to carry out these analyses. David Cooke received support from the Research and Development Directorate of the Greater Glasgow Primary Care NHS Trust. Christine Michie received support from the Economic and Social Research Council grant Ref. No. L133222704.

References

Af Klinteberg, B., Humble, K., & Schalling, D. (1992). Personality and psychopathy of males with a history of early criminal behaviour. *European Journal of Personality, 6*, 245–266.

Alarcon, R. D., Foulks, E. F., & Vakkur, M. (1998). *Personality disorders and culture: Clinical and conceptual interactions*. New York: John Wiley & Son, Inc.

Bentler, P. M., & Wu, E. J. C. (1995). *EQS for Windows*. Encino, CA: Multivarate Software Inc.

Byrne, B. M. (1994). *Structural equation modeling with EQS and EQS/Windows*. London: Sage Publications, Inc.

Compton, W. M., Helzer, J. E., Hwu, H. G., Yeh, E. K., McEvoy, L., Tipp, J. E., et al. (1991). New methods in cross-cultural psychiatry: psychiatric illness in Taiwan and the United States. *American Journal of Psychiatry, 148*, 1697–1704.

Cooke, D. J. (1996). Psychopathic personality in different cultures. What do we know? What do we need to find out? *Journal of Personality Disorders, 10*(1), 23–40.

Cooke, D. J., Forth, A., & Hare, R. D. (1998). *Psychopathy: Theory, research and implications for society*. Kluwer Academic Publishers.

Cooke, D. J., Kosson, D. S., & Michie, C. (2001). Psychopathy and ethnicity: Structural, item and test generalizability of the Psychopathy Checklist Revised (PCL-R) in Caucasian and African–American participants. *Psychological Assessment, 13*, 531–542.

Cooke, D. J., & Michie, C. (1997). An item response theory evaluation of Hare's Psychopathy Checklist. *Psychological Assessment, 9*, 2–13.

Cooke, D. J., & Michie, C. (1999). Psychopathy across cultures: North America and Scotland Compared. *Journal of Abnormal Psychology, 108*, 55–68.

Cooke, D. J., & Michie, C. (2001). Refining the construct of psychopathy: Towards a hierarchical model. *Psychological Assessment, 13*, 171–188.

Cooke, D. J., & Michie, C. (2002). Towards valid cross-cultural measures of risk. In R. R. Corrado, R. Roesch, & S. D. Hart (Eds.), *Multi-problem youth: A foundation for comparative research on need, interventions and outcomes*. Amsterdam: IOS Press.

Cooke, D. J., Michie, C., & Hart, S. D. (in press) Facets of clinical psychopathy: towards clearer measurement. In Christopher Patrick (Ed.), *Handbook of psychopathic personality disorder*. Guilford: New York.

Cooke, D. J., Michie, C., Hart, S. D., & Clark, D. (2004). Reconstructing psychopathy: Clarifying the significance of antisocial and socially deviant behavior in the diagnosis of psychopathic personality disorder. *Journal of Personality Disorders, 18*, 337–357.

Cooke, D. J., Michie, C., Hart, S. D., & Clark, D. (submitted for publication). Assessing psychopathy in the United Kingdom: Concerns about cross-cultural generalisability.

Cooke, D. J., Michie, C., & Ryan, J. (2001). *Evaluating risk for violence: A preliminary study of the HCR-20, PCL-R and VRAG in a Scottish Prison sample*. Edinburgh: Scotland Office.

Cross, S. E., & Markus, H. R. (1999). The cultural constitution of personality. In L. A. Pervin & P. O. John (Eds.), *Handbook of personality* (pp. 378–396). New York: Guilford.

Darke, S., Kaye, S., Finlay-Jones, R., & Hall, W. (1998). Factor structure of psychopathy among methodone maintenance patients. *Journal of Personality Disorders, 12*, 162–171.

Embretson, S. E., & Reise, S. P. (2000). *Item response theory for psychologists*. Mahwah, NJ: Lawrence Erlbaum, Associates.

Hare, R. D. (2003). *Manual for the Hare Psychopathy Checklist-Revised* (3rd ed.). Toronto: Multi-Health Systems, Inc.

Hart, S. D., Cox, D. N., & Hare, R. D. (1995). *The Hare Psychopathy Checklist: Screening Version* (1st ed.). Toronto: Multi-Health Systems Inc.

Howard, R., Payamal, L. T., & Neo, L. H. (1997). Response modulation deficits in psychopaths: A failure to confirm and a reconsideration of the Patterson–Newman model. *Personality and Individual Differences, 22*, 707–717.

Lopez, S. T., & Gaurnaccia, P. J. J. (2000). Cultural psychopathology: Uncovering the social world of mental illness. *Annual Review of Psychology, 5*, 571–598.

Loranger, A. M. (1999). *International personality disorder examination.* Odessa, FL: Psychological Assessment Resources.

Lykken, D. T. (1995). *The antisocial personalities* (1st ed.). Hillsdale: Lawrence Erlbaum.

Lyon, D., & Ogloff, J. R. P. (2000). Legal and ethical issues in psychopathy assessment. In C. B. Gacono (Ed.), *The clinical and forensic assessment of psychopathy* (pp. 139–173). Mahwah, NJ: Lawrence Erlbaum Associates.

Meredith, W., & Millsap, E. E. (1992). On the misuse of manifest variables in the detection of measurement bias. *Psychometrika, 57*, 289–311.

Millsap, R. E. (1997). Invariance in measurement and prediction: Their relationship in the single-factor case. *Psychological Methods, 2*, 248–260.

Paris, J. (1998). Personality disorders in sociocultural perspective. *Journal of Personality Disorders, 12*, 289–301.

Pham, T. H. (1998). Evaluation psychométrique du questionnaire de la psychopathie de Hare auprès d'une population carcérale belge. *L'Encephale, 24*, 435–441.

Quinsey, V. L., Harris, G. T., Rice, M. E., & Cormier, C. A. (1998). *Violent offenders: appraising and managing risk.* (1st ed.). Washington, DC: American Psychological Press.

Raju, N. S., Linden, W. J., & Fleer, P. F. (1995). Van der IRT-based internal measures of differential functioning of items and tests. *Applied Psychological Measurement, 19*, 353–368.

Robins, L. N., Tipp, J., & Przybeck, T. (1991). Psychiatric disorders in America. In L. N. Robins & D. A. Regier (Eds.), *Antisocial personality disorder* (pp. 258–290). Free Press.

Rogler, L. H. (1999). Methodological sources of cultural insensitivity in mental health. *American Psychologist, 54*, 424–433.

Skeem, J. L., Mulvey, E. P., & Grisso, T. (2003). Applicability of the traditional and revised models of psychopathy to the psychopathy checklist: Screening version (PCL:SV). *Psychological Assessment, 15*, 41–55.

Steadman, H., Silver, E., Monahan, J., Appelbaum, P., Robbins, P. C., Mulvey, E. P., et al. (2000). A classification tree approach to the development of acturial violence risk assessment tools. *Law and Human Behavior, 24*, 83–100.

Susser, M. (1973). *Causal thinking in the health sciences.* New York: Oxford University Press.

Tanzer, N. K. (1995). Cross-cultural bias in Likert-type inventories: Perfect matching factor structures and still biased? *European Journal of Psychological Assessment, 11*, 194–201.

Tengstrom, A., Grann, M., Langstrom, N., & Kullgren, G. (2000). Psychopathy (PCL-R) as a predictor of violent recidivism among criminal offenders with schizophrenia. *Law and Human Behavior, 24*, 45–58.

Thissen, D. (1991). *Multilog user's guide (version 6)* (1st ed.). Mooresville, IN: Scientific Software.

Waller, N. G., Thompson, J. S., & Wenk, E. (2000). Using IRT to separate measurement bias from true group difference on homogenous and heterogenous scales: An illustration with the MMPI. *Psychological Methods, 5*, 125–146.

Weisz, J. R., Suwanlert, S., Chaiyasit, W., & Walter, B. R. (1987). Over-and undercontrolled referral problems among children and adolescents from Thailand and the United States: The Wat and Wai of cultural differences. *Journal of Consulting and Clinical Psychology, 55*, 719–726.

Webster, C. D., Douglas, K., Eaves, D., & Hart, S. D. (1997). *HCR-20 Assessing risk for violence* (2nd ed.). Vancouver: Simon Fraser University.

Widiger, T. A., Cadoret, R., Hare, R. D., Robins, L. N., Rutherford, M. J., Zanarini, M., et al. (1996). DSM-IV antisocial personality disorder field trial. *Journal of Abnormal Psychology, 105*, 3–16.

[4]

The Characteristics of Persistent Sexual Offenders: A Meta-Analysis of Recidivism Studies

R. Karl Hanson and Kelly E. Morton-Bourgon
Public Safety and Emergency Preparedness Canada

A meta-analysis of 82 recidivism studies (1,620 findings from 29,450 sexual offenders) identified deviant sexual preferences and antisocial orientation as the major predictors of sexual recidivism for both adult and adolescent sexual offenders. Antisocial orientation was the major predictor of violent recidivism and general (any) recidivism. The review also identified some dynamic risk factors that have the potential of being useful treatment targets (e.g., sexual preoccupations, general self-regulation problems). Many of the variables commonly addressed in sex offender treatment programs (e.g., psychological distress, denial of sex crime, victim empathy, stated motivation for treatment) had little or no relationship with sexual or violent recidivism.

Keywords: sexual offenders, recidivism, forensic, meta-analysis

Sexual offenses are among the crimes that invoke the most public concern. Community surveys have found that 5% to 20% of men admit to at least one instance of sexual aggression (Grotpellier & Elliott, 2002; Koss, 1987; Lisak & Miller, 2002), and official records indicate that 1% to 2% of the adult male population will eventually be convicted of a sexual crime (California Office of the Attorney General, 2004; P. Marshall, 1997). The observed sexual recidivism rate is typically 10% to 15% after 5 years (Hanson & Bussière, 1998), but for some offenders, the rate is much higher (Harris et al., 2003). Identifying the characteristics of persistent sexual offenders is important for understanding this highly troubling behavioral disorder, as well as for the practical task of administrating policies directed toward high risk sexual offenders (e.g., treatment, civil commitment, community notification).

There is now a general consensus that sexual recidivism is associated with at least two broad factors: (a) deviant sexual interests and (b) antisocial orientation/lifestyle instability (Hanson & Bussière, 1998; Quinsey, Lalumière, Rice, & Harris, 1995; Roberts, Doren, & Thornton, 2002). Deviant sexual interests refer to enduring attractions to sexual acts that are illegal (e.g., sex with children, rape) or highly unusual (e.g., fetishism, autoerotic asphyxia). Although all sexual offending is socially deviant, men who commit such acts do not necessarily have enduring preferences for such behavior (Hudson & Ward, 1997; W. L. Marshall, 1997).

Antisocial orientation refers to antisocial personality, antisocial traits (such as impulsivity, substance abuse, unemployment), and a history of rule violation. There is a strong association between rule violation and impulsive, reckless behavior, such as excessive drinking, frequent moves, fights, and unsafe work practices (Caspi et al., 1994; Gottfredson & Hirschi, 1990). Antisocial orientation facilitates sexual offending because individuals will not commit sexual crimes unless they are (a) willing to hurt others, (b) can convince themselves that they are not harming their victims, or (c) feel unable to stop themselves. Rapists are more likely than child molesters to have an antisocial orientation (Firestone, Bradford, Greenberg, & Serran, 2000; see review by West, 1983), but indicators of hostility and lifestyle instability are associated with sexual recidivism in both groups (Prentky, Knight, Lee, & Cerce, 1995; Rice, Quinsey, & Harris, 1991).

Contemporary theories posit that a variety of factors are associated with the development of sexual offending (Knight & Sims-Knight, 2003; Malamuth, 2003; Ward & Siegert, 2002). These models suggest that adverse family environments provide the breeding grounds for sexual offending. Lacking nurturance and guidance, the potential sexual offender develops problems in social functioning (e.g., mistrust, hostility, and insecure attachment) that, in turn, are associated with social rejection, loneliness, negative peer associations and delinquent behavior. The form of sexuality that develops in the context of pervasive intimacy deficits is likely to be impersonal and selfish and may even be adversarial. Further contributing to the risk of sexual offending are beliefs that permit nonconsenting sex. Attitudes allowing nonconsenting sex can develop through the individuals' trying to understand their own

---

R. Karl Hanson and Kelly Morton-Bourgon, Public Safety and Emergency Preparedness Canada.

Kelly Morton-Bourgon is now with the Department of Justice, Canada, Ottawa.

The views expressed are those of the authors and are not necessarily those of Public Safety and Emergency Preparedness Canada. We thank the following researchers who provided raw data or findings not included in other reports: S. Brown, H. Gretton, G. Harris, N. Långström, C. Langton, R. Lieb, J. Marques, M. Miner, L. Motiuk, T. Nicholaichuk, J. Proulx, J. Reddon, M. Rice, G. Schiller, L. Studer, L. Song, and D. Thornton. We greatly appreciate the help of R. Broadhurst, R. Dempster, R. Kropp, L. Hartwell, A. Hills, N. Morvan and L. Rasmussen in locating unpublished documents. We also thank Dale Arnold, Jim Bonta, Guy Bourgon, Don Grubin, Amy Phenix, Vern Quinsey, Marnie Rice and David Thornton, who provided comments on an earlier version of this study.

Correspondence concerning this article should be addressed to R. Karl Hanson, Corrections Research, Public Safety and Emergency Preparedness Canada, 340 Laurier Avenue West, Ottawa, Ontario K1A 0P8, Canada. E-mail: Karl.Hanson@psepc-sppcc.gc.ca

experiences and adopting the attitudes of their significant others (friends, family, abusers).

Such a model suggests that, apart from sexual deviancy and lifestyle instability, there may be three additional characteristics of persistent sexual offenders: (a) negative family background, (b) problems forming affectionate bonds with friends and lovers, and (c) attitudes tolerant of sexual assault. Examination of the most commonly used rating scales for sexual offenders indicate that these factors have considerable credibility among those conducting sexual offender evaluations (Beech, Fisher, & Thornton, 2003).

The research evidence addressing some of these factors is surprisingly weak. Hanson and Bussière's (1998) meta-analytic review found that the average correlation between sexual recidivism and sexual abuse as a child was $r = -.01$ (based on 5 studies), and the correlation between recividism and deviant sexual attitudes was $r = .09$ (4 studies). The relationship between sexual recidivism and intimacy deficits (apart from marital status) has not been the target of a systemic review.

Recidivism studies are important because sexual offenders are likely to have many problems, not all of which are related to sexual offending. For example, sexual offenders are at increased risk for anxiety and depression (Raymond, Coleman, Ohlerking, Christensen, & Miner, 1999), but such problems have not been associated with sexual recidivism (Hanson & Bussière, 1998). Similarly, Hanson and Bussière's quantitative review found that sexual recidivism was unrelated to the seriousness of the index offense (e.g., victim injury, intercourse) and clinical presentation variables (e.g., denial, victim empathy, motivation for treatment).

Hanson and Bussière's (1998) meta-analysis made an important contribution by summarizing the available evidence concerning recidivism risk factors for sexual offenders. Most of their findings, however, concerned static, historical factors. Static factors are useful for long-term recidivism prediction, but those interested in understanding (and changing) recidivism risk are interested in dynamic (changeable) risk factors, also called "criminogenic needs" (Andrews & Bonta, 2003), "stable dynamic risk factors" (Hanson & Harris, 2000b) or "causal psychological risk factors" (Beech & Ward, 2004).

The purpose of the present study was to update Hanson and Bussière's (1998) meta-analysis in light of the ongoing research on sexual-offender risk assessment. Rather than repeat all the variables from Hanson and Bussière, in the present study, we considered only findings that (a) were considered important to the understanding and management of sexual offenders and (b) were weak or controversial in the earlier review (e.g., denial, victim damage). The review focused on sexual recidivism but also considered nonsexual violent and general (any) recidivism. Sexual offenders are more likely to reoffend with a nonsexual offense than with a sexual offense (Hanson & Bussière), and an important question is whether the predictors of sexual recidivism are substantially different from the predictors of nonsexual recidivism.

Method

Sample

Computer searches of PsycLIT, the National Criminal Justice Reference Service of the United States, and the library of Public Safety and Emergency Preparedness Canada were conducted by using the following key terms: *child molester, exhibitionism, exhibitionist, failure, frotteur, incest, indecent exposure, paraphilias(c), pedophile, pedophilia, predict(ion), rape, rapist, recidivate, recidivism, recidivist, relapse, reoffend, reoffense, sex(ual) offender, sexual assault, sexual deviant.* Additional sources included the reference lists of empirical studies and previous reviews, recent issues of relevant journals (e.g., *Criminal Justice and Behavior, Sexual Abuse: A Journal of Research and Treatment*), and letters sent to 34 established researchers in the field of sexual offender recidivism.

Included were studies that examined offenders who were released after an index sexual offense and for whom the recidivism rate (sexual, violent, or any) was reported after a follow-up period. Researchers assessing offender characteristics were blind to recidivism status. Studies needed to include sufficient statistical information, and at least 5 subjects for all marginal totals were required for dichotomous variables.

As of January, 2003, our search yielded 115 usable documents (e.g., published articles, books, government reports, conference presentations). In 15 cases, the analyses were based on raw data or analyses provided by the original researchers. When the same data set was reported in several articles, all the results from these articles were considered to come from the same study. Consequently, the 115 documents represented 82 different studies (country of origin: 35 United States; 26 Canada; 12 United Kingdom; 2 Austria; 2 Sweden; 2 Australia; and 1 each from France, the Netherlands, and Denmark). Of these studies, 41 (50%) were unpublished. The studies were produced between 1943 and 2003 (median = 1996); the average sample size was 359 (median = 174, range = 12–1,407). Thirty-five studies were the same as those included in Hanson and Bussière's (1998) review, 10 studies contained updated information (e.g., longer follow-up periods, new analyses), and 37 studies were new.

Most of the studies examined mixed groups of adult sexual offenders (72 mixed-offense types, 7 child molesters, 2 rapists, 1 exhibitionist; 67 predominantly adults, 15 adolescents; all male). All the offenders had committed offenses that meet contemporary definitions of sexual crimes (i.e., old studies containing homosexuals were excluded). Most of the offenders were released from institutions (41 institution only, 17 community only, 22 institution and community, and 2 unknown). The offenders in 31 studies came from treatment programs. When demographic information was presented, the offenders were predominantly Caucasian (in 40 of 43 studies).

Effect sizes were recorded for four outcome criteria: (a) any sexual recidivism (vs. no recidivism or only nonsexual recidivism—605 effect sizes); (b) violent nonsexual recidivism (vs. no recidivism, sexual recidivism, or nonviolent recidivism—248 effect sizes); (c) any violent recidivism—sexual or nonsexual—(vs. no recidivism or only nonviolent recidivism—339 effect sizes); and (d) any recidivism (vs. no recidivism—428 effect sizes).

The most common sources of recidivism information were national criminal justice records (48), provincial or state records (32), records from treatment programs (18) and self-reports (13). Other sources (e.g., child-protection records, parole files) were used in 20 studies. In 34 studies, multiple sources were used. The source of the recidivism information for 10 studies was unknown. The recidivism criterion was arrest in 25 studies, reconviction in 24 studies, and reincarceration in 3 studies. Twenty-six studies used multiple criteria (e.g., arrest, parole violations, noncriminal justice-system reports). Recidivism was assessed solely from self-reports in 2 studies, and, in 2 studies, the recidivism criterion was unknown. The follow-up period ranged from 12 months to 330 months, with a mean of 76.0 months ($SD = 56.8$).

Coding Procedure

Each study was coded separately by the two authors, who used a standard list of variables and explicit coding rules (available on request). Variables were first coded into specific individual variables (e.g., sexual interest in boys), which were then subsumed into general categories (e.g., sexual deviancy). The general categories were as follows:

1. *Sexual deviancy*: deviant sexual interests, such as children, rape, and other paraphilias, as well as sexual preoccupations and gender dysphoria);

2. *Antisocial orientation*: antisocial personality (e.g., antisocial personality disorder, psychopathy, Minnesota Multiphasic Personality Inventory Scale 4), antisocial traits (e.g., lifestyle instability, substance abuse, hostility), and a history of rule violation (e.g., childhood criminality, history of nonsexual crime, violation of conditional release);

3. *Sexual attitudes*: tolerance of sexual crime, support for adult–child sex, and low sex knowledge;

4. *Intimacy deficits*: poor social skills, negative social influences, conflicts in intimate relationships, emotional identification with children, and loneliness;

5. *Adverse childhood environment*: conflicts with and separation from parents, neglect, and physical and sexual abuse;

6. *General psychological problems*: internalization of psychological problems (e.g., anxiety and low self-esteem, as well as major mental illness); and

7. *Clinical presentation*: denial, minimization, lack of victim empathy, low motivation for treatment, and poor progress.

Only one finding per individual variable was coded per sample on the basis of (a) sample size and (b) completeness of information. If the sample sizes and descriptive detail were equivalent, the median value was used. Because many of the variables were intended to be dynamic (changeable), posttreatment findings were privileged over pretreatment findings except when the posttreatment finding was based on an insufficient number of cases.

Interrater reliability was calculated for approximately 10% of the sample ($n = 10$), by using kappa for dichotomous and categorical variables and two-way random effects model intraclass correlation coefficients, or ICC (type absolute agreement) for ordinal and interval variables (Design 2 in Orwin, 1994). The agreement for the sample characteristics (e.g., adults or adolescents, treated or not) was perfect for 14 variables, excellent ($\kappa > .80$; ICC $> .85$) for 6 variables, and fair ($\kappa > .50$) for 3 variables: Did the recidivism criteria include parole violations, arrests, or nonjustice system reports? Kappa was low (–.11) for 1 variable (did the recidivism criteria include reconvictions?); for 8 of the 10 studies, the raters agreed that the researchers counted convictions, but each rater identified a different study where he or she thought conviction records had not been consulted.

The interrater reliability of the effect sizes was .83 for a single rater and .90 for the average of two raters. In the 10 reliability studies, Rater 1 identified 134 findings, and Rater 2 identified 131 findings, with agreement on 245 of the 265 findings (92.5%). The actual agreement would be greater because judges conferred on their final rating. Most differences involved simple omissions or clerical errors.

Index of Predictive Accuracy

The effect size indicator was the standardized mean difference, d, defined as follows: $d = (M_1 - M_2)/S_w$, where M_1 is the mean of the deviant group, M_2 is the mean of the nondeviant group, and S_w is the pooled-within standard deviation (Hasselblad & Hedges, 1995). In other words, d measures the average difference between the recidivists and the nonrecidivists, and compares this difference to how much recidivists differ from each other, and how much nonrecidivists differ from each other. The formula for calculating d can be found in Hanson and Morton-Bourgon (2004).

The d statistic was selected because it is less influenced by recidivism base rates than correlation coefficients—the other statistic commonly used in meta-analyses. According to Cohen (1988), d values of .20 are considered "small;" those of .50, "medium;" and .those of .80, "large." The value of d is approximately twice as large as the correlation coefficient calculated from the same data. When the 95% confidence interval for d does not contain zero, it can be considered statistically significant at $p < .05$. When the confidence intervals for two predictors do not overlap, they can be considered significantly different from each other ($p < .05$).

Aggregation of Findings

Two methods were used to summarize the findings: median values (Slavin, 1995) and weighted mean values (Hedges & Olkin, 1985). The averaged d value, $d.$, was calculated by weighing each d_i by the inverse of its variance:

$$d. = \left(\sum_{i=1}^{k} w_i d_i\right) / \left(\sum_{i=1}^{k} w_i\right),$$

where k is the number of findings, $w_i = 1/v_i$, and v_i is the variance of the individual d_i (fixed effect model). The variance of the weighted mean was used to calculate 95% confidence intervals:

$$Var(d.) = 1/\left(\sum_{i=1}^{k} w_i\right);\ 95\%\ \text{C.I.} = d. \pm (\text{Var}[d.])^{1/2}.$$

Weighting d values by the inverse of their variance means that findings from small samples are given less weight than findings from large samples.

When d_i was calculated from 2×2 tables, the variance of d_i was estimated by using Formula 6 from Hasselblad and Hedges (1995):

$$Var(d_i) = \frac{3}{\pi^2}\left(\frac{1}{a+.5} + \frac{1}{b+.5} + \frac{1}{c+.5} + \frac{1}{d+.5}\right).$$

When d_i was calculated from other statistics (t, ROC areas, means, etc.), the variance of d_i was estimated by using Formula 3 from Hasselblad and Hedges (1995):

$$Var(d_i) = \left[\frac{N_1 + N_2}{N_1 N_2} + \frac{d_i^2}{2(N_1 + N_2)}\right].$$

To test the generalizability of effects across studies, Hedges and Olkin's (1985) Q statistic was used:

$$Q = \sum_{i=1}^{k} w_i (d_i - d.)^2.$$

The Q statistic is distributed as a χ^2 with $k - 1$ degrees of freedom (k is the number of studies). A significant Q statistic indicates that there is more variability across studies than would be expected by chance. Outliers were excluded from each category if the single extreme value accounted for more than 50% of the total variance (Q).

Results

On average, the observed sexual recidivism rate was 13.7% ($n = 19{,}267$; 73 studies), the violent nonsexual recidivism rate was 14.3% ($n = 6{,}928$; 24 studies), the violent recidivism rate (including sexual and nonsexual violence) was 14.3% ($n = 11{,}361$; 29 studies) and the general (any) recidivism rate was 36.2% ($n = 12{,}708$; 56 studies). Studies that specified in advance the number of recidivists and nonrecidivists were excluded from the rate calculations (e.g., Dempster, 1998). The average follow-up time was 5–6 years. These figures should be considered underestimates because not all offenses are detected.

The 82 studies produced 1,620 effect sizes (total of 29,450 sexual offenders). The average effect size for the published studies (M = .23, SD = .40, n = 555) was the same as in the unpublished studies (M = .22, SD = .35, n = 1,065), $t(1618)$ = .50, p = .62. The correlation between sample size and effect size was positive (r = .12, n = 1,620, $p < .001$). (A negative correlation is expected when there is selective reporting of significant findings.) The correlation remained significantly positive after removing 103 d values estimated as zero because they were reported as nonsignificant.

Effect sizes were not related to publication date (r = .001) or to the thoroughness with which researchers tracked recidivism information (r = .026). The thoroughness of the recidivism search was rated on a 7-point scale (1 = *self-report only*, 4 = *one method searches*, and 7 = *multiple sources including national criminal records*). The effect sizes were the same whether recidivism was measured by arrests (M = .23, SD = .34, n = 1,001) or convictions (M = .21, SD = .39, n = 542; $t(1541)$ = 1.14, p = .25). The effect sizes for adult offenders (M = .23, SD = .36, n = 1,319) were similar to effect sizes for adolescents (M = .21, SD = .37, n = 301; $t(1618)$ = 1.11, p = .27). The coding did not permit comparisons between rapists and child molesters.

Comparisons Across Categories of Risk Predictors

Table 1 presents the association with recidivism for the seven broad categories of risk factors. These broad comparisons were based on one individual finding per study (see coding manual and Hanson and Morton-Bourgon (2004) for further information about the individual predictors). The strongest predictors of sexual recidivism were those related to sexual deviancy ($d.$ = .30) and antisocial orientation ($d.$ = .23). The general category of sexual attitudes was also significantly related to sexual recidivism, but the effect was small ($d.$ = .17, 95% confidence interval of .04 to .28) and contained significant variability. The effects were not significant for child molester attitudes, low sex knowledge, or other deviant sexual attitudes (e.g., prudish attitudes toward masturbation).

The general category of intimacy deficits showed a small, significant relationship to sexual recidivism ($d.$ = .15), with substantial variation among its subcomponents. Of the subcomponents of intimacy deficits, relatively larger effects were found for conflicts in intimate relationships ($d.$ = .36, 4 studies) and emotional identification with children ($d.$ = .42, 3 studies) than for social skills deficits ($d.$ = −.07, 6 studies) or loneliness ($d.$ = .03, 6 studies). The general categories of adverse childhood environment ($d.$ = .09), general psychological problems ($d.$ = .02), and clinical presentation ($d.$ = −.02) had little or no relationship with sexual recidivism.

Antisocial orientation (antisocial personality, antisocial traits, history of rule violation) was the major predictor of violent nonsexual recidivism ($d.$ = .51), violent (including sexual) recidivism ($d.$ = .54) and any recidivism ($d.$ = .52). Almost all of the individual indicators of antisocial orientation were significantly related to nonsexual violent, violent, and general recidivism; most of the relationships were moderate to large. Among the strongest individual predictors of any recidivism were general problems with self-regulation ($d.$ = .75, 6 studies, which included measures of impulsivity, lifestyle instability, and Factor 2 of the Psychopathy Checklist Revised, or PCL-R (Hare et al., 1990), a history of nonviolent crime ($d.$ = .68, 9 studies), psychopathy (PCL-R total scores; $d.$ = .67, 9 studies), and a history of nonsexual crime ($d.$ = .63, 8 studies).

Few variables other than antisocial orientation were predictive of nonsexual violent or general (any) recidivism. Sexual attitudes showed a small relationship with general recidivism ($d.$ = .24). Sexual deviancy was unrelated to violent nonsexual recidivism ($d.$ = −.05) and general (any) recidivism ($d.$ = .04).

The same major predictors were found for adolescent sex offenders as for adult sexual offenders. For adolescent sex offenders, sexual recidivism was predicted by sexual deviance ($d.$ = .36 ± .24, 95% confidence interval of .12 to .60, 7 studies; n = 734) and antisocial orientation ($d.$ = .19 ± .17, 14 studies; n = 1,958). Antisocial orientation also predicted violent nonsexual recidivism ($d.$ = .33 ± .19, 5 studies; n = 825), any violent recidivism ($d.$ = .46 ± .26, 3 studies; n = 559), and any recidivism ($d.$ = .41 ± .13, 10 studies; n = 1,400) among adolescent sex offenders.

Possible Dynamic Risk Factors for Sexual Recidivism

Table 2 presents some of the most promising targets for intervention. All of these findings were based on at least 5 studies with a combined sample of at least 1,000, with no significant variability between studies. The most confidence can be placed in those findings with narrow confidence intervals (large sample size). Readers should be cautioned, however, that the findings based on

Table 1
Factors Associated With Recidivism Among Sexual Offenders

	Type of recidivism			
Category	Sexual	Violent nonsexual	Violent	Any
Sexual deviancy	.30 ± .08 (5,053; 32)	−.05 ± .17 (1,385; 10)	.19 ± .08 (3,155; 17)	.04 ± .08 (6,555; 19)
Antisocial orientation	.23 ± .04 (23,012; 65)	.51 ± .07 (8,283; 24)	.54 ± .05 (13,065; 28)	.52 ± .04 (15,988; 43)
Sexual attitudes	.16 ± .12 (2,370; 14)	.17 ± .22 (732; 6)	.14 ± .11 (1,598; 9)	.24 ± .10 (1,053; 9)
Intimacy deficits	.15 ± .11 (2,852; 22)	.12 ± .21 (822; 6)	.12 ± .12 (1,197; 8)	.10 ± .10 (1,715; 15)
Adverse childhood environment	.09 ± .08 (7,259; 27)	−.02 ± .17 (2,256; 7)	.14 ± .08 (5,041; 14)	.11 ± .07 (5,044; 15)
General psychological problems	.02 ± .10 (3,208; 19)	.21 ± .14 (2,089; 8)	.00 ± .10 (1,974; 10)	−.04 ± .11 (1,658; 11)
Clinical presentation	−.02 ± .09 (5,094; 24)	.16 ± .20 (2,090; 5)	.09 ± .09 (3,849; 12)	.12 ± .08 (4,714; 18)

Note. Values are averaged d values, followed by their 95% confidence interval and (in parentheses) the total sample size and the number of studies (k).

Table 2
Selected Predictors of Sexual Recidivism

Variable	Mean *d*	Median *d*	*Q*	Total (*k*)
Possible dynamic risk factors				
Any deviant sexual interest	.31 ± .10	.36	21.91	2,769 (16)
Sexual preoccupations	.39 ± .16	.51	8.31	1,119 (6)
Antisocial personality disorder	.21 ± .10	.29	13.01	3,267 (12)
Psychopathy Checklist—Revised	.29 ± .09	.25	14.36	2,783 (13)
General self-regulation problems	.37 ± .11	.34	22.85	2,411 (15)
Employment instability	.22 ± .09	.15	20.88	5,357 (15)
Hostility	.17 ± .13	.16	12.69	1,960 (9)
Potentially misleading risk factors				
Force/violence in sex offending	.09 ± .07	.00	29.28	7,221 (25)
Neglect or abuse during childhood	.10 ± .09	.00	27.43	5,490 (18)
Sexual abuse during childhood	.09 ± .10	.02	24.44	5,711 (17)
Loneliness	.03 ± .13	.02	5.79	1,810 (6)
Low self-esteem	.04 ± .16	.03	10.12	1,424 (10)
Lack of victim empathy	−.08 ± .13	−.01	0.92	1,745 (5)
Denial of sexual crime	.02 ± .17	−.02	11.72	1,780 (9)
Low motivation for treatment at intake	−.08 ± .13	−.04	13.83	1,786 (12)
Poor progress in treatment (post)	.14 ± .17	.11	9.35	1,118 (7)

Note. Each mean is followed by its 95% confidence interval. Total is number of subjects; *k* is the number of studies. All *Q* values were not significant, $p > .05$.

the minimum inclusion criteria (5 studies, 1,000 subjects) could still be substantially changed by new, large studies with divergent results.

The promising dynamic risk factors included variables related to sexual deviancy (any deviant sexual interest, sexual preoccupations), antisocial personality (antisocial personality disorder, psychopathy as measured by PCL-R), and antisocial traits (general self-regulation problems, employment instability, hostility). The potentially misleading risk factors were negative family background, internalization of psychological problems, and poor clinical presentation (e.g., denial, low motivation for treatment).

The different approaches used to assess deviant sexual interests included self-report ($d. = .38 \pm .18$, 5 studies; $n = 780$), phallometric assessments ($d. = .24 \pm .12$, 13 studies; $n = 2{,}180$), offense history ($d. = .15 \pm .18$, 3 studies; $n = 1{,}042$), and structured clinical ratings relying on multiple sources of information ($d. = .42 \pm .19$, 8 studies; $n = 947$), such as the Sexual Deviance item from Sexual Violence Risk–20 (Boer, Hart, Kropp, & Webster, 1997). For the 6 studies that presented dichotomous ratings of sexual deviancy, 65.5% of the sexual recidivists ($n = 261$) were classified as sexual deviant compared with 42.3% of the nonrecidivists ($n = 749$). Sexual preoccupations were assessed through either self-report questionnaires ($d. = .35 \pm .18$, 3 studies; $n = 3{,}911$) or structured clinical ratings ($d. = .68 \pm .45$, 3 studies; $n = 208$). The structured clinical ratings showed greater predictive accuracy than the other assessment approaches, but the confidence intervals overlapped for all measures.

Discussion

Most sexual offenders were not caught for another sexual offense (13.7%); on average, they were more likely to recidivate with a nonsexual offense than a sexual offense (overall recidivism rate of 36.2%). The major predictors of general (any) and violent recidivism were variables related to antisocial orientation, such as antisocial personality, antisocial traits, and a history of rule violation. These are the same risk factors that predict general and violent recidivism among mentally disordered offenders (Bonta, Law, & Hanson, 1998) and unselected groups of offenders (Gendreau, Little, & Goggin, 1996).

The variables that predicted sexual recidivism were similar, but not identical, to the predictors of nonsexual recidivism. Sexual deviancy and antisocial orientation were the major predictors of sexual recidivism for both adult and adolescent sexual offenders. Sexual deviancy was unrelated to nonsexual recidivism. For the general categories of deviant sexual attitudes and intimacy deficits, some of the individual variables were related to sexual recidivism (e.g., emotional identification with children, conflicts in intimate relationships) and some were not (e.g., loneliness). Such variability suggests that further research is needed to uncover those aspects of attitudes and social functioning most associated with persistent sexual offending.

The present results also suggest that the factors that initiate sexual offending may not be the same as the factors associated with persistence. Negative family backgrounds and internalization of psychological problems are common among sexual offenders (Lee, Jackson, Pattison, & Ward, 2002; Raymond et al., 1999; Smallbone & Dadds, 1998), but these factors were unrelated to sexual recidivism. The prototypic sexual recidivist is not upset or lonely; instead, he leads an unstable, antisocial lifestyle and ruminates on sexually deviant themes. There is some evidence, however, that sexual offenders are more likely than other groups to respond to stress through sexual acts and fantasies (deviant or otherwise; Cortoni & Marshall, 2001; McKibben, Proulx, & Lusignan, 1994) thereby creating discrete time periods where they are at increased risk of sexual recidivism (Hanson & Harris, 2000b).

The distinction between sexual recidivists and nonrecidivists invites comparisons with Moffitt's (1993) distinction between adolescence-limited and life-course persistent delinquents. In Moffitt's typology, the life-course persistent offenders have behavior problems in childhood, engage in interpersonal violence, and have many sexual partners (Sluyter et al., 2003)—all characteristics that predicted sexual and nonsexual recidivism in the present study. These characteristics can be considered common manifestations of low self-control (e.g., Gottfredson & Hirschi, 1990), but they have also been considered as an evolutionary adaptation to stressful childhood environments (Belsky, Steinberg, & Draper, 1991; Moffit, Caspi, Belsky, & Silva, 1992). The substantial overlap in the characteristics of persistent sexual and persistent nonsexual offenders suggests that those concerned with the assessment and management of sexual offenders could profit from the substantial literature on the assessment and treatment of general criminal offenders (e.g., Andrews & Bonta, 2003; Gendreau, French, & Gionet, 2004).

For those involved in applied risk assessments with sexual offenders, the review confirms sexual deviancy and antisocial orientation as major predictors of sexual recidivism and extends the range of relevant variables to include some potentially changeable characteristics: sexual preoccupations, lifestyle instability/impulsivity, pro-offending attitudes, and intimacy deficits. Readers will notice, however, that the predictive accuracy of most of the characteristics was small. Consequently, prudent evaluators need to consider a range of potential risk factors in an overall evaluation. The best methods for combining risk factors into an overall evaluation remain an active topic of scientific debate (Berlin, Galbreath, Geary, & McGlone, 2003; Hanson, Morton, & Harris, 2003).

Another outstanding research question is whether changes on the potentially dynamic factors are actually associated with reductions in recidivism risk. In general, evaluations of treatment progress showed little relationship to recidivism, with an average *d*. of .14. Nevertheless, there were some recent examples in which ratings of progress in treatment were significantly related to recidivism (Beech, Erikson, Friendship, & Ditchfield, 2001, $d = .50$; Marques, Day, Wiederanders, & Nelson, 2002, $d = .55$). Both of these studies used highly structured approaches to evaluating treatment gains and were informed by recent empirical research.

Evaluators may also note that many of the variables used in clinical assessments had little or no relationship with recidivism (e.g., denial, low victim empathy, low motivation for treatment). The lack of relationship may be linked to the difficulty of assessing sincere remorse in criminal justice settings. It is also possible that evaluators looking for risk factors have little to gain from listening to offenders' attempts to justify their transgressions. Psychotherapists often consider full disclosure desirable, and courts are lenient toward those who show remorse; few people, however, are inclined to completely reveal their faults and transgressions. Research has even suggested that full disclosure of negative personal characteristics is associated with negative social outcomes, including poor progress in psychotherapy (Kelly, 2000). Consequently, resistance to being labeled a sexual offender may not be associated with increased recidivism risk, even though it does create barriers to engagement in treatment. Offenders who minimize their crimes are at least indicating that sexual offending is wrong.

The present findings may also be useful to those wishing to improve treatment programs for sexual offenders. On average, sexual offenders who attend treatment are less likely to recidivate than are comparison groups (Hall, 1995; Hanson et al., 2002), but it is easy to locate well-controlled studies that find no effect for sexual offender treatment (e.g., Marques, Wiederanders, Day, Nelson, & van Ommeren, 2005). For general offenders, treatment is effective only when it targets criminogenic needs (i.e., characteristics associated with offending; Dowden & Andrews, 2000). A review of the core treatment targets of sexual offender treatment programs (McGrath, Cumming, & Burchard, 2003, Table 9.1) suggests that most programs direct considerable resources toward characteristics that have little or no relationship with recidivism (e.g., offense responsibility, victim awareness, and empathy). An important question is whether programs that target the major predictors of sexual offense recidivism (e.g., lifestyle instability, deviant sexual interests, sexual preoccupations) are more effective than programs that target other factors.

Meta-analyses provide broad overviews and can easily neglect potentially important differences between studies. The definitions of constructs varied across studies, as did the samples. The present study focused on mixed groups of sexual offenders, and there was no effort to identify distinct predictors for specific subgroups (e.g., rapists, exhibitionists). Nevertheless, the findings were remarkably consistent. For 70% of the individual findings, the amount of variability across studies was no more than would be expected by chance ($p < .05$). Furthermore, there was substantial consistency within many of the categories of predictors, with almost all of the variables being significant (e.g., sexual deviancy, history of rule violation) or nonsignificant (e.g., general psychological problems, clinical presentation; see Hanson & Morton-Bourgon, 2004). There is still substantial variability across studies that remains to be explained, but it appears that research is getting closer to identifying the constructs that are, and are not, related to recidivism among sexual offenders. Hopefully these research gains can be used to promote effective interventions and just social policies for sexual offenders.

References

References marked with an asterisk were included in the meta-analysis

*Abel, G. G., Mittelman, M., Becker, J. V., Rathner, J., & Rouleau, J. L. (1988). Predicting child molesters' response to treatment. In R. A. Prentky & V. L. Quinsey (Eds.), *Human sexual aggression: Current prespectives* (pp. 223–234). New York: New York Academy of Science.

*Allam, J. (1999). *Effective practice in work with sex offenders: A reconviction study comparing treated and untreated offenders.* Birmingham, West Midlands, England: West Midlands Probation Service Sex Offender Unit.

Andrews, D. A., & Bonta, J. (2003). *The psychology of criminal conduct* (3rd ed.). Cincinnati, OH: Anderson.

*Barbaree, H. E., & Marshall, W. L. (1988). Deviant sexual arousal, offense history, and demographic variables as predictors of reoffense among child molesters. *Behavioural Sciences & the Law, 6,* 267–280.

*Barbaree, H. E., & Seto, M. C. (1998). *The ongoing follow-up of sex offenders treated at the Warkworth Sexual Behaviour Clinic* (Research Rep.). Toronto, Canada: Forensic Program, Centre for Addiction and Mental Health.

*Barbaree, H. E., Seto, M. C., Langton, C. M., & F. E. Peacock, E. J. (2001). Evaluating the predictive accuracy of six risk assessment instruments for adult sex offenders. *Criminal Justice and Behavior, 28,* 490–521.

*Barbaree, H. E., Seto, M. C., & Maric, A. (1996). *Working papers in impulsivity research: Sex offender characteristics, response to treatment, and correctional release decisions at the Warkworth Sexual Behaviour Clinic* (Research Rep.). Toronto, Canada: Forensic Division, Clarke Institute of Psychiatry.

*Beech, A., Erikson, M., Friendship, C., & Ditchfield, J. (2001). *A six-year follow-up of men going through probation-based sex offender treatment programmes* (Findings #144). London: Home Office.

Beech, A. R., Fisher, D. D., & Thornton, D. (2003). Risk assessment of sex offenders. *Professional Psychology: Research and Practice, 34,* 339–352.

Beech, A., & Ward, T. (2004). The integration of etiology and risk in sexual offenders: A theoretical framework. *Aggression and Violent Behavior, 10,* 31–63.

Belsky, J., Steinberg, L., & Draper, P. (1991). Childhood experiences, interpersonal development, and reproductive strategy: An evolutionary theory of socialization. *Child Development, 62,* 647–670.

*Berger, P. (2002, September). *The role of personality disorders and paraphilias as predictors of relapse in male sexual offenders.* Paper presented at the 7th conference of the International Association for the Treatment of Sexual Offenders, Vienna.

Berlin, F. S., Galbreath, N. W., Geary, B., & McClone, G. (2003). The use of actuarials at civil commitment hearings to predict the likelihood of future sexual violence. *Sexual Abuse: A Journal of Research and Treatment, 15,* 377–382.

Boer, D. P., Hart, S. D., Kropp, P. R., & Webster, C. D. (1997). *Manual for the Sexual Violence Risk – 20: Professional guidelines for assessing risk of sexual violence.* Vancouver: The British Columbia Institute Against Family Violence.

*Bonta, J., & Hanson, R. K. (1995). [Ten year recidivism data for offenders released from the Correctional Service of Canada in 1983/1984]. Unpublished raw data.

Bonta, J., Law, M., & Hanson, R. K. (1998). The prediction of criminal and violent recidivism among mentally disordered offenders: A meta-analysis. *Psychological Bulletin, 123,* 123–142.

*Bradford, J., Firestone, P., Fernandez, M., Curry, S., & Larose, M. (1997). *Predictors of recidivism in a population of Canadian sex offenders: Psychological, physiological, and offense factors.* Unpublished manuscript.

*Broadhurst, R. (1999). *Probabilities of sex offender recidivism: A survival analysis.* Unpublished manuscript.

*Broadhurst, R., & Loh, N. (2003). The probabilities of sex offender rearrest. *Criminal Behaviour and Mental Health, 13,* 121–139.

*Broadhurst, R., & Maller, R. A. (1992). The recidivism of sex offenders in the Western Australian prison population. *British Journal of Criminology, 32,* 54–80.

*Buffington-Vollum, J., Edens, J. F., Johnson, D. W., & Johnson, J. K. (2002). Psychopathy as a predictor of institutional misbehaviour among sex offenders: A prospective replication. *Criminal Justice and Behavior, 29,* 497–511.

California Office of the Attorney General. (2004). *Sex offender registration statistics as of June 1, 2004.* Retrieved June 28, 2004, from http://caag.state.ca.us/megan/pdf/5_04pie1.pdf

Caspi, A., Moffit, T. E., Silva, P. A., Stouthamer-Loeber, M., Krueger, R. F., & Schmutte, P. S. (1994). Are some people crime-prone? Replications of the personality-crime relationship across countries, genders, races, and methods. *Criminology, 32,* 163–195.

*Christiansen, K. O., Elers-Nielsen, M., Le Maire, L., & Sturup, G. K. (1965). Recidivism among sexual offenders. *Scandinavian Studies in Criminology, 1,* 55–85.

Cohen, J. (1988). *Statistical power analysis for the behavioral sciences* (2nd ed.). Hillsdale, NJ: Erlbaum.

*Cooper, H. (2000). *Long-term follow-up of a community-based treatment program for adolescent sex offenders.* Unpublished master's thesis, Lakehead University, Thunder Bay, Ontario, Canada.

Cortoni, F., & Marshall, W. L. (2001). Sex as a coping strategy and its relationship to juvenile sexual history and intimacy in sexual offenders. *Sexual Abuse: A Journal of Research and Treatment, 13,* 27–43.

*Davis, G. L., Hoffman, R. G., & Stacken, N. (1991, August). *2–4 Year post-incarceration follow-up of treated sex offenders.* Paper presented at the 99th meeting of the American Psychological Association, San Francisco.

*Dempster, R. J. (1998). *Prediction of sexually violent recidivism: A comparison of risk assessment instruments.* Unpublished master's thesis, Simon Fraser University, British Columbia, Canada.

*Dempster, R. J., & Hart, S. D. (2002). The relative utility of fixed and variable risk factors in discriminating sexual recidivists and nonrecidivists. *Sexual Abuse: A Journal of Research and Treatment, 14*(2), 121–138.

*Dix, G. E. (1976). Differential processing of abnormal sex offenders: Utilization of California's mentally disordered sex offender program. *Journal of Criminal Law & Criminology, 67,* 233–243.

*Doshay, L. J. (1943). *The boy sex offender and his later career.* Montclair, NJ: Patterson Smith.

Dowden, C., & Andrews, D. A. (2000). Effective correctional treatment and violent reoffending: A meta-analysis. *Canadian Journal of Criminology, 42,* 449–467.

*Dwyer, S. M. (1997). Treatment outcome study: Seventeen years after sexual offender treatment. *Sexual Abuse: A Journal of Research and Treatment, 9,* 149–160.

*Epperson, D. L., Kaul, J. D., & Hesselton, D. (1998). *Minnesota Sex Offender Screening Tool–Revised (MnSOST–R): Development, performance, and recommended risk level cut scores.* Iowa State University & Minnesota Department of Corrections.

*Epperson, D. L., Kaul, J. D., & Huot, S. J. (1995, October). *Predicting risk of recidivism for incarcerated sex offenders: Updated development on the Sex Offender Screening Tool (SOST).* Paper presented at the 14th annual Research and Treatment Conference of the Association for the Treatment of Sexual Abusers, New Orleans, LA.

*Federoff, J. P., Wisner-Carlson, R., Dean, S., & Berlin, F. S. (1992). Medroxy-progesterone acetate in the treatment of paraphilic sexual disorders. *Journal of Offender Rehabilitation, 18,* 109–123.

Firestone, P., Bradford, J. M., Greenberg, D. M., & Serran, G. A. (2000). The relationship between deviant sexual arousal and psychopathy in incest offenders, extrafamilial child molesters, and rapists. *Journal of the American Academy of Psychiatry and the Law, 28,* 303–308.

*Firestone, P., Bradford, J. M., McCoy, M., Greenberg, D. M., Curry, S., & Larose, M. R. (1998). Recidivism in convicted rapists. *Journal of the American Academy of Psychiatry & Law, 26*(2), 185–200.

*Fischer, D. R. (2000). *Sex offender risk assessment validation study.* Phoenix, AZ: Arizona Department of Corrections.

*Fitch, J. H. (1962). Men convicted of sexual offences against children: A descriptive follow-up study. *British Journal of Criminology, 3,* 18–37.

*Frisbie, L. V., & Dondis, E. H. (1965). *Recidivism among treated sex offenders* (California Mental Health Monograph No. 5). Sacramento: State of California Department of Mental Hygiene.

Gendreau, P., French, S. A., & Gionet, A. (2004). What works (what doesn't work): The principles of effective correctional treatment. *Journal of Community Corrections, 13,* 4–6, 27–30.

Gendreau, P., Little, T., & Goggin, C. (1996). A meta-analysis of the predictors of adult offender recidivism: What works! *Criminology, 34,* 575–607.

*Gfellner, B. M. (2000). *Adult sex offenders in treatment programs: Predictors of success and recidivism* (Research Rep. to the Sex Offender Treatment Advisory Group (SOTAG). Brandon, Manitoba, Canada.

Gottfredson, M. R., & Hirschi, T. (1990). *A general theory of crime.* Stanford, CA: Stanford University Press.

*Greenberg, D. M., Da Silva, J., & Loh, N. (2002). *Evaluation of the Western Australian sex offender treatment unit (1987–1999): A quantitative analysis.* Perth: University of Western Australia, Forensic Research Unit, Department of Psychiatry and Behavioural Sciences.

*Greenberg, D. M., Firestone, P., Bradford, J. M., & Broom, I. (2000). Infantophiles. In L. B. Schlesinger (Ed.), *Serial offenders: Current thought, recent findings* (pp. 229–246). New York: CRC Press.

*Gretton, H. M. (1995). [The relationship between phallometric assessment and recidivism among 185 juvenile sex offenders]. Unpublished raw data.

*Gretton, H. M., McBride, M., Hare, R. D., O'Shaughnessy, R., & Kumka, G. (2001). Psychopathy and recidivism in adolescent sex offenders. *Criminal Justice and Behavior, 28,* 427–499.

Grotpellier, J. K., & Elliott, D. S. (2002). *Violent sexual offending.* Boulder: Center for the Study and Prevention of Violence, University of Colorado.

*Hall, G. C. N. (1988). Criminal behavior as a function of clinical and actuarial variables in a sexual offender population. *Journal of Consulting and Clinical Psychology, 56,* 773–775.

Hall, G. C. N. (1995). Sexual offender recidivism revisited: A meta-analysis of recent treatment studies. *Journal of Consulting and Clinical Psychology, 63,* 802–809.

*Hanson, R. K. (2002). [Evaluation of Manitoba's Secondary Risk Assessment]. Unpublished raw data.

Hanson, R. K., & Bussière, M. T. (1998). Predicting relapse: A meta-analysis of sexual offender recidivism studies. *Journal of Consulting and Clinical Psychology, 66,* 348–362.

Hanson, R. K., Gordon, A., Harris, A. J. R., Marques, J. K., Murphy, W., Quinsey, V. L., & Seto, M. C. (2002). First report of the Collaborative Outcome Data Project on the effectiveness of psychological treatment for sex offenders. *Sexual Abuse: A Journal of Research and Treatment, 14,* 169–194.

*Hanson, R. K., & Harris, A. J. R. (2000a). [Dynamic predictors of sexual recidivism based on comparing 208 recidivists and 201 non-recidivists on community supervision]. Unpublished raw data.

Hanson, R. K., & Harris, A. J. R. (2000b). Where should we intervene? Dynamic predictors of sex offense recidivism. *Criminal Justice and Behavior, 27,* 6–35.

Hanson, R. K., Morton, K. E., & Harris, A. J. R. (2003). Sexual offender recidivism risk: What we know and what we need to know. In R. A. Prentky, E. S. Janus, & M. C. Seto (Eds.), *Annals of the New York Academy of Sciences: Vol. 989. Sexually coercive behavior: Understanding and management* (pp. 154–166). New York: New York Academy of Sciences.

Hanson, R. K., & Morton-Bourgon, K. E. (2004). *Predictors of sexual recidivism: An updated meta-analysis.* (Research Rep. No. 2004–02). Ottawa, Canada: Public Safety and Emergency Preparedness Canada.

*Hanson, R. K., Steffy, R. A., Scott, H., & Gauthier, R. (1993). [Long-term recidivism of child molesters released from Millbrook Institution between 1958 & 1974]. Unpublished raw data.

Hare, R. D., Harpur, T. J., Hakstian, A. R., Forth, A. E., Hart, S. D., & Newman, J. P. (1990). The Revised Psychopathy Checklist: Reliability and factor structure. *Psychological Assessment, 2,* 338–341.

*Harris, G. T., Rice, M. E., Quinsey, V. L., Lalumiere, M. L., Boer, D., & Lang, C. (2003). A multi-site comparison of actuarial risk instruments for sex offenders. *Psychological Assessment, 15,* 413–425.

Hasselblad, V., & Hedges, L. V. (1995). Meta-analysis of screening and diagnostic tests. *Psychological Bulletin, 117,* 167–178.

*Haynes, A. K., Yates, P. M., Nicholaichuk, T., Gu, D., & Bolton, R. (2000, June). *Sexual deviancy, risk and recidivism: The relationship between deviant arousal, the RRASOR and sexual recidivism.* Paper presented at the annual conference of the Canadian Psychological Association, Ottawa, Ontario, Canada.

*Hecker, J., Scoular, J., Righthand, S., & Nangle, D. (2002, October). *Predictive validity of the J-SOAP over 10-plus years: Implications for risk assessment.* Poster presented at the 21st annual conference of the Association for the Treatment of Sexual Abusers, Montreal, Quebec, Canada.

Hedges, L. V., & Olkin, I. (1985). *Statistical methods for meta-analysis.* New York: Academic Press.

*Hildebrand, M., de Ruiter, C., & de Vogel, V. (2004). Psychopathy and sexual deviance in treated rapists: Association with (sexual) recidivism. *Sexual Abuse: A Journal of Research and Treatment, 16,* 1–24.

*Hood, R., Shute, S., Feilzer, M., & Wilcox, A. (2002). Sex offenders emerging from long-term imprisonment: A study of their long-term reconviction rates and of parole board members' judgments of their risk. *British Journal of Criminology, 42,* 371–394.

*Hudson, S. M., Wales, D. S., Bakker, L., & Ward, T. (2002). Dynamic risk factors: The Kia Marama evaluation. *Sexual Abuse: A Journal of Research and Treatment, 14,* 103–119.

Hudson, S. M., & Ward, T. (1997). Rape: Psychopathology and theory. In D. R. Laws & W. O'Donohue (Eds.), *Sexual deviance: Theory, assessment and treatment* (pp. 332–355). New York: Guilford Press.

*Kahn, T. J., & Chambers, H. J. (1991). Assessing reoffense risk with juvenile sexual offenders. *Child Welfare, 70,* 333–345.

Kelly, A. E. (2000). Helping construct desirable identities: A self-presentational view of psychotherapy. *Psychological Bulletin, 126,* 475–494.

*Khanna, A., Brown, P., Malcolm, P. B., & Williams, S. M. (1989, March). *Outcome data on sex offenders assessed and treated at Regional Treatment Centre (Ontario).* Paper presented at the annual meeting of the Special Needs Offenders Conference, Ottawa, Ontario, Canada.

Knight, R. A., & Sims-Knight, J. E. (2003). The developmental antecedents of sexual coercion against women: Testing alternative hypotheses with structural equation modeling. In R. A. Prentky, E. S. Janus, & M. C. Seto (Eds.), *Annals of the New York Academy of Sciences: Vol. 989. Sexually coercive behavior: Understanding and management* (pp. 72–85). New York: New York Academy of Sciences.

Koss, M. P. (1987). Hidden rape: Sexual aggression and victimization in a national sample of students in higher education. In A. W. Burgess (Ed.), *Rape and sexual assault II* (pp. 3–25). New York: Garland.

*Lab, S. P., Shields, G., & Schondel, C. (1993). Research note: An evaluation of juvenile sexual offender treatment. *Crime and Delinquency, 39,* 543–553.

*Langevin, R., & Fedoroff, J. P. (2000). *25 year recidivism study of sex offenders.* Unpublished manuscript.

*Långström, N. (2002a). Long-term follow-up of criminal recidivism in young offenders: Temporal patterns and risk factors. *Psychology, Crime & the Law, 8,* 41–58.

*Långström, N. (2002b). [Relationship of denial to recidivism among 46 juvenile sex offenders in Sweden]. Unpublished raw data.

*Långström, N., & Grann, M. (2000). Risk for criminal recidivism among young sex offenders. *Journal of Interpersonal Violence, 15,* 855–871.

*Långström, N., Sjöstedt, G., & Grann, M. (2004). Psychiatric disorders and recidivism among sexual offenders. *Sexual Abuse: A Journal of Research and Treatment, 16,* 139–150.

*Langton, C. M. (2003a). *Contrasting approaches to risk assessment with adult male sexual offenders: An evaluation of recidivism prediction schemes and the utility of supplementary clinical information for enhancing predictive accuracy.* Unpublished doctoral dissertation, Institute of Medical Science, University of Toronto, Toronto, Ontario, Canada.

*Langton, C. M. (2003b). [The relationship between progress in treatment and recidivism among 444 sexual offenders released from Warkworth Institution]. Unpublished raw data.

Lee, J., Jackson, H., Pattison, P., & Ward, T. (2002). Developmental risk factors for sexual offending. *Child Abuse & Neglect, 26,* 73–92.

Lisak, D., & Miller, P. M. (2002). Repeat rape and multiple offending among undetected rapists. *Violence and Victims, 17,* 73–84.

*Mair, K. J., & Wilson, D. (1994). *Prevalence, prediction and perseveration of sexual reoffending in a sample identified through court records.* Unpublished manuscript.

*Mair, K. J., & Wilson, D. (1995). *Sexual reconviction over time in Scottish sex offenders identified through court records.* Unpublished manuscript.

Malamuth, N. M. (2003). Criminal and noncriminal sexual aggressors:

Integrating psychopathy in heirarchical-mediational confluence model. In R. A. Prentky, E. S. Janus, & M. C. Seto (Eds.), *Annals of the New York Academy of Sciences: Vol. 989. Sexually coercive behavior: Understanding and management* (pp. 33–58). New York: New York Academy of Sciences.

*Marques, J. K., & Day, D. M. (1996). [SOTEP follow-up data for 1995]. Unpublished raw data.

*Marques, J. K., Day, D. M., Wiederanders, M., & Nelson, C. (2002, October). *Main effects and beyond: New findings from California's Sex Offender Treatment & Evaluation Project (SOTEP).* Paper presented at the 21st annual conference of the Association for the Treatment of Sexual Abusers, Montreal, Quebec, Canada.

Marques, J. K., Wiederanders, M., Day, D. M., Nelson, C., & van Ommeren, A. (2005). Effects of a relapse prevention program on sexual recidivism: Final results from California's Sex Offender Treatment and Evaluation Project (SOTEP). *Sexual Abuse: A Journal of Research and Treatment, 17,* 79–107.

Marshall, P. (1997). *The prevalence of convictions for sexual offending* (Research Finding No. 55). London: Research and Statistics Directorate, Home Office.

Marshall, W. L. (1997). Pedophilia: Psychopathology and theory. In D. R. Laws & W. O'Donohue (Eds.), *Sexual deviance: Theory, assessment and treatment* (pp. 152–174). New York: Guilford Press.

*Marshall, W. L., & Barbaree, H. E. (1988). The long-term evaluation of a behavioral treatment program for child molesters. *Behaviour, Research and Therapy, 26,* 499–511.

*McBride, M., Gretton, H., Hare, R. D. (1995, October). *Familial risk factors, psychopathy and recidivism in adolescent sexual offenders.* Paper presented at the annual conference of the Association for the Treatment of Sexual Abusers, New Orleans, LA.

McGrath, R. J., Cumming, G. F., & Burchard, B. L. (2003). *Current practices and trends in sexual abuser management.* Brandon, VT: Safer Society.

*McGrath, R. J., Cumming, G., Livingston, J. A., & Hoke, S. E. (2003). Outcome of a treatment program for adult sex offenders: From prison to community. *Journal of Interpersonal Violence, 18*(1), 3–17.

McKibben, A., Proulx, J., & Lusignan, R. (1994). Relationships between conflict, affect and deviant sexual behaviours in rapists and pedophiles. *Behaviour Research and Therapy, 13,* 571–575.

*Meyer, L. C., & Romero, J. (1980). *A ten-year follow-up of sex offender recidivism.* Unpublished manuscript.

*Meyer, W. J., Cole, C., & Emory, E. (1992). Depo Provera treatment for sex offending behaviour: An evaluation of outcome. *Bulletin of the American Academy of Psychiatry and Law, 20,* 249–259.

*Miner, M. H. (2002). [Factors associated with recidivism among 129 juvenile sex offenders released from Minnesota Corrections]. Unpublished raw data.

*Minnesota Department of Corrections. (1999). *Community-based sex offender program evaluation project: 1999 report to the legislature.* St. Paul, MN: Author.

Moffitt, T. E. (1993). "Life-course-persistent" and "adolescence-limited" antisocial behavior: A developmental taxomony. *Psychological Review, 100,* 893–910.

Moffitt, T. E., Caspi, A., Belsky, J., & Silva, P. A. (1992). Childhood experience and the onset of menarche: A test of a sociobiological model. *Child Development, 63,* 47–58.

*Mohr, J. W., Turner, R. E., & Jerry, M. B. (1964). *Pedophilia and exhibitionism.* Toronto, Canada: University of Toronto Press.

*Money, J., & Bennett, R. G. (1981). Post adolescent paraphilic sex offenders: Antiandrogenic and counseling therapy follow-up. *International Journal of Mental Health, 10,* 122–133.

*Morton, K. E. (2003). [Recidivism prediction in a sample of male adolescent sexual offenders assessed at a community sexual offender treatment program]. Unpublished raw data.

*Motiuk, L. L., & Brown, S. L. (1995). [Survival time for sexual offenders released from the Correctional Services of Canada in 1991 & 1994]. Unpublished raw data.

*Mulloy, R., & Smiley, W. C. (1996). *Recidivism and treated sex offenders.* Paper presented at the International Congress of Psychologists, Montreal, Quebec, Canada.

*Nunes, K. L., Serran, G. A., Firestone, P., Greenberg, D. M., & Bradford, J. M. (2000, November). *A comparison of child molesters who deny vs. those who admit their offenses.* Paper presented at the annual conference for the Association for the Treatment of Sexual Abusers, San Diego, CA.

*Nutbrown, V., & Stasiak, E. (1987). *A retrospective analysis of O. C. I. cost effectiveness 1977–81* (Ontario Correctional Institute Research Monograph No. 2). Brampton, Ontario, Canada: Ontario Ministry of Correctional Services.

*Ohio Department of Rehabilitation and Correction. (2001). *Ten-year recidivism follow-up of 1989 sex offender releases.* Columbus, OH: Author.

Orwin, R. G. (1994). Evaluating coding decisions. In H. Cooper & L. V. Hedges (Eds.), *The handbook of research synthesis* (pp. 139–162). New York: Russell Sage Foundation.

*Pacht, A. R., & Roberts, L. M. (1968). Factors related to parole experience and the deviated sex offender. *Correctional Psychologist, 3,* 8–11.

*Perkins, D. (1987). A psychological treatment programme for sex offenders. In B. J. McGurk, D. M. Thornton, and M. Williams (Eds.), *Applying psychology to imprisonment: Theory and practice* (pp. 191–249). London: Her Majesty's Stationery Office.

*Prentky, R., Harris, B., Frizzell, K., & Righthand, S. (2000). An actuarial procedure for assessing risk with juvenile sex offenders. *Sexual Abuse: A Journal of Research and Treatment, 12,* 71–93.

*Prentky, R., Knight, R. A., & Lee, A. F. S. (1997). Risk factors associated with recidivism among extrafamilial child molesters. *Journal of Consulting and Clinical Psychology, 65,* 141–149.

*Prentky, R. A., Knight, R. A., Lee, A. F., & Cerce, D. D. (1995). Predictive validity of lifestyle impulsivity for rapists. *Criminal Justice and Behavior, 22,* 106–128.

*Proulx, J., Pellerin, B., McKibben, A., Aubut, J., & Ouimet, M. (1995). [Static and dynamic predictors in sexual aggressors]. Unpublished raw data.

*Quinsey, V. L., Khanna, A., & Malcolm, P. B. (1998). A retrospective evaluation of the Regional Treatment Centre sex offender treatment program. *Journal of Interpersonal Violence, 13,* 621–644.

Quinsey, V. L., Lalumière, M. L., Rice, M. E., & Harris, G. T. (1995). Predicting sexual offenses. In J. C. Campbell (Ed.), *Assessing dangerousness: Violence by sexual offenders, batterers, and child abusers* (pp. 114–137). Thousand Oaks, CA: Sage.

*Quinsey, V. L., Rice, M. E., & Harris, G. T. (1995). Actuarial prediction of sexual recidivism. *Journal of Interpersonal Violence, 10,* 85–105.

*Rabinowitz-Greenberg, S. R. (1999). *Predictors of recidivism in a population of Canadian exhibitionists: Psychological, phallometric and offense factors.* Unpublished doctoral dissertation, University of Ottawa, Ottawa, Canada.

*Radzinowicz, L. (1957). *Sexual offenses: A report of the Cambridge Department of Criminal Science.* London: MacMillan.

*Rasmussen, L. A. (1999). Factors related to recidivism among juvenile sexual offenders. *Sexual Abuse: A Journal of Research and Treatment, 11,* 69–85.

Raymond, N. C., Coleman, E., Ohlerking, R., Christensen, G. A., & Miner, M. (1999). Psychiatric comorbidity in pedophilic sex offenders. *American Journal of Psychiatry, 156,* 786–788.

*Reddon, J. R., Studer, L., & Estrada, L. (1996). [Recidivism data from the Pheonix Program for sex offender treatment]. Unpublished raw data.

*Rice, M. E., Harris, G. T., & Quinsey, V. L. (1990). A follow-up of rapists assessed in a maximum security psychiatric facility. *Journal of Interpersonal Violence, 5,* 435–448.

*Rice, M. E., Quinsey, V. L., & Harris, G. T. (1989). Predicting sexual recidivism among treated and untreated extrafamilial child molesters released from a maximum security psychiatric institution (Penetanguishene Mental Health Centre Research Report, Vol. VI (3)). Penetanguishene, Ontario, Canada.

*Rice, M. E., Quinsey, V. L., & Harris, G. T. (1991). Sexual recidivism among child molesters released from a maximum security psychiatric institution. *Journal of Consulting and Clinical Psychology, 59,* 381–386.

Roberts, C. F., Doren, D. M., & Thornton, D. (2002). Dimensions associated with assessments of sex offender recidivism risk. *Criminal Justice and Behavior, 29,* 569–589.

*Rooth, F. G., & Marks, I. M. (1974). Persistent exhibitionism: Short-term response to aversion, self-regulation, and relaxation treatments. *Archives of Sexual Behavior, 3,* 227–249.

*Ryan, G., & Miyoshi, T. (1990). Summary of a pilot follow-up study of adolescent sexual perpetrators after treatment. *Interchange, 1,* 6–8.

*Santman, J. (1998). *A taxonomic model of juvenile sexual offender recidivism.* Unpublished doctoral dissertation, CA School of Professional Psychology, Fresno, CA.

*Schram, D. D., & Milloy, C. D. (1995). *Community notification: A study of offender characteristics and recidivism.* Olympia, WA: Washington State Institute for Public Policy.

*Serin, R. C., Mailloux, D. L., & Malcolm, P. B. (2001). Psychopathy, deviant sexual arousal and recidivism among sexual offenders. *Journal of Interpersonal Violence, 16,* 234–246.

*Sjöstedt, G., & Långström, N. (2001). Actuarial assessment of sex offender recidivism risk: A cross-validation of the RRASOR and the Static-99 in Sweden. *Law and Human Behaviour, 25,* 629–645.

*Sjöstedt, G., & Långström, N. (2002). Assessment of risk for criminal recidivism among rapists: A comparison of four different measures. *Psychology, Crime & the Law, 8,* 25–40.

Slavin, R. E. (1995). Best evidence synthesis: An intelligent alternative to meta-analysis. *Journal of Clinical Epidemiology, 48,* 9–18.

Sluyter, F., Arseneault, L., Moffitt, T. E., Veenema, A. H., de Boer, S., & Koolhaas, J. M. (2003). Toward an animal model for antisocial behavior: Parallels between mice and humans. *Behavior Genetics, 33,* 563–574.

Smallbone, S. W., & Dadds, M. R. (1998). Childhood attachment and adult attachment in incarcerated adult male sex offenders. *Journal of Interpersonal Violence, 13,* 555–573.

*Smith, W. R., & Monastersky, C. (1986). Assessing juvenile sexual offenders' risk for reoffending. *Criminal Justice and Behavior, 13,* 115–140.

*Song, L., & Lieb, R. (1994). [Recidivism data for the study of Washington State's sentencing alternative for sex offenders]. Unpublished raw data.

*Soothill, K. L., Jack, A., & Gibbens, T. C. N. (1976). Rape: A 22-year cohort study. *Medicine, Science, and the Law, 16,* 62–69.

*Soothill, K. L., Way, C. K., & Gibbens, T. C. N. (1980). Rape acquittals. *Modern Law Review, 43,* 159–172.

*Sturup, G. K. (1953). Sexual offenders and their treatment in Denmark and the other Scandinavian countries. *International Review of Criminal Policy, 4,* 1–19.

*Sturup, G. K. (1960). Sex offenses: The Scandinavian experience. *Law and Contemporary Problems, 25,* 361–375.

*Thornton, D. (1997). [A 16-year follow-up of 563 sexual offenders from HM Prison Service in 1979]. Unpublished raw data.

*Thornton, D. (2002). [Factors associated with sexual recidivism in a sample of treated sex offenders]. Unpublished raw data.

*Tough, S. E. (2001). *Validation of two standardized risk assessments (RRASOR, 1997; Static-99, 1999) on a sample of adult males who are developmentally disabled with significant cognitive deficits.* Unpublished master's thesis, University of Toronto, Toronto, Ontario, Canada.

*Tracy, F., Donnelly, H., Morgenbesser, L., & MacDonald, D. (1983). Program evaluation: Recidivism research involving sex offenders. In J. G. Greer & I. R. Stuart (Eds.), *The sexual aggressor: Current perspectives on treatment* (pp. 198–213). New York: Van Nostrand Reinhold.

*Waite, D., Pinkerton, R., Wieckowski, E., McGarvey, E., & Brown, G. L. (2002, October). *Tracking treatment outcome among juvenile sexual offenders: A nine year follow-up study.* Paper presented at the 21st annual conference of the Association for the Treatment of Sexual Abusers, Montreal, Quebec, Canada.

Ward, T., & Siegert, R. J. (2002). Toward a comprehensive theory of child sexual abuse: A theory knitting perspective. *Psychology, Crime, & Law, 8,* 319–351.

*Weaver, C., & Fox, C. (1984). The Berkeley Sex Offenders Group: A seven-year evaluation. *Probation Journal, 31,* 143–146.

West, D. J. (1983). Sex offenses and offending. In M. Tonry & N. Morris (Eds.). *Crime and justice: An annual review of research* (pp. 183–233). Chicago: University of Chicago Press.

*Wing, S. W. (1984). *A study of reoffenses by treated sex offenders at Western State Hospital.* Unpublished manuscript.

*Witte, T., Di Placido, C., Gu, D., & Wong, S. (2002, May). *Criminal Sentiments Scale: Predictive validity in a sample of sexual offenders primarily composed of rapists.* Poster presented at the 63rd annual convention of the Canadian Psychological Association, Vancouver, British Columbia, Canada.

*Witte, T., Di Placido, C., & Wong, S. (2001). *How dangerous are dangerous sex offenders? An estimation of recidivism and level of risk using a matched control group.* Saskatoon, Saskatchewan, Canada: Regional Psychiatric Centre.

*Worling, J. R. (2001). Personality-based typology of adolescent male sexual offenders: Differences in recidivism rates, victim-selection characteristics, and personal victimization histories. *Sexual Abuse: A Journal of Research and Treatment, 13,* 149–166.

Received July 20, 2004
Revision received May 2, 2005
Accepted May 4, 2005 ■

[5]

The Competence of Criminal Defendants: A Theoretical Reformulation

Richard J. Bonnie, LL.B

"Competence" of criminal defendants is best viewed not as an open-textured single construct but rather as two related but separable constructs-a foundational concept of competence to assist counsel, and a contextualized concept of decisional competence. This approach has several advantages. First, it provides a useful explanatory framework for the settled features of existing law. Second, it helps to clarify the issues in areas where the law is unsettled or controversial, such as the circumstances under which incompetence bars adjudication and the abilities required for decisional competence. Third, it exposes the similarities between competencies in criminal defense and competencies in other legal contexts, and thereby helps to link what have been discrete literatures in both law and behavioral science. Fourth, because this approach is derived from a theoretical analysis of the purposes of the pertinent legal rules, it provides a framework for defining the "psycho-legal abilities" that are encompassed by each of the two competence constructs. In this respect, a relatively simple reconceptualization has surprisingly concrete implications for designing a program of empirical research and, eventually, for improving the scientific basis of competence assessments in criminal cases.

I. INTRODUCTION

The proposition that a defendant's incompetence bars adjudication is deeply rooted in the common law[1] has been constitutionalized by the United States Supreme

Address reprint requests to R. J. Bonnie, LL.B at University of Virginia School of Law, Charlottesville, VA 22901, USA. John S. Battle Professor of Law and Director, Institute of Law, Psychiatry and Public Policy, University of Virginia. This research was supported by the John D. and Catherine T. MacArthur Foundation Research Network on Mental Health and the Law.

I am grateful to all members of the Network for helping me develop the ideas expressed in this paper. I owe a special debt to John Monahan, Tom Grisso, Elyn Sans and Ken Hoge, who commented extensively on earlier drafts. I am also indebted to Mary Porto, UVA Law School Class of 1991, Eric Fishman, Class of 1992 and Laurie Meehan, Class of 1993, for their invaluable research assistance.

[1] WILLIAM BLACKSTONE, COMMENTARIES 24, 395 (9th ed. 1783).

Court,[2] and is taken as axiomatic in the administration of criminal justice. The Supreme Court has adopted prophylactic procedural requirements to induce trial judges to order mental evaluations,[3] and to hold hearings,[4] whenever significant doubts are raised regarding the defendant's mental competence.[5] In addition, a defense attorney's failure to seek a mental evaluation in doubtful cases is likely to invalidate any resulting conviction.[6] These rules are designed to accomplish the dual purposes of assuring a fair adjudication and of preserving finality by having all doubts regarding the defendant's mental condition raised and resolved as early in the process as possible. Available data suggest that pretrial competence evaluations are sought in between two and eight percent of felony cases.[7]

Given the operational requirements of everyday processing of criminal cases, it is not surprising that an abundant literature has emerged to assist forensic mental health practitioners who are called upon to evaluate a defendant's competence.[8] Efforts have been made to develop structured protocols for assessing the psychological capacities thought to be relevant to the ultimate legal judgment,[9] but they have been only modestly successful because the concept of competence is so ill-defined; it has aptly been characterized as an "open construct" with little determinate content independent of the context in which the competence issue is raised.[10]

The most widely used interview protocols include "checklists" of behaviors and functions which are rated by the interviewer and which may or may not be assembled into a total score.[11] If the items are summed, the quantitative rating is only an indicator, not a measure, of the defendant's competence; the interviewers are expected to weight the items subjectively in making their ultimate judgment. Thus, the available instruments do little more than structure the interview and focus the

[2] Pate v. Robinson, 383 U.S. 375, 378 (1966) (noting and apparently endorsing the government's stipulation "that the conviction of an accused person [who] is legally incompetent violates due process. . . .").

[3] Drope v. Missouri, 420 U.S. 162 (1975).

[4] Pate v. Robinson, 383 U.S. 375 (1966).

[5] The word "competence" is out of vogue in the mental disability field. A variety of factors account for this: The term has a global connotation which is normatively undesirable. The implication that incompetence is a personal characteristic suppresses its situational and interactive aspects. Finally, the term is ultimately a legal conclusion with inescapably moral dimensions. Notwithstanding all of this, I am using the term, uncritically, as a shorthand for the functional incapacities of criminal defendants that trigger the application of various legal rules in a criminal case. In so doing, I should not be understood as endorsing the naive idea that "competence" is an objective, clinically measurable phenomenon. In referring to the "objective" aspects of judgments about competence, I will use the terms abilities and capacities interchangeably.

[6] *See generally* AMERICAN BAR ASSOCIATION CRIMINAL JUSTICE MENTAL HEALTH STANDARDS Std. 7–4.2(c) and accompanying commentary (1986) (hereinafter ABA STANDARDS).

[7] Steven K. Hoge, Richard J. Bonnie, Norman Poythress and John Monahan, *Attorney-Client Decision-Making in Criminal Cases: Client Competence and Participation as Perceived by Their Attorneys*, 10 Behavioral Sciences and the Law, 385 (1992).

[8] *See generally* Gary Melton, John Petrilla, Norman Poythress and Christopher Slobogin, PSYCHOLOGICAL EVALUATIONS FOR THE COURTS 66–92 (1987); Thomas Grisso, EVALUATING COMPETENCIES 62–78 (1986).

[9] Thomas Grisso, EVALUATING COMPETENCIES 78–112 (1986).

[10] Ronald Roesch and Stephen L. Golding, COMPETENCY TO STAND TRIAL 10–13 (1980).

[11] Grisso reviews and discusses the mostly widely used instruments in EVALUATING COMPETENCIES at 78–104. The Competency to Stand Trial Assessment Instrument (CAI) developed by Louis A. McGarry and Associates Laboratory of Community Psychiatry, Harvard Medical School, is described in COMPETENCY TO STAND TRIAL AND MENTAL ILLNESS (1974); The Interdisciplinary Fitness Interview (IFI) developed by Stephen Golding and Ronald Roesch, is described in Stephen L. Golding, Ronald Roesch, and Jan Schreiber, *Assessment and Conceptualization of Competency to Stand Trial: Preliminary Data on the Interdisciplinary Fitness Interview*, 8 LAW AND HUMAN BEHAVIOR, 321 (1984).

interviewer's attention on a series of items thought to be relevant to a highly individualized assessment. The items listed in the most widely used protocols have usually been distilled from appellate opinions and interviews with judges; they have not been derived either from a theory of competence or from empirical study of the difficulties encountered by attorneys representing defendants with mental disabilities. Abilities thought to be relevant to competence have not been systematically studied in normal populations of criminal defendants.

The problem, I suggest, is that the legal formulations which clinicians and judges are trying to operationalize are not firmly anchored in a shared understanding about why (in)competence matters. What is missing, in a word, is a theory. This is not the fault of forensic researchers. The leading theoretical accounts in the legal literature tend to focus more on the disutility of the legal rules barring adjudication[12] than on the meaning of incompetence in relation to the social purposes the rules are supposed to serve.[13]

The need for theoretical attention to the concept of competence in relation to criminal defense[14] is perhaps best illustrated by the inadequacy of the legal vocabulary itself. An umbrella phase—"competence to stand trial"—is commonly used to refer to an array of contextual inquiries that bear very little relationship with one another, either functionally or sequentially. This same term is used, for example, to refer to assessments conducted immediately after arrest—before any attorney has been appointed—to ascertain whether the process should be permitted to go forward at all, and is also used to refer to assessments conducted on the eve of a trial to ascertain the likely impact of stress on the defendant's ability to participate in the proceeding.

Moreover, as is commonly observed, the phrase "competence to stand trial" is actually misleading in a fundamental way because it implies, incorrectly, that competence assessment is primarily directed at trial participation. Because more than 90% of defendants plead guilty, trial participation is entirely hypothetical in most cases. The relevant dimensions of a defendant's "competence" in most situations are his or her capacity to assist counsel conduct an adequate investigation of the case and to make whatever decisions a defendant is required or expected to make in order to defend and/or resolve the case without a trial.

Explicit attention to guilty pleas exposes a puzzling and controversial feature of the current law—the relation between the legal "tests" for competence to plead guilty and competence to stand trial. Consider two cases. In one, suppose a defendant's auditory hallucinations and attentional deficits make it impossible for him to sustain his attention in a courtroom for more than a few minutes. Assume further,

---

[12] The "incompetence plea" bars adjudication adverse to the defendant, not adjudication *per se*. Thus, one-way, "innocence-only" procedures are permissible. *See, e.g.* ILL. REV. STAT., ch. 38, §§ 104–17–18 (Supp. 1991); CAL. PENAL CODE § 1368 (West, 1992). For convenience of reference, however, I will characterize the rule as one which "bars adjudication."

[13] *See e.g.*, Robert A. Burt and Norval Morris, *A Proposal for Abolition of the Incompetency Plea*, 40 U. CHI. L. REV. 66 (1972) (hereinafter Burt and Morris); Bruce J. Winick, *Incompetency to Stand Trial: An Assessment of Costs and Benefits and a Proposal for Reform*, 39 RUTGERS L. REV. 243 (1987) (hereinafter Winick).

[14] The paucity of theoretical literature on the components of competence in the criminal process is somewhat puzzling in light of the pervasive attention that has been given to the analogous construct in other contexts, especially in relation to treatment decision-making. The most elaborate theoretical account of the reasons for the competence doctrine appears in Note, *Incompetency to Stand Trial*, 81 HARV. L. REV. 454, 457–59 (1967).

however, that his understanding of the charges and the criminal process are unimpaired, he is able to provide pertinent information to his attorney regarding the evidence in the case, and he is able to understand the relevant considerations in deciding whether to accept a proffered plea agreement. In this case, it might be said that the defendant is competent to plead guilty even though he might not be able to stand trial.

In a contrasting case, suppose a defendant is able to communicate rationally with counsel, to pay attention in court, and to understand the nature and purpose of a criminal prosecution and the roles of all the participants. In this case, however, suppose that the defendant is unable, due to mental retardation, to understand the differences between greater and lesser-included charges, and is unable to understand the probability assessments that are relevant to deciding whether to accept a plea agreement or, if the case is tried, to have a bench trial instead of a jury trial. In this case, it might be said that the defendant is competent to stand trial, but not competent to plead guilty ot waive a jury trial.[15]

These two cases expose the following question: is "competence" of criminal defendants a single construct or more than one construct? The case law addressing this question is in a state of confusion. When asked to rule that the "test" for competence to plead guilty is "higher" than the "test" for competence to stand trial, most courts have insisted that competence to stand trial/plead guilty is a single construct.[16] On the other hand, some courts have reached a different conclusion in the context of arguments that a defendant who is admittedly competent to plead guilty or to stand trial on a not guilty plea, might *not* be competent to decide whether to plead insanity.[17]

In this paper I argue that competence in the criminal process is best viewed as two related but separable constructs, not as an open-textured single construct. Specifically, I draw a distinction between a foundational concept of competence to assist counsel,[18] and a contextualized concept of decisional competence. As I will show, this approach is grounded securely in a proper theoretical understanding of the purposes of the legal rules relating to defendant competence, and it is generally compatible with the settled features of current law. At a minimum then, this reconceptualization provides a useful explanatory framework for existing law. But I think it offers three additional advantages. First, it helps to clarify the issues in areas where the law is unsettled or controversial, especially in relation to decisional competence. Second, it exposes the similarities between competencies in criminal defense and competencies in other legal contexts, and thereby helps to link what, until now, have been discrete literatures in both law and behavioral science. Third, because this approach is derived from a theoretical analysis of the purposes of the pertinent

[15] One can argue, as a matter of policy, that this is not a sound result, and that such a defendant should not be denied the advantages of plea bargaining or of a bench trial. If this view is accepted, the legal basis for a valid waiver can be established either (i) by holding that 'competence' to plead guilty or waive jury trial does not require the abilities to understand the differences among charges or to weigh advantages and disadvantages of waiving constitutional rights, or (ii) by allowing surrogate decision-making by the attorney, or a third party. These issues are discussed *infra*.

[16] *See, e.g.*, Allard v. Helgemoe, 572 F.2d 1, 3 (1st Cir. 1978), and cases cited therein. *Contra* Seiling v. Eyman, 478 F.2d 211 (9th Cir. 1973).

[17] *See. e.g.*, Frendak v. United States, 408 A.2d 364 (D.C. 1979).

[18] In an earlier version of this paper, I referred to this foundational construct as "competence to proceed," a phrase occasionally used as a synonym for "competence to stand trial" in its generic sense. However, I chose to use "competence to assist counsel" to better convey the functional content of the concept.

legal rules, it provides a framework for defining the "psycho-legal abilities" that are encompassed by each of the two competence constructs. In this respect, what seems to be a relatively simple reconceptualization has surprisingly concrete implications for designing a program of empirical research and, eventually, for improving the scientific basis of competence assessments in criminal cases.

II. WHY (IN)COMPETENCE MATTERS

A review of cases and commentary yields three conceptually independent rationales for barring adjudication on grounds of a defendant's incompetence. I will label them *dignity*, *reliability*, and *autonomy*.

A person who lacks a rudimentary understanding of the nature and purpose of the proceedings against her is a not a "fit" subject for criminal prosecution and punishment. To proceed against such a person offends the moral *dignity* of the process because it treats the defendant not as an accountable person, but as an object of the state's effort to carry out its promises. The dignity rationale is implicated only in cases involving defendants who lack a meaningful moral understanding of wrongdoing and punishment, or the nature of a criminal prosecution.[19]

Beyond the minimal demands of the dignity rationale, the bar against adverse adjudication in cases involving incompetent defendants serves as a prophylactic protection against erroneous convictions. Just as the assistance of competent counsel is regarded as a prerequisite of reliable adjudication, so too is the participation of a competent defendant. As stated by Weihofen in 1954, a mentally impaired defendant might be unfairly convicted if he "alone has knowledge" of certain facts but does "not appreciate the value of such facts, or the propriety of communicating them to his counsel."[20] To proceed against a defendant who lacks the capacity to recognize and communicate relevant information to his or her attorney and to the court would be unfair to the defendant and would undermine society's independent interest in the *reliability* of its criminal process. This is what the Supreme Court had in mind when it stated that the bar against trying the incompetent defendant "is fundamental to an adversary system of justice."[21]

As critics of the existing legal arrangements have correctly noted,[22] the bar against prosecuting incompetent defendants evolved at a time when the defendant was

[19] Lists of purposes served by the incompetence doctrine typically include the need to preserve the decorum of the courtroom and the dignity of the trial process. *See, e.g.* Note, *Incompetency to Stand Trial, supra note* 14 at 458. However, I do not regard this as a viable rationale for a bar against adjudication. As I note at pages 315–316 *infra*, a disruptive defendant can be removed from the courtroom if necessary and an otherwise competent defendant can waive his or her right to be present. Moreover, judicial tolerance for "disturbing" behavior in the courtroom should be very high in plea proceedings and bench trials. In short, the "dignity" rationale for the incompetence doctrine refers to the inherent morality of the process carried out in the courtroom, not to its outward appearances.

[20] Henry Weihofen, *Mental Disorder as a Criminal Defense* 429–30 (1954). *See also* 4 WILLIAM BLACKSTONE, COMMENTARIES 24: "If a man in his sound memory commits a capital offense, and before arraignment for it, he becomes mad, he ought not to be arraigned for it; because he is not able to plead to it with that advice and caution that he ought. And if, after he has pleaded, the prisoner becomes mad, he shall not be tried: for how can he make his defense? If, after he be tried and found guilty, he loses his senses before judgment, judgment shall not be pronounced; and if, after judgment, he becomes of nonsane memory, execution shall be stayed."

[21] Drope v. Missouri, 420 U.S. 162, 172 (1975).

[22] E.G. Winick, *supra* note 13, at 260.

responsible for mounting his own defense. Indeed, assistance of counsel was actually precluded in felony and treason cases until the mid-eighteenth century.[23] Today, in contrast, assistance of counsel is available as a matter of constitutional right in all serious criminal cases.[24] Although representation by counsel does not render the traditional rules obsolete, the construct of incompetence itself must be operationalized in the context of the attorney-client relationship. Thus, to the extent that the meaning of incompetence is derived from its instrumental function, it refers to the capacity to provide whatever assistance counsel requires in order to explore and present an adequate defense.[25]

A third dimension of the competence construct, which is conceptually independent of the two dimensions thus far discussed, is derived from legal rules which establish that certain decisions regarding the defense or disposition of the case must be made by (or are within the prerogative of) the defendant him or herself. Some construct of "decisional competence" is an inherent, though derivative, feature of any legal doctrine that prescribes a norm of client *autonomy*. In theory, at least, it is possible to imagine a system of criminal adjudication which leaves no room for client self-determination—one which bars self-representation, which does not permit guilty pleas, and in which all decisions regarding the conduct and defense of the case are made by counsel, not by the defendant.[26] Under these legal arrangements, a defendant's decisional competence would not be relevant. But this is not our system.

In our system, some decisions regarding the defense or disposition of the case are committed, by law, to the defendant and not to the attorney. According to all authorities, these include decisions regarding the plea, and, if the case is to be tried, whether it should be tried before a jury, whether the defendant will be present, and whether the defendant will testify.[27] In more general terms, the defendant is permitted, if not required, to make decisions regarding the objectives of representation, including the basic theory of defense.[28] For some of these decisions (i.e., those involving waivers of constitutional rights), the principle of self-determination is reinforced by the obligation imposed on courts to assure that the defendant's decision is knowingly, intelligently, and voluntarily made.[29] Not surprisingly,

[23] Faretta v. California, 422 U.S. 806, 823 (1975).

[24] Argersinger v. Hamlin, 407 U.S. 25 (1972); Gideon v. Wainwright, 372 U.S. 335 (1963).

[25] *See, e.g.*, Dusky v. United States, 362 U.S. 402 (1960) ("[T]he test will be whether [the defendant] has sufficient present ability to consult with his lawyer with a reasonable degree of rational understanding–and whether he has a rational as well as factual understanding of the proceedings against him"); Drope v. Missouri, 420 U.S. 162, 171 (1975) ("It has long been accepted that a person whose mental condition is such he lacks the capacity to understand the nature and object of the proceedings against him, to consult with counsel, and to assist in preparing his defense may not be subjected to trial").

[26] Faretta v. California, 422 U.S. 806 (1975), holding that a defendant is constitutionally entitled to waive assistance of counsel and to represent him or herself, was, after all, a 6–3 decision.

[27] *See, e.g.*, Brookhart v. Janis, 384 U.S. 1 (1966) (whether to plead guilty); Rock v. Arkansas, 483 U.S. 44 (1987) (whether to testify); Adams v. United States *ex rel.* McCann, 317 U.S. 269, (1942) (waiver of jury trial). *See generally* ABA STANDARDS *supra* note 5, Standard 4–5.2(a); MODELRULES OF PROFESSIONAL CONDUCT Rule 1.2(a) (1983).

[28] See ABA Standard 4–5.2(a); Model Rule 1.2(a). In contrast "decisions on what witnesses to call, whether and how to conduct cross-examination, what jurors to accept or strike, what trial motions should be made, and all other strategic and tactical decisions are the exclusive province of the lawyer after consultation with the client." ABA Standard 4–5.2(b). *See also* Jones v. Barnes, 463 U.S. 745 (1983), regarding lawyer's prerogative to decide what issues to raise on appeal. The distinction between "objectives" and "means" of representation is, of course, indeterminate at the margins.

[29] *See, e.g.*, Boykin v. Alabama, 395 U.S. 238 (1969); Johnson v. Zerbst, 304 U.S. 458 (1938).

judicial scrutiny is likely to be most intensive when the defendant decides to represent himself.[30]

III. THE TWO DIMENSIONS OF COMPETENCE IN THE CRIMINAL PROCESS

Against this theoretical backdrop, I want to suggest a simple and, I think, relatively uncontroversial conceptual vocabulary that reflects a sensible understanding of the main purposes served by competence determinations in the criminal process. In explicating this vocabulary, I want to emphasize that the language I am proposing carries no implications regarding the psychological abilities that should be encompassed within a legal "test" of competence and, specifically, regarding the "level" of competence that should be required in any specific context. Although I have views on these issues, the vocabulary itself is meant to be normatively neutral.[31]

The key conceptual distinction I want to draw is between a foundational concept of "competence to assist counsel" and a contextualized concept of "decisional competence." By "competence to assist counsel," I mean to refer to the minimum conditions required for participating in one's own defense. Although there is some room for debate about what the law "is" in this context, most courts and commentators refer to (i) capacity to understand the charges, the purpose of the criminal process and the adversary system, especially the role of defense counsel; (ii) capacity to appreciate one's situation as a defendant in a criminal prosecution; and (iii) ability to recognize and relate pertinent information to counsel concerning the facts of the case.[32] As I am defining the concept, however, it does *not* encompass the ability to make decisions that may be confronted in the case or the defendant's likely behavioral functioning at trial.

As customarily defined, these components serve both the dignity and reliability rationales described above. The capacities required to assure the dignity of the process would seem to include the ability to understand the nature of wrongdoing and punishment and the purpose and effect of a criminal prosecution and conviction, together with the ability to relate this understanding to one's own situation as a defendant. The capacities required to assure the reliability of the outcome would seem to include the ability to understand the role of the defense attorney and to apply that understanding to one's own situation, and the ability to recognize and relate pertinent information in a coherent manner.

The capacities required to preserve the dignity of the process and to assure

[30] Westbrook v. Arizona, 384 U.S. 150 (1966).

[31] The vocabulary is obviously not normatively neutral to the extent that it assumes that (in)competence matters in the ways described in the previous section.

[32] This is, of course, an elaboration of the "test" articulated in Dusky v. United States, 362 U.S. 402 (1960). In addition, the concept may also encompass a "motivational" component pertaining to capacity to cooperate with one's attorney, thereby enabling the attorney to perform her assigned role in the process. *Cf.* State v. Johnson, 133 Wisc. 2d 207, 395 N.W.2d 176 (1986). However, this additional feature is not necessary to encompass delusional beliefs pertaining to the role of counsel because they are included within the concept of appreciation. Other clinical problems which interfere with motivation to cooperate present difficulties in distinguishing between "can't" and "won't"; the possibility that failure to cooperate or assist could be construed as "inability" to cooperate or assist raises serious moral hazard problems. *See e.g.* Commonwealth v. Logan, 549 A.2d 531, 539 (Pa. 1988). These issues—whether competence to assist counsel should include a motivational component and, if so, how it should be operationalized—need more systematic attention than they have thus far received.

reliability are conceptually distinct. Although they probably overlap a great deal empirically, abundant clinical experience demonstrates that they are not congruent, and that the ability to perform one set of tasks does not necessarily predict ability to perform the other. Many mentally disabled defendants who understand the process and their own situations are unable to assist counsel; and, conversely, a delusional defendant may be able to understand counsel's role and to relate relevant information but may believe that the criminal prosecution is serving a benevolent divine plan and has no punitive purpose or effect. Despite the conceptual and empirical divergence of these two clusters of capacities, however, it is sensible to combine them in a single foundational construct because both of these rationales (dignity and reliability) underlie the traditional bar against prosecution and conviction of incompetent defendants.[33]

In most cases, questions about "competence to assist counsel" arise at the outset of the process—before significant interactions with counsel have occurred and before strategic decisions regarding defense of the case have been encountered or considered. This has two implications: first, for defendants regarded initially as incompetent, restorative intervention achieves sufficient improvement to permit the procedural bar to be lifted in most cases; second, determinations of competence in borderline cases (either upon initial assessment or upon restoration) are best regarded as provisional.

A defendant who is (provisionally) competent to assist counsel may not be competent to make specific decisions[34] that are encountered as the process unfolds.[35] Decision-making involves cognitive tasks in addition to those required for assisting in one's defense, as defined above, including abilities to understand and choose among alternative courses of action. Which abilities should be regarded as *necessary* for legally valid decision-making, and therefore included within a "test" of decisional competence, must be derived from a normative conception of client autonomy in criminal defense. For the moment, however, my interest is not in the precise content of the "test", but rather in whether decision-making capacity, however, defined,

[33] This assertion describes present law. However, the reliability and dignity rationales can be disentwined. As will be discussed *infra*, it is possible to imagine a system in which prosecution could proceed against a defendant unable to assist counsel if reliable adjudication could otherwise be assured. *See* Burt and Morris, *supra* note 13, at 93–95. If prosecutions were permitted in such cases, then the foundational dimension of competence would include only those capacities necessary to assure the dignity of the process.

It should also be noted that the dignity rationale does have independent and exclusive force in relation to the variety of companion common-law doctrines (carried forward in many contemporary statutes) that barred the *sentencing* of a defendant who became incompetent after conviction, and that barred the *execution of sentence* against a prisoner who became incompetent after pronouncement of judgment. In fact, as I have noted elsewhere, the ban on executing the "presently incompetent," now constitutionalized in Ford v. Wainwright, 477 U.S. 399 (1986), can only be understood in dignitarian terms. *See* Richard J. Bonnie, *Dilemmas in Administering the Death Penalty: Conscientious Abstention, Professional Ethics and the Needs of the Legal System, 14* LAW AND HUMAN BEHAVIOR 67, 86–88 (1990).

[34] As noted earlier, the relevant "decisions" are those which are committed, by law, to the competent defendant and not to the lawyer—or, to state it the other way, those that counsel is not permitted to make on his/her own—whether they are made prior to trial, at trial, or in lieu of trial.

[35] The question also arises whether a defendant who is unable to assist counsel, as defined here, may nonetheless be decisionally competent. Although the question is solely of theoretical interest—because inability to assist counsel bars adjudication—the relation between abilities required for assisting counsel and for decision-making should be explored empirically.

is best understood as a component of a single construct of competence in the criminal process or rather as a separate construct.

Competence in the criminal process might be sensibly understood as a single construct if a generally applicable test of decision-making ability could be defined and folded into a unitary test of adjudicative competence (or whatever it would be called). This approach would promote efficiency in assessment because it would not require contextualized application and would resolve all potential disputes about competence at one time. Despite these practical advantages, however, the "single construct" approach has two serious normative disadvantages. First, it is fundamentally incompatible with the contemporary understanding of the contextual nature of legal incompetence. It is now axiomatic that a person may be competent for one purpose, such as decision-making about medical treatment, but not about others, such as the management of financial affairs. Tests of competence, and the procedures required to resolve doubts about competence, vary from context to context, depending upon both normative and practical considerations. Adherence to the idea that a criminal defendant is competent for all decision-making purposes, or for none, would be anomalous in the face of such a pervasive understanding.

A second problem with the single construct approach is that it unnecessarily links the finding of decisional incompetence to the procedural bar against adjudication. Prosecution of a defendant who is not competent to assist counsel, as defined above, should be categorically barred to preserve the moral dignity of the criminal process and to avoid an unacceptable risk of unreliable convictions. However, more flexible responses—such as surrogate decision-making or specifically tailored default rules—should be available to deal with deficiencies in decisional competence. If the defendant is able to assist counsel, a bar against adjudication is not necessarily advantageous to either the defendant or society. Yet, if competence is a unitary construct, adjudication is categorically prohibited in such cases. In no other legal context does a finding of decisional incompetence have such paralyzing consequences.

In one context at least—waiver of counsel, and choosing to represent oneself—decisional competence is by all accounts a separate construct.[36] A defendant who is competent to proceed to adjudication *with* counsel may not be allowed to proceed to adjudication *without* representation. In upholding the defendant's constitutional right to represent herself, in *Faretta v. California*,[37] the Supreme Court explicitly recognized that self-representation increased the danger of unreliable adjudication.[38] *Faretta* holds, in effect, that autonomy can trump reliability.[39] However, courts have uniformly concluded, in the wake of *Faretta*, that autonomy prevails *only* if

[36] I am focusing here only on the *decision-making abilities* required for effecting a legally valid waiver of one's right to be represented by counsel in favor of self-representation, i.e., to exercise one's "*Faretta*-right." I am not referring to whatever performance abilities may be required, in addition to decisional competence, for self-representation at a trial. Nor does this discussion have any bearing on the abilities required to waive one's right to counsel during a custodial interrogation.

[37] Faretta v. California, 422 U.S. 806 (1975).

[38] *Id.* at 834 ("It is undeniable that in most criminal prosecutions defendants could better defend with counsel's guidance than with their own unskilled efforts.").

[39] *Id.* at 834. ("[The defendant] must be personally free to decide whether in his particular case counsel is to his advantage. And although he may conduct his own defense ultimately to his own detriment, his choice must be honored out of 'that respect for the individual which is the lifeblood of the law'.")

the defendant satisfies a more demanding test of decisional competence than would otherwise be required for adjudication with counsel.[40]

Faretta and its progeny reflect an explicit trade-off between autonomy and reliability in cases involving defendants who want to represent themselves. It is clear, however, that these considerations may also conflict in cases involving defendants who are represented by counsel. Thus, we should expect the test for decisional competence to be especially demanding in situations where reliability is seriously threatened, such as when a defendant wants to plead guilty against his lawyer's advice,[41] or rejects the most plausible theory of defense in favor of a theory which the attorney believes to be unsupportable.

Moreover, autonomy is more at stake in some decisional contexts than in others. Decisions whether or not to raise an insanity defense, or whether or not to seek leniency in a capital prosecution, inevitably implicate the personal values of the defendant. Other decisions, such as whether to waive indictment or preliminary hearing, are primarily matters of "legal judgment" and are so unlikely to implicate the defendant's personal values that the attorney may be allowed to make them without the defendant's participation at all; and, even if client participation is required, it may be required only if the decision goes in one direction (i.e., to waive the right), and one would not expect the test for competence to be especially demanding.

Even when autonomy is clearly at stake, paternalistic concerns are more prominent in some decisional contexts than in others, and attorneys and courts may be expected to take steps to resolve doubts about competence that would not be required in other contexts. For example, the attorney may be obligated to raise in court whatever genuine doubts she has about a client who instructs her not to present a case in mitigation at a capital sentencing proceeding,[42] but may not be obligated to raise these concerns about a defendant who has assented to her recommendation that a jury trial be waived in favor of a bench trial.[43]

In short, decisions which defendants are expected or permitted to make in the course of criminal defense are normatively diverse. As *Faretta* demonstrates, a single criterion of decisional competence is not likely to fit every decisional context. There may be practical reasons to deploy a single test of decisional competence, but any such criterion is bound to produce undesirable results, either by respecting client prerogatives in cases where doing so endangers reliability, or by barring adjudication

[40] *See e.g.*, State v. Harding, 137 Ariz 278, 670 P.2d 383 (1983); People v. Burnett, 188 Cal. App. 3d 1314, 234 Cal. Rptr. 67 (Cal. App. 1st Dist. 1987). These rulings had been presaged by Arizona v. Westbrook, 384 U.S. 150 (1966). At a minimum, it is clear that the defendant must have the capacity to understand and weigh the risks and benefits of self-representation, including the risk that the defendant might be erroneously convicted due to deficiencies of his self-representation. The society's independent interest is not sacrificed entirely in the situation, however, because a valid *Faretta* waiver may require the "mental ability to present a rudimentary defense" or "some minimal ability to present a personal defense." *See* People v. Burnett, *supra*, 234 Cal. Rptr. at 73–78.

[41] Concerns about reliability may be so compelling that the defendant is denied the prerogative to decide to plead guilty, even if he is competent. *See, e.g.*, CAL PENAL CODE § 1018 (West 1992) (precluding a defendant from pleading guilty to a capital offense without the consent of his or her lawyer). However, the same concerns which underlie the California statute might yield an alternative rule which respects the defendant's prerogative to reject counsel's advice but only if the defendant meets a demanding test of competence.

[42] *See e.g.*, Fisher v. State, 739 P.2d 523, 525 (Okla, Crim. App. 1987); Commonwealth v. Crawley, 514 Pa. 539, 526 A.2d 334, 340 n.1 (Pa. 1987). *See* my discussion of this problem in *The Dignity of the Condemned*, 74 VA L. REV. 1363, 1388–89 (1988).

[43] *Cf.* McCarlo v. State, 677 P.2d 1268 (Alaska Ct. App. 1984).

in cases in which the mentally impaired defendant is not called upon to waive any constitutional rights or to make any other significant decisions.

In summary, rules relating to a defendant's decisional competence are derived from the rules allocating decision-making prerogatives in criminal defense. Client autonomy may be displaced entirely in some contexts, in which case competence does not come into play at all. When client participation is permitted or required by law, however, competence is prerequisite to validity. My sole claim at this point is that the normative diversity of decisional contexts in criminal defense strongly implies that the criteria for decisional competence, and the procedures required for raising and resolving doubts, are likely to vary from one context to another.

The criteria for decisional competence, the procedures for resolving doubts about competence, and the legal responses to incompetence can be sensibly formulated only in the context of a more general theory concerning client autonomy in the attorney-client relationship. Insofar as the theory aims to describe the existing legal rules, it must explain why certain decisions are allocated to the [competent] defendant rather than to counsel,[44] and why counsel generally has no legally enforceable obligation, analogous to the physician's duty in medicine, to facilitate informed client decision-making.[45] Recognizing that legal rules cannot assure autonomous action, even for competent persons, what function do they actually serve?[46] Development of such a theory would exceed the ambition of this paper, but I will venture some tentative assertions in support of what I will characterize as a "weak" theory of client self-determination: attorneys are obligated to inform clients of their prerogative to make binding decisions regarding defense and disposition of the case. However, clients need not personally make such decisions in any authentic sense, and the attorneys' obligation to inform is generally contingent upon the client's desire to be informed. In my view, it is only in the context of such a theory that one can make sense of the law governing decisional (in)competence in the criminal process.

The next two sections of the paper will elaborate on the theoretical implications of the distinction I have drawn between competence to assist counsel and decisional competence. I should note, at this point, that these two concepts, as defined above, seem to embrace the full range of competencies in the criminal process. I am presently inclined to regard competence to plead guilty and competence to stand trial as being particular elaborations of these foundational concepts. However, as will appear below, these are provisional opinions which may be modified in light of empirical investigation and further theoretical discourse.

---

[44] For example, should the attorney be permitted, or even obligated, to introduce mitigating evidence in a capital case over the defendant's objection? See my discussion of this issue in *The Dignity of the Condemned*, 74 VA. L. REV. 1363 (1988). Should the attorney be permitted to seek a lesser included offense instruction over the defendant's objection? *Cf.* State v. Johnson, 133 Wisc. 2d 207, 395 N.W.2d 176 (1986).

[45] In response to a perceived pattern of attorney dominance in the attorney-client relationship, several commentators have proposed that the informed consent doctrine be implanted in the law of attorney-client relations. *See, e.g.*, Marcy Strauss, "*Toward a Revised Model of the Attorney-Client Relationship: The Argument for Autonomy*, 65 N.C. L. REV. 315 (1987); Susan R. Martyn, *Informed Consent in the Practice of Law*, 48 GEO. WASH. L. REV. 307 (1980); Mark Spiegel, *Lawyering and Client Decision-Making: Informed Consent and the Legal Profession*, 128 U. PENN. L. REV. 41 (1979). To date, however, facilitation of informed client decision-making remains an aspirational ethical norm rather than a legal duty.

[46] *See generally*, Ruth R. Faden and Tom L. Beauchamp, A HISTORY AND THEORY OF INFORMED CONSENT 274–297 (1986).

IV. COMPETENCE TO ASSIST COUNSEL

One of the most important advantages of separating decisional competence from the baseline construct of competence to assist counsel is that it permits tailored responses to cases involving decisional incompetence that are not possible when abilities relating to decision-making are folded into a single construct of adjudicative competence. Discrete tests of decisional competence can be defined to fit particular decision-making contexts and, most importantly, a finding of decisional incompetence need not bar adjudication. Only incompetence to assist counsel bars adjudication. It follows, however, that the components of competence to assist counsel must be defined and applied with its preclusive effect in mind.

An important ambiguity regarding competence to assist counsel is whether application of this construct is in any way dependent on the particular defendant's situation. This issue has both practical and theoretical dimensions. On the one hand, viewing competence to assist counsel in absolute terms has many practical advantages. Most importantly, definitive assessments could be made early in the process against a single normatively-derived standard and need not be focused on the circumstances of the particular defendant's case (which are not likely to be evident to the evaluator in any event). Moreover, in theoretical terms, the capacities required to preserve the moral dignity of the criminal process can be formulated and assessed without reference to the facts of a particular defendant's case.

On the other hand, an absolute standard is bound to be either underinclusive or overinclusive in terms of the ultimate concern with reliability of the outcome. If the threshold of competence to assist counsel is set too low, deficient interactions between attorney and client could lead to erroneous convictions. If the threshold is set too high, to take account of the demands presented by the most intricate case, some defendants will be unnecessarily found incompetent and hospitalized, and some reliable convictions will be unnecessarily barred.[47] Thus, reliability concerns would suggest that "competence to assist counsel" must be sufficiently linked to the particular defendant's situation to take into account the complexity of the charges and the attorney's actual need for information.[48]

An analogous problem is raised when a defendant has amnesia for the time of the offense. Under the prevailing judicial practice, the legal significance of a (genuine) claim of amnesia is determined in light of the strength of the evidence in the particular case; adjudication is barred only if there is a significant possibility that the defendant would have been able to produce evidence raising a reasonable doubt about guilt.[49] The reliability judgment is made on a case-by-case basis.

Burt and Morris, who propose abolition of the "incompetence plea," argue that the more flexible amnesia rule should displace the *per se* rule now being applied in cases of mental "incompetence."[50] Adjudication should be permitted, they argue, as long as the procedures are suitably designed to redress the disadvantages

[47] It bears emphasis, see note 12 *supra*, that incompetence only bars adjudication adverse to the defendant, so we are concerned exclusively with the risk of erroneous convictions.

[48] This is the common understanding reflected in the forensic literature on assessment of competence in criminal defendants. *See, e.g.*, Thomas Grisso, EVALUATING COMPETENCIES 76–77 (1986). In Grisso's terminology, assessment of competence to assist counsel has "interactive" dimensions. *Id.* at 18–26.

[49] *See, e.g.*, Wilson v. United States, 391 F.2d 460 (D.C. Cir. 1968).

[50] Burt and Morris, *supra* note 12, at 82–83.

attributable to the defendant's mental disability. In my view, the analogy between amnesia and other mental disabilities would be apt if reliability were the only relevant consideration. However, the Burt and Morris proposal fails to take account of the widely-shared intuition that adjudication of guilt is morally inappropriate unless the defendant has a basic understanding of the process to which he is being subjected. At the least, the moral dignity of the criminal process requires a categorical bar against adjudication in some cases. If this much is acknowledged, little is lost, and much is gained, by including within the foundational test of competence certain *minimum* capacities required for assisting counsel.

From a normative standpoint, then, a two-step approach would seem to provide a sensible resolution. An "absolute" level of capacity to assist counsel should be required in all cases. (The components of the test should probably include an *actual* understanding of the nature and purpose of the criminal process and the essence of the wrongful act embedded in the criminal charge, appreciation of one's own situation as a criminal defendant, and a capacity to recognize and relate relevant information to the attorney.)[51] In addition, however, adjudication should be barred, even for defendants who meet these minimum requirements, if their disabilities—in relation to understanding the charges or communicating with counsel—raise serious doubts about the reliability of the process in the particular case.

I suspect that prevailing clinical and judicial practice conforms to this two-step model. By law, courts and attorneys are currently required to refer defendants for evaluation whenever a *bona fide* doubt about mental capacity, regardless of context, is raised.[52] The threshold for referral is set very low in order to cleanse all cases of doubts about competence. Most defendants are found competent by the evaluators and most others are restored to competence after a short period of treatment. But a small proportion of defendants cannot be said to be clearly competent, even after a reasonable period of treatment. In these borderline cases, I suspect that the standard practice is to return the defendants to court, as "competent," if they meet a fairly low standard. The case will then proceed unless the *attorney* raises further doubts, thereby reflecting a genuine concern about the adequacy of the defendant's assistance in the particular case.

This observation implies that the attorney is best situated to know whether the defendant's impairments compromise defense of the case. In some situations this might lead an attorney to question the competence of a client who has (provisionally) been "found" competent at any earlier stage of the case. In other situations, however, an attorney might see no reason to question the "competence" of a clearly impaired

[51] Understanding of the charge is often included in the definition of competence to assist counsel, and forensic specialists typically emphasize that this is one of the interactive aspects of competence assessment. That is, a defendant who is able to understand some charges may not be able to understand more complex charges. As I will indicate below, however, my tentative view is that ability to understand the specific charges in one's own case is *not* an independent prerequisite for competence to assist counsel. All that is necessary in this regard is the ability to relate pertinent information to the attorney (who, one hopes, does understand the charges). A defendant's inability to understand the subleties of the charge may become pertinent later on in the process if the defendant seeks to plead guilty because the incapacity may affect the reliability of the admissions embedded in the plea. See pages 311–312 *infra*. I have discussed this issue in Richard J. Bonnie, *The Competence of Criminal Defendants With Mental Retardation to Participate in Their Own Defense*, 81 J. CRIM. L. AND CRIMINOL. 419, 435–42 (1990).

[52] *See* ABA CRIMINAL JUSTICE MENTAL HEALTH STANDARDS, Std. 7–4.2(c) and accompanying commentary (1986).

client because, in the attorney's judgment, the defendant's impairments do not affect his or her ability to develop a defense.

One of the most interesting (and controversial) issues about competence to assist counsel concerns the circumstances under which the attorney is obligated to raise the issue and seek an evaluation.[53] The prevailing view obligates the attorney to raise the issue formally whenever he has a "good faith doubt" about the client's competence, notwithstanding his view that such a course is not in the client's best interests. Imposing this obligation on the attorney, as well as on the prosecution and the trial court, is generally thought to be a necessary corollary of the procedural bar against adjudication in cases involving incompetent defendants.[54]

I disagree. Even if disposition of cases against defendants who are unable to assist counsel is constitutionally barred, it does not follow that the issue must be raised in formal judicial proceedings. The constitutional values at stake can be protected by other procedural arrangements, such as *ex parte* judicial review of counsel's decision not to raise the issue, a second opinion by a disinterested lawyer, or consultation with a forensic mental health professional. These approaches would substitute the attorney's informed judgment about the client's competence (in relation to the actual need for client participation in the particular case) for the formal evaluation (and, possibly, adjudication) which are now thought to be required.[55]

In sum, I am proposing that the law explicitly confer authority on attorneys to make the decisions which they now must make in the shadow of an ambiguous obligation to seek judicial resolution. When the attorney concludes that the client lacks the necessary capacities to assist counsel, and if adequate clinical intervention is not otherwise available, the attorney may be obligated, as a last resort, to seek a judicial determination of incompetence and an order of commitment. But whether such a procedure is necessary should be left to the defense attorney.[56]

The central role which defense attorneys inevitably play in deciding how to respond to clients with mental disabilities calls attention to a more general point which underlies many of the ideas developed in this paper. Issues relating to adequacy of attorney performance often masquerade as issues of client competence. If the primary objective is to assure that the interests of mentally disabled defendants are adequately protected, attention should be focused less on whether a particular defendant is or is not competent than on whether the attorney has taken appropriate steps to identify client impairments, to seek clinical assistance in assessing and responding to these impairments, and in assuring that any persisting impairments do not compromise preparation or presentation of a reasonable defense. If courts doubt the capacities of attorneys to carry out these obligations, then the problem most needing attention is raising the level of attorney representation, not "restoring" the competence of defendants.

---

[53] *See generally* Paul A. Chernoff and William G. Schaffer, *Defending the Mentally Ill: Ethical Quicksand,* 10 AM. CR. L. REV. 505 (1972); RODNEY J. UPHOFF, *The Role of the Criminal Defense Lawyer in Representing the Mentally Impaired Defendant: Zealous Advocate or Officer of the Court,* 1988 WISC. L. REV. 65.

[54] *See, e.g.*, ABA CRIMINAL JUSTICE MENTAL HEALTH STANDARDS, Std. 7–4.2, and accompanying commentary.

[55] It would follow also that the process of evaluation and treatment should be more fully within the attorney's control. Bruce Winick has proposed that continuances be routinely granted upon request of counsel and that judicial involvement be otherwise severely limited. *See* Winick, *supra* note 13, at 281–87.

[56] Deficient performance by the attorney would, of course, invalidate a defendant's conviction if it amounts to constitutionally deficient representation under Strickland v. Washington, 466 U.S. 668 (1984).

V. DECISIONAL COMPETENCE

As noted above, decisional competence is conceptually and clinically distinct from competence to assist counsel. Although the relevant psychological capacities may overlap, decision-making about defense strategy encompasses conceptual abilities, cognitive skills, and capacities for rational thinking that are not required for assisting counsel. The key question is how demanding the test for decisional competence should be in any given context. Although forensic experts have not yet conceptualized the clinical content of alternative tests of decisional competence in the context of criminal defense, the formulations developed by Appelbaum and Grisso in their continuing research on decisional competence for medical treatment can be used as a starting point.[57]

The least demanding "test" of competence is the ability to *communicate a preference*. A defendant who is unable to express a choice or who is unable to maintain a stable preference, is not competent to decide whatever questions the client may be permitted or required to decide. The mere ability to express a preference, however, is not likely to be regarded as a sufficient measure of competence in many legal contexts, and is especially unsuitable in the context of criminal defense. Moreover, a bare expression of a preference, without any understanding, is hardly an exercise of self-determination.[58]

The ability to *understand relevant information* about a particular decision is the criterion most often utilized in both treatment settings and criminal defense. This "test" involves the basic idea that clients who cannot understand the relevant considerations after they have been conveyed, or who cannot understand their own prerogatives as a "decision–maker," are not competent to decide whether to accept or reject the attorney's advice. This test, which is purely cognitive, can be varied in its stringency according to which considerations are regarded as relevant, and therefore must be understood by the defendant.

A defendant who is able to comprehend relevant information may be unable to *appreciate the significance of that information* in his or her own case. Problems in appreciating the situation and its consequences may arise due to limitations in cognitive capacity, to disturbances of thought, or to affective disorders. Problems in appreciation are most often evident in cases involving psychotic defendants who deny their illness, or whose beliefs about the desirability or undesirability of a difficult course of action are pathologically distorted by delusions or affective impairment. Whether the test of competence should be more demanding than "understanding" in order to take into account defects in appreciation is perhaps the most critical question faced in both treatment settings and criminal defense.

A defendant who is able to understand information relevant to a decision and is able to appreciate the "meaning" of the decision in his or her situation may nonetheless lack the capacity to use logical processes to compare the benefits and risks of the decisional options. Appelbaum and Grisso[59] use the phrase *rational*

[57] *See generally* Paul S. Appelbaum and Thomas Grisso, *Assessing Patients' Capacities to Consent to Treatment*, 319 NEW ENGLAND J. MED. 1635 (1988).

[58] Simple "assent" to an attorney's recommendation may be all the law requires in some contexts, but it would be more accurate to say in such cases that the law does not insist the defendant's personal participation in the decision at all, and that the defendant's incompetence is therefore without legal significance.

[59] *Id.*

manipulation of information to refer to the process of weighing information to reach a decision. What is important here is the decisional *process*, not its *outcome*, although an outcome considered by others to be irrational obviously may signal a problem with the defendant's reasoning process. A defendant's capacity to weigh information in order to make rational choices, consistent with starting premises and assigned values, may be impaired by psychotic thought disorder, delirium and dementia, extreme phobia or panic, anxiety, euphoria and depression.

As this summary of alternative clinical criteria demonstrates, the legal "test" for decisional competence can be made more or less demanding. What is expected of defendants in relation to decision-making should be anchored in a practical understanding of the attorney-client relationship, and in a theory of client autonomy in criminal defense. In addition, the choice of a test of competence in a particular decision-making context should take into account the consequences, for the defendant and society, of determinations of competence and incompetence in that particular context.

One of the reasons why the law governing decisional competence in criminal defense is so ill-defined is that the law governing allocation of decision-making between attorneys and clients is unclear. The literature on decision-making in criminal defense is sparse and is in marked contrast to the literature on treatment decision-making and the physician–patient relationship. In that context, the literature on decisional competence is fully integrated into a sophisticated literature on patient autonomy and informed consent. In an effort to define decisional competence, theoreticians have sought to link the various "tests" of competence employed by courts and described above to the concept of autonomy and the functions of legal regulation.[60]

In light of the thin theoretical literature on the topic, my comments on decisional competence in criminal defense are meant to be tentative and speculative. I mainly want to sketch the general outline of current legal doctrine and to call attention to what strikes me as the issue most in need of theoretical discussion—whether the "test" of decisional competence is less demanding where the client chooses to follow her attorney's recommendation than when she decides to reject it.

Decisions in Criminal Defense

Many types of decisions can arise during the course of defending a criminal case. Most of these, such as decisions concerning investigation, discovery, pretrial motions and trial and appellate strategy, are made by counsel alone without the defendant's direct participation. Although many of these decisions may, in effect, waive constitutional rights, they do not require personal participation by the defendant; counsel acts on the defendant's behalf, and binds the defendant, subject of course to Sixth Amendment standards of adequate representation.[61] However, a defendant's personal participation is legally and ethically required in several specific contexts. Most clearly, waivers of several constitutional protections must be made personally by the defendant. These include waiver of the cluster of rights effected

[60] *See, e.g.*, Paul S. Appelbaum, Charles W. Lidz and Alan Meisel, INFORMED CONSENT: LEGAL THEORY AND CLINICAL PRACTICE (1987).

[61] *See, e.g.*, Smith v. Murray, 477 U.S. 527 (1986) (waiver of constitutional objection to admissibility of psychiatric testimony due to failure to preserve it on direct appeal).

by a guilty plea,[62] the right to jury trial,[63] the right to testify,[64] and the right to be present at trial.[65]

It is important to emphasize that the constitutional requirement of personal waiver of the particular right does not necessarily entail the broader proposition that the attorney has an enforceable duty to elicit a decision by the client to invoke the right. That is, the principle of self-determination underlying the waiver cases is one-directional. When a decision is made by counsel to assert, rather than waive, these constitutional rights, no definitive rule of law appears to require client participation[66] even though applicable standards of professional practice and ethical guidelines obligate the attorney to elicit client decision-making on these issues.[67]

The client prerogatives to define the basic objectives of representation and to select the main theory of defense lie at the core of the idea that the client is the principal (and the attorney, the agent) in legal representation. Clearly this implies that the attorney is bound to accede to the client's wishes in regard to these fundamental choices. But the distinction between "objectives" and "means" of representation[68] is not particularly helpful in defining the decision-making prerogatives of attorney and client. For example, some otherwise tactical decisions, involving professional risk-benefit judgment, may implicate deeply held personal values of the defendant. Because the defense of insanity implicates a defendant's personal values more clearly than any other defensive theory, the decision (not) to invoke the insanity defense is now generally held to belong to the client,[69] but other defensive claims may also have substantial personal meaning in particular cases.[70]

Although my views remain tentative, I am inclined to believe that a sorting of decisions into two categories—a sphere of client decisions and a residual category of decisions within attorney control—is neither sensible in theory nor compatible with judicial practice. On the one hand, the legally enforced sphere of client control must far fall short of what might be widely regarded as the preferred professional practice. To say that an attorney ought to promote client participation on all important decisions regarding defense of the case is *not* to say that convictions should be overturned because the attorney failed to do so. Further, to say that a decision to waive a jury trial must be made personally by the client is not to say that a decision to have a jury trial must be made by the client. Respect for client autonomy may require that the defendant be afforded an *opportunity to decide*, but in the absence of a client's insistence on waiving a jury trial, the attorney is probably free to request one.

62 Boykin v. Alabama, 395 U.S. 238, 242 (1969).

63 Adams v. United States ex rel. McCann, 317 U.S. 269, 278 (1942).

64 *See, e.g.*, United States v. Teague, 953 F.2d 1525 (*en banc*) (11th Cir. 1992).

65 Taylor v. Illinois, 484 U.S. 400, 418, n.24 (1988) (*dictum*).

66 *See, e.g.*, Johnson v. Duckworth, 793 F.2d 898 (7th Cir.), *cert. den.* 479 U.S. 937 (1986) (rejection of prosecution's plea offer by attorney without personal participation by the client does not constitute ineffective assistance of counsel under circumstances of this case).

67 *See, e.g.*, AMERICAN LAW INSTITUTE, RESTATEMENT OF THE LAW, THE LAW GOVERNING LAWYERS, PRELIMINARY DRAFT No. 6, § 31 Comment e, and Reporters Note, pp. 92–96 (July 25, 1990).

68 Model Rules of Professional Conduct, Rule 1.2(a).

69 For an elaborate discussion of the general allocation of decision-making prerogatives in the course of addressing the insanity plea, see Treece v. State, 313 Md. 665, 547 A.2d 1054 (1988).

70 If the client insists on raising a defense of entrapment, should the client's preferences be ignored? Moreover, cross-examining a prosecution witness, which is clearly a matter of tactics, also implicates the defendant's Sixth Amendment right of confrontation. If the attorney would not otherwise cross-examine a witness, should the client's contrary instructions be followed?

On the other hand, the attorney is probably obligated to adhere to the preferences of an insistent client even on matters relating to legal strategy and tactics. To say that the attorney has no presumptive obligation to secure an informed client decision on whether to raise an entrapment defense, or to seek a lesser-included defense instruction, or to forego cross-examining a key prosecution witness, is *not* to say that the attorney should be free to ignore the client's objections to such decisions.

Strands of Decisional Competence

How, then, does decisional competence fit into this picture of attorney-client decision-making in criminal cases? Although the case-law is complicated by variations in doctrinal formulation, several principles emerge fairly clearly.

At a minimum, the defendant must have the *abilities required to effect a valid waiver of constitutional rights*. In most contexts, the criteria for a valid waiver pertain to understanding the right and the consequences of waiving it. The definition of what must be understood may be made more or less inclusive. For example, it is clear that a defendant who waives a right to a jury trial must be able to understand that the decision about his guilt or innocence will be made by a judge rather than by a group of people from the community.[71] But the defendant probably does not have to be able to understand the selection process, including the concept of peremptory challenges.[72] Similar questions can be raised about the waivers embedded in guilty pleas, waiver of the right to testify, and waivers of other rights.

Competence to effect a valid waiver is not the exclusive measure of decisional competence in the criminal process because the legal criteria for a valid waiver do not encompass the person's reasons for deciding to waive.[73] Yet, even the least demanding approaches to decisional competence in other legal contexts include some dimension of gross irrationality.[74] The question, in criminal defense as in other contexts, is what *abilities required for rational choice* should be regarded as necessary for decisional competence.

Consider a possibly innocent defendant who insists on accepting a plea bargain, against counsel's advice, because he believes that the devil will prevent all defense witnesses from appearing at his trial. Or consider a defendant who insists on waiving a jury trial, against counsel's advice, because he believes that the judge and he have the same "earth mother." Each of these defendants may have sufficient understanding of the rights being waived to effect a valid waiver. Yet, I am confident that no court would regard these defendants as decisionally competent.[75]

In each of these hypothetical cases, the defendant insists on acting contrary to counsel's advice for irrational reasons. The client's competence is often put in issue in cases of this kind, and a substantial body of case law has emerged. (In contrast,

---

[71] *See, e.g.*, United States v. DeRobertis, 715 F.2d 1174, 1180 (7th Cir. 1983).

[72] *See, e.g.*, United States ex rel Wandick v. Chrans, 869 F.2d 1084 (7th Cir. 1989).

[73] The defendant's reasons for choosing to waive the particular right are pertinent to the validity of the waiver only if the defendant is succumbing to coercive threats.

[74] *See generally* Stephen J. Morse, *Crazy Behavior, Morals and Science: An Analysis of Mental Health Law*, 51 S. CAL L. REV. 527 (1978); Elyn R. Saks, *Competency to Refuse Treatment*, 69 N.C.L. REV. 945 (1991).

[75] I am assuming in all illustrative cases that the defendant is competent to assist counsel as defined above.

the client's decisional competence is rarely put in issue when he or she is acceding to the attorney's advice.)[76] The case law reveals a good deal of judicial sparring over whether competence is, or is not, a unitary construct and whether the test for competence to waive counsel, or "waive" an insanity plea, is different from, or "higher" than, the test for competence to stand trial. I am prepared to argue, however, that this doctrinal disagreement tends to obscure a common pattern which lies beneath the surface in these cases. Regardless of their doctrinal approach, the courts tend to be uneasy with a test of competence which focuses exclusively on cognitive understanding, and they tend to apply a more inclusive "rational choice" formula.

The line of cases involving defendants who decline to raise the insanity defense is illustrative. Under the prevailing view, articulated in *Frendak v. United States*,[77] the "competent" defendant is entitled to decline to invoke the insanity defense, notwithstanding the possibility that the defense might be meritorious, in recognition of the fact that there are rational grounds for declining to invoke the defense (e.g., to avoid stigmatization and indeterminate hospitalization that may exceed the likely prison sentence).[78] The pertinent question, of course, is what "competence" means in this context. On the surface, we find confusion. Some courts hold or imply that a defendant who is competent to stand trial is, by definition, competent to "waive" an insanity plea.[79] Others, following *Frendak*, hold that a defendant who is competent to plead guilty and competent to be tried on a not-guilty plea may not be competent to decide *not* to invoke an insanity defense.[80] Some courts seem completely bewildered by the problem.[81]

All of these cases involve delusional defendants. In some cases, the delusions so fully infect the defendant's understanding of his situation and of the purpose of the criminal prosecution, that the defendant is not competent to assist counsel, and the decisional competence issue has no independent significance. (Under the usual doctrinal analysis, such defendants are not "competent" to stand trial and are, therefore, not competent to "waive" the insanity defense).[82]

In the remaining cases, however, the defendant's delusions do not interfere with the ability to appreciate the nature and purpose of the prosecution or the roles of the participants. To use the *Dusky* language, these defendants have a "factual and rational" understanding of the proceedings. In addition, they are able to understand the nature of an insanity plea and the consequences of raising it or declining to raise it. The problem in these cases concerns their reasons for choosing to forego

[76] The exception concerns defendants with mental retardation. This is why the cases concerning the proper test for competence to plead guilty have usually involved defendants with mental retardation. *See, e.g.*, Allard v. Helgemoe, 572 F.2d 1 (1st Cir. 1978); United States v. Masthers, 539 F.2d 721 (D.C. Cir. 1976).

[77] 408 A.2d 364 (D.C. 1979).

[78] Before *Frendak*, the prevailing approach permitted imposition of the insanity defense, regardless of the defendant's preferences, in order to preserve the moral integrity of the law (or, more cynically, to permit indeterminate confinement at the prosecution's behest). For present purposes, the important point is that the principle of self-determination did not apply, and the outcome therefore did not turn on the defendant's decisional competence, as it does under *Frendak*.

[79] *See, e.g.*, State v. Hahn, 41 Wash. App. 876, 707 P.2d 699 (Ct. App. I, 1986).

[80] United States v. Marble, 940 F.2d 1543 (D.C.Cir. 1991). *See e.g.*, State v. Khan, 175 N.J. Super. 72, 417 A.2d 585 (Sup.Ct. App. Div. 1980).

[81] State v. Fayle, 658 P.2d 218 (Ariz. Ct. App. 1983).

[82] *See, e.g.*, United States v. Blohm, 579 F. Supp. 495 (S.D.N.Y. 1983); *cf.* United States v. Riggin, 732 F. Supp. 958 (S.D. Ind. 1990).

the defense—virtually always the same crazy reasons which underlie the insanity claim itself. In short, these defendants are competent to assist counsel, and would be competent to make any other decision that might arise (such as whether to have a jury trial) that did not tap into the delusion. The question is whether, under such circumstances, the defendant should be regarded as competent to make the particular decision affected by the delusion.

The issue then is what test of decisional competence should be used. One possibility is an "understanding" test under which the defendant's choice is respected as long as he or she understands the risks and benefits of raising or not raising the defense. This formulation would eschew the paternalistic tendencies which inhere in an appreciation formula—questioning whether the defendant's reasons reflect a rational understanding of his or her situation. The alternative is to invoke an appreciation standard, which rests on a judgment that the defendant lacks the capacity to be the best judge of his or her own best interests.

The cases reveal a judicial inclination toward an appreciation test in these cases. They reach this result by various routes. The *Frendak* court held that "competence to stand trial" does not include decisional competence and went on to hold that competency to "waive" an insanity plea requires ability to make a "voluntary and intelligent decision" to forego the defense.[83] Other courts have held that competence to stand trial includes decisional competence, and therefore includes competence to waive the insanity defense. In the context of these delusional defendants, however, they have nonetheless allowed the defendant's decision to be overridden—either by using a "rational choice" formulation for competence to stand trial,[84] or by finding the defendant's accompanying waiver of counsel was incompetent.[85] Whatever the doctrinal path, the courts have, in effect, adopted a demanding standard of decisional competence in order to facilitate the outcome which the attorney and the court believe to be in the defendant's best interests.[86]

In sum, it appears that decisional competence cases in criminal defense tend to fit a pattern which has been observed in treatment cases: the test of competence seems to be more demanding in cases where the defendant is refusing to adhere to the attorney's advice than in cases where the defendant is following the attorney's recommendation. Understanding, perhaps even at a minimal level, may be sufficient

[83] 408 A.2d at 380.

[84] *See e.g.*, State v. Jones, 99 Wash. 2d 735, 664 P.2d 1216 (1983).

[85] *See, e.g.*, State v. Hahn, 41 Wash. App. 876, 707 P.2d 699 (1986) (invalidating waiver of counsel of delusional defendant who withdrew insanity plea); *cf.* State v. Bauer, 310 Minn. 103, 245 N.W.2d 848 (1976).

[86] This same pattern is evident in cases involving capital defendants who decline to authorize their attorneys to introduce mitigating evidence. Here again, it appears that those courts which obligate the attorneys to adhere to the competent client's instructions (some do not) tend to adopt an "elevated" standard of competence—one which distinguishes between a preference for a death sentence that reflects a rational choice among alternatives and one that reflects the distorting effects of psychopathology.

Although the reported cases raising "right to refuse" issues involve defendants who decline to raise the insanity defense and capital defendants who decline to introduce mitigating evidence, the problem presumably arises in other contexts—e.g., defendants who insist on pleading guilty when counsel believes the case should be tried, and defendants who insist on testifying in support of an unsupportable defense (e.g., self-defense or choice of evils) where the lawyer believes that another strategy would be preferable. An interesting puzzle is presented by defendants who *refuse* to plead guilty for "crazy" reasons even though counsel has arranged a favorable plea bargain. Although I assume that the problem arises in non-capital cases, the form it often takes in capital cases is that the attorney arranges a plea in return for a life sentence while the defendant prefers a "walk or burn" strategy.

for assent, but a competent refusal requires appreciation and, perhaps, capacity for rational manipulation.[87]

VI. COMPETENCE AND GUILTY PLEAS

In the two previous sections of the article, I have described the concepts of competence to assist counsel and decisional competence. In the two concluding sections, I will comment on the implications of this conceptual approach for guilty pleas and trials.

Guilty pleas implicate both reliability and autonomy concerns.[88] First, the admissions embedded in a guilty plea may not be reliable. To the extent that reliability is the underlying concern, a finding that the defendant is competent to make the requisite admissions is a necessary condition for a fair adjudication *if* the adjudication is to be accomplished by a guilty plea. Second, even if the reliability of the defendant's admissions is not in doubt, the defendant may be regarded as "incompetent" to plead guilty (and to waive his or her constitutional rights) because the conditions of "autonomy" are lacking. Because decisional competence in this sense is *not* a prerequisite for a reliable adjudication, the "test" for competence to plead guilty, when viewed from this perspective, depends entirely on the theory of autonomy that is or should be reflected in the law.

Reliability

Insofar as reliability is the underlying concern, the capacities required for competent guilty pleas are substantially congruent with those required for competence to assist counsel. The defendant must have a sufficient understanding of the charges, in lay terms, and a sufficient understanding of what happened at the time of the offense, to "understand and agree that he performed some acts and that those acts are unlawful."[89] Whether the acts admitted by the defendant provide a sufficient foundation for the plea is a legal judgment which must be made initially by the attorney and then by the court. In *this* respect, the "test" for competence to plead guilty is not "higher" than the test for competence to assist counsel; however, this formulation of the issue misses the key point—the fact that the defendant has been "found" to be competent to assist counsel (or to "stand trial," in the usual phrase) does not, in itself, establish the reliability of the admissions that may subsequently be embedded in a guilty plea. This matter requires careful attention by counsel and independent scrutiny by the court at the time of the plea in order to assure that the defendant's admissions, when taken together with other evidence, provide a reliable foundation for the plea.

---

[87] Whether the criteria for competence to say "yes" and "no" should differ is a matter of debate in the literature on biomedical ethics. *See, e.g.*, Mark R. Wicclair, *Patient Decision-Making Capacity and Risk*, 5 BIOETHICS 91 (1991); Dan W. Brock, *Decision-making Competence and Risk*, 5 BIOETHICS 105 (1991); Elyn R. Saks, *Competency to Refuse Treatment*, 69 N.C.L. REV. 945 (1991).

[88] Obviously, guilty pleas by mentally impaired defendants might also implicate the moral dignity of the process. First, a defendant who lacks a meaningful understanding of wrongdoing and punishment or the nature and consequences of an admission of guilt is not a fit subject for the imposition of criminal punishment. Second, the proceedings at which such a defendant appears would be a ceremonial farce. I have not highlighted this concern in the text, however, because the reliability of the plea would be in doubt in such cases.

[89] Allard v. Helgemoe, 572 F.2d 1, 6 (1st Cir. 1978).

Cases may arise in which the reliability of the defendant's admissions is so much in doubt that a guilty plea should not be accepted. If the defendant's capacity to assist counsel is sufficient to resolve the case at a trial, it might be tempting to conclude that the "test" for competence to plead guilty is "higher" than the test for competence to stand trial. However, this result need not be explained in terms of a deficiency of "competence". A court is permitted, and may be required, to reject a proffered guilty plea that lacks an adequate factual foundation. In some cases, the questionable reliability of the admissions embedded in the guilty plea may erode what otherwise would be an adequate foundation, and the court would properly be exercising its discretionary prerogative to reject the plea. Careful judicial monitoring of the reliability of guilty pleas by mentally impaired defendants also provides a check on ineffective assistance of counsel. In general, then, I would argue that the reliability of guilty pleas should be carefully scrutinized, but not by elevating the criteria for competence.

Autonomy

The controversy regarding the proper "test" for competence to plead guilty has turned on different conceptions of decisional competence which, in turn, reflect different conceptions of the conditions of autonomous decision-making. At the risk of over-simplification, there appear to be two views. Under one view, the standard of competence derives exclusively from the constitutional requirements for a "valid" plea: the defendant must understand the "critical elements" of the offense to which he is pleading guilty, the nature of the right he is surrendering, and the consequences of the plea in relation to conviction and punishment.[90] Under this view, mental impairments which might affect the choice between pleading guilty and going to trial—the defendant's reasons and her reasoning process—are not relevant. To use the vocabulary suggested earlier, the exclusive focus is on the "waiver" strand of decisional competence rather than the "rational choice" strand.[91]

In contrast, under the contending view, the test for competence to plead guilty includes dimensions which are not required for a valid plea. In the predominant formulation, the defendant must be able to "make a reasoned choice among alternatives", a test that presumably requires ability to understand the risks and benefits of the alternative courses of action, the ability to apply that information to one's own situation, and the ability to weigh these considerations in a rational manner.[92]

The debate has usually been phrased in terms of whether the test for competence to plead guilty is "higher" than the test for competence to stand trial. The underlying assumption is that the "reasoned choice" test is higher than the test for trial competence, while the "valid plea" approach is congruent with the test for trial competence. It should be clear, however, that the relation between the guilty plea test and the trial competence test depends on what level of decision-making capacity is encompassed within the criteria for "standing trial". On the one hand, if the

[90] *See, e.g.*, Henderson v. Morgan, 426 U.S. 637 (1976).

[91] *See, e.g.*, State v. Bailey, 464 N.W.2d 626 (S.D. 1991); State ex rel. Wilson v. Hendrick, 379 S.E.2d 493 (1989).

[92] *See, e.g.*, State v. Bishop, 162 Ariz. 103, 781 P.2d 581 (1989); Chavez v. United States, 656 F.2d 512 (9th Cir. 1981).

defendant who stands trial must have the ability to make reasoned choices regarding the theory of the defense, whether to testify, whether to waive a jury trial, and other trial decisions, then the "reasoned choice" test for competence to plead guilty is the same as the generic legal test for trial competence. On the other hand, if the ability to make reasoned choices is not required for either trials or guilty pleas, then even the "valid plea" test for competence to plead guilty may be more demanding, in practical application, than the test for competence to stand trial. This is so because the level of understanding required for a valid guilty plea, which surrenders virtually all constitutional safeguards, would presumably be higher than the level of understanding required for waiving any of the trial protections.

As I noted earlier, the appropriate test for decisional competence turns on many considerations, and there is no reason, *a priori*, to assume that the criteria should be the same in all decision-making contexts in criminal defense. In the context of guilty pleas, the legal system has a compelling interest in assuring reliability of the admissions embedded in a plea entered by a person with mental disability, and in assuring that the defendant understands the essential nature of the rights being waived and the consequences of the plea. In relation to autonomy, however, the guilty plea provides a vivid context for exploring the proposition that the test for competence might sensibly differ according to whether the plea is entered with, or against, the advice of counsel.

If the defendant insists on pleading guilty *against* counsel's advice, I am inclined to argue that this choice should be honored only if the defendant has a rational understanding of the meaning and consequences of the plea, and is able to make a reasoned choice between pleading guilty and going to trial in relation to her own values. However, if the plea is entered *with* counsel's advice, the defendant should ordinarily be regarded as competent if she has sufficient understanding to effect a valid waiver. Alleged mental impairments or deficits bearing on the defendant's reasons for pleading guilty should not matter unless the defendant denies guilt,[93] or unless none of the defendant's reasons for pleading guilty has any plausible grounding in reality (i.e., unless all of the defendant's reasons rest on patently false beliefs about the world).[94]

Differential tests of competence to accept and refuse counsel's advice admittedly raise puzzling ethical issues. I am inclined nonetheless toward this paternalistic pos-

[93] In effect, I mean to require a more demanding standard of competence to offer an *Alford* plea. I do so in part because of underlying concerns about reliability of such pleas.

[94] For a similar "gross delusion" test in connection with treatment decision-making, see Elyn R. Saks, *Competency to Refuse Treatment*, 69 N.C.L. REV. 945 (1991). Professor Saks emphatically rejects the concept of "different levels" of competence for accepting and refusing treatment.

The exception for gross delusions is rooted in the dignity rationale for the competence requirement. When the disposition of a serious criminal case occurs as a result of a guilty plea, the defendant must be the primary actor in the process of adjudicating guilt. We do not allow counsel to enter the plea on the defendant's behalf. Nor do we permit guilty pleas to be entered in absentia. For the process to retain its moral dignity, the defendant must be seen as a subject, as a person capable of choosing to stand up against the state. If the defendant is to say "convict me, I will not stand up against you," the surrender must have meaning in relation to the prosecution itself. Consider, for example, a defendant who pleads guilty for no reason other than a false belief that the courtroom will explode if he goes to trial. The decision to plead guilty has no link to the evidence, to the concept of guilt or to the real personal costs of a criminal trial. In a sense, I am arguing that a minimum capacity for rational decision-making is required to protect the moral dignity of the process *if the proceedings is to be terminated by a plea of guilt*. (I tend to think this is not necessary for any trial-related "decisions" by counsel to which the defendant accedes.)

ition because the consequences of the "same test" approach are normatively unattractive. On the one hand, a "paternalistic" (i.e., more demanding) test of competence for "refusals" is justified by the same considerations that account for the more demanding standard for competence to waive counsel and for the California statute which precludes a capital defendant from pleading guilty without counsel's consent. On the other hand, a more demanding standard for "consents" would be undesirable because it would deny defendants with mental disabilities the advantages of plea bargaining.

Admittedly, defendants with mental disability can also be victimized by the plea bargaining process, especially if they are poorly represented by defense counsel. But this is a quality assurance problem, not an autonomy problem. If attention to "competence" should be enhanced in this context, it should be directed toward the competence of counsel, not the competence of the defendant. Thus, courts should carefully scrutinize the factual foundation for the plea and should be willing to use other devices for monitoring the performance and advice of counsel, such as second opinions.

VII. COMPETENCE AND TRIALS

Although I regard "trial competence" as a purely derivative application of the two concepts already discussed, it requires separate elaboration to clarify terminology and also to demonstrate how these concepts become operationalized in the context of trial proceedings.[95] In the small proportion of cases that are actually tried, the defendant must be competent to participate, to the extent necessary to assure a fair trial, in his own defense.

First, the defendant must be *competent to assist counsel* in the sense described above—capable of understanding the proceedings and of engaging in rational communication with counsel. This is "*competence to stand trial*" in its precise sense and a focus on the trial setting emphasizes the dynamic and sequential dimensions of competence assessment. A defendant who was regarded as sufficiently competent during earlier stages of the process (or who was restored to competence) may deteriorate under the stresses of a trial. This aspect of competence assessment appears to be generally recognized and incorporated in assessment protocols.[96]

Second, numerous decisions requiring the defendant's participation can arise at trial if they have not been anticipated and resolved beforehand during the course of pre-trial interactions with the attorney. Although any doubts regarding a defendant's decisional competence should ordinarily be resolved earlier in the process, no such prior determination can be regarded as conclusive, as the Supreme Court has made clear.[97] For example, a defendant convicted of a capital crime may seek to preclude his attorney from introducing mitigating evidence or arguing for leniency at the sentencing phase of the trial. In states where appellate courts have held that the attorney is obligated to adhere to the defendant's wishes, they have also directed trial judges to make contemporaneous assessments of the defendants' competence.[98]

[95] I mean to include here the sentencing phase of the trial in capital cases and any other proceedings involving an evidentiary hearing aside from adjudications of competence.

[96] *See generally*, Thomas Grisso, EVALUATING COMPETENCIES 62–112 (1986).

[97] Drope v. Missouri, 420 U.S. 162 (1975); Pate v. Robinson, 383 U.S. 375 (1966).

[98] I have discussed this problem in "The Dignity of the Condemned", 74 VA. L. REV. 1363 (1988).

Other decisional competence issues can arise in relation to defendants who insist on testifying over their attorneys' objections.[99]

The Disruptive Defendant

Does trial competence entail a capacity in addition to those required for competence to assist counsel and decisional competence—that is, the capacity to control one's behavior in the courtroom? There are numerous cases involving disruptive defendants, and many of the protocols for forensic assessment of competence to stand trial refer to the defendant's ability to avoid disruptive behavior. My provisional view is that this problem collapses into a problem of decisional competence, and should not be regarded as a separate component of trial competence.

There are two different theoretical accounts of the law permitting courts to remove disruptive defendants. On one account, the social interest in trying the case can override the defendant's right to be present.[100] On this view, a defendant's right to be present at trial is not unqualified, and may be trumped even if it is not waived. It would follow from this analysis that the ability to behave oneself is *not* a necessary feature of trial competence, and that an otherwise competent mentally ill, disruptive defendant may be tried, in his absence, without violating either his right to be present or his right not to be tried while incompetent. Assuming that the ejected defendant is competent to assist counsel, remote cameras and the opportunity to communicate with counsel provide sufficient safeguards against unreliable conviction.

Exclusion of the disruptive defendant does implicate the competence doctrine under an alternative account of the existing law, which holds that the ejected defendant has waived his right to be present. Under the usual scenario, the disruptive defendant is warned about the consequences of further disruption, and having defied the warning, is said to have waived his right to be present.[101] On this account, a mentally ill defendant who is "unable" to refrain from disruptive behavior could not be said to have chosen to waive his right to be present. Thus, trying him in his absence would violate his right to be present even if it did not violate his right not to be tried while incompetent.

It is possible to move in either of two directions at this point. One could accept the proposition that the capacity to behave in the courtroom is a component of trial competence, thereby adding a dimension to "competence to stand trial" that is not encompassed within either of the two constructs defined in this paper. Or one could argue, as I am inclined to do, that the difficulty presented by the disruptive

[99] Some decisions may also be required as part of the sentencing process itself such as the exercise (or waiver) of the right of allocution. *See, e.g.*, Wotjowicz v. United States, 550 F.2d 786 (2d Cir. 1977).

Decisional competence is also pertinent in connection with the filing or withdrawing of post-conviction proceedings. This problem arises virtually exclusively in capital cases. Ordinarily, the decision whether or not to appeal (or seek habeas relief) belongs to the convicted defendant. However, as I have noted elsewhere, "The Dignity of the Condemned", 74 VA. L. REV. 1363 (1988), some courts have held that the principle of client self-determination does not apply in capital cases; in the context of direct appeal at least, the attorney is directed to file the appeal without the client's authorization. In other states, though, the principle of self-determination applies on direct appeal; and in all states (and in the federal courts) it appears to apply to collateral proceedings. Thus, in these situations, the prisoner's refusal to authorize the "appeal" must be honored unless the prisoner is not competent to decide. Not surprisingly, the meaning of competence in this context has been widely litigated in recent years.

[100] *See generally*, Wayne R. LaFave & Jerold H. Israel, CRIMINAL PROCEDURE 1012–13 (2d ed. 1992).

[101] This was the situation in Illinois v. Allen, 397 U.S. 337 (1970). *See also* Scurr v. Moore, 647 F.2d 854 (8th Cir. 1981).

defendant is better viewed as a problem of decisional competence rather than volitional incapacity. To say that the defendant is "unable to desist" merely recapitulates the persistent conceptual and operational problems presented by the volitional inquiry, which should be avoided in this context as well as others.[102] Instead, the issue should be cast in terms of competence to waive the right to be present. The court should assure that the defendant understands the consequences of further disruption. Only if the defendant is not able to understand would the trial have to be suspended.

VIII. CONCLUSION

The conceptual vocabulary proposed in this paper disaggregates two functionally distinct features of the "open construct," typically called "competence to stand trial." Competence to assist counsel and decisional competence appear to map the relevant portion of the legal landscape,[103] and "fit" existing legal doctrine fairly well. This conceptualization has several important advantages. First, it facilitates greater determinacy in the articulation of legal criteria, and therefore better definition of the psychological capacities that are relevant to these criteria. As a result, it should be possible to develop assessment instruments more useful than those now available. Second, it isolates, for independent study, the decision-making dimensions of competence in criminal defense, and exposes the analogies between decision-making within the attorney–client relationship and within the doctor–patient relationship. This move will help to link the literatures in these two fields and to clarify the similarities and differences between decision-making in these two settings.

---

[102] I am not referring to epilepsy and other disorders in which the person's movements or outbursts are outside the conscious physical control of the defendant. In those situations, the defendant could not fairly be excluded under any theory, and certainly would not be decisionally competent during the period of dyscontrol.

[103] They do not map the whole legal landscape pertaining to competence in the criminal process. However, the other competence concepts are either conceptually independent or peripheral to this paper. The subject of this paper is the competence of a criminal defendant to participate in his or her own defense. For example, I have not included "competence to confess or waive *Miranda* rights" (even though this is a form of "decisional competence") because the issue always arises retrospectively before counsel has become involved. This is not to say that protocols developed for assessing "competence to waive *Miranda* rights" would not be useful in relation to other forms of decisional competence involving waivers (such as guilty pleas) or *vice versa*. *See* Thomas Grisso, *Waiver of Rights to Silence and Legal Counsel*, in EVALUATING COMPETENCIES 113–55 (1986).

Also, I have not mentioned the dimensions of competence that do not pertain to the adjudicatory process, such as competence to "be sentenced" (an empty set if there ever was one) or competency "to be executed." As I noted earlier, I believe these constructs reflect essentially "dignitarian" aims (treating the defendant or prisoner with respect as a person) rather than the instrumental ones served by the competence constructs relating to the adjudicatory process.

[6]

An Investigation of the Construct of Competence: A Comparison of the FIT, the MacCAT-CA, and the MacCAT-T

Patricia A. Zapf[1,3] **and Ronald Roesch**[2]

The 1990s witnessed Supreme Court decisions in both Canada and the United States on issues of competence that went against longstanding case law, psychological research, and common sense. These decisions held that there is to be one standard for all types of criminal competencies. The present research attempts to investigate whether this is an appropriate assumption and thus tests whether there are one or more constructs that underlie different types of competence. Two divergent types of competence were examined, competence to stand trial (both Canadian and American conceptualizations) and competence to consent to treatment, to determine if these different types of competence share a common underlying construct. Confirmatory factor analysis was used to test this question and results indicate that there is a common construct that underlies different types of competence.

KEY WORDS: competency to stand trial; consent to treatment; construct of competence; adjudicative competence.

Issues of competence and incompetence are relevant in many domains. Much research has been conducted on incompetence in both criminal and civil legal contexts and it has become widely accepted in the psychological and legal literatures that competence is not a static concept and that it varies with time and specific abilities (Appelbaum & Grisso, 1988, 1995; Bonnie, 1993; Burra, Kimberly, & Miura, 1980; Grisso & Appelbaum, 1995; Grisso, Appelbaum, Mulvey, & Fletcher, 1995; Meisel, Roth, & Lidz, 1977; Perlin, 1996; Roesch & Golding, 1980; Roesch, Hart, & Zapf, 1996; Roth, Meisel, & Lidz, 1977). That is, an individual may be considered competent with respect to one type of ability but incompetent with respect to another. These researchers and commentators have argued that mental incompetence

[1]Department of Psychology, Doctoral Program in Forensic Psychology, John Jay College of Criminal Justice, The City University of New York, New York.
[2]Department of Psychology, Mental Health, Law, and Policy Institute, Simon Fraser University, Burnaby, British Columbia, Canada.
[3]To whom correspondence should be addressed at Department of Psychology, John Jay College of Criminal Justice, The City University of New York, New York 10019; e-mail: pzapf@jjay.cuny.edu.

is context-specific and therefore must be determined with respect to the situation in which it arises as an issue. Supreme Court decisions made in both the United States and Canada in the 1990s, however, appear to have made a move in the direction of re-examining the notion of competence as being context-specific.

In *Regina v. Whittle* (1994), the Supreme Court of Canada ruled that there is to be only one standard for competency regardless of the specific abilities to be performed by an accused. The Supreme Court of Canada concluded that there is no difference between the abilities needed to be found fit to waive counsel, to stand trial, to confess, or to plead guilty. The Court ruled that different standards of competency should not be applied for different aspects of criminal proceedings and that the test to be used is one of "limited cognitive capacity" (p. 567) in each of these circumstances.

Similarly, in *Godinez v. Moran* (1993), the United States Supreme Court held that the standard for the various types of competency (i.e., competency to plead guilty, to waive counsel, to stand trial) should be considered the same. Justice Thomas wrote for the majority:

> While the decision to plead guilty is undeniably a profound one, it is no more complicated than the sum total of decisions that a defendant may be called upon to make during the course of a trial.... Nor do we think that a defendant who waives his right to the assistance of counsel must be more competent than the defendant who does not, since there is no reason to believe that the decision to waive counsel requires an appreciably higher level of mental functioning than the decision to waive other constitutional rights. (p. 2686)

In his dissent, Justice Blackmun noted that the "majority's analysis is contrary to both common sense and long-standing case law" (p. 2691). He reasoned that competency cannot be considered in a vacuum, separate from its specific legal context. Justice Blackmun argued that "competency for one purpose does not necessarily translate to competency for another purpose" (p. 2694) and noted that prior Supreme Court cases have "required competency evaluations to be specifically tailored to the context and purpose of a proceeding" (p. 2694).

Perlin (1996) argued that the decision made by the Court in *Godinez* was detrimental to both the court process as well as to the rights and dignity of the accused. He argued that this was illustrated in the case of Colin Ferguson, a mentally disturbed individual who killed six people on the Long Island Rail Road and was allowed to represent himself at trial because the court, following the *Godinez* decision, ruled that he was generally competent. Perlin wrote that the "Ferguson spectacle was the inevitable denouement of the *Godinez* decision" (p. 61) and that this case will "drive whatever debate develops over competence questions" (p. 80).

These two Supreme Court decisions (*Whittle* and *Godinez*), in light of all the accumulated research on the issue of competency, beg the question of whether there is one construct or ability that underlies different types of competencies. The present research investigates this question by examining the relations between two divergent types of competencies—competency to stand trial and competence to consent to treatment.[4] In order to set the foundation for this research, the standards for

[4]The rationale for choosing competency to stand trial and competency to make treatment decisions was twofold. First, questions regarding these two types of competencies often co-occur in forensic

competence to stand trial in both Canada and the United States will be reviewed and the differences between these two systems highlighted. A discussion of competence to consent to treatment will follow.

Competence to Stand Trial

It has been a generally accepted legal principle in Western jurisprudence that incompetent individuals should not be allowed to proceed with a trial (Blackstone, 1783; *Frith's Case*, 1790). Although both the United States and Canada have their roots in English common law, case law in the two jurisdictions has led to somewhat different conceptualizations of competence to stand trial.

Canadian Conceptualization of Fitness to Stand Trial

In Canada, the issue of competence to stand trial has been interpreted as meaning that individuals charged with a criminal offence must be able to understand the nature of the proceedings and assist counsel in order to participate in their own defence and have a fair trial (see *Regina v. Pritchard*, 1836; *The Queen v. Berry*, 1876). Prior to 1992 there was no codified definition of the term unfit to stand trial. The criteria that were used were taken from case law.

In 1992, the *Criminal Code of Canada* (1985) was amended. Many changes were made to the legal procedures related to the determination of fitness to stand trial. Explicit guidelines were set out in Section 2, which include a definition as well as standards for the determination of fitness to stand trial. *Unfit to stand trial* is a legal term that is now defined as follows—a defendant is unfit to stand trial if he or she is:

> Unable on account of mental disorder to conduct a defence at any stage of the proceedings before a verdict is rendered or to instruct counsel to do so, and, in particular, unable on account of mental disorder to (a) understand the nature or object of the proceedings, (b) understand the possible consequences of the proceedings, or (c) communicate with counsel (C. C. C., S. 2, 1992).

Since 1992 there have been finer distinctions made in case law with respect to these three standards. In *Regina v. Taylor* (1992) the Ontario Court of Appeal decided "the test to be applied in determining the accused's ability to communicate with counsel is one of limited cognitive capacity" (p. 553). This means that it is not necessary that accused individuals be able to act in their own best interests, but rather, must only be able to recount the necessary facts pertaining to the offence to counsel so that counsel can present a proper defence. The appellate judge in *Taylor* decided that the "'limited cognitive capacity' test strikes an effective balance between the objective of the fitness rules and the constitutional right of the accused to choose his own defence and to have a fair trial within a reasonable time" (p. 567). This case serves to narrow the criteria used to assess fitness to stand trial.

patients who have been remanded for assessment of criminal competency. Second, these two types of competencies are very diverse (encompass both criminal and civil domains) and thus if no common underlying construct can be found for these two competencies, we can begin to narrow our focus to only those competencies within one domain or the other (i.e., criminal or civil).

American Conceptualization of Competence to Stand Trial

Although the Canadian and American criminal justice systems are both grounded in English common law, the two countries have somewhat different legal systems. In the United States, each state has its own Criminal Code and, therefore, its own provisions for determining competence to stand trial. Unlike the situation in Canada where the standard for fitness to stand trial was only recently codified, the modern standard for competency to stand trial in the United States was established by the Supreme Court in *Dusky v. United States* (1960). Although the exact wording is different from state to state, each state uses some variation of the *Dusky* standard to define competence to stand trial (Favole, 1983). The Court, in *Dusky*, held that for a defendant to be considered competent to stand trial, he or she must have "sufficient present ability to consult with his attorney with a reasonable degree of rational understanding" and "a rational as well as factual understanding of the proceedings against him" (p. 402). This decision reflects the need for a defendant to have both understanding as well as rationality. This appears to be a stricter test of competence than that currently being used in Canada (as explained in the next section).

Differences Between the USA and Canada

There appear to be certain fundamental differences between the current American and Canadian conceptualizations of competence to stand trial. The scopes of the standards for competency are different between the USA and Canada. The American conceptualization takes into consideration the rationality of the defendant whereas the Canadian system does not. In *Taylor* (1992), the Canadian court ruled that the test to be used in determining fitness was one of limited cognitive capacity. This is in contrast to the decision of the US court in *Dusky* (1960), which reflected the need to take into consideration the rationality of the defendant when making a determination of competency. The Canadian conceptualization appears to have a more narrow scope than does the American conceptualization and, therefore, takes into account fewer abilities than does the American conceptualization of competence to stand trial. Specifically, there is no use of the word "appreciate" in the Canadian conceptualization of fitness to stand trial. Accused individuals in Canada must only be able to understand the nature and object of the proceedings as well as the possible consequences of those proceedings. In some States, an accused individual must be able to appreciate the personal relevance of the proceedings (see Roesch & Golding, 1980). Thus, it would appear that the US has a stricter standard of criminal competency than does Canada.

Treatment Competence

Until recent decades, there had been no consensually agreed upon or legally defined means for determining competency to give informed consent. Beginning with the work of Roth and colleagues (Roth et al., 1977), however, a consensus has evolved as to the tests that are generally applied by the courts in making a determination of competency to consent to treatment (Appelbaum & Grisso, 1995). The article that reawakened modern interest in legal standards of competence to consent to treatment (Roth et al., 1977) stated that the search for a single test of competency was "a search for the Holy Grail" (p. 283). Although various authors have used different terminology at different points in time, there currently are four commonly accepted basic competence-related abilities that are discussed in the literature as tests of competence (see Appelbaum & Grisso, 1988, 1995; Appelbaum, Lidz, & Meisel, 1987; Appelbaum & Roth, 1982; Roth et al., 1977). These competence-related abilities can be arranged in hierarchical order and an inverse relationship exists between the amount of protection afforded by each test and the degree of independence granted to the patient. In increasing order of stringency, the four tests are (1) the ability to communicate a choice, (2) the ability to understand relevant information, (3) the ability to appreciate the nature of the situation and its likely consequences, and (4) the ability to rationally manipulate information.

The courts do not apply a single standard in all cases, but rather, choose from this small number of possibilities when selecting the tests that will be used in particular cases (Bonnie, 1993; Grisso, 1986, 2002; Tepper & Elwork, 1984). These tests may be used individually or in combination depending upon the determination of the court in a specific jurisdiction (Appelbaum & Grisso, 1995; Stanley, 1987). Additionally, the tests are flexible and can be applied somewhat differently in each case. One consequence of this flexibility is that the tests are often tailored to fit the needs of the situation. Roth and colleagues (Roth et al., 1977) have argued that the situation is often determined by two conditions: whether the patient is refusing or consenting to treatment, and whether the risk/benefit ratio is high or low.

The careful reader will note that the tests used to determine an individual's competency to consent to treatment are similar in nature to those defined by the courts as being important for determining an individual's competency to stand trial. That is, in both of these very different contexts, the abilities to understand, appreciate, and reason have been defined by various courts (as well as various scholars, researchers, and commentators) as being important to the issue of competency.

The Present Research

The present research addressed the issue of whether there is one or more construct or ability that underlies different types of competence. Two divergent types of competencies were examined—competence to stand trial and competence to consent to treatment—to determine if competencies within two completely different contexts would show a common underlying construct. These two competencies were selected as previous research (Zapf & Roesch, 1997, 1998) has indicated that questions of treatment competence and competence to stand trial often co-occur in samples of forensic psychiatric patients. Individuals who are remanded by the courts to an inpatient facility for an evaluation of their competence to stand trial are often asked to consent to treatment while on remand. The majority of individuals (76%) remanded to one Canadian facility, the Forensic Psychiatric Institute in British Columbia, either refuse treatment or are considered to be incompetent to consent to treatment as they are then certified under the Mental Health Act and subsequently treated with psychotropic medications (Zapf & Roesch, 1998).

By examining treatment competence and competence to stand trial in a sample of forensic patients we may be better able to answer the question of whether there are specific constructs or abilities that underlie both types of competence in two very different domains (i.e., criminal and civil).

The goal of the present research was to investigate the construct of competence in two different domains and the specific abilities required of different competencies. Three different instruments, which purport to measure competence-related abilities in three legal contexts, were examined in relation to each other: the Fitness Interview Test (Canadian conceptualization of fitness to stand trial as set out in Section 2 of the *Criminal Code of Canada*), the MacArthur Competence Assessment Tool—Criminal Adjudication (American conceptualization of competence to stand trial as set out in *Dusky v. United States* [1960]), and the MacArthur Competence Assessment Tool—Treatment (treatment competence as described by Paul Appelbaum and his colleagues [Appelbaum et al., 1987; Appelbaum & Grisso, 1988, 1995; Appelbaum & Roth, 1982; Roth et al., 1977]).

METHOD

Participants

Participants were 100 males remanded to the Forensic Psychiatric Institute (FPI) in British Columbia for evaluations of fitness to stand trial. Each new admission was given a copy of the consent form and had the consent form read to him by one of the two interviewers. The potential participant was then asked if he would like to take part in the study and given the opportunity to ask questions. Those individuals who agreed to participate were then asked to sign the consent form and were given a copy to keep.[5]

Each participant was given $5 as remuneration for participation in the study. This amount was thought to be small enough that it would not be an enticement for participation in the study, yet provide some compensation for the participant's time.

There were 186 males remanded to FPI for fitness evaluations during the time period of the study and the researchers contacted 165 of them to ask for their participation in the study.[6] Of those contacted, 105 (63.6%) agreed to take part in the study whereas 53 (32.1%) refused to participate. Five individuals agreed to take part but the researchers were unable to complete the interviews with these individuals due to scheduling difficulties. Seven individuals could not speak English well enough to participate in this study.

Most of the participants (69.1%) were single, White (72%), and unemployed (78.3%) at the time of admission to FPI. The average age at the time of admission

[5]By applying a standard of assent rather than competence to consent to research in order to establish eligibility for participation, we attempted to minimize the restrictions on variability in competence-related abilities, which would necessarily be introduced by the adoption of the higher standard for participation. Medical staff at the forensic facility gave consent for all individuals who participated.

[6]The researchers were unable to contact 21 of the men remanded during this time period as these individuals were placed directly into segregation and were not taken out of segregation while at FPI or were discharged from FPI within a few days of admission.

to FPI was 34.49 ($SD = 10.23$ years). According to file information, 85.1% of the remands had previous contact with mental health services, 75.5% had previously been hospitalized for psychiatric problems, and 66% were currently diagnosed with a psychotic disorder. As well, 90.4% of the remands had previous criminal histories, 46.7% had previously been in prison, and 67% were currently remanded to FPI on charges of violence (i.e., offences perpetrated against persons).

Instruments

Three measures of competence were used in this study: the Fitness Interview Test (revised edition) (FIT; Roesch, Zapf, Eaves, & Webster, 1998), the MacArthur Competence Assessment Tool—Criminal Adjudication (MacCAT-CA; Hoge, Bonnie, Poythress, & Monahan, 1999; Poythress et al., 1999), and the MacArthur Competence Assessment Tool—Treatment (MacCAT-T; Grisso & Appelbaum, 1998a, 1998b).

Fitness Interview Test

The FIT is a semistructured interview that takes approximately 30 min to administer and assesses the three areas specified in Section 2 of the 1992 revision of the *Criminal Code* with respect to fitness to stand trial. That is, the ability to understand the nature and object of the proceedings, the ability to understand the possible consequences of the proceedings, and the ability to communicate with counsel.

Each of these three sections is broken down into specific questions that tap into different psycholegal abilities involved in fitness to stand trial. The first section (6 items) assesses the accused's understanding of the arrest process, the nature and severity of current charges, the role of key players, legal processes, pleas, and court procedure. The second section (3 items) assesses the accused's appreciation of the range and nature of possible penalties, appraisal of available legal defences, and appraisal of likely outcome. The final section (7 items) assesses the accused's capacity to communicate facts to the lawyer, relate to the lawyer, plan legal strategy, engage in his or her own defence, challenge prosecution witnesses, testify relevantly, and manage courtroom behavior. Each of the items is rated as 0, 1, or 2 indicating no impairment, some/mild impairment, and severe impairment, respectively.

Research has indicated that the FIT has adequate psychometric properties. With respect to reliability, Viljoen, Roesch, and Zapf (2002) found that the average interrater reliability of the FIT for overall determination of fitness was .98. Reliability for sections was lower, and ranged from .54 to .70 for groups of raters. Predictive validity of the FIT has been established (see Boddy, Roesch, Zapf, & Eaves, 2000; Zapf & Roesch, 1997; Zapf, Roesch, & Viljoen, 2001) and evidence of the construct validity of the FIT is seen in the reasonably high agreement (chance-corrected $\kappa = .51$) between the FIT and the MacArthur Competency Assessment Tool—Criminal Adjudication (see Zapf & Roesch, 2001).

MacArthur Competence Assessment Tool—Criminal Adjudication

The MacCAT-CA was developed between 1989 and 1996 by the MacArthur Foundation Research Network on Mental Health and the Law to assess the abilities that are included in the legal definition of competence to stand trial in the United States. A comprehensive research instrument was developed, pilot tested, and refined and a large field study conducted (Hoge, Bonnie, et al., 1997; Hoge, Poythress, et al., 1997; Otto et al., 1998). The MacCAT-CA was developed from this comprehensive research instrument and assesses three main abilities—understanding, reasoning, and appreciation.

The MacCAT-CA consists of 22 items that are broken down into three sections, each measuring one of the main competence-related abilities set out in the U.S. standards for competence to stand trial. The MacCAT-CA begins with a vignette that establishes the context for the first 16 items. The first section (8 items) assesses the defendant's ability to understand information about the legal system and the process of adjudication. The second section (8 items) assesses the defendant's ability to reason and the final section (6 items) assesses the defendant's ability to appreciate his or her own legal circumstances and situation. Each item is scored on a 3-point scale (0, 1, or 2) according to standardized criteria.

The psychometric properties of the MacCAT-CA were established in a large-scale study funded by NIMH (see Otto et al., 1998). The results indicated that the MacCAT-CA demonstrates good reliability and validity. Specifically, internal consistency for the three sections ranged from .81 to .88 (Cronbach's alpha = .81 for Reasoning, .85 for Understanding, .88 for Appreciation), interrater reliability ranged from very good to excellent for each of the three sections (intraclass $R = .75$ for Appreciation, .85 for Reasoning, .90 for Understanding), and support for the construct validity of the MacCAT-CA was "found in the pattern of correlations between the MacCAT-CA measures and select clinical variables" (p. 439).

MacArthur Competence Assessment Tool—Treatment

The MacCAT-T was developed between 1988 and 1995 by the MacArthur Foundation Research Network on Mental Health and the Law to assess the specific abilities that comprise legal competence to consent to treatment. This research drew upon developments in the law and clinical literature on informed consent for medical treatment. A series of comprehensive research instruments was developed, pilot tested, and refined and then a field study was conducted to test these research instruments with four groups—persons with schizophrenia, persons with depression, persons with angina, and a nonill control group (see Appelbaum & Grisso, 1995; Grisso et al., 1995; Grisso & Appelbaum, 1995, 1998). The MacCAT-T was developed from these comprehensive research instruments and is designed to measure four abilities: the ability to communicate a choice, the ability to understand relevant information, the ability to appreciate the nature of the situation and its likely consequences, and the ability to manipulate information rationally.

The MacCAT-T is an interview that combines disclosure of information regarding disorder and treatment with an assessment of the patient's ability to use this information in deciding to accept or refuse the disclosed treatments. In preparation for this interview the clinician reviews the patient's file to determine the diagnoses, symptoms, and possible treatment options that are relevant to the patient. The interview is tailored specifically to the individual being assessed.

Published information on the psychometric properties of the MacCAT-T indicates that it shows good interrater reliability, with ICCs ranging from .82 to .99 and Pearson correlations ranging from .59 to .99 for summary scores. In general, the understanding section shows the highest interrater reliability and the appreciation section the lowest (see Grisso & Appelbaum, 1998a, 1998b). Additionally, initial indications of validity for the MacCAT-T were favorable (Grisso, Appelbaum, & Hill-Fotouhi, 1997).

Procedure

Assessment Information

Individuals who chose to participate in this study were administered four assessment instruments (FIT, BPRS,[7] CAT-T,[8] and the MacCAT-CA in this order) by one of two senior clinical psychology graduate students from Simon Fraser University. The majority of participants completed all four assessment instruments in one assessment session (up to 2 hr in duration). All participants completed the four assessment instruments within two assessment sessions. Only the results of the three competence assessment instruments (FIT, MacCAT-CA, MacCAT-T) were used in the present study.

No names were associated with the information collected. All procedures were approved by the appropriate university and institutional ethics review boards and were in accordance with current ethical principles.

File Information and Data Coding

Basic demographic information—age, ethnicity, current diagnoses, mental health history, outcome of the inpatient evaluation, and so forth—were collected on every participant. No names were associated with the file information that was collected.

RESULTS

Before beginning a discussion of the results for each specific model, the criteria that were used to determine whether or not each model was considered an appropriate fit for the data will be explained. First, a model was rejected outright if problems in convergence were encountered. LISREL 8.30 incorporates an admissibility check

[7]Participants were administered the Brief Psychiatric Rating Scale (BPRS: Overall & Gorham, 1962) as this research was part of a larger research study. The BPRS will not be described in this paper nor will any of results pertaining to it be discussed.

[8]For the purposes of this research, the MacCAT-T was tailored to a diagnosis of psychotic disorder and administered in a standardized fashion to each of the participants. Previous research conducted with the same population at FPI (Zapf & Roesch, 1997, 1998) indicated that the most prevalent type of disorder among defendants remanded for fitness evaluations (54%) was psychotic disorder, specifically, Schizophrenia.

whereby a solution is found nonadmissible if convergence has not been reached after 20 iterations. As most of the models being tested had a large number of parameters it was not uncommon for the solution to be found nonadmissible after only 20 iterations. For the purposes of these analyses, if a model did not pass the admissibility test the number of iterations was increased to three times the number of parameters in the model being tested.[9] If convergence was not reached after this increase in iterations, the model was rejected. Second, a model was rejected outright if the estimates produced were out-of-bounds. Specifically, if negative error variances or correlations greater than 1 were encountered the solution was considered to be anomalous and therefore unacceptable (Long, 1983a; Schwarzer, 1986). If convergence occurred within the maximum allowable number of iterations and the estimates produced were in-bounds, then an examination of the parameters and goodness of fit statistics determined whether or not the model was considered to have fit the data.

Several relevant indices of goodness of fit for each model are reported as each index addresses a slightly different issue, and good-fitting models will produce consistent results across many indices (Ullman, 2001). Specifically, for each model, we report (a) absolute fit indices (χ^2, χ^2/df, GFI index, AGFI index), (b) relative fit indices (CFI, NFI), (c) parsimoniousness fit indices (AIC, CAIC), and (d) noncentrality-based indices (RMSEA) (for overviews, see Bentler, 1995; Church & Burke, 1993; Kline, 1998; MacCallum & Austin, 2000; Ullman, 2001).

In terms of the absolute fit indices, the chi-square is a test of independence and therefore a *non*significant chi-square is indicative of a confirmation of the model (i.e., the data fit the model). The chi-square is very sensitive to sample size and, therefore, some authors (e.g., Carmines & McIver, 1981; Long, 1983b; Schwarzer, 1986) have suggested that the ratio between the chi-square statistic and the degrees of freedom should be used as an indicator of the goodness of fit of a model. Large values of chi-square relative to the degrees of freedom indicate that the model is not a good fit of the data (Long, 1983b). For the purposes of these analyses, if the chi-square statistic was greater than approximately twice the degrees of freedom it was considered to be unacceptable (see Carmines & McIver, 1981).

We weighed the adjusted goodness of fit index (AGFI; Jöreskog & Sörbom, 1989) more than the GFI in our decision regarding whether or not to reject a model. The AGFI is a measure of how much better the model fits the data than no model at all. This index does not depend on sample size explicitly and is adjusted for the degrees of freedom (Jöreskog & Sörbom, 1993b). For the purposes of these analyses, if the AGFI was below 0.80 then it was considered to be unacceptable (see Bollen, 1989; Hair, Anderson, Tatham, & Grablowsky, 1995).

Relative fit indices such as the comparative fit index (CFI) and the normed fit index (NFI) are difficult to interpret; however, minimum values of .90 for these statistics are conventionally required to indicate adequate, satisfactory, or acceptable fit (Byrne, 1994). This is the cutoff for these statistics that we used in deciding whether or not to reject a model.

[9]This is the maximum number of iterations allowed when testing a model using confirmatory factor analysis (Jöreskog & Sörbom, 1993b, p. 182).

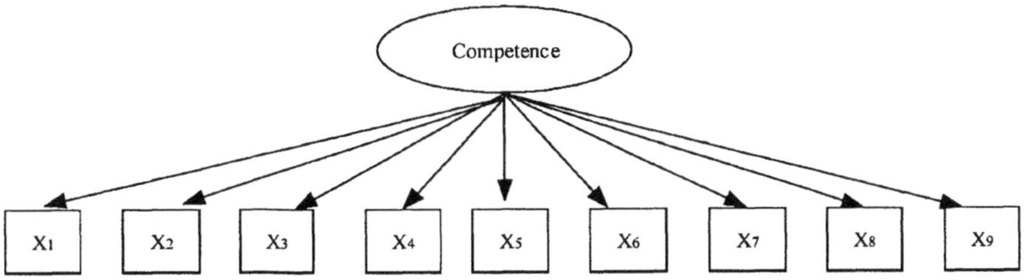

Fig. 1. Unidimensional model (one latent variable†, nine observed variables‡). $\chi^2 = 154.8$ $df = 27$ RMSEA = .219. †Latent variables are denoted by ellipses. ‡Observed variables are denoted by boxes. X_1–X_3 correspond to understanding nature/object, understanding consequences, communicate with counsel sections of the FIT, respectively. X_4–X_6 correspond to the understanding, appreciation, reasoning sections of the MacCAT-CA, respectively. X_7–X_9 correspond to the understanding, appreciation, reasoning, sections of the MacCAT-T, respectively.

Parsimonious fit indices and noncentrality-based indices are reported and the root mean square error of approximation (RMSEA) was considered to be reflective of an inadequate fit if it was greater than .10, an adequate fit if it was between .05 and .10, and a reasonably good fit if it was less than .05 (see Byrne, 1994; Ullman, 2001).

To answer the question of whether there are one or more constructs that underlie different types of competence, a series of eight *a priori* structural models was developed and these models were tested using confirmatory factor analysis with LISREL 8.30 (Jöreskog & Sörbom, 1993a, 1993b). Three combinations of instruments were tested: (1) all three of the competence instruments (FIT, MacCAT-CA, MacCAT-T; Figs. 1–3), (2) the two criminal competence instruments (FIT, MacCAT-CA; Figs. 5–6), and (3) the two MacArthur instruments (MacCAT-CA, MacCAT-T; Figs. 7–9). The results will be discussed in terms of the strict testing of each of the proposed *a priori* models for each group of instruments. After the results have been discussed for each of the *a priori* models, a discussion of some exploratory results (i.e., confirmatory factor analyses with models that were not specified *a priori*) using the modification indices will follow. All indices for each of the models tested are found in Table 1.

The FIT, the MacCAT-CA, and the MacCAT-T

The first three models (Figs. 1–3) pertain to the FIT, the MacCAT-CA, and the MacCAT-T as a group. Each of these three models takes into consideration nine observed variables (as indicated by the boxes labeled X_1 through X_9). The variables labeled X_1–X_3 relate to the total scores for the three sections of the FIT (Understand the Nature/Object of the Proceedings, Understand the Possible Consequences of the Proceedings, Communicate with Counsel), respectively, variables labeled X_4–X_6 relate to the total scores for the understanding, appreciation, and reasoning components of the MacCAT-CA, respectively, and variables labeled X_7–X_9 relate to the total scores for the understanding, appreciation, and reasoning components of the MacCAT-T, respectively. In addition to the observed variables, each of these

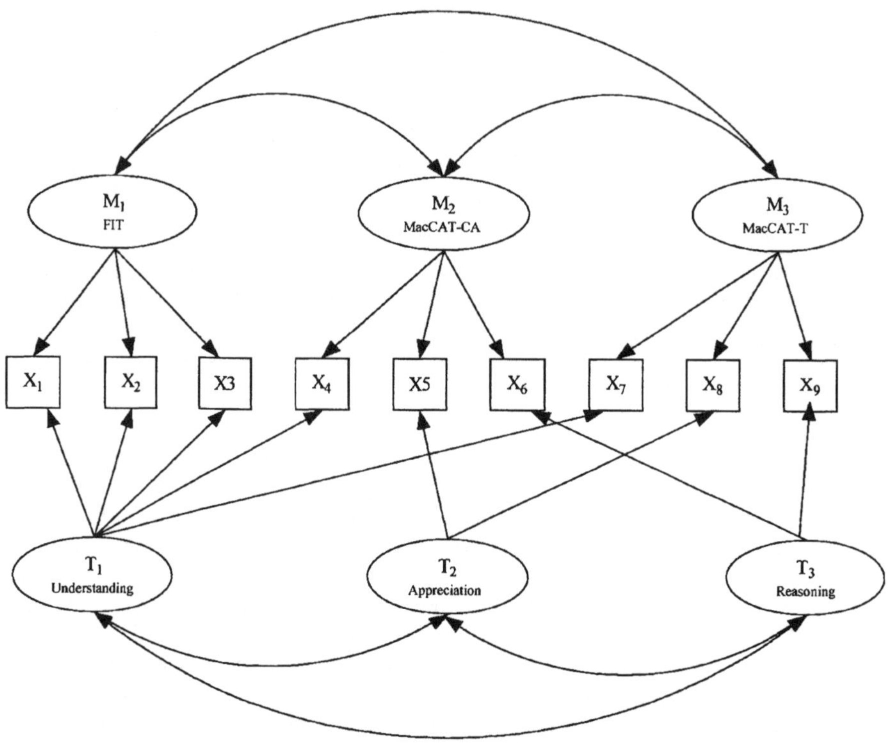

Fig. 2. Full model (three latent "method" variables, three latent "trait" variables). Model did not converge.

models proposes a number of latent variables as indicated by the ellipses. The unidirectional arrows pointing to the observed variables from the latent variables are indicative of the causal effect of the latent variables on the observed variables. The curved bidirectional arrows between latent variables indicate that those latent variables are correlated. Each observed variable has associated with it (not diagramed) a uniqueness factor or error variance. For the purposes of testing each of the *a priori* models, the error variances were assumed to be uncorrelated.

The first model (see Fig. 1) is a test of unidimensionality. That is, it is a test of the hypothesis that each of the nine observed variables used in this research is a measure of the same underlying construct (i.e., competence). This model was rejected as the results of the analyses indicate that this model does not fit the data well, χ^2 (27, N = 100) = 154.8, $p < .001$, AGFI = 0.57, CFI = .84, NFI = .81, and RMSEA = .219.

The second model (see Fig. 2) is the most general model wherein there are three methods (FIT, MacCAT-CA, MacCAT-T) and three traits (Understanding, Appreciation, Reasoning) that attempt to explain the scores obtained on the observed variables. This model was rejected outright as it did not yield a solution after the maximum allowable number of iterations (even using more liberal criteria than

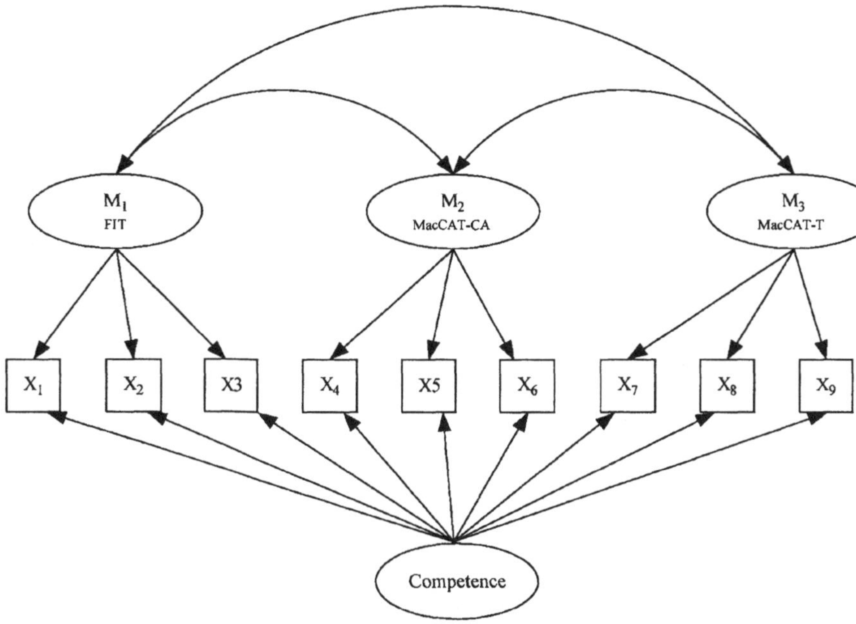

Fig. 3. Reduced model (three latent "method" variables, one latent "trait" variable). $\chi^2 = 26.72$ $df = 15$ RMSEA = .089.

that recommended by Jöreskog & Sörbom, 1993b, p. 182). A solution was forced by placing no limit on the number of iterations and convergence occurred after 108 iterations. This solution, however, was artificial as evidenced by negative error variances for two of the observed variables.

The final model (see Fig. 3) that was tested incorporates the same three methods as the second model (FIT, MacCAT-CA, MacCAT-T) but only one underlying trait (Competence) in attempting to explain the scores obtained on the observed variables. This third model is derived from the second model by fixing the correlations between the three traits to 1 and therefore is considered to be a nested

Table 1. Goodness of Fit Indices for Models Tested

Model	χ^2	*df*	χ^2/df	CFI	NFI	GFI	AGFI	AIC	CAIC	RMSEA
Model 1.1	154.8	27	5.73	.84	.81	.74	.57	190.8	255.7	.219
Model 1.2[a]	—	—	—	—	—	—	—	—	—	—
Model 1.3	26.72	15	1.78	.98	.96	.94	.83	86.72	194.87	.089
Model 2.1	40.92	9	4.55	.93	.92	.88	.72	64.92	108.18	.189
Model 2.2[a]	—	—	—	—	—	—	—	—	—	—
Model 3.1	26.04	9	2.89	.94	.91	.92	.81	50.04	93.31	.138
Model 3.2[a]	—	—	—	—	—	—	—	—	—	—
Model 3.3[a]	—	—	—	—	—	—	—	—	—	—
Modified Model 1.3	20.33	14	1.45	.99	.97	.96	.86	82.33	194.09	.068

[a]Model did not converge.

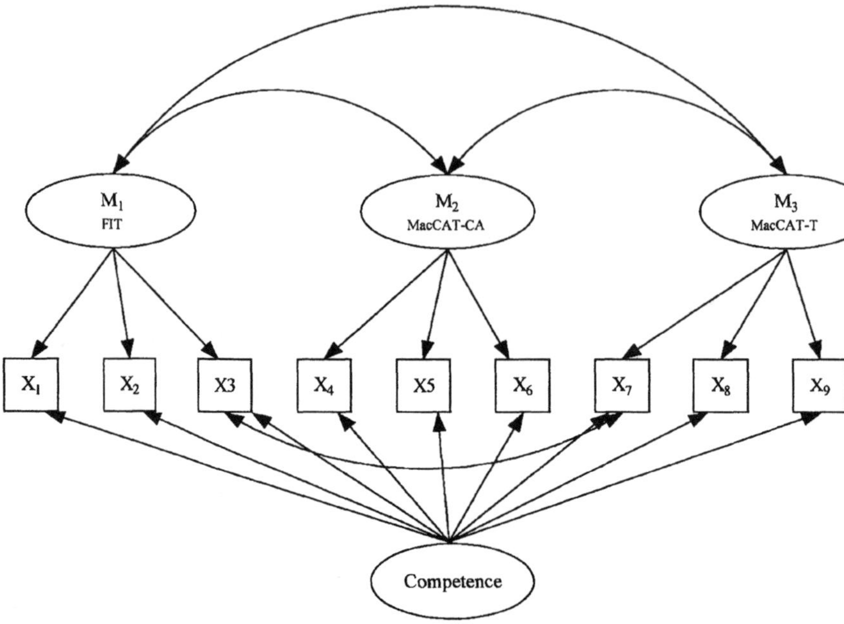

Fig. 4. Modified model 1.3 (allowing for the errors between X_3 and X_7 to correlate). $\chi^2 = 20.33$ $df = 14$ RMSEA = .068.

model.[10] This model was accepted as it fit the data reasonably well, χ^2 (15, N = 100) = 26.72, $p < .01$, $AGFI = 0.83$, $CFI = .98$, $NFI = .96$, and $RMSEA = .089$.

The factor loadings for the observed variables on the underlying trait variable (i.e., competence) were (X_1–X_9 respectively): −1.22, −0.41, −1.21, −3.06, −0.53, −2.37, −1.14, −0.37, −0.90. The correlation between the FIT and the MacCAT-CA was .88, between the FIT and the MacCAT-T was .64, and between the MacCAT-CA and the MacCAT-T was .75. The loadings for each of the observed variables on its respective method variable were: 1.91, 1.33, 2.34 (X_1–X_3 respectively on the FIT); 1.54, 2.25, 1.79 (X_4–X_6 respectively on the MacCAT-CA); and 0.83, 0.94, 1.34 (X_7–X_9 respectively on the MacCAT-T).

A modified version of this model (see Fig. 4) is presented in the section on exploratory results below.

The FIT and the MacCAT-CA

The next two models (Figs. 5–6) are a subset of models derived from the previous set. These two models incorporate the six observed variables related to the FIT (X_1–X_3) and the MacCAT-CA (X_4–X_6).

[10] Although this model is a nested model, a difference in chi-square test could not be performed between the two models as there was no solution for model 1.2.

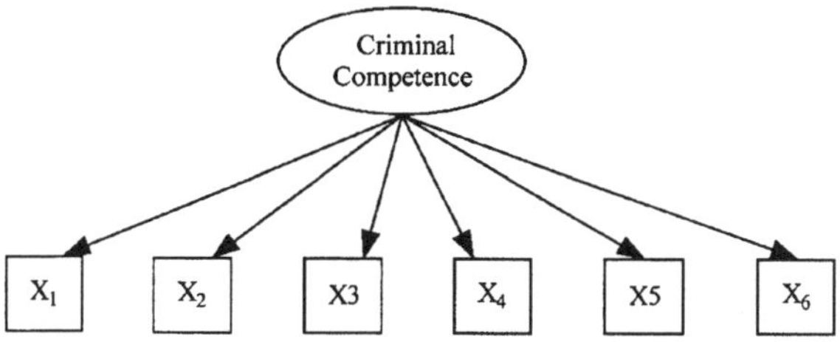

Fig. 5. Unidimensional model with FIT (X_1–X_3) and MacCAT-CA (X_4–X_6) only. $\chi^2 = 40.92$ $df=$ 9 RMSEA = .189.

The first model (see Fig. 5) is a test of unidimensionality. That is, a test of the hypothesis that the components of both the FIT and the MacCAT-CA are measuring the same construct (i.e., criminal competence). The nine-variable model of this type (Fig. 1) was rejected and, therefore, it is logical to test a subset of the variables from this model. This model was rejected as the results of the analyses indicate that this model does not fit the data well, χ^2 $(9, N = 100) = 40.92, p < .001$, AGFI = 0.72, CFI = .93, NFI = .92, and RMSEA = .189.

The second model (see Fig. 6) did not converge due to problems of identification. This model is a subset of the nine-variable model of this same type (Fig. 3), which was accepted, therefore this more comprehensive model can be used to interpret the variables (see Long 1983a, 1983b).

The MacCAT-CA and the MacCAT-T

The last three models (Figs. 7–9) are also a subset of models derived from the first set of models. Each of these three models takes into consideration the six observed variables related to the two MacArthur instruments, the MacCAT-CA

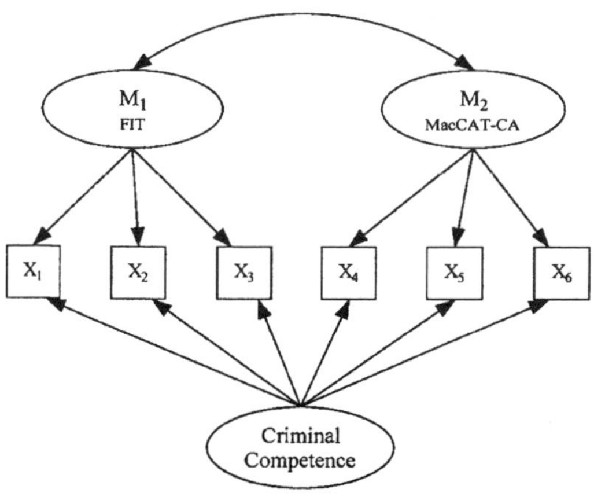

Fig. 6. Expanded model (two latent "method" variables, one latent "trait" variable). Model did not converge.

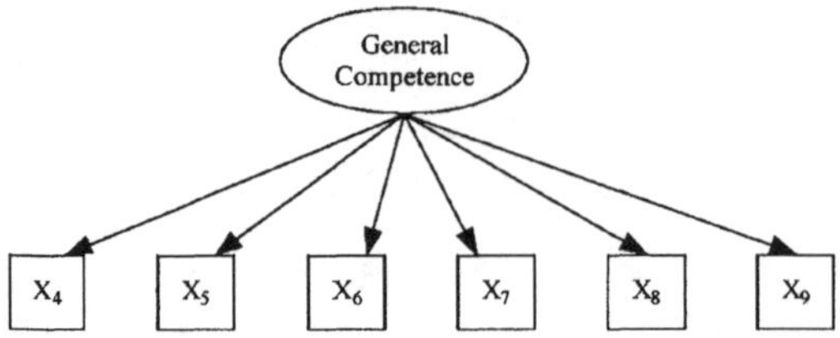

Fig. 7. Unidimensional model with MacCAT-CA (X_4–X_6) and MacCAT-T (X_7–X_9) only. $\chi^2 = 26.04$ $df = 14$ RMSEA = .138.

(X_4–X_6) and the MacCAT-T (X_7–X_9). These two instruments were developed based on the same theoretical foundation (i.e., Bonnie, 1992, 1993) and purport to measure the same three abilities (i.e., understanding, appreciation, reasoning).

The first model (see Fig. 7) is a test of unidimensionality. That is, a test of the hypothesis that the components of these two instruments are measuring the same underlying construct (i.e., competence). It is logical to test this model as the more comprehensive nine-variable model (Fig. 1) was rejected and therefore, it is possible that this six-variable version may be accepted. This model was rejected as the results of

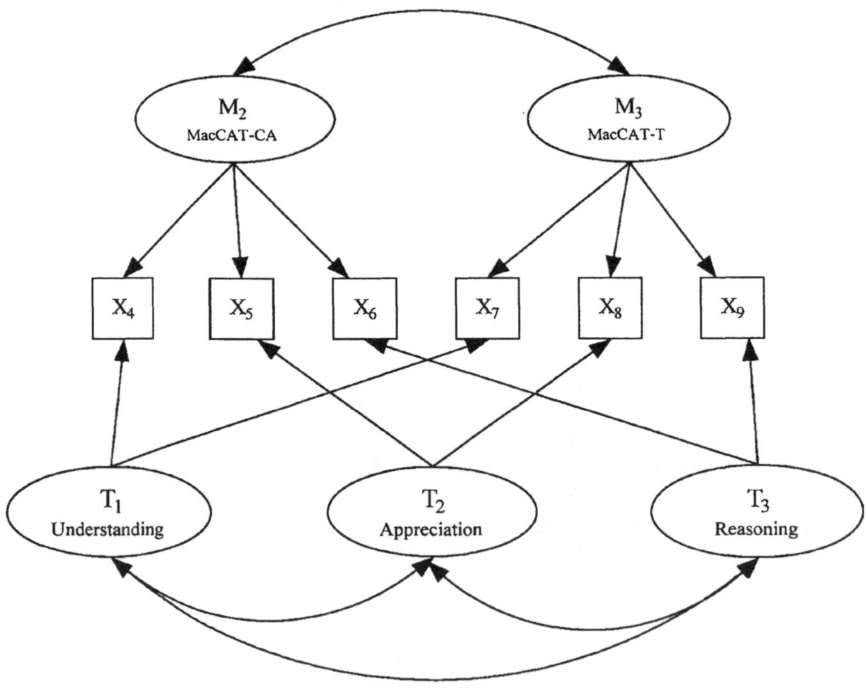

Fig. 8. Full model (two latent "method" variables, three latent "trait" variables). Model did not converge.

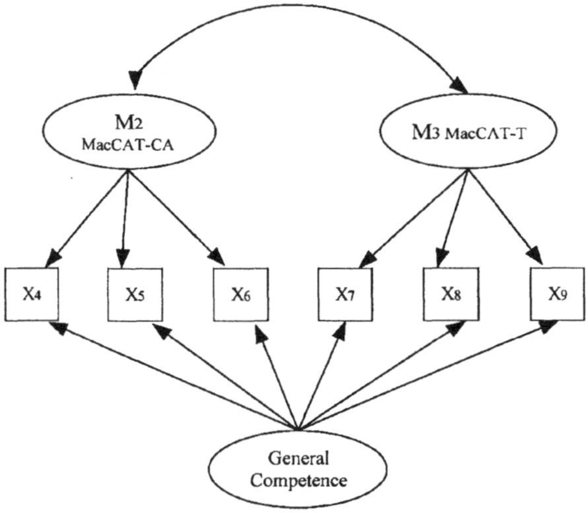

Fig. 9. Reduced model (two latent "method" variables, one latent "trait" variable). Model did not converge.

the analyses indicate that this model does not fit the data well, χ^2 (9, $N = 100$) = 26.04, $p < .01$, AGFI = 0.81, CFI = .94, NFI = .91, and RMSEA = .138.

The second model (see Fig. 8) is a subset of the nine-variable model of this same type (Fig. 2) and includes two methods (MacCAT-CA and MacCAT-T) and three traits (Understanding, Appreciation, Reasoning). It is logical to test this less comprehensive six-variable model as the more comprehensive nine-variable model was rejected. This model was rejected outright as the solution did not converge after the maximum allowable number of iterations. When a solution was forced, convergence occurred at 127 iterations, however the estimates given were anomalous (negative error variance and correlations greater than 1).

The final model (see Fig. 9) did not converge due to problems of identification; however, as this model is a subset of the nine-variable model of this same type (Fig. 3), this more comprehensive model can be used to interpret the variables.

Exploratory Results of Structural Equation Modeling Using the Modification Indices

After the *a priori* models were tested and either accepted or rejected, exploratory analyses using some of the suggested modification indices were performed. The results of these analyses are purely for the purpose of attempting to gain further understanding of the observed variables.

Model 1.3 Modified

Different variations of this model were tested, taking the modification indices into consideration, in an attempt to improve upon the fit of the original model.

When the errors of two of the observed variables (X_3 and X_7) were allowed to correlate, this modified model (see Fig. 4) fit the data well, χ^2 (14, $N = 100$) = 20.33, $p = .08$, AGFI = 0.86, CFI = .99, NFI = .97, and RMSEA = .068 and yielded a significantly better fit of the data than did the original model, χ^2 (1 *df*) = 6.39, $p < .025$. These variables (X_3 and X_7) correlated at the level of 0.51.

The factor loadings for each of the observed variables on the underlying trait variable were (X_1–X_9, respectively): 1.00, 0.92, 1.79, 0.45, 1.91, 0.94, 0.27, 0.61, 0.75. The correlation between the FIT and the MacCAT-CA was .82, between the FIT and the MacCAT-T was .67, and between the MacCAT-CA and the MacCAT-T was .86. The loadings for each of the observed variables on its respective method variable were: 2.15, 0.99, 1.92 (X_1–X_3, respectively on the FIT); 3.40, 1.24, 2.83 (X_4–X_6, respectively on the MacCAT-CA); and 1.39, 0.70, 1.38 (X_7–X_9, respectively on the MacCAT-T).

DISCUSSION

The results of these analyses appear to lend support to the notion that there is one common construct that underlies these two different types of competence. Model 1.3 demonstrates that each of the observed variables used in this research load onto some common underlying construct. Further examination of this model indicates that each of the observed variables load in a negative direction on this common underlying construct. That is, there is a negative or inverse relationship between the observed variables and the underlying construct (i.e., higher scores on the observed variables are associated with lower levels of the construct). If this underlying construct were to be termed *competence*, higher scores on the competence assessment instruments are associated with lower levels of competence (i.e., incompetence).

Model 1.3 was modified to allow the errors of two of the observed variables (X_7 and X_3) to correlate. This modified version of the model fit the data significantly better than the original model; therefore, this modified model will be discussed in detail.

The observed variables that have the highest factor loadings on the common underlying construct are the "Communicate with Counsel" section of the FIT (X_3) and the "Appreciation" section of the MacCAT-CA (X_5). Both of these variables require an individual to apply abstract knowledge to their own personal situation. The Communicate with Counsel section of the FIT asks questions such as whether or not an individual would accept certain plea bargains, what an individual would do if someone were to tell lies about him or her in court, how an individual thinks he or she can best be defended against the charges he or she is facing, and what an individual would do if he or she disagreed with his or her lawyer. The Appreciation section of the MacCAT-CA asks questions such as how likely an individual thinks he or she is to be found guilty, how much punishment an individual thinks he or she may get if found guilty, how likely an individual is to accept a plea bargain, and how likely it is that an individual will be treated fairly by the legal system. Both of these variables (X_3 and X_5) require an individual to think about his or her own situation and to apply any relevant knowledge that he or she might have to that situation.

It appears that this ability (or lack thereof) makes an important contribution to an individual's overall level of competence (or incompetence).

The fit of the original model (Model 1.3) was significantly improved by allowing the errors of two of the observed variables (X_3 and X_7) to correlate. These variables both, to some extent, appear to tap into an individual's ability to communicate and, therefore, are both affected by severity of mental illness. The "Understanding" section of the MacCAT-T (X_7) requires that an individual be able to listen to, attend, process, and reiterate presented information. The "Communicate with Counsel" section of the FIT (X_3), in addition to asking an individual about certain specific situations (as previously discussed) also explicitly asks an individual about his or her ability to communicate. This item asks an individual whether he or she has any emotional problems (e.g., becoming angry, anxious, agitated) or communication difficulties (e.g., concentrating, talking, keeping on track) that would interfere with his or her ability to talk to a lawyer or testify in court. Since these two variables (X_7 and X_3) both appear to tap into an individual's ability to communicate but to different degrees it seems logical that they would correlate positively at a moderate level.

An examination of the factor loadings for each of the observed variables on their respective instruments (X_1–X_3 on the FIT; X_4–X_6 on the MacCAT- CA; X_7–X_9 on the MacCAT-T) reveals that X_2, X_5, and X_8 all load lower than their respective counterparts. That is, the "Understand the Possible Consequences" section (X_2) loads lower on the FIT than do the "Understand the Nature/Object of the Proceedings" or the "Communicate with Counsel" sections. As well, the "Appreciation" section (X_5) loads lower on the MacCAT-CA than do the "Understanding" or "Reasoning" sections, and the "Appreciation" section (X_8) loads lower on the MacCAT-T than do the "Understanding" or "Reasoning" sections. It appears that all three of these variables (X_2, X_5, X_8) attempt to measure an individual's appreciation in terms of asking questions surrounding personal involvement in specific situations. Perhaps part of the reason why these variables load lowest on their respective instruments is because of the difficulty in measuring an individual's appreciation of his or her personal situation via a standardized structured interview format.

One issue that needs to be discussed with respect to the analysis of Model 1.3 and the modified version of this model is the conflation between methods and traits in the method variables. All of the *a priori* models (with the exception of the unidimensional models—1.1, 2.1, 3.1) were structured in terms of a multitrait multimethod approach wherein there were a certain number of method variables (diagramed in ellipses above the observed variables) and a certain number of trait variables (diagramed in ellipses below the observed variables) that were included in each model to explain the scores obtained on the observed variables. It should be noted, however, that although this approach was used as a means by which to structure the models, neither the data collected nor the results obtained represent a true multitrait multimethod approach. There is an inherent conflation of method and trait variance in each of the method variables (FIT, MacCAT-CA, MacCAT-T).[11] That is, each of the instruments uses a somewhat different

[11] Because of this conflation, the squared multiple correlations obtained could not be decomposed further into trait and method variances as there would be no way to interpret these data.

methodology and measures a somewhat different type of competence than the others.

An examination of the correlations between these three instruments indicates that they all correlate at a moderate to high level. The correlation between the FIT and the MacCAT-CA is .82, the correlation between the FIT and the MacCAT-T is .67, and the correlation between the MacCAT-CA and the MacCAT-T is .86. These correlations make intuitive sense as the FIT and MacCAT-CA are both measures of criminal competence and, therefore, ask similar types of questions but get at somewhat different abilities by virtue of one being a measure of the Canadian criteria and the other being a measure of the American criteria. A lower correlation between the FIT and MacCAT-T can be explained by the fact that these two instruments use somewhat different formats and measure two different types of competence, although they assess some of the same psycholegal abilities. A strong correlation between the two MacArthur instruments can be explained by the fact that both of these instruments were based on the same theoretical foundation and purport to measure the same psycholegal abilities in a similar manner.

The results of the other significant exploratory analyses indicate that a strong negative correlation between X_4 and X_8 occurs when the test of unidimensionality was performed for the observed variables associated with the MacCAT-CA and the MacCAT-T (Model 3.1). That is, there is a strong inverse relationship between performance on the "Understanding" section of the MacCAT-CA (X_4) and the "Appreciation" section of the MacCAT-T (X_8): Individuals who obtain lower scores on the understanding section of the MacCAT-CA are more able to appreciate that they have a mental disorder and that treatment would help control the symptoms of this disorder. While at first counterintuitive, this relationship could possibly be explained in terms of severity of mental illness. Those individuals who obtained lower scores on the Understanding section of the MacCAT-CA were unable to concentrate and hold information in working memory, suggesting that they may have been severely mentally ill. Perhaps these severely ill individuals were better able to appreciate that they were experiencing symptoms of mental disorder (i.e., psychosis) and/or that medication may help to control these symptoms.[12]

Turning briefly to the issue of unidimensionality, it should be noted that the models that tested for this (Model 1.1, 2.1, 3.1) were all rejected. These results indicate that the different sections of the FIT, the MacCAT-CA, and the MacCAT-T are not all measures of the same construct. Since these instruments each purport to measure a number of different psycholegal abilities, a finding of unidimensionality would have been surprising. These results cannot be interpreted as support for the assumption that the different sections of these instruments each measure different psycholegal abilities; however, the results do not disconfirm this assumption.

[12]Anecdotally, many of the individuals who were grossly psychotic at the time of interview were able to identify that they had difficulty concentrating after this symptom of mental disorder had been presented during the administration of the MacCAT-T.

SUMMARY AND CONCLUSIONS

To summarize, it appears that there is some common construct that underlies these different types of competence. Exactly what this construct is may never be known. For now, we can only speculate as to what it might be. For the purposes of this research the common underlying construct was called competence (incompetence), however, this is simply a matter of syntax. Other possibilities include psychoticism, general cognitive ability, or conceptual disorganization. More research needs to be conducted to further specify what this underlying construct is.

It is important to note, however, that the fact that there is some common construct underlying these different types of competence does not mean that competence is a global all-or-nothing characteristic. It is obvious from this research (i.e., individuals performed differently on each of the three instruments) as well as from the body of previous psychological literature and research that an individual may be competent for one specific purpose and incompetent for another. Therefore, competence needs to be assessed in direct relation to the specific context in which it is considered.

Supreme Court decisions in Canada (*R. v. Whittle*) and the United States (*Godinez v. Moran*) have started to move away from this context-specific view of competence. It seems that the courts have begun to recognize the potential burden of having to assess competence in relation to each specific context in which it arises as an issue. Perhaps these decisions are an attempt to halt this process before it gets out of hand. How specific do evaluations of competence really have to be? The challenge lies in finding a balance between evaluations that are manageable for the courts and the protection of the rights of the individuals involved while preserving the integrity of the legal process.

DIRECTIONS FOR FUTURE RESEARCH

The accepted models should be treated as provisional and cross-validation procedures need to be performed in order to determine the appropriateness of these models (as discussed in Cudeck & Browne, 1983) for further use. In addition to cross-validation of the models, future research in this area could include larger sample sizes. Bollen (1989) recommended using sample sizes of 100 or more for this type of analysis in order to achieve convergence. Perhaps the reason that some of the models in this research did not reach convergence was because the sample size was toward the lower end of the desired range.

The method/trait conflation in the method variables was a source of additional *noise* in this research. Future research efforts could attempt to reduce or eliminate this method/trait conflation. This would result in a more precise picture of competence. In addition, a true multitrait multimethod approach would be useful in terms of allowing for a meaningful decomposition of variances into method and trait variances, thereby further delineating this picture of competence.

Finally, more of this same type of research is needed in order to attempt to define and further refine this common construct that underlies different types of competence. Much of the empirical research that has been conducted in the area of competence has focused on the assessment of competence and related issues. The work that has been done on the conceptualization of competence has been mainly theoretical in nature. This research attempts to investigate the construct of competence through empirical means, thereby forging a nexus between the theoretical and the empirical.

ACKNOWLEDGMENTS

This research was supported by a grant awarded to R. Roesch from the Social Sciences and Humanities Research Council of Canada. This research was part of the first author's dissertation and was supported by grants awarded to P. A. Zapf from the British Columbia Health Research Foundation, the Social Sciences and Humanities Research Council of Canada, the American Psychology—Law Society, and the American Academy of Forensic Psychology. The authors would like to thank Dr. Derek Eaves for his cooperation and support of this research and Karen E. Whittemore for her contribution as a research assistant.

REFERENCES

Appelbaum, P. S., & Grisso, T. (1988). Assessing patients' capacities to consent to treatment. *The New England Journal of Medicine, 319,* 1635–1638.

Appelbaum, P. S., & Grisso, T. (1995). The MacArthur treatment competence study. I: Mental illness and competence to consent to treatment. *Law and Human Behavior, 19,* 105–126.

Appelbaum, P. S., Lidz, C. W., & Meisel, A. (1987). *Informed consent: Legal theory and clinical practice.* New York: Oxford University Press.

Appelbaum, P. S., & Roth, L. H. (1982). Competency to consent to research: A psychiatric overview. *Archives of General Psychiatry, 39,* 951–958.

Bentler, P. (1995). *EQS structural equation program model.* Encino, CA: Multivariate Software.

Blackstone, W. (1783). *Commentaries on the laws of England* (9th ed.). London: W. Strahan.

Boddy, J., Roesch, R., Zapf, P., & Eaves, D. (2000, March). *Characteristics of defendants remanded for fitness assessments.* Poster presented at the American Psychology and Law Society Conference, New Orleans, LA.

Bollen, K. A. (1989). *Structural equations with latent variables.* New York: Wiley.

Bonnie, R. J. (1992). The competence of criminal defendants: A theoretical reformulation. *Behavioral Sciences and the Law, 10,* 291–316.

Bonnie, R. J. (1993). The competence of criminal defendants: Beyond Dusky and Drope. *University of Miami Law Review, 47,* 539–601.

Burra, P., Kimberley, R., & Miura, C. (1980). Mental competence and consent to treatment. *Canadian Journal of Psychiatry, 25,* 251–253.

Byrne, B. (1994). *Structural equation modeling with EQS and EQS/Windows: Basic concepts, applications, and programming.* Thousand Oaks, CA: Sage.

Carmines, E. G., & McIver, J. P. (1981). Analyzing models with unobserved variables: Analysis of covariance structures. In G. W. Bohrnstedt & E. F. Borgatta (Eds.), *Social measurement: Current issues* (pp. 65–115). Beverly Hills, CA: Sage.

Church, A., & Burke, P. (1993). Exploratory and confirmatory tests of the Big Five and Tellegen's Three- and Four-Dimensional models. *Journal of Personality and Social Psychology, 66,* 83–114.

Criminal Code of Canada, R. S. C., C-46 (1985).

Cudeck, R., & Browne, M. W. (1983). Cross-validation of covariance structures. *Multivariate Behavioral Research, 18,* 147–167.

Dusky v. United States, 362 U. S. 402 (1960).

Favole, R. J. (1983). Mental disability in the American criminal process: A four issue survey. In J. Monahan & H. J. Steadman (Eds.), *Mentally disordered offenders: Perspectives from law and social science.* New York: Plenum.

Frith's Case, 22 How. St. Tr. 307 (1790).
Godinez v. Moran, 113 S. Ct. 2680 (1993).
Grisso, T. (1986). *Evaluating competencies: Forensic assessments and instruments.* New York: Plenum.
Grisso, T. (2002). *Evaluating competencies: Forensic assessments and instruments* (2nd ed.). New York: Plenum.
Grisso, T., & Appelbaum, P. (1998a). *Assessing competence to consent to treatment: A guide for physicians and other health care professionals.* New York: Oxford University Press.
Grisso, T., & Appelbaum, P. (1998b). *MacArthur Competence Assessment Tool for Treatment (MacCAT-T).* Sarasota, FL: Professional Resource.
Grisso, T., & Appelbaum, P. S. (1995). The MacArthur treatment competence study. III: Abilities of patients to consent to psychiatric and medical treatments. *Law and Human Behavior, 19,* 149–174.
Grisso, T., Appelbaum, P. S., & Hill-Fotouhi, C. (1997). The MacCAT-T: A clinical tool to assess patients' capacities to make treatment decisions. *Psychiatric Services, 48,* 1415–1419.
Grisso, T., Appelbaum, P. S., Mulvey, E. P., & Fletcher, K. (1995). The MacArthur treatment competence study. II: Measures of abilities related to competence to consent to treatment. *Law and Human Behavior, 19,* 127–148.
Hair, J. F., Jr., Anderson, R. E., Tatham, R. L., & Grablowsky, B. J. (1995). *Multivariate data analysis: With readings.* Englewood Cliffs, NJ: Prentice Hall.
Hoge, S. K., Bonnie, R. J., Poythress, N., & Monahan, J. (1999). *The MacArthur Competence Assessment Tool—Criminal Adjudication.* Odessa, FL: Psychological Assessment Resources.
Hoge, S. K., Bonnie, R. J., Poythress, N., Monahan, J., Eisenberg, M., & Feucht-Haviar, T. (1997). The MacArthur Adjudicative Competence Study: Development and validation of a research instrument. *Law and Human Behavior, 21,* 141–179.
Hoge, S. K., Poythress, N., Bonnie, R. J., Monahan, J., Eisenberg, M., & Feucht-Haviar, T. (1997). The MacArthur competence study: Diagnosis, psychopathology, and competence-related abilities. *Behavioral Sciences and the Law, 15,* 329–345.
Jöreskog, K. G., & Sörbom, D. (1989). *LISREL 7—A guide to the program and applications* (2nd ed.). Chicago: SPSS.
Jöreskog, K. G., & Sörbom, D. (1993a). *New features in LISREL 8.* Chicago: Scientific Software.
Jöreskog, K. G., & Sörbom, D. (1993b). *LISREL 8: Structural equation modeling with the SIMPLIS command language.* Chicago: Scientific Software.
Kline, R. (1998). *Principles and practice of structural equation modeling.* New York: Guilford.
Long, J. S. (1983a). *Confirmatory factor analysis: A preface to LISREL.* Beverly Hills, CA: Sage.
Long, J. S. (1983b). *Çovariance structure models : An introduction to LISREL.* Beverly Hills, CA: Sage.
MacCallum, R., & Austin, J. (2000). Applications of structural equation modeling in psychological research. *Annual Review of Psychology, 51,* 201–226.
Meisel, A., Roth, L. H., & Lidz, C. W. (1977). Toward a model of the legal doctrine of informed consent. *American Journal of Psychiatry, 134,* 285–289.
Otto, R. K., Poythress, N. G., Nicholson, R. A., Edens, J. F., Monahan, J., Bonnie, R. J., Hoge, S. K., & Eisenberg, M. (1998). Psychometric properties of the MacArthur Competence Assessment Tool—Criminal Adjudication (MacCAT-CA). *Psychological Assessment, 10,* 435–443.
Overall, J. E., & Gorham, D. R. (1962). The Brief Psychiatric Rating Scale. *Psychological Reports, 10,* 799–812.
Perlin, M. L. (1996). "Dignity was the first to leave": Godinez v. Moran, Colin Ferguson, and the trial of mentally disabled criminal defendants. *Behavioral Sciences and the Law, 14,* 61–81.
Poythress, N., Nicholson, R., Otto, R. K., Edens, J. F., Bonnie, R. J., Monahan, J., & Hoge, S. K. (1999). *The MacArthur Competence Assessment Tool—Criminal Adjudication: Professional manual.* Odessa, FL: Psychological Assessment Resources.
Regina v. Pritchard, 7 Car. & P. 304, 173 E. R. 135 (1836).
Regina v. Taylor, 77 C. C. C. (3d) 551 (Ont. C. A.) (1992).
Regina v. Whittle, 2 S. C. R. 914 (1994).
Roesch, R., & Golding, S. L. (1980). *Competency to stand trial.* Urbana, IL: University of Illinois Press.
Roesch, R., Hart, S. D., & Zapf, P. A. (1996). Conceptualizing and assessing competency to stand trial: Implications and applications of the MacArthur treatment competence model. *Psychology, Public Policy, and Law, 2,* 96–113.
Roesch, R., Zapf, P. A., Eaves, D., & Webster, C. D. (1998). *The Fitness Interview Test* (Rev. ed.). Burnaby, British Columbia: Mental Health, Law, & Policy Institute, Simon Fraser University.
Roth, L. H., Meisel, A., & Lidz, C. W. (1977). Tests of competency to consent to treatment. *American Journal of Psychiatry, 134,* 279–284.

Schwarzer, R. (1986). Evaluation of convergent and discriminant validity by use of structural equations. In A. Angleitner & J. S. Wiggins (Eds.), *Personality assessment via questionnaires: Current issues in theory and measurement* (pp. 191–213). Berlin: Springer-Verlag.

Stanley, B. (1987). Informed consent in treatment and research. In I. B. Weiner & A. K. Hess (Eds.), *Handbook of forensic psychology* (pp. 63–85). New York: Wiley.

Tepper, A., & Elwork, A. (1984). Competence to consent to treatment as a psycholegal construct. *Law and Human Behavior, 8,* 205–223.

The Queen v. Berry, 1 Q. B. D. 447 (1876).

Ullman, J. (2001). Structural equation modeling. In B. G. Tabachnick & L. S. Fidell (Eds.), *Using multivariate statistics* (4th ed., pp. 653–771). Boston: Allyn and Bacon.

Viljoen, J. L., Roesch, R., & Zapf, P. A. (2002). Interrater reliability of the Fitness Interview Test across four professional groups. *Canadian Journal of Psychiatry, 47,* 945–952.

Zapf, P. A., & Roesch, R. (1997). Assessing fitness to stand trial: A comparison of institution-based evaluations and a brief screening interview. *Canadian Journal of Community Mental Health, 16,* 53–66.

Zapf, P. A., & Roesch, R. (1998). Fitness to stand trial: Characteristics of remands since the 1992 Criminal Code amendments. *Canadian Journal of Psychiatry, 43,* 287–293.

Zapf, P. A., & Roesch, R. (2001). A comparison of the MacCAT-CA and the FIT for making determinations of competency to stand trial. *International Journal of Law and Psychiatry, 24,* 81–92.

Zapf, P. A., Roesch, R., & Viljoen, J. (2001). The utility of the Fitness Interview Test for assessing fitness to stand trial. *Canadian Journal of Psychiatry, 46,* 426–432.

Part II
Civil Forensic Assessment

[7]

Legal protection in psychiatry: balancing the rights and needs of patients and society

J Legemaate

Department of Health Policy and Management, Erasmus University, PO Box 1738, 3000 DR Rotterdam, The Netherlands

Summary - Attention to the legal position of psychiatric patients has greatly increased during the last 25 years. The criteria for a civil commitment have been tightened and procedural guarantees have increased. In many countries major changes and improvements in the area of mental health law took place. In this paper the main developments are discussed. Attention is given to the legal protection in case of civil commitment, to the legal position of the involuntarily admitted patient during his stay in hospital and to the relationship between patients' rights and the availability of mental health care. Furthermore the impact of legal intentions to the field of psychiatry is discussed. It is argued that legal interventions should be closely monitored, in order to prevent negative consequences. Legal interventions may be necessary, but this instrument should be used with great caution.

mental health law / patients' rights / legal protection

INTRODUCTION

Attention to the legal position of psychiatric patients has greatly increased during the last 25 years. As a result, among other things, the legislation with respect to involuntary admission to psychiatric hospitals has been revised in a large number of European countries [6]. Under the influence of both the jurisprudence of the European Court of Human Rights in Strasbourg [3] and the United Nations guidelines concerning the protection of persons with mental illness of 1991 [7] the patient's legal position has improved. The criteria for a civil commitment have been made more stringent, the procedural guarantees have increased. Legal aid was introduced for patients and nowadays we pay attention to the patient's legal position during his involuntary stay in hospital. It appears that the position of mental patients has been strengthened considerably. In this paper I will summarise and comment on the main legal developments in the area. Furthermore I will look into the relationship between patients' rights on the one hand and the availability of mental health facilities on the other. Finally I will discuss the impact of legal interventions in the field of psychiatry and the necessity to closely monitor the legislative developments in this area, in order to be able to balance the rights and needs of both mental patients and society.

LEGAL BACKGROUND

Until the beginning of the 1970s the procedure and criteria for involuntary admission were dominated primarily by medical considerations [4, 6]. The large international emancipation and democratisation movements in the 1960s played an important role in the improvement of individual legal rights for various categories of the socially disadvantaged. With regard to psychiatric patients one of the results was the new insight that the requirement of 'due process of law' was also applicable to their involuntary admission to a hospital. Another view being advocated was that patients could only be restricted in exercising their civil rights in cases which serve a compelling interest of the government, and even then, only if and when there was no less-restrictive alternative available to serve that interest. In these requirements of proportionality and subsidiarity which limitations on the legal rights of the mental patient must meet, the image of the patient as a *citizen with rights* emerged [4]. It was stipulated that the concept of citizenship with rights constitutes the core of legal protection and should be applied in constitutional states as a principle upon which the legal regulation of involuntary admission must be based.

The concept of citizenship with rights entails that all citizens, no matter where they reside, whether in freedom or in freedom-restricting institutions, must be allowed to continue to participate optimally in the law and in the application of the fundamental principles and values of justice. This means that those who are institutionalised in a psychiatric hospital must continue to enjoy their constitutional rights and other substantive civil rights and that, insofar as this is not always possible, they must be maximally accommodated in the needs for justice which are specifically inherent to the institutionalisation itself. The primary aim of legal protection is to award and strengthen procedural rights and possibilities, since these enable the individual to exercise his rights and to contest decisions made with regard to him. This strengthening of individual autonomy and independence can be seen as one of the preconditions for an acceptable 'environment' as it should exist in a welfare state which is also concerned with the well-fare and well-being of its citizens, and a fortiori when involuntary admission in a psychiatric hospital is involved. As a result the discussion is no longer limited to the criteria and procedure for involuntary admission. Nowadays it includes the patient's legal rights during his stay in hospital (hereafter referred to as the patient's internal legal position) as well. In the legislation effected in the previous century hardly any attention was paid to the internal legal position, but in the course of this century we increasingly realised that there were no good reasons for the automatic linkage of involuntary admission and incompetency. The shift from general to specific incompetence made it clear that a psychiatric disorder and/or an involuntary admission does not automatically render a patient incompetent to take decisions on certain matters. It has become necessary to develop a framework for the patient's internal legal position, addressing issues like information, consent, refusal of treatment and privacy.

The discussion about the legal position of psychiatric patients usually focuses on the triangle of autonomy, beneficence and the protection of society. This triangle represents the pluralistic set of objectives of what we understand to be 'mental health': here the tension between protecting society and the protection of the individual's rights is evident. It is customary to present the notions of autonomy, beneficence and protection of society in the form of contrasts. This is quite obvious in the case of an involuntary commitment. By speaking about involuntary admission in terms of contrasts it becomes clear that there are conflicting values and interests at stake. Generally speaking, however, we run a considerable risk of polarisation and a hardening in points of view by analysing solely in terms of contrasts. It is, for instance, not desirable to construct a black-and-white choice between beneficence and autonomy. It is much more a matter of degrees, a question of more or less. Wherever beneficence is overly dominant, one should aim at more autonomy. Patient, therapist and society have nothing to gain from a strong antithesis between these elements, but only by an optimal symbiosis between them. One should aim at a balance between justice and welfare. To what extent this balance is reached primarily in a legal way or by other means will depend on the conditions existing in each jurisdiction, such as legal tradition, cultural views, health care system and so on. When judging the impact of legal interventions one should always take this into account. I will come back to this issue later on.

LEGAL PROTECTION IN THE CASE OF CIVIL COMMITMENT

Originally, involuntary admission mainly had the character of a measure for the patient's own good in order to alleviate his suffering and protect him against himself [5, 6]. Nowadays, the central point is that civil commitment is a form of deprivation of freedom to which one may only proceed if this is strictly necessary. Procedural guarantees have been accentuated and the same holds true for the criteria on the basis of which involuntary admission is possible. Internationally speaking, a decision making model in which an independent decision maker, such as a judge, plays an important part is increasingly used (cf, the new Belgian law). In Europe the developments I am referring to are to a large degree the result of a strongly increased orientation on the European Convention of Human Rights. Section 5 of the Convention states that the deprivation of freedom of mental patients should take place 'in accordance with a procedure prescribed by law'. In a number of important decisions the European Court has described in fuller detail the legal guarantees which the patient may derive from these and other provisions of the Convention. In the past few years new legislation has come into effect in the Netherlands, Belgium, France and Austria as a result of this jurisprudence. Similar developments have taken place in the United States and Canada, in the latter case due to the enactment of the Canadian Charter of Rights and Freedoms. Of course, these developments are showing oscillations now and again, for instance with regard to the interpretation of the dangerous criterion in both the European and the American legislation and jurisprudence.

It is a well-known fact that the juridification of civil commitment has not passed off without any problems. From the circles of therapists in particular objections are raised to legal requirements which are considered to be an impediment for adequate therapy to patients with mental disorders. And yet, it seems that gradually among lawyers as well as therapists a certain degree of consensus is coming into being about the carefulness, including independent decision making, to be taken into account when decisions concerning deprivation of freedom are at stake. One of the advantages of this development is that it becomes possible to make a clear distinction between the responsibilities of the professionals involved. Whereas formerly the therapist was the one who technically of actually decided on involuntary admission, in modern legislation he is increasingly allotted the role of adviser. As a result his relationship with the patient is becoming less encumbered and we are getting better perspectives for reaching therapeutic results. The latter is all the more important as an involuntary admission definitely does not mark the best possible start of a successful patient-therapist relationship.

THE INTERNAL LEGAL POSITION OF THE INVOLUNTARILY ADMITTED PATIENT

As I mentioned before the changes with respect to the patient's legal position have not been restricted to civil commitment, but they have also had their effects on the legal position of the involuntarily admitted patient during his stay in hospital, the so-called 'internal legal position' of the patient [4, 5]. Nowadays we agree that a psychiatric disorder does not make a patient automatically and/or completely incompetent to take decisions on certain matters. As a result jurisprudence and most of the legislation are no longer confined to issues pertaining to the procedures and criteria for civil commitment. It has become necessary to develop a framework for the internal legal position, paying attention to the patient's right to information, the requirement of consent, the decision making process in respect to incompetency, the use of restraints and restrictions of freedom of movement, the right of access to records, etc. In the 1970s the lead was taken by the American jurisprudence but nowadays practically every new law in this field has a chapter on the internal legal position. However, we still have modern exceptions to this rule. The recent Belgian and French Acts still do not address the patient's internal legal position.

The most controversial result of this development is the right of the involuntarily admitted patient to refuse treatment. By now this right has been recognised on a large scale but its range has by no means been completely crystallised. A great deal of reluctance is, for instance, shown in the English Mental Health Act 1983, which only gives the patient a very limited right to refuse treatment. The Dutch Act of 1994 goes a bit further and includes the possibility of treating involuntarily admitted but competent patients when they present a serious danger in the hospital. At the other end of the spectrum we find the jurisdictions where involuntarily admitted patients who are competent to decide about treatment have an absolute right to refuse (among others Massachusetts, Ontario, and to a certain extent Austria). In the jurisdictions just mentioned the possibilities to apply involuntary treatment in a hospital are restricted to incompetent patients and patients causing an acute emergency. This development is in line with the views in legal literature wherein objections are increasingly being raised to involuntary treatment of competent psychiatric patients. A much heard argument is that it is a matter of discrimination on the grounds of mental disorder now that involuntary treatment of competent patients in general health care is usually considered to be unacceptable.

As a result of the right to refuse treatment the objectives of civil commitment and the position of the psychiatric hospital have come into a different perspective. Even though a large number of therapists has, in the mean time, accepted the fact that psychiatric patients do not lose their autonomy as a result of admission, they are drawing our attention to the negative effects to which an excessive right to refuse treatment may lead: unnecessary suffering, prolongation of hospitalisation and risks for fellow-patients and staff members. Research into the extent in which patients make use of this right, however, has shown that in practice the scale of the problem appears to be limited. In view of the pressure on the patient inherent in an involuntary admission to co-operate in the treatment, it is an illusion to think that the right to refuse treatment will enable the patient to make a free choice. The value of this right is mainly that it provides the patient a position to negotiate. Therapists will be expected to motivate their decisions conscientiously and to aim at a consensus with the patient for as far as this is possible. Looking at it from this angle, we may, in principle, speak of a development with positive aspects from both a legal and a therapeutical viewpoint. It is worth mentioning that the American psychiatrists who fiercely opposed the right-to-refuse-treatment-movement in their country nowadays tend to underline that having a legally regulated right to refuse treatment improves the patient's self-image and, as a result, the patient's compliance [1].

It is to be expected that in the years to come the focus

will shift more and more from the involuntary admission process to the patient's internal legal position. Both the 1994 Recommendation of the Parliamentary Assembly of the Council of Europe and the UN 'Principles' of December 1991 accentuate the importance of the patient's internal legal position. Its decision in the case of Herczegfalvy v Austria (1992) indicates that also the European Court will look at defects in the regulation of the patient's internal legal position scrupulously. Legislators in several countries have not yet adequately dealt with this issue.

PATIENTS' RIGHTS AND THE AVAILABILITY OF MENTAL HEALTH CARE

It is completely clear that major developments have taken place in the area of patients' rights regarding involuntary admission and the right to refuse treatment. These rights reflect important and internationally accepted fundamental standards and can in principle be applied all over the world. It is important to note, however, that the fundamental rights I mentioned should not be isolated from the quality and quantity of the mental health care available to the patient. What is the use of having a strong legal position concerning your individual rights when at the same time adequate mental health care is not available? What if a government invests a lot of energy in preparing modern legislation, but refuses to develop or adequately fund mental health facilities? In most western countries such a contradiction may seem out-dated. In other parts of Europe, however, we can identify countries in which creating legislation on patients' rights is given priority, while at the same time the restructuring of the often inadequate and badly organised mental health care is set behind. Let me give an example. The research-group I am part of was closely involved in a European PHARE-project aimed at developing health legislation in Albania, some time before last year's turmoil brought this country to complete chaos [2]. The Albanian authorities were interested very much in the development of western-style legislation, including mental health legislation, which incorporated all the internationals standards and human rights. But there was no health care structure to which the proposed legislation could be connected. I am not using this Albanian example to criticise this unfortunate country. The point I want to make is that in situations in which mental health care is poorly structured or perhaps even non-existent one should always do two things at the same time: defining and implementing patients' rights and realising mental health care of good quality. And if at any given moment it is unavoidable to make a (temporary) choice between the two the latter should be given priority. Having good mental health care while not having rights in my opinion is less dramatic than having rights but not having good mental health care. It is important that international standards and guidelines concerning mental health and mentally ill persons underline the importance of connecting the issue of individual rights on the one hand and the availability of mental health facilities on the other. We see this for instance in the 1991 UN-principles. UN-Principle 14 rightly stipulates that a mental health facility should have access to the same level of resources as any other health establishment. When the need for having adequate legislation is over-emphasised the development of good mental health facilities may be jeopardised. Over-emphasising the importance of legislation may even be done on purpose, to conceal defects regarding the availability and quality of mental health care itself. In some parts of the former USSR this kind of window-dressing has become quite popular.

THE LIMITS OF THE LAW

This brings me to the final issue I want to address, which is the impact of legal interventions in the field of psychiatry. Legal action in this area is both useful and necessary, but it is important not to overestimate the impact of legal interventions and to be constantly aware of the limits of the law. The law may increase the awareness of a society concerning fundamental principles or values, but it functions quite poorly in the area of changing undesirable behaviour. A few years ago the well-known American psychiatrist Paul Appelbaum addressed this issue [1]. Looking back at the legal developments in the United States in the 1970s and 1980s Appelbaum concludes that daily practices often develop themselves rather independent from the intentions of legislators and courts. Consequences of legal reform were much more limited than partisans on either side anticipated, Appelbaum shows us. He makes it clear that a law is doomed to fail, it its contents does not reflect, at least to a certain extent, the moral views of the professionals who have to implement the act: "Law represents an embodiment of the moral sentiments of a community. When those sentiments can be honoured only by violating the terms of the law, a tension is created between law and morality" ([1] p 56). In the long run such a tension will undermine the legitimacy of the law. It is absolutely necessary to monitor and assess the impact of legal interventions. Not to set aside the rule of law, but to connect as carefully as possible normative concepts and the needs and characteristics of daily practice. In the Netherlands we have tried to remedy these kind of problems by introducing a policy aimed at the evaluation of legislation. Most of the recent health care legislation in the Netherlands obliges the legislator to evaluate the Act and to present the results of the evaluation to Parliament. In 1994 the Dutch Lunacy Act of 1884 was replaced by the Act on Formal Admissions to a Psychiatric Hospital. In December 1996 the results of the first evaluation of the new Act were published. The evaluation appeared to have been carried out a little bit too soon, but nevertheless generated empirical information indicating the necessity of changing some parts of the new Act. In November 1997 the Dutch government informed Parliament about its official position regarding the evaluation results. It is to be expected that after a parliamentary debate some sections of the Act will be revised. Such a process of evaluation is one of the means to identify and remedy tensions between theory and practice. As a result both the quality of mental health care and the quality of legislation may improve.

CONCLUSIONS

Since the early part of the 1970s attention for the psychiatric patient's legal position has increased substantially. The case law of the European Court on Human Rights revealed that the legislation on involuntary admission in a number of European countries did not meet all the safeguards and requirements of the European Convention. In many countries the legislator decided to adjust the domestic legislation. In at least nine European countries the legislation was revised in the period 1978–1992. In most of these countries this revision was inspired to a large extent by the desire to improve the patient's legal position. For as far as this goes, we can speak of a development on a European level. In some countries major changes or improvements took place. After 140 years the Belgium legislator replaced a law based on a 'medical model' decision making (inspired by the famous French law of 1838) by a much more legally oriented approach. In The Netherlands the legislator stuck to the principles already apparent in the previous century (such as decision making by a judge) but added an important chapter on the patient's internal legal position to the new law.

Generally speaking, the revised legal regulations are an improvement in comparison with the legislation previously prevailing in the countries concerned. But if we compare the individual countries with each other, then great differences are to be found with respect to the starting-points and the extent to which the patient is offered legal protection. These differences concern the criteria as well as the decision-making procedure (physician or judge) and the other legal guarantees (whether there is legal aid, periodic reviewing or not). There are also major differences on the point of the internal legal position, an issue–as I mentioned earlier–that will be accentuated in the years to come. It is clear that the European Convention does not necessarily lead to a harmonisation of European legislation. Both the Convention and the case law of the European Court leave room for different national approaches. This reflects the relevance of the national, cultural, legal and health care characteristics of each jurisdiction. But even though there can be a great variation in the extent to which and in the manner in which the patient is offered legal protection, the actual practice in the various countries may be similar in many ways. For example, the percentages of patients admitted voluntarily and involuntarily show approximately the same ratio in almost all countries. In England/Wales (medically oriented process of decision making) the percentage of patients admitted involuntarily is less than in The Netherlands (legally oriented process of decision making). This finding makes it clear that the balance between medical and legal decision making approaches is not the only relevant aspect. Not only legal and medical factors play a role, but other social forces as well. This may vary from the policy regarding financial responsibility (is that a national or a regional responsibility) to the availability of community-based alternative. Also the general attitude in society with regard to mental illness and legal protection is important. These phenomena call for further research into the relevant national circumstances and characteristics. An overview of legislative developments is an important but incomplete source of information, as far as the developments in actual practice are concerned. The law does not reveal possible gaps between legislation and actual practice. The reasons underlying these gaps, and the way in which they influence the implementation of the law, require empirical research, for instance in the context of the evaluation of legislation. Legal interventions may be necessary, but this instrument should be used with great caution. A policy based on both the importance and the limits of legal interventions provides the best starting-point for future changes in mental health law, to the advantage of both patients and society.

REFERENCES

1 Appelbaum PS. *Almost a revolution - mental health law and the limits of change*. New York: Oxford University Press; 1994

2 Den Exter AP et al. Health care legislation in central and eastern Europe. *Rev Cent Eastern Eur Law* 1997 ; 23 : 117-32

3 Harding TW. The application of the European Convention of Human Rights to the field of psychiatry. *Int J Law Psychiatry* 1989 ; 12 : 245-62

4 Kelk C, Legemaate J. *Rechtsbescherming in de psychiatry - Een rechtsvergelijkend perspectief [Legal protection in psychiatry - a comparative perspective]*. Utrecht: Kluwer; 1990

5 Legemaate J. Compulsion and patients' rights in psychiatry: an international perspective. In: Casselman J et al, eds. *Law and mental health*. Leuven: 1992. p 94-103

6 Legemaate J. Involuntary admission to a psychiatric hospital: recent European developments. European Journal of Health Law 1995; 2: 15-32.

[8]

The MacArthur Treatment Competence Study. I

Mental Illness and Competence to Consent to Treatment*

Paul S. Appelbaum and Thomas Grisso

This is the first of three papers reporting the results of the MacArthur Treatment Competence Study, a project designed to develop reliable and valid information with which to address clinical and policy questions regarding the abilities of persons with mental illness to make decisions about psychiatric treatment. Four commonly applied legal standards for determining decision-making competence are described: abilities to communicate a choice, understand relevant information, appreciate the nature of the situation and its likely consequences, and rationally manipulate information. Previous research related to the capacities of persons with mental illness in relation to these standards is reviewed and critiqued. The principles underlying the design of the MacArthur Treatment Competence Study are described.

The legal doctrine of informed consent to treatment is aimed at promoting a meaningful role for patients in making decisions about their care. Conceived in U.S. courts in the 1950s, under the influence of common law rules proscribing unwanted intrusions on bodily integrity, informed consent law was fully developed over the two subsequent decades. Since then, informed consent has become a

---

* This work was supported by the Research Network on Mental Health and the Law, John D. and Catherine T. MacArthur Foundation. The authors are grateful to the members of the Network for their assistance in the conceptual development of this project and for their comments on an earlier draft of this paper: Shirley Abrahamson, Richard Bonnie, Pamela Hyde, John Monahan, Stephen Morse, Ed Mulvey, Loren Roth, Paul Slovic, Henry Steadman, and David Wexler. Address correspondence to either author at Department of Psychiatry, University of Massachusetts Medical School, Worcester, MA 01655.

nearly universal prerequisite to the initiation of medical diagnostic and treatment procedures (Appelbaum, Lidz, & Meisel, 1987). Its principles have been applied to a range of other clinical interventions, from psychotherapy to release of confidential information (Appelbaum & Gutheil, 1991).

Informed consent law has established three requirements for valid consent to treatment. First, care-givers, usually patients' physicians, are responsible for providing patients with information regarding the nature and purpose of the recommended procedure, probable benefits, likely risks, and the alternatives to the proposed treatment—including the option of forgoing treatment altogether—along with their benefits and risks. In most jurisdictions, the amount and precise details of the information to be disclosed are determined by what a reasonable person would find material to a decision about treatment (Merz & Fischoff, 1990). Second, patients must have the opportunity to make decisions in the absence of coercion by those providing their care. This requirement for a voluntary decision is the least well-analyzed and least frequently litigated component of informed consent law (Faden & Beauchamp, 1986).

Finally, patients must be competent to make treatment decisions. Since informed consent law is aimed at encouraging patients' participation in the decision-making process, its rationale is undermined when patients' incapacities preclude them from playing a meaningful role. In those cases in which mental disabilities result in substantial decision-making impairment, a substitute decision maker will be called upon to protect patients' interests (Meisel, 1979).

This article and the two articles that follow (Grisso, Appelbaum, Mulvey, & Fletcher, 1995; Grisso & Appelbaum, 1995) focus on the requirement that patients be competent to give valid consent to treatment and, in particular, on the role that mental illness may play in impairing decision-making abilities. The first article in this series explores recent changes in how medicine and law have responded to persons with mental illness who may be legally incompetent to make decisions about their medical and psychiatric treatment, reviews what is known about the impact of mental illness on decision-making abilities related to legal competence, and describes the design of the MacArthur Treatment Competence Study, an effort to develop standardized means of assessing decision-making abilities in the context of consent to treatment. In the second article (Grisso et al., 1995), the measures developed for the study are described and their psychometric properties are detailed. The final article (Grisso & Appelbaum, 1995) reports the results of an application of these instruments to samples of patients with mental illness and medical illness and non-ill control groups, with consideration of the implications of these findings for policy regarding consent to treatment.

Mental Illness, Competence, and Consent to Treatment

Consent and Persons with Mental Illness

Before the development of informed consent law, relations between patients and physicians had been governed for centuries by the requirement that patients' simple consent be sought for medical interventions (Appelbaum et al., 1987; *Slater v. Baker & Stapleton*, 1767). That is, physicians were obligated, on pain of liability for battery, to inform patients of the nature of the proposed intervention and to obtain their agreement before proceeding. Until recent years, however, persons with mental illness had been dealt with as exceptions to the usual requirements for consent.

Nineteenth-century medicine, for example, expressed the belief that mental illness invariably destroyed decision-making capacities, rendering patients unable to make valid decisions of any kind (Ray, 1864). Thus, although statutes authorizing involuntary hospitalization of persons with mental illness became widespread in the 1830s and 1840s, it was not until 1881 that the first state (Massachusetts) codified a procedure for voluntary hospitalization (Brakel, 1985). Families usually made the decision to hospitalize persons with mental illness in the nineteenth century, and their consent to treatment generally was accepted as valid. Indigent persons without involved families often were hospitalized by authority of the overseers of the poor (Appelbaum & Kemp, 1982). Whether patients were committed involuntarily or admitted themselves voluntarily, the question of consent to treatment once hospitalized seems not to have been raised.

With the growth of informed consent law after the middle of the twentieth century, the assumption that people with mental illness were uniformly deficient in decision-making abilities and should be considered legally incompetent began to be called into question (Shapiro, 1974). Advocates argued that persons with mental illness, like persons with mental retardation, often suffered selective impairment of decision-making abilities or none at all, with retention of competence for many purposes. It was unfair, therefore, to deprive them of decision-making rights, especially about treatment, without an individualized determination of their residual capacities. By the late 1970s, courts began to accept this argument, frequently imposing requirements that a formal hearing occur at which persons with mental illness are found incompetent before treatment can take place over their objections (e.g., *Goedeke v. State*, 1979; *In re the Mental Health of K. K. B.*, 1980; *Jarvis v. Levine*, 1988; *Riese v. St. Mary's Hospital*, 1987; *Rivers v. Katz, 1986; Rogers v. Okin*, 1979; *State ex rel. Jones v. Gerhardstein*, 1987). Conversely, if patients were found to lack the requisite abilities, several courts suggested that their agreements to undergo hospitalization or treatment may be considered invalid (*Rogers v. Commissioner*, 1983; *Zinermon v. Burch*, 1990).

Patients' "right to refuse treatment," the rubric under which this issue was usually discussed, became a highly contentious matter, particularly as applied to involuntarily committed mental patients (Appelbaum, 1988, 1994). Many mental health professionals argued against the new rules on the basis that their nineteenth-century predecessors had been correct: Severe mental illness almost always destroyed decision-making abilities, particularly with regard to treatment of the disorder itself. Thus, they contended, most patients with severe mental illness were not able to recognize the existence of their illness and their need for care (American Psychiatric Association, 1980). Others objected to the imposition of formal legal proceedings for determining competence. They maintained that if not universal, serious deficiencies in decisional abilities were sufficiently frequent among patients that the burden of preparing for and attending court hearings would be overwhelming (Mills, Yesavage, & Gutheil, 1983; Rachlin, 1975).[1] Reliable and valid means of assessing the decision-making abilities of persons with mental illness, and means of comparing them to groups of people without mental illness, became crucial to the resolution of these controversies.

Simultaneously, the introduction of requirements for individualized assessment of decision-making capacities, especially in treatment settings, underscored the critical need for clearly defined standards and procedures for making determinations concerning competence (Cutter & Shelp, 1991; McKinnon, Cournos, & Stanley, 1989). Clinicians required guidance in weighing whether to accept patients' consent or refusal on the basis that their competent wishes should be respected or to challenge them in the belief that patients were incompetent to make decisions. When general medical or surgical treatment was in question, the clinician's judgment, perhaps augmented by a colleague's consultation, was likely to be determinative; commonly accepted practice calls for physicians to abide by the family's wishes in such cases, without legal formalities (President's Commission, 1982). With regard to psychiatric treatment, for which many states require judicial or administrative review of competence determinations, a new set of nonclinical decision makers was now also in need of assistance in reaching conclusions about patients' competence.

Legal Standards for Assessing Decision-Making Competence

Despite the conceptual importance of competence as the touchstone for determining whether a person's decisions will be set aside, until recently relatively little attention has been given to the legal standards to be employed in determining competence. Indeed, the most influential scholar of competence prior to this generation suggested that, in practice, when a party's competence was challenged, courts often focused more on the reasonableness of the contract in question than on the decision-making abilities of the alleged incompetent person (Green, 1944). Even the article that reawakened modern interest in legal standards of competence to consent to treatment despaired of identifying a single operative standard as "a search for the holy grail" (Roth, Meisel, & Lidz, 1977).

The work of Roth and his colleagues (1977), however, has led to an evolving consensus on the standards that are generally applied by the courts when determining competence to consent to treatment (Annas & Densberger, 1984; Bonnie, 1993; Drane, 1984; Grisso, 1986; McKinnon, Cournos, & Stanley, 1989; Tepper & Elwork, 1984). Their critical insight was that courts did not apply a single standard in all cases, but generally chose from a small number of possibilities in selecting the standards to be used in particular instances. Depending on the facts of a case and precedent in that jurisdiction, court decisions might be based on one standard or some combination of standards. As refined in subsequent work (Appelbaum &

[1] Opposition to the right to refuse treatment was not always centered on the question of patients' decision-making capacities. Some commentators argued that competence was irrelevant in the case of involuntarily committed patients: Whatever gave the state right to deprive them of liberty (i.e., the police power or the parens patriae function) also provided sufficient basis for nonconsensual treatment aimed at restoring liberty (Appelbaum, 1994).

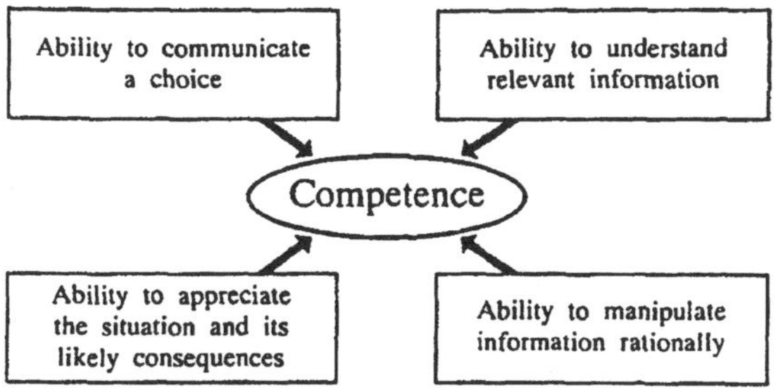

Fig. 1. Structure of competence to consent to treatment.

Roth, 1982; Appelbaum & Grisso, 1988), four legal standards for determining competence have been identified.[2] Each standard implicates a set of decision-making abilities that must be considered to assess whether the standard has been met (Grisso, 1986).

Ability to communicate a choice is the first, and least stringent, standard that ordinarily is applied. When patients are unable, as a result of illness, to reach a decision or to indicate to their caregivers what course of treatment they desire, they uniformly will be considered incompetent (*Matter of Conroy*, 1985; *Matter of O'Brien*, 1986; President's Commission, 1982). Indeed, so self-evident is this standard that courts often fail to mention it explicitly, taking the incompetence of noncommunicative patients as a matter of course (*Superintendent of Belchertown State School v. Saikewicz*, 1977). Some patients are able to express choices, but their decisions vacillate to such an extent that a course of treatment cannot be implemented before they change their minds again. They also may be considered not to have met this standard. Although maximally protective of individual decision-making rights, a standard that focuses only on the ability to communicate a choice recognizes decisions as valid regardless of the process by which they are reached.

The second and most common component of judicial standards for competence is the *ability to understand relevant information*, a standard that emphasizes the importance of patients' comprehension of information related to the issue at hand. This requirement is often overtly derived from contract law (White & De-

[2] The original article by Roth et al. (1977) included two standards not discussed here and omitted one that has become accepted since. Roth and colleagues distinguished between ability to understand relevant information and actual understanding; rather than representing separate standards, however, these can be seen as the statement of a standard (i.e., one must have the ability to understand) and specification of how achievement of that standard will be measured (i.e., the patient must actually understand the information). Their paper also pointed to reasonable outcome of the patient's choice as an alternate standard. As they themselves acknowledged, however, this is less a standard of decision-making competence than it is a way of voiding patients' decisions on grounds other than the process by which the decision was made. Although, as suggested by Green (1944), the choice made may have an important influence on judicial decisions, it is not, strictly speaking, a standard of judging patients' competence. Finally, the original paper omitted mention of appreciation of the nature of the situation and potential consequences, a standard described by Appelbaum and Roth (1982).

nise, 1991), where it serves as the basis for determinations of competence to contract. Its application is seen in *Grannum v. Berard* (1967), a case in which a patient challenged the validity of a consent he had given for nasal surgery, alleging that he had been incompetent because of the effects of the medications he was receiving. The court held that "The [test of] mental competency or capacity of an individual to execute an agreement . . . [is] whether the person . . . possessed sufficient mind or reason to enable him to understand the nature, the terms and the effect of the transaction" (p. 814). In treatment situations, the information that must be understood is generally that which must be disclosed to the patient under the law of informed consent.

A third legal standard is the *ability to appreciate the nature of the situation and its likely consequences*. This standard differs from an ability to understand information in requiring that patients be able to apply the information abstractly understood to their own situation. Thus, patients who understand that their physicians believe they are ill, but, in the face of objective evidence to the contrary, deny that this is so, or who understand that an effective treatment exists, but refuse to believe that it is likely to help them, will be said to lack appreciation. Use of the appreciation standard is demonstrated in two contrasting Massachusetts cases. In *Lane v. Candura* (1978), the appellate court overturned a finding of incompetence concerning a woman who was refusing amputation of a gangrenous leg. The court upheld her right to make that choice, finding that she "appreciat[ed] the nature and consequences of her act" (p. 1236), specifically that she was suffering from gangrene and likely would die without surgery. In contrast, the state's Supreme Judicial Court ruled incompetent a man suffering from schizophrenia whose refusal to take medication was based on denial that he was mentally ill, which prevented him from "appreciat[ing] the need to control his illness with antipsychotic medication," or "the risks associated with refusing it" (p. 1286) (*Guardianship of John Roe,* 1992).

Finally, courts also have applied the standard of *ability to manipulate information rationally* in determining decision-making competence. This standard emphasizes patients' abilities to employ logical processes to compare the benefits and risks of treatment options. Even in the presence of good understanding and appreciation, decision making still might be impaired if patients fail to process information logically. Conversely, the rational manipulation standard might be met even by patients who have impaired understanding or defective appreciation if their reasoning processes are intact. Some courts have shied away from embracing this standard because of an apparent confusion regarding interpretation of the term *irrational*. A decision sometimes has been called irrational merely because the patient's choice was unconventional (which is not a sufficient basis by itself to consider the decision maker incompetent) (*In re Milton,* 1987; *In re Yetter,* 1973). In contrast, the "irrationality" to which this standard properly refers pertains to illogic in the processing of information, not the choice that eventually is made. An example of a court adopting this standard is found in *Riese v. St. Mary's Hospital* (1987), a California case dealing with mental patients' right to refuse treatment. After endorsing understanding and appreciation standards, the court indicated that legal competence also required an ability to "knowingly and intelligently evaluate the information . . . and otherwise participate in the treatment decision by means of rational thought processes" (p. 254).

As suggested by the *Riese* decision, courts often create compound legal standards for their jurisdictions. The New Jersey Supreme Court in *Matter of Conroy* (1985), for example, held that "[a] patient may be incompetent because he lacks the ability to understand the information conveyed, to evaluate the options, or to communicate a decision" (p. 1241), apparently combining understanding, rational manipulation, and communicating standards. Even in cases where courts cite one standard or some combination of standards, it is difficult to know the extent to which their decisions are being narrowly tailored to the facts of a particular case and whether additional standards might be included in other fact situations. Thus, faced with a patient who denied the existence of his or her disorder, New Jersey courts might determine that the ability to "evaluate the options," required by *Conroy*, goes beyond the rational manipulation standard that it appears to endorse and includes an appreciation standard as well.

In addition to helping clinicians and judges clarify the basis for their competence decisions, this conceptualization of operative standards for legal competence laid the groundwork for empirical examination of policy-relevant questions.[3] Indeed, almost all of that empirical literature postdates the original Roth et al. (1977) paper, and much of it refers explicitly to their work. For our purposes here, it is important to determine what that literature tells us about the relationship between mental illness and the psychological abilities relevant to competence to make decisions about treatment, and what questions the previous studies have left unanswered.

Research on Mental Illness and Decision-making Capacities

Mental illnesses involve alterations of mental functioning, including attention, perception, cognition, and mood, all of which might be expected to affect decision making. We review here those studies that explicitly have attempted to ascertain the impact of mental illness on abilities related to one or more of the four legal standards for decision-making competence described above. Several considerations should be kept in mind in assessing these data.

First, mental illness is not a homogeneous category. Patterns of deficits in cognitive functioning would be expected to differ across diagnostic groups. Thus, studies of patients with schizophrenia might yield quite different findings than studies of depressed patients. The care with which diagnostic determinations are made will affect the composition of subject groups and, thus, the results of the study. Meaningful conclusions are likely to be made only within well-defined diagnostic categories.

Second, the impact of symptoms of mental illness on mental functioning may

[3] Although this model was formulated explicitly to describe competence judgments related to consent for treatment, it may well be more broadly applicable to decision-making competence in general. For an effort to apply the model to defendants' competence to make decisions related to their defense, see Bonnie (1993).

fluctuate with the severity of the disorder. Acutely ill patients who recently have been hospitalized may show greater degrees of impairment than patients who have undergone a course of treatment and are about to be discharged; samples recruited in the community may manifest still higher levels of function. Comparisons among studies must take this issue into account. Independent measures of symptom severity are crucial in characterizing the populations under examination.

Third, considerable variability is introduced into these data by the lack of standardized means of measuring the dependent variables. Investigators frequently devise their own measures of understanding, appreciation, and rational manipulation, with varying (and often unspecified) psychometric properties. Adoption of standardized measures has been impeded by the difficulty of translating legal standards for decision-making competence into psychological constructs that lend themselves to consistent operationalization (Grisso, 1986).

Finally, sampling problems are omnipresent. Researchers investigating the decision-making abilities of people with mental illness must begin by asking them to decide whether or not to participate in the research study. Patients who lack even minimal abilities to consent to participation or who are so disorganized as to be unable to complete the study protocols almost always must be excluded. Thus, the very population of greatest interest—persons whose decision making is manifestly impaired—tends to be selectively eliminated from most studies. This problem is somewhat mitigated by the use of a relatively low threshold of abilities for determining subjects' competence to consent to participation in studies with little or no risk; most investigators require minimal understanding of the consent disclosure. Nonetheless, almost all existing data systematically underestimate the prevalence and degree of impairment in more severely ill populations, because of the necessary exclusion of the most severely impaired patients.

Ability to Communicate a Choice

Relatively few studies have examined the abilities of people with mental illness to reach and communicate choices, perhaps in part because of the methodologic issues referred to above: Unless patients' abilities in this area are intact, they cannot decide whether to participate in the study itself, nor can they indicate their willingness to do so. In reporting their data, unfortunately, most investigators fail to separate potential subjects who did not respond to their requests to join the study from those who refused to participate. Some data, however, offer rough approximations regarding the frequency of severe impairments in reaching and communicating choices.

Appelbaum, Mirkin, and Bateman (1981) evaluated decision-making capacities in a group of 75 diagnostically heterogeneous, but primarily schizophrenic (62%), inpatients, who were admitted consecutively to a community mental health center. They found that 7 patients (9%) were mute or catatonic when approached about participating in the study (although one was deaf and another spoke no English, lowering the probable incidence of truly incapable subjects to 6.7%). Another inpatient study, using a sample mostly suffering from mood disorders, presented subjects with two vignettes requiring resolution of dilemmas not involving treatment (Radford, Mann, & Kalucy, 1986). Seven of 39 subjects (18%) were noted to be "incapable of deciding."

This dearth of information regarding the distribution of abilities to communicate a choice can be remedied in two ways. Clinical populations can be observed in naturalistic settings to ascertain the incidence of actual failures to communicate choices (e.g., patients in an emergency room for whom admission is being recommended or potential subjects being approached for participation in research). Alternatively, hypothetical choices can be placed before research subjects, as in the study of Radford et al. (1986). The latter strategy affords a greater degree of control over the decision task and offers more opportunities to collect data on predictive variables, whereas the former is less likely to result in the exclusion of the most severely impaired subjects from the sample.

Ability to Understand Relevant Information

Studies of comprehension of relevant information can be divided into two categories. The first group comprises surveys of what people with mental illness know about their treatment (Appelbaum et al., 1981; Hoffman & Srinivasan, 1992; Jaffe, 1986; Linden & Chaskel, 1981; Norko, Billick, McCarrick, & Schwartz, 1990; Olin & Olin, 1975; Soskis, 1978; Soskis & Jaffe, 1979). In general, the findings in these studies are similar to those of Geller (1982), who surveyed all 281 patients in a state hospital on a single day regarding knowledge of their medications. Sixty-nine percent of patients could not name even one medication they took, and 59% did not know how often their medications were administered. Fewer than one half of the patients surveyed knew what the medications were supposed to do.

Although this group of studies reveals an alarming lack of knowledge regarding treatment, the relationship to impaired ability to understand is unclear. The method assumes that patients have been given the information being sought, which other studies suggest often is not the case (Benson, 1983; Lidz et al., 1984). Even if the information was revealed (for example, in consent forms patients were asked to sign), patients may not have attended to the disclosure, or their comprehension may have been limited by poor literacy skills, not mental illness (Berg & Hammitt, 1980; Coles, 1978). In some cases, disclosure may have occurred at such a remote time that, although once understood, the information was long since forgotten. Finally, the relation of mental illness to subjects' poor understanding remains unclear without an evaluation of the performance of subjects without mental illness.

In the second group of studies on abilities to understand, some of these problems were reduced by observation of the disclosure (Benson, Roth, Appelbaum, Lidz, & Winslade, 1988; Lidz et al., 1984) or presentation of a standardized disclosure (Beck, 1988; Beck & Staffin, 1986; Benson et al., 1988; Grossman & Summers, 1980; Irwin et al., 1985; Janofsky, McCarthy, & Folstein, 1992; Kleinman, Schacter, & Koritar, 1989; Munetz & Roth, 1985; Palmer & Wohl, 1972; Roth et al. 1982). Results from Irwin et al. (1985) demonstrate both the usual findings of this group of studies and the methodologic problems common to many efforts. Forty-seven psychotic inpatients were assessed, of whom two thirds had schizophrenic and the remainder affective disorders. Information about antipsychotic medication was read to each subject, followed by a series of questions. Most patients claimed they understood the information, but 19% to 43% were classified as having poor comprehension (depending on the criteria used), and only 26% to 60% as having substantial comprehension. Most of the other studies in this category report similar degrees of deficits.

Unfortunately, the procedures used in the study compromise the degree of assurance with which its findings can be endorsed. The disclosure was read to subjects, obviating the problem of poor reading skills, but its level of complexity was not measured in any standard way. Scoring appears to have been performed in a nonblind fashion by the interviewer, with no efforts reported to establish reliability. Criteria for scoring of responses are not specified. Thus, subsequent researchers desiring to replicate this study would be unable to do so.

Implicit in many of the studies of understanding is the assumption that detected impairments can be attributed to mental illness. Other factors, however, such as the stress associated with any illness, might compromise understanding even in persons without mental illness. A few studies have compared the performance of samples with and without mental illness. Jaffe (1986), for example, found no differences in understanding (without controlled disclosure) between two groups of 16 outpatients, one treated for mental disorder and the other for a physical condition. The sample, however, was small, and the scoring criteria were vague and of uncertain reliability. Nonetheless, similar results appeared in comparisons of elderly depressed patients with nonpsychiatrically ill older persons after information disclosure (Stanley, Stanley, Guido, & Garvin, 1988) and in two studies of inpatients with mental and medical illnesses (Janofsky et al., 1992; Soskis, 1978).

On the other hand, examinations of the correlates of poor performance within groups with mental illness have revealed significant relationships with various kinds of symptomatology. Thought disorder (Irwin et al., 1985), evidence of organic impairment (Janofsky et al., 1992), psychosis (Roth et al., 1982), and a diagnosis of schizophrenia as opposed to depression (Benson et al., 1988) all predicted poorer performance. Thus, suggestive evidence exists both supporting and refuting the impact of mental illnesses on ability to understand relevant information.

To avoid the problems of most earlier studies, future research on understanding in mentally ill persons should use standardized disclosures of predetermined levels of complexity, structured probes, and scoring procedures of known reliability. Analyses should control for diagnosis, symptomatology, and sociodemographic factors that might affect comprehension (e.g., age, education, social class). If causal relationships are to be established with mental disorders, control groups without mental illness must be included.

Ability to Appreciate the Nature of the Situation and Its Likely Consequences

Competent decision making according to the appreciation standard requires recognition that one is suffering from a disorder and that the generally accepted risks and benefits of treatment apply to one's own situation. An enormous literature exists in this area, perhaps because failures in appreciation often are considered to be core components of the major psychiatric disorders. (Efforts also have been made to assess appreciation in medical patients—e.g., Levine et al., 1986—a literature that will not be reviewed here.)

Many studies document impairments in the abilities of patients with schizophrenia to appreciate that they are ill (usually termed *denial* or *lack of insight*) (Amador et al., 1993; Appelbaum et al., 1981; Brooks, Deane, & Hugel, 1968; Davidhizar & Wehlage, 1984; Greenfield, Strauss, Bowers, & Mandelkern, 1989; Heinrichs, Cohen, & Carpenter, 1985; Hoffman & Srinivasan, 1992; Lin, Spiga, & Fortsch, 1979; Markova & Berrios, 1992; McEvoy, Aland, Wilson, Guy, & Hawkins, 1981; McEvoy, Appelbaum, Apperson, Geller, & Freter, 1989; McEvoy, Apperson et al., 1989; McEvoy, Freter et al., 1989; McEvoy, Schooler, Friedman, Steingard, & Allen, 1993; Munetz & Roth, 1985; Norko et al., 1990; Takai, Uematsu, Ueki, Sone, & Kaiya, 1992; Van Putten, Crumpton, & Yale, 1961; Walker & Rossiter, 1989; Wing, Monck, Brown, & Carstairs, 1964). Indeed, lack of insight was identified as the most common symptom in the core group of schizophrenics in the World Health Organization's International Pilot Study of Schizophrenia (Carpenter, Bartko, Carpenter, & Strauss, 1976), a finding confirmed in another multinational study by Wilson, Ban, and Guy (1986). Nonetheless, when dichotomous judgments have been made, the percentage of patients with schizophrenia reported as lacking insight has varied widely, from 97% (Carpenter et al., 1976) to as little as 27% (Wing et al., 1964), despite similar measures of the concept.

Recent studies have separated insight into subcomponents, looking at the ability to acknowledge current problems as a separate dimension from acknowledgment of problems in the past or the possibility of problems in the future (Amador et al., 1993; McEvoy, Apperson et al., 1989). Conflicting results have been reported on the degree of correlation among these dimensions. Recognition of the presence of abnormal mental events has been distinguished conceptually from identification of those events as symptoms of a mental disorder, although these characteristics seem to be highly correlated (Amador et al., 1993; Greenfield et al., 1989). Investigators also have examined the ability of patients with schizophrenia to appreciate their need for treatment in the present and the future (Lin et al., 1979; McEvoy et al., 1981; McEvoy, Apperson et al., 1989), both of which generally have been found to be impaired.

Patients with depression are the other major group whose degree of appreciation has been subject to extensive study. The association of depression with feelings of hopelessness and helplessness (American Psychiatric Association, 1987) has led investigators to wonder whether people with depression might have impaired appreciation of likely consequences of a situation, focusing too one-sidedly on negative outcomes (Ackermann & DeRubeis, 1991). Research was stimulated by early findings suggesting that depression, paradoxically, might contribute to more realistic assessments, stripping away the illusions that contribute to false optimism in nondepressed populations (Taylor, 1989). Reviews of this literature have pointed to conflicting findings in this regard, as well as the tendency to use subjects who display symptoms of dysphoria but do not meet criteria for clinical depression (Ackermann & DeRubeis, 1991).

Indeed, results from the small number of studies with clinical populations support Taylor's hypothesis: Mild depression may be associated with depressive realism, but severe depression is characterized by overt cognitive distortions (Taylor, 1989). Morgado, Smith, Lecrubier, and Widlocher (1991), for example, assessed 25 patients with major depression on a scale of social adjustment, comparing the data with patients' self-reports. When depressed, but not when recovered, patients markedly overreported maladjustment. Unfortunately, we are unaware of studies directly examining decision making relative to treatment of patients with depression.

Limited investigations have examined the relationship of impairments of appreciation in groups with mental illness to the presence or severity of the mental illness itself. Comparisons with populations without mental illness are almost entirely lacking. In one study, a mixed group of psychiatric inpatients was shown to be significantly less likely to acknowledge mental problems at admission, but not at discharge, compared with medically ill controls (Small, Messina, & Small, 1964). Several studies have examined correlations between impaired appreciation and severity of symptoms, with results both supporting (Markova & Berrios, 1992; Takai et al., 1992) and refuting (Amador et al., 1993; McEvoy, Apperson et al., 1989) the presence of a relationship between them. Much attention has been given to the relationships among insight into illness, compliance, and outcome of treatment. Most studies, although not all, have suggested that better compliance and more positive outcomes are associated with greater insight (Amador, Strauss, Yale, & Gorman, 1991).

Recent efforts to develop valid and reliable measures of appreciation have improved the quality of work in this area (Amador et al., 1993; McEvoy, Apperson et al., 1989). Most studies, however, have attempted to illuminate the phenomenology of mental illness, rather than to provide information about functioning relative to decision-making competence. Thus, they generally fail to provide comprehensive assessments of the relevant aspects of appreciation. Insight into the presence of illness has been studied extensively, whereas appreciation of the risks and benefits of treatment rarely has been examined. The majority of work has been done with patients with schizophrenia, although there are reasons to suspect impaired appreciation in other diagnostic groups as well. The differences in appreciation between groups with and without mental illness, and the relationship between particular symptoms and failures in appreciation, remain to be determined.

Ability to Manipulate Information Rationally

Rational manipulation of information by persons with mental illness has not been studied extensively. In contrast to understanding, examination of this ability requires more complex methods than merely asking for recall of disclosed information. Compared with appreciation, which has always been thought to affect compliance and therefore outcome, its clinical relevance seems weaker. Nonetheless, some investigators have developed paradigms for assessing rational manipulation of information in various diagnostic and symptomatic groups.

Focusing on persons with schizophrenia, Rosenfeld, Turkheimer, and Gardner (1992) devised a gambling paradigm to assess reasoning. Inpatients and outpatients with schizophrenia were compared with nonschizophrenic siblings or parents. Subjects were asked to indicate their choices between two possible bets displayed graphically on a computer screen; the options differed in probability of winning, amount that could be won, and amount that might be lost. Inpatients were significantly less likely to conform to a rational choice model (one that maximized gain and minimized loss) than were outpatients and controls. Predictors included severity of symptoms and IQ measures.

Reasoning also has been examined in patients with depression, but no consistent results have been obtained across studies. Compared with nondepressed controls, subjects with depression were found to show greater decisional stress, lower decisional self-esteem, and more dysfunctional decisional response styles, all of which correlated with degree of depressive symptoms; subjects with depression in Australia and Japan showed similar results, although nondepressed controls in Australia differed significantly from those in Japan (Radford, Mann & Kalucy, 1986; Radford, Nakane, Ohta, Mann, & Kalucy, 1991). Another study measuring quality of reasoning about treatment choices in subjects with and without depression found no differences between the groups (Stanley, Stanley, Guido, & Garvin, 1988). A vignette study, in which subjects were asked to make hypothetical decisions, showed significant differences in choices between depressed and nondepressed groups (Lee & Ganzini, 1992). In a study that stimulated much of the work on "depressive realism," Costello (1983) asked women with depression to decide at what level of expected utility they would favor risky choices over more certain ones. She concluded that they performed closer to a rational choice model than did nondepressed controls, who favored risk-prone judgments.

Mixed diagnostic groups were examined by Stanley et al. (1982), who asked subjects whether they would consent to participate in hypothetical research projects. Forty percent of acutely hospitalized patients said they would agree to participate in high-risk/low-benefit research, whereas up to 32% refused low-risk/high-benefit participation. A second study that compared performance of psychiatric inpatients with medical inpatients, however, found no differences in choices between the groups (Stanley, Stanley, Lautin, Kane, & Schwartz, 1981).

Finally, the impact of particular symptoms on rational decision making has been explored. Delusional subjects with schizophrenia were asked to guess which of two jars colored beads were being drawn from, knowing the distribution of colors in each jar (Huq, Garety & Hemsley, 1988). They required fewer trials before reaching a decision and expressed higher certainty in their choices than did nondeluded patients and nonpatient controls. This would seem to suggest that deluded subjects were likely to jump to conclusions based on limited data; the way in which the task was constructed, however, allows the inference that the nondeluded subjects may have been overcautious and the deluded group closer to a rational choice model. Nonetheless, at least a subgroup of deluded subjects seemed to decide more impulsively than normals. Similarly, in another study by the same research group, persons with paranoid schizophrenia were more likely than nonparanoid patients and normal controls to report illusory correlations between word pairs (Brennan & Hemsley, 1984). The investigators suggested that paranoid patients integrated new information rapidly into preexisting explanatory schemata, short-circuiting an inductive reasoning process.

Overall, studies of rational manipulation of information often have used tasks that do not resemble treatment decision making, resulting in uncertainty about the application of these findings to clinical decision-making competence. Indeed, some of the tests used, relying for example on Bayesian models, may be so complex that ordinary people could not be expected to perform adequately (e.g., Costello, 1983). In many cases, the outcome of patients' choices has been used as a proxy for their rational thought processes, an equation that may be fallacious; failures in understanding and appreciation, as well as values different from the norm, might equally well explain deviations from a rational choice model. The need in future work is for clinically relevant tasks of appropriate complexity that focus on thought processes, rather than outcomes.

Relationship Among Standards

Most investigators have limited themselves to examining psychological functions related to one standard of decision-making competence: understanding, appreciation, or rational manipulation. The few exceptions usually involve concurrent measures of understanding and appreciation (e.g., Linden & Chaskell, 1981; Munetz & Roth, 1985), or focused on samples without mental illness (e.g., normal children compared with adults; Weithorn & Campbell, 1982). No investigators, however, have explored the relationships among these standards. Unexamined questions include the extent to which the standards have similar associations with diagnostic and symptomatic entities, the relative stringency of each standard, in particular whether one is subsumed by another, and the effects of applying several standards simultaneously. Because courts frequently employ compound standards, this latter question has important clinical and legal relevance.

Design of the MacArthur Treatment Competence Study

The MacArthur Treatment Competence Study was designed to develop reliable and valid information with which to address clinical and policy questions regarding the abilities of persons with mental illness to make decisions about psychiatric treatment: Do persons with mental illness differ from nonmentally-ill persons in their decision-making abilities, particularly as they relate to legal standards of competence? Are whatever impairments may be detected common to all persons with mental illness, or do they vary in type and magnitude? If the latter, what clinical and demographic characteristics are associated with particular patterns of impairment?

Methods were sought of addressing these questions that would yield more interpretable findings than earlier studies. This required the development of reliable and valid measures of decision-making abilities conceptually related to the four major legal standards for competence to consent to treatment. These measures then were applied to clinical populations to generate data on the comparative functioning of persons with and without mental illness.

Development of Dependent Measures

Based on our understanding of the limitations of previous research, criteria were established to guide the development of our measures to assess abilities related to each of the four standards of competence. Six of these criteria were formulated.

The functions being assessed should have close conceptual relationships with the appropriate standards of competence. Tasks should not be drawn reflexively from standard psychological approaches (e.g., standard IQ measures). These may have little relevance to the ways in which the law has thought about the abilities required to consent to treatment. Moreover, the tasks themselves may tap general cognitive abilities that only imperfectly reflect the specific functions required for decision making. Measurement tasks should be derived from a study of the legal standards, with the goal of identifying functional abilities that the courts are likely to consider relevant.

The content of the instruments should be relevant to the decision being studied (i.e., whether or not to proceed with treatment). As a legal construct, competence is now generally recognized to be task-specific (Faden & Beauchamp, 1986). Performance on measures designed to assess decision making in one domain (e.g., gambling paradigms) may lack relevance to the question of subjects' performance in the treatment context. This is because content in other domains may differ in familiarity, complexity, and the degree to which it motivates subjects to perform. Even if the correspondence in performance across content domains is high, measures that target decisions other than those related to treatment will lack face validity with clinicians and, even more importantly, with the courts.

The content of the instruments should be meaningful to the persons being studied. Research participants may perform differently when faced with content that relates directly to their own situation (i.e., when it concerns treatments for their own disorder) than with content that is personally irrelevant (e.g., hypothetical descriptions of research projects in which they will never actually be asked to participate). Performance may be heightened by greater motivation to reach a good decision about a personally relevant issue or reduced by the overwhelming anxiety that attends their consideration of their own situation. Because the net effect of these factors is unpredictable, content should focus on information relevant to research participants' own situations, insofar as possible. Persons with different disorders may require different versions of the instruments.

Content should be sufficiently standardized that comparisons within and across research groups are possible. At the limit, maximum validity might be obtained by individualizing the content to focus on the precise details of persons' own situations. A compromise is required, however, that allows stimuli to be standardized to the extent that valid comparisons are possible. Content should be selected so as to be generally relevant to all members of a diagnostic group and to allow parallel versions to be generated for other diagnostic groups.

Measures must have objective criteria for scoring that can be applied in a reliable fashion. A consistent problem with previous research has been the absence of objective scoring criteria, often leading to an inability to demonstrate reliability and making replication problematic. Development of reliable methods for assessing competence-related functions would be a major contribution in its own right.

Instruments should be practical for use in a research setting and potentially adaptable for clinical use. The instruments must be brief enough to allow administration of all experimental measures and several measures of independent variables in a single sitting, with patients with severe mental and physical illnesses. This has been less of an issue in previous research, in which investigators rarely have attempted to measure abilities related to more than one legal standard at a time. Moreover, to ensure adequate sample size at acceptable cost, the instruments should be capable of being employed by interviewers without extensive clinical training. They should be designed to allow them, if they are successful as research instruments, to be adapted for routine use in clinical practice.

The instruments developed according to these criteria were tested and refined during the pilot phase of the study (Grisso & Appelbaum, 1991). A full description of the instruments is provided in the second article in this series (Grisso et al., 1995).

Selection of Diagnostic Groups for Study

In recognition of the heterogeneity of mental disorders, two mental illnesses were chosen for study: *schizophrenia,* because it is among the most severe of mental illnesses and is known to have an adverse effect on cognitive functioning (Gold & Harvey, 1993), and because questions of decision-making competence frequently arise among persons with the disorder; and *major depression,* because it is the most common of the major mental illnesses, and in its severe forms may also raise questions of competence. The majority of previous studies of abilities related to legal competence has involved these two disorders, permitting comparison of results with previous findings.

Persons with mental illness are called upon to make treatment-related decisions at multiple points in the course of their illnesses. The study focused on decision-making capacities soon after admission to an inpatient facility. Although it would be of interest to assess functioning at other points in time (e.g., during outpatient treatment), the postadmission period was selected for initial study because it was thought to maximize the possibility of including a range of impairments, including severely disordered patients. In addition, decision making by inpatients is the focus of recent controversies over the implementation of a right to refuse treatment, and those decisions frequently are made during the first few days of hospitalization.

A third group—medically ill patients—was included to allow inferences to be drawn regarding the effects of mental illness, as opposed to the impact on performance of illness *per se* and of the stress associated with hospitalization. The selection of a hospitalized, medically ill sample was constrained by the need to identify a patient group that resembled the two groups with mental illness in several ways: a high incidence of hospitalization, considerable chronicity, frequent treatment with medication, and availability during hospitalization for interview. To allow inferences to be drawn regarding the effect of mental illness *per se* on decision making, it was important that neither the medical disorder nor the treatment typically result in mental impairment. Patients with ischemic heart disease (angina pectoris) were selected as the group that best met these criteria.

Selection of Comparison Groups

Many of the earlier studies designated levels of performance that were said to constitute competent or incompetent functioning. There are several difficulties with this approach. A priori determination of any particular level of performance as a proxy for legal competence or incompetence is likely to be highly arbitrary. The law specifies no particular level of ability for competence when determined according to any of the four legal standards. Moreover, the requisite level of ability is likely to vary as a function of case-specific circumstances (e.g., the degree of intrusiveness or risk associated with the treatment) (Drane, 1984; Grisso, 1986). Functioning of a person with mental illness might be considered inadequate when it deviates substantially from the level that is usually manifested in the population at large. Controls without mental illness, therefore, were included in our design to assess the degree to which the performance of participants without mental illness corresponds to the functioning of the general population.

Sociodemographic factors, such as education and occupation, may be related to performance on cognitive tasks, and a random sample of the general population is likely to differ substantially from groups with mental and medical illnesses on these variables. In addition, groups with medical illness and mental illness are likely to differ from each other on variables other than mental illness that might affect cognitive functioning. Therefore, for each diagnostic group, we recruited a non-ill control group matched with it on age, gender, race, education, and highest occupation. The schizophrenia and depression modules of the Diagnostic Interview Schedule Screening Interview were administered to exclude from the control groups persons who met criteria for those disorders (Marcus, Robins, Bucholz, & Przybeck, 1987).

The study design is shown in Figure 2, which describes the main comparisons (solid-line arrows) and secondary comparisons (dotted-line arrows) to be made.

Other Design Features

Data were collected at three sites (Worcester, MA, Pittsburgh, PA, and Kansas City, MO) to maximize the generalizability of the results by avoiding bias resulting from peculiarities at a single study site. Each site was responsible for collecting 75% of one of the hospitalized groups and its matched controls, and 25% of a second hospitalized group and its controls (see Figure 2). Patients with schizophrenia were recruited in Kansas City and Worcester, patients with depression in Pittsburgh and Kansas City, and ischemic heart disease (angina pectoris) patients in Worcester and Pittsburgh. The degree to which competence-related functioning changes over time is of relevance theoretically, as well as from a policy perspective. Therefore, our design called for between one quarter and one

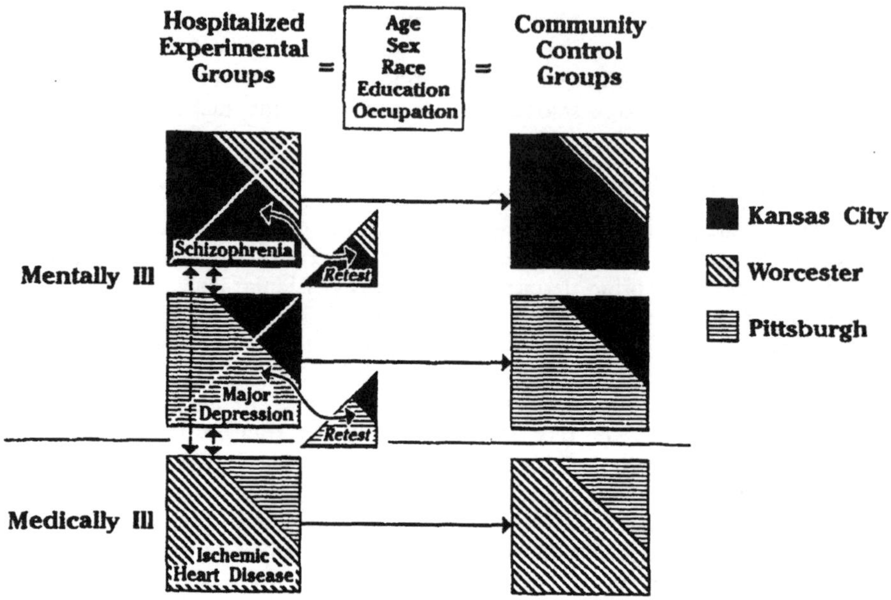

Fig. 2. Design of study.

third of the groups with mental illness to be retested two weeks after the initial evaluation.

CONCLUSION

The MacArthur Treatment Competence Study was designed to minimize many of the problems of previous research in developing and testing measures of patients' abilities related to legal standards of decision-making competence. The following article (Grisso et al., 1995) describes the psychometric characteristics of the instruments developed for this purpose. Initial application of the measures was aimed at shedding light on the degree to which patients with mental illness function differently from medically ill patients and nonpatient controls. These data are contained in the third article in this series (Grisso & Appelbaum, 1995), where we also explore the implications of our results for the question of whether different policies with regard to informed consent can be justified for mentally ill people.

REFERENCES

Ackermann, R., & DeRubeis, R. J. (1991). Is depressive realism real? *Clinical Psychology Review, 11*, 565–584.

Amador, X. F., Strauss, D. H., Yale, S. A., Flaum, M. M., Endicott, J., & Gorman, J. M. (1993). Assessment of insight in psychosis. *American Journal of Psychiatry, 150*, 873–879.

Amador, X. F., Strauss, D. H., Yale, S. A., & Gorman, J. M. (1991). Awareness of illness in schizophrenia. *Schizophrenia Bulletin, 17,* 113–132.

American Psychiatric Association (1980). Brief *amicus curiae,* Rogers v. Okin, 634 F.2d 650 (1st Cir. 1980).

American Psychiatric Association (1987). *Diagnostic and statistical manual, 3rd ed.* Washington, DC: APA.

Annas, G. J., & Densberger, J. E. (1984). Competence to refuse medical treatment: Autonomy vs. paternalism. *University of Toledo Law Review, 15,* 561–596.

Appelbaum, P. S. (1988). The right to refuse treatment with antipsychotic medications: Retrospect and prospect. *American Journal of Psychiatry, 145,* 413–419.

Appelbaum, P. S. (1994). *Almost a revolution: Mental health law and the limits of change.* New York: Oxford University Press.

Appelbaum, P. S., & Grisso, T. (1988). Assessing patients' capacities to consent to treatment. *New England Journal of Medicine, 319,* 1635–1638.

Appelbaum, P. S., & Gutheil, T. G. (1991). *Clinical handbook of psychiatry and the law.* Baltimore: Williams & Wilkins.

Appelbaum, P. S., & Kemp, K. N. (1982). The evolution of commitment law in the nineteenth century: A reinterpretation. *Law and Human Behavior, 6,* 343–354.

Appelbaum, P. S., Lidz, C. W., & Meisel, A. (1987). *Informed consent: Legal theory and clinical practice.* New York: Oxford University Press.

Appelbaum, P. S., Mirkin, S. A., & Bateman, A. L. (1981). Empirical assessment of competency to consent to psychiatric hospitalization. *American Journal of Psychiatry, 138,* 1170–1176.

Appelbaum, P. S., & Roth, L. H. (1982). Competency to consent to research: A psychiatric overview. *Archives of General Psychiatry, 39,* 951–958.

Beck, J. C. (1988). Determining competency to assent to neuroleptic drug treatment. *Hospital and Community Psychiatry, 39,* 1106–1108.

Beck, J. C., & Staffin, R. D. (1986). Patients' competency to give informed consent to medication. *Hospital and Community Psychiatry, 37,* 400–402.

Benson, P. R. (1983). Informed consent: Drug information disclosed to patients prescribed antipsychotic medication. *Journal of Nervous and Mental Disease, 172,* 642–652.

Benson, P. R., Roth, L. H., Appelbaum, P. S., Lidz, C. W., & Winslade, W. J. (1988). Information disclosure, subject understanding, and informed consent in psychiatric research. *Law and Human Behavior, 12,* 455–476.

Berg, A., & Hammitt, K. B. (1980). Assessing the psychiatric patient's ability to meet the literacy demands of hospitalization. *Hospital & Community Psychiatry, 31,* 266–268.

Bonnie, R. J. (1993). The competence of criminal defendants: Beyond Dusky and Drope. *University of Miami Law Review, 47,* 539–601.

Brakel, S. J. (1985). Voluntary hospitalization. In S. J. Brakel, J. Parry, & B. Weiner (Eds.), *The mentally disabled and the law, 2nd ed.* Chicago: American Bar Foundation.

Brennan, J. H., & Hemsley, D. R. (1984). Illusory correlations in paranoid and nonparanoid schizophrenia. *British Journal of Clinical Psychology, 23,* 225–226.

Brooks, G. W., Deane, W. N., & Hugel, R. W. (1968). Some aspects of the subjective experience of schizophrenia. *Diseases of the Nervous System, 29*(suppl. 5), 78–82.

Carpenter, W. T., Bartko, J. J., Carpenter, C. L., & Strauss, J. S. (1976). Another view of schizophrenia subtypes: A report from the International Pilot Study of Schizophrenia. *Archives of General Psychiatry, 33,* 508–516.

Coles, G. S., Roth, L., & Pollack, I. W. (1978). Literacy skills of long-term hospitalized mental patients. *Hospital & Community Psychiatry, 29,* 512–516.

Costello, E. J. (1983). Information processing for decision making in depressed women: A study of subjective expected utilities. *Journal of Affective Disorders, 5,* 239–251.

Cutter, M. A. G., & Shelp, E. E. (1991). *Competency: A study of informal competency determinations in primary care.* Dordrecht: Kluwer Academic Publishers.

Davidhizar, R., & Wehlage, D. (1984). Can the client with chronic schizophrenia consent to nursing research? *Journal of Advanced Nursing, 9,* 381–390.

Drane, J. F. (1984). Competency to give an informed consent: A model for making clinical assessments. *Journal of the American Medical Association, 252*, 925–927.

Faden, R., & Beauchamp, T. (1986). *A history and theory of informed consent*. New York: Oxford University Press.

Geller, J. L. (1982). State hospital patients and their medication—Do they know what they take? *American Journal of Psychiatry, 139*, 611–615.

Goedecke v. State, Dep't of Institutions, 603 P.2d 123 (Colo. 1979).

Gold, J.M., & Harvey, P.D. (1993). Cognitive deficits in schizophrenia. *Psychiatric Clinics of North America, 16*, 295–312.

Grannum v. Berard, 422 P.2d 812 (Wash. 1967).

Green, M. (1944). Proof of mental incompetency and the unexpressed major premise. *Yale Law Journal, 53*, 271–311.

Greenfeld, D., Strauss, J. S., Bowers, M. B., & Mandelkern, M. (1989). Insight and interpretation of illness in recovery from psychosis. *Schizophrenia Bulletin, 15*, 245–252.

Grisso, T. (1986). *Evaluating competencies: Forensic assessments and instruments*. New York: Plenum Press.

Grisso, T., & Appelbaum, P. S. (1991). Mentally ill and non-mentally-ill patients' abilities to understand informed consent disclosures for medication: Preliminary data. *Law and Human Behavior, 15*, 377–388.

Grisso, T., & Appelbaum, P. S., & Mulvey, E. P., & Fletcher, K. (1995). The MacArthur Treatment Competence Study. II: Measures of abilities related to competence to consent to treatment. *Law and Human Behavior, 19*, 127–148.

Grisso, T., & Appelbaum, P. S. (1995). The MacArthur Treatment Competence Study. III: Abilities of patients to consent to psychiatric and medical treatments. *Law and Human Behavior, 19*, 149–174.

Grossman, L., & Summers, F. (1980). A study of the capacity of schizophrenic patients to give informed consent. *Hospital & Community Psychiatry, 31*, 205–206.

Guardianship of John Roe, 583 N.E. 2d 1282 (Mass. 1992).

Heinrichs, D. W., Cohen, B. P., & Carpenter, W. T. (1985). Early insight and the management of schizophrenic decompensation. *Journal of Nervous and Mental Disease, 173*, 133–138.

Hoffman, B. F., & Srinivasan, J. (1992). A study of competence to consent to treatment in a psychiatric hospital. *Canadian Journal of Psychiatry, 37*, 179–182.

Huq, S. F., Garety, P. A., & Hemsley, D. R. (1988). Probabilistic judgements in deluded and non-deluded subjects. *Quarterly Journal of Experimental Psychology, 40A*, 801–812.

In re the Mental Health of K. K. B., 609 P.2d 747 (Okla. 1980).

In re Milton, 505 N.E.2d 255 (Ohio 1987).

In re Yetter, 52 Pa.D&C 619 (1973).

Irwin, M., Lovitz, A., Marder, S., Mintz, J., Winslade, W. J., Van Putten, T., & Mills, M. J. (1985). Psychotic patients' understanding of informed consent. *American Journal of Psychiatry, 142*, 1351–1354.

Jaffe, R. (1986). Problems of long-term informed consent. *Bulletin of the American Academy of Psychiatry and the Law, 14*, 163–169.

Janofsky, J. S., McCarthy, R. J., & Folstein, M. F. (1992). The Hopkins competency assessment test: A brief method for evaluating patients' capacity to give informed consent. *Hospital and Community Psychiatry, 43*, 132–136.

Jarvis, v. Levine, 418 N.W.2d 139 (Minn. 1988).

Kleinman, I., Schacter, D., & Koritar, E. (1989). Informed consent and tardive dyskinesia. *American Journal of Psychiatry, 146*, 902–904.

Lane v. Candura, 376 N.E.2d 1232 (Mass. App. 1978).

Lee, M. A., & Ganzini, L. (1992). Depression in the elderly: Effect on patient attitudes toward life-sustaining therapy. *Journal of the American Geriatrics Society, 40*, 983–988.

Levine, J., Warrenburg, S., Kerns, R., Schwartz, G., Fontana, A., Gradman, A., Smith, S., Allen, S., & Cascione, R. (1989). The role of denial in recovery from coronary heart disease. *Psychosomatic Medicine, 49*, 109–117.

Lidz, C. W., Meisel, A., Zerubavel, E., Carter, M., Sestak, R. M., & Roth, L. H. (1984). *Informed consent: A study of decisionmaking in psychiatry*. New York: Guilford Press.

Lin, I. F., Spiga, R., & Fortsch, W. (1979). *Journal of Clinical Psychiatry, 40,* 430–432.

Linden, M., & Chaskel, R. (1981). Information and consent in schizophrenic patients in long-term treatment. *Schizophrenia Bulletin, 3,* 372–378.

Marcus, S. C., Robins, L. N., Bucholz, K. K., & Przybeck, T. R. (1989). Diagnostic interview schedule screening instrument (DISSI). St. Louis, MO: Department of Psychiatry, Washington University School of Medicine.

Markova, I. S., & Berrios, G. E. (1992). The assessment of insight in clinical psychiatry: A new scale. *Acta Psychiatria Scandinavica, 86,* 159–164.

Matter of Conroy, 486 A.2d 1209 (N.J. 1985).

Matter of O'Brien, 517 N.Y.S.2d 346 (Sup.Ct. 1986).

McEvoy, J. P., Aland, J., Wilson, W. H., Guy, W., & Hawkins, L. (1981). Measuring chronic schizophrenic patients' attitudes toward their illness and treatment. *Hospital & Community Psychiatry, 32,* 856–858.

McEvoy, J. P., Appelbaum, P. S., Apperson, L. J., Geller, J. L., & Freter, S. (1989). Why must some schizophrenic patients be involuntarily committed? The role of insight. *Comprehensive Psychiatry, 30,* 13–17.

McEvoy, J. P., Apperson, L. J., Appelbaum, P. S., Ortlip, P., Brecosky, J., Hammill, K., Geller, J. L., & Roth, L. (1989). Insight in schizophrenia: Its relationship to acute psychopathology. *Journal of Nervous and Mental Disease, 177,* 43–47.

McEvoy, J. P., Freter, S., Everett, G., Geller, J. L., Appelbaum, P., Apperson, L. J., & Roth, L. (1989). Insight and the clinical outcome of schizophrenic patients. *Journal of Nervous and Mental Disease, 177,* 48–51.

McEvoy, J. P., Schooler, N. R., Friedman, E., Steingard, S., & Allen, M. (1993). Use of psychopathology vignettes by patients with schizophrenia or schizoaffective disorder and by mental health professionals to judge patients' insight. *American Journal of Psychiatry, 150,* 1649–1653.

McKinnon, K., Cournos, F., & Stanley, B. (1989). *Rivers* in practice: Clinicians' assessments of patients' decision-making capacity. *Hospital and Community Psychiatry, 40,* 1159–1162.

Meisel, A. (1979). The exceptions to the informed consent doctrine: Striking a balance between competing values in medical decision making. *Wisconsin Law Review, 1979,* 413–488.

Merz, J. F., & Fischoff, B. (1990). Informed consent does not mean rational consent: Cognitive limitations on decision making. *Journal of Legal Medicine, 11,* 321–350.

Mills, M. J., Yesavage, J. A., & Gutheil, T. G. (1983). Continuing case law development in the right to refuse treatment. *American Journal of Psychiatry, 140,* 715–719.

Morgado, A., Smith, M., Lecrubier, Y., & Widlocher, D. (1991). Depressed subjects unwittingly overreport poor social adjustment which they reappraise when recovered. *Journal of Nervous and Mental Disease, 179,* 614–619.

Munetz, M. R., & Roth, L. H. (1985). Informing patients about tardive dyskinesia. *Archives of General Psychiatry, 42,* 866–871.

Norko, M. A., Billick, S. B., McCarrick, R. G., & Schwartz, M. A. (1990). A clinical study of competency to consent to voluntary psychiatric hospitalization. *American Journal of Forensic Psychiatry, 11, 3–15.*

Olin, G. B., & Olin, H. S. (1975). Informed consent in voluntary mental hospital admissions. *American Journal of Psychiatry, 132,* 938–941.

Palmer, A. B., & Wohl, J. (1972). Voluntary admission forms: Does the patient know what he's signing? *Hospital & Community Psychiatry, 23,* 38–40.

President's Commission for the Study of Ethical Problems in Medicine and Biomedical and Behavioral Research (1982). *Making health care decisions*. Vol. 1. Washington, DC: U.S. Government Printing Office.

Rachlin, S. (1975). One right too many. *Bulletin of the American Academy of Psychiatry and the Law, 3,* 99–102.

Radford, M. H. B., Mann, L., & Kalucy, R. S. (1986). Psychiatric disturbance and decision-making. *Australian and New Zealand Journal of Psychiatry, 20,* 210–217.

Radford, M. H. B., Nakane, Y., Ohta, Y., Mann, L., & Kalucy, R. S. (1991). Decision making in clinically depressed patients: a transcultural social psychological study. *Journal of Nervous and Mental Disease, 179,* 711–719.

Ray, I. (1864). American legislation on insanity. *American Journal of Insanity, 20,* 21–62.

Riese v. St. Mary's Hospital & Medical Center, 243 Cal. Rptr. 241 (Ct.App. 1987).

Rivers v. Katz, 495 N.E.2d 337 (N.Y. 1986).

Rogers v. Commissioner, Dep't of Mental Health, 458 N.E.2d 308 (Mass. 1983).

Rogers v. Okin, 478 F.Supp. 1342 (D.Mass. 1979).

Rosenfeld, B., Turkheimer, E., & Gardner, W. (1992). Decision making in a schizophrenic population. *Law and Human Behavior, 16,* 651–662.

Roth, L. H., Lidz, C. W., Meisel, A., Soloff, P. H., Kaufman, K., Spiker, D. G., & Foster, F. G. (1982). Competency to decide about treatment or research: An overview of some empirical data. *International Journal of Law and Psychiatry, 5,* 29–50.

Roth, L. H., Meisel, A., & Lidz, C. W. (1977). Tests of competency to consent to treatment. *American Journal of Psychiatry, 134,* 279–284.

Shapiro, M. H. (1974). Legislating the control of physician control: Autonomy and the coercive use of organic therapies. *Southern California Law Review, 47,* 237–356.

Slater v. Baker & Stapleton, 95 Eng. Rep. 860 (K.B. 1767).

Small, I. F., Messina, J. A., & Small, J. G. (1964). The meaning of hospitalization: A comparison of attitudes of medical and psychiatric patients. *Journal of Nervous and Mental Diseases, 139,* 575–580.

Soskis, D. A. (1978). Schizophrenic and medical inpatients as informed drug consumers. *Archives of General Psychiatry, 35,* 645–647.

Soskis, D. A., & Jaffe, R. L. (1979). Communicating with patients about antipsychotic drugs. *Comprehensive Psychiatry, 20,* 126–131.

Stanley, B., Stanley, M., Guido, J., & Garvin, L. (1988). The functional competency of elderly at risk. *The Gerontologist, 28,* 53–58.

Stanley, B., Stanley, M., Lautin, A., Kane, J., & Schwartz, N. (1981). Preliminary findings on psychiatric patients as research participants: A population at risk? *American Journal of Psychiatry, 138,* 669–671.

Stanley, B., Stanley, M., Peselow, E., Wolkin, A., Deutsch, S., Platt, L., Speicher, J., Golash, L., & Kaufman, M. (1982). The effects of psychotropic drugs on informed consent. *Psychopharmacology Bulletin, 18,* 102–104.

State ex rel. Jones v. Gerhardstein, 416 N.W.2d 883 (Wis. 1987).

Superintendent of Belchertown State School v. Saikewicz, 370 N.E.2d 417 (Mass. 1977).

Takai, A., Uematsu, M., Ueki, H., Sone, K., & Kaiya, H. (1992). Insight and its related factors in chronic schizophrenic patients: A preliminary study. *European Journal of Psychiatry, 6,* 159–170.

Taylor, S. E. (1989). *Positive illusions: Creative self-deception and the healthy mind.* New York: Basic Books.

Tepper, A., & Elwork, A. (1984). Competence to consent to treatment as a psycholegal construct. *Law and Human Behavior, 8,* 205–223.

Van Putten, T., Crumpton, E., & Yale, C. (1976). Drug refusal in schizophrenia and the wish to be crazy. *Archives of General Psychiatry, 33,* 1443–1446.

Walker, E. F., & Rossiter, J. (1989). Schizophrenic patients' self-perceptions: Legal and clinical implications. *Journal of Psychiatry & Law, 17,* 55–73.

Weithorn, L., & Campbell, S. (1982). The competency of children and adolescents to make informed treatment decisions. *Child Development, 53,* 1589–1599.

White, P. D., & Denise, S. H. (1991). Medical treatment decisions and competency in the eyes of the law: A brief survey. In M. A. G. Cutter & E. E. Shelp (Eds.), *Competency: A study of informal competency determinations in primary care.* Dordrecht: Kluwer Academic Publishers.

Wilson, W. H., Ban, T. A., & Guy, W. (1986). Flexible system criteria in chronic schizophrenia. *Comprehensive Psychiatry, 27,* 259–265.

Wing, J. K., Monck, E., Brown, G. W., & Carstairs, G. M. (1964). Morbidity in the community of schizophrenic patients discharged from London mental hospitals in 1959. *British Journal of Psychiatry, 110,* 10–21.

Zinermon v. Burch, 494 U.S. 113 (1990).

[9]

Mental Disorder, Violence, and Gender

Pamela Clark Robbins,[1,4] John Monahan,[2] and Eric Silver[3]

Recent studies have reported comparable rates of violence among men and women with mental disorder, raising important issues for clinical risk assessment. This study examines the relationship between gender and violence using data from the MacArthur Violence Risk Assessment Study. Patients in acute psychiatric wards were interviewed 5 times over the year following their discharge to the community. Results showed some differences between men and women in the violence committed immediately following discharge, with rates for men being higher. But the prevalence of violence over the 1 year was similar for female and male discharged patients. However, there were substantial gender differences in the situational context of the violence committed. Men were more likely to have been drinking or using street drugs, and less likely to have been adhering to prescribed psychotropic medication, prior to committing violence. The violence committed by men was more likely to result in serious injury than the violence committed by women, and men were more likely than women to be arrested after committing a violent act. Women were more likely to target family members and to be violent in the home.

KEY WORDS: mental disorder; violence; gender; rares; MacArthur Risk Assessment Study.

That women commit violent acts at a much lower rate than men is a staple in criminology. Women make up 51% of the population of the United States but only 11% of the people arrested for violent crime (Reiss & Roth, 1993). The United States appears to be approximately in the middle of the international distribution of gender ratios in arrest rates for violence, which vary from 5-1 to 50-1 (Wilson & Herrnstein, 1985). Although gender differences are sometimes less for self-report than for official report (Steffensmeier & Allen, 1996), national crime survey findings closely parallel the arrest record data: 14% of violent offenders were reported by their victims to be women or girls (Greenfeld & Snell, 1999). As Sampson and Lauritsen (1994, p. 19) concluded, "sex is one of the strongest demographic correlates of violent offending."

[1]Policy Research Associates, Inc., Delmar, New York.
[2]School of Law, University of Virginia, Charlottesville, Virginia.
[3]Department of Sociology, The Pennsylvania State University, College Park, Pennsylvania.
[4]To whom correspondence should be addressed at Policy Research Associates, Inc., Delmar, New York; e-mail: probbins@prainc.com.

It is against the background of this fundamental tenet of criminology that the results of several recent studies of violence by men and women with mental disorder are so striking. Recent studies of persons discharged from short-term psychiatric facilities by Lidz, Mulvey, and Gardner (1993), Newhill, Mulvey, and Lidz (1995), and Hiday, Swartz, and Swanson (1998) found no significant differences in the rates of community violence by male and female patients. Similar results have been reported for violence within mental hospitals (Binder & McNiel, 1990; Lam, McNiel, & Binder, 2000). Indeed, the underestimation of the likelihood of violence by women patients has been suggested as a major factor underlying the lack of validity that plagues clinical violence risk assessment (Coontz, Lidz, & Mulvey, 1994; Lidz et al., 1993; McNiel & Binder, 1995). The hypothesis that mental disorder has more of an effect on the violence-potential of women than of men has also received support in the epidemiological literature (Brennan, Mednick, & Hodgins, 2000; Hodgins, 1992; Swanson, Holzer, Ganju, & Jono, 1990). Even where gender differences in violence are not eliminated, the magnitude of those differences appears strongly attenuated when the samples consist of men and women with mental disorder, as compared to when they consist of men and women without it (Stueve & Link, 1998).

This paper assesses gender differences in violence among people with mental disorder. It improves upon previous studies on this topic in three ways. First, an atypically large and representative sample of patients discharged from acute psychiatric facilities is assessed. Second, the criterion measure consists of triangulated information sources that yield a more sensitive indicator of violence (and other aggressive acts) in the community than measures previously reported. Third, descriptive information essential for understanding violence in context is provided (Steadman & Silver, 2000). More specifically, the prevalence of violence by gender is presented at two levels of seriousness (violence and other aggressive acts) over the course of five follow-up periods. The observed violence and other aggressive acts is characterized by the type of act, the relationship between the offender and victim, and the location where it transpired. The sequelae of violence is also discussed. In addition, the effect of two demonstrated risk factors for violence—diagnosis and substance abuse—is disaggregated by gender.

Although gender differences have been described indirectly in other publications arising from the MacArthur Violence Risk Assessment Study, this paper goes beyond the data previously reported. The results published to date from the MacArthur data have focused on the overall prevalence of violence among recently released psychiatric patients when compared to the community (Steadman et al., 1998), and specific topic areas related to violence such as delusions (Appelbaum, Robbins, & Monahan, 2000; Appelbaum, Robbins, & Roth, 1999), violent thoughts (Grisso, Davis, Vesselinov, Appelbaum, & Monahan, 2000), and neighborhood contextual factors (Silver, 2000). Other work has been published on a classification tree methodology for assessing risk in the next 20 weeks for persons admitted to short-term acute psychiatric units (Monahan et al., 2000; Steadman et al., 2000). And most recently, a strategy for employing multiple models as a technique for improving risk classifications has been presented (Banks et al., 2002). But in the framework of the other MacArthur publications, the topic of gender differences has not been fully analyzed, and the differences by gender in terms of the targets, and locations of violence have not been fully described. In addition, prior studies using MacArthur data have focused primarily on the first 20 weeks following discharge and therefore have not addressed differences for all follow-ups; nor have these studies attempted to explain the reported gender differences.

METHOD

Patient Enrollment and Data Collection

A complete description of the MacArthur Violence Risk Assessment Study is available elsewhere (Steadman et al., 1998). In brief, admissions were sampled from acute psychiatric inpatient facilities at three sites: Western Psychiatric Institute and Clinic (Pittsburgh, PA); Western Missouri Mental Health Center (Kansas City, MO); Worcester State Hospital and the University of Massachusetts Medical Center (Worcester, MA). Selection criteria for research patients were (a) civil admissions; (b) between the ages of 18 and 40; (c) English-speaking; (d) White, or African American ethnicity (or Hispanic in Worcester only); and (e) a chart diagnosis of schizophrenia, schizophreniform, schizoaffective, depression, dysthymia, mania, brief reactive psychosis, delusional disorder, alcohol or drug abuse or dependence, or a personality disorder. After complete description of the study to the subjects, written informed consent was obtained.

Hospital data collection was conducted in two parts: an interview by a research interviewer to obtain background data, and an interview by a research clinician (PhD or MA/MSW in psychology or social work) to confirm the chart diagnosis using the *DSM-IIIR* Checklist.

Patients were recontacted in the community by the research interviewers and interviewed up to five times (every 10 weeks) over 1 year from the date of discharge. A collateral informant who knew of the patient's behavior in the community was also interviewed on the same schedule. Arrest and rehospitalization records provided the third source of information about the patients' behavior in the community.

Subjects and collaterals were asked whether the subject had engaged in several categories of aggressive behavior in the past 10 weeks. If a positive response was given, the subject or collateral was asked to list the number of times the behavior occurred. Detailed information was obtained about each act, including the target and location.

Acts were divided into two categories of seriousness: *violence* (battery that resulted in physical injury; sexual assaults; assaultive acts that involved the use of a weapon; or threats made with a weapon in hand) and *other aggressive acts* (battery that did not result in physical injury). Acts reported by any information source were reviewed by two independent coders to obtain a single reconciled report of violence. Only the most serious act for each incident was coded.

RESULTS

Sample Description

A complete characterization of the sample is presented in Steadman et al. (1998) and we will here describe only relevant gender comparisons. We approached a quota sample of 994 men and 701 women to participate. The refusal rate was 29.9% for men and 27.8% for women. The final sample given a hospital interview consisted of 667 men and 469 women. The male sample was 68.8% White, 29.5% African American, and 1.6% Hispanic. The female sample was 69.5% White, 28.4% African American, and 2.1% Hispanic. The mean age of the male patients was 29.6 and of the female patients was 29.9. The median length of hospitalization at the three sites for enrolled male patients was 9 days and for enrolled female patients was 10 days. Diagnostic differences between men and women are presented below.

Prevalence of Violence and Other Aggressive Acts

The proportion of patients with at least one act of violence during the 1-year follow-up was 29.7% for men and 24.6% for women (see Table 1). It is important to note that the significant difference between the proportion violent for the men and the women occurred only at the first follow-up period, immediately following discharge from the hospital, and any differences observed in the other follow-ups were not significant. The proportion of patients with at least one other aggressive act only during the 1-year follow-up was 30.1% for men and 37.0% for women, a statistically significant difference ($\chi^2 = 4.9$, $df = 1$, $p < .05$). This finding was significant for the first and fifth follow-ups (see Table 1). (To avoid double counting, patients with both violence and an other aggressive act are counted as "violent" in computing these rates.) Adding together these two levels of seriousness would yield a 1-year total prevalence rate of "violence or other aggressive acts" of 59.8% for men and 61.6% for women.

Types, Targets, and Locations of Violence

For both men and women, the acts that were coded as violence were primarily "kick/bite/choke/hit–beat up" and "weapon threat/weapon use," and the acts that

Table 1. Prevalence of Violence and Other Aggressive Acts in 1 Year by Gender (Person Level)

	Violence (%)		Other aggressive acts (%)	
	Men ($n = 548$)	Women ($n = 403$)	Men ($n = 548$)	Women ($n = 403$)
First follow-up	16.3**	9.7	22.0*	29.6
Second follow-up	10.8	9.6	21.6	24.2
Third follow-up	7.5	6.2	17.8	20.0
Fourth follow-up	7.8	7.4	18.0	17.9
Fifth follow-up	7.8	4.6	11.6*	17.3
One-year aggregate	29.7	24.6	30.1*	37.0

Note. A confirmatory random effects model for violence was built (SAS PROC MIXED) with two hierarchical levels: person level and time level (follow-ups 1 through 5). The model included autoregressive covariance term (AR(1) = 0.16) with chi-square for the null model of 62.68, $p < .0001$. Type 1 sequential test we performed with significant time effect of follow-up 1 through 5 ($p < .0001$) and gender ($p = .0111$). Next, the interaction term of follow-up 1 and gender was significant ($p = .0180$) and the other interaction term of the rest of the follow-ups not significant. The results from the random effects models for other aggressive acts were very similar with the interaction term for follow-up 1 and gender marginally significant at $p = .0935$ and not significant for the rest of the follow-ups, including follow-up 5. Difference of proportions test (Fisher's exact): male versus female: $^{*}p < .05$. $^{**}p < .01$. $^{***}p < .001$.

Table 2. Types, Targets, and Locations of Violence and Other Aggressive Acts in 1 Year by Gender

	Violence (%)		Other aggressive acts (%)	
	Men	Women	Men	Women
A. Types of violence and other aggressive acts (incident level)				
n	393	215	1,339	1,329
Throw object, push, grab, shove, or slap	9.9*	15.8	68.2***	79.9
Kick, bite, choke, hit, beat up	52.4*	43.7	25.5***	18.5
Forced sex	4.3	7.0	0.0	0.0
Weapon use or threat with weapon in hand	28.2	31.2	0.0	0.0
Other, type unknown	5.1	2.3	6.3***	1.6
B. Targets of violence and other aggressive acts (incident level)				
n	348	210	1,163	1,203
Family	39.9***	69.5	48.8***	74.6
Spouse	10.6***	44.3	14.6***	31.8
Girlfriend/boyfriend	17.2**	8.1	11.0***	19.2
Parental figure	3.2	1.4	3.6	3.5
Child	0.3***	6.2	4.4***	9.0
Other family	8.6	9.5	15.1**	11.2
Friend, acquaintance	40.5***	26.2	33.6***	20.9
Stranger	19.5***	4.3	17.6***	4.4
C. Locations of violence and other aggressive acts (incident level)				
n	344	208	1,163	1,199
Subject's home	35.8***	55.8	53.1***	68.2
Other residence	28.8*	20.7	15.0	12.8
Street/outdoors	25.9***	14.4	20.5***	9.5
Bar	4.9	3.8	4.7	4.1
Outpatient clinic	0.9	0.5	1.5	0.8
Workplace	0.3	1.0	2.6***	0.8
Other	3.5	3.8	2.5	3.8

Note. Difference of proportions test: Male versus female: $^{*}p < .05$. $^{**}p < .01$. $^{***}p < .001$.

were coded as other aggressive acts were primarily "throwing objects/push/grab/shove/slap" (Table 2, Panel A). "Throwing objects/push/grab/shove/slap" constituted a significantly higher proportion of women's than of men's violence and a significantly higher proportion of women's than of men's other aggressive acts. "Kick/bite/choke/hit–beat up" constituted a significantly higher portion of men's than of women's violence, and a significantly higher proportion of men's than of women's other aggressive acts.

The targets of both violence and other aggressive acts committed by the total sample were most often family members, followed by friends and acquaintances but this differed significantly by gender. For both violence and other aggressive acts, the targets of women were significantly more likely than the targets of men to be family members, and the targets of men were significantly more likely than the targets of women to be friends and acquaintances, or to be strangers (Table 2, Panel B).

The locations of both violence and other aggressive acts committed by men and by women were most often in the subject's home, in the home of another, or outdoors/on the street (Table 2, Panel C). For both violence and other aggressive acts, the locations of women were significantly more likely than the locations of men

Table 3. Description of Violent Incidents by Gender

Incident descriptors	Gender[a]	
	Women ($n = 215$)	Men ($n = 393$)
% Alcohol consumption by patient prior to incident	36.7***	62.2
% Street drug consumption by patient prior to incident	15.8**	26.4
% Subject taking medications as prescribed	23.5***	16.6
% Resulting in patient's arrest	6.1***	20.6
% Resulting in someone going to doctor/hospital	13.0***	29.6
% Resulting in patient's rehospitalization	4.9	7.6

Note. Chi-square test. ** $p < .01$. *** $p < .001$.
[a] *ns* vary because of missing data.

to be the subject's home, and the locations of men were significantly more likely than the locations of women to be outdoors/on the street.

To eliminate any bias that may have been introduced in these analyses due to the fact that some of the patients committed multiple acts of violence or other aggressive acts, we reanalyzed the data looking only at the most serious act for each individual. The reanalysis generally supported the findings reported above (e.g., there were significant differences between men and women in the choice of target, with men more likely to target strangers and less likely to target spouses and children, and in the location of the violence, with men more likely to have outdoor incidents).

Table 3 provides descriptive data on the contexts preceding and following the violent incidents of men and women (these data were not collected for the other aggressive acts). As shown, violent acts by women were less likely to have been preceded by alcohol or drug consumption and more likely to occur while psychiatric medications were being taken. In addition, violent acts by women were less likely to result in arrest and less likely to result in someone being sent for medical treatment.

In a previous paper (Steadman et al., 1998), we demonstrated that violence was not equally distributed across the five follow-ups, but rather heavily concentrated in the first two (i.e., the first 20-weeks after hospital discharge). Our efforts to identify risk factors for violence among persons discharged from psychiatric facilities, therefore, have focused on the first 20-week period (Banks et al., 2002; Monahan et al., 2000; Steadman et al., 2000). The remaining analyses in this paper will also focus on the first 20 weeks given the prior work and the finding that this is the time period where men were found to be more violent than women. During this period, at least one violent act was committed by 21.4% of men and by 15.2% of women, a significant difference ($\chi^2 = 5.7$, $df = 1$, $p < .05$). At least one "other aggressive act" (and no violent act) only was committed by 27.1% of men and by 35.2% of women, also a significant difference ($\chi^2 = 7.0$, $df = 1$, $p < .01$). Adding together these two levels of seriousness would yield first 20-week total prevalence rate of "violence or other aggressive acts" of 48.5% for men and 50.4% for women, a difference that is not statistically significant.

Table 4. Primary Diagnosis by Gender

	All patients		% With co-occurring substance abuse	
Primary diagnosis	Women (n = 469)	Men (n = 667)	Women (%)	Men (%)
Depression	47.3***	35.4	36.5***	63.5
Schizophrenia	15.4*	18.4	37.5	43.1
Bipolar	14.5	12.4	27.9*	45.8
Other Psychosis	1.9**	4.6	33.3	48.4
Personality only	2.3	1.5	0.0	0.0
Alcohol/drug	18.6***	27.6	*na*	*na*

Note. Difference of proportions test: Male versus female: *$p < .05$. **$p < .01$. ***$p < .001$.

In addition, diagnosis and, particularly, a co-occurring diagnosis of alcohol or drug abuse/dependence have been shown to be among the strongest risk factors for violence during the first 20-week period (Steadman et al., 1998). As shown in Table 4, women were more likely than men to be diagnosed with depression, and men were more likely than women to be diagnosed with primary alcohol or drug abuse disorders. In addition, we find that men with depression were significantly more likely than women with depression also to have a co-occurring substance abuse disorder. Similarly, men with bipolar disorder were significantly more likely than women with bipolar disorder also to have a co-occurring substance abuse disorder. No significant differences in co-occurring substance abuse disorders were found between men and women with schizophrenia. When all primary diagnoses listed in Table 4, excluding alcohol/drug, are combined, men were significantly more likely ($p < .001$) to have a co-occurring substance abuse diagnosis (52.2%) than were women (34.0%).

In Table 5, descriptive data on the effect of diagnosis and substance abuse on violence during the first 2 follow-ups is disaggregated by gender. Those patients with co-occurring substance abuse diagnoses were usually more likely to be violent with some differences within gender and diagnostic group. To analyze these data, we estimated a series of logistic regression equations with gender, primary diagnosis,

Table 5. Percent Violent in F1-2 by Primary Diagnosis and Co-Occurring Substance Abuse/Dependence, for Men and Women

				No co-occurring substance abuse		Co-occurring substance abuse	
Diagnosis	Gender	N	% Violent	N	% Violent	N	% Violent
Depression	Women	193	15.0	123	7.3	70	28.6
	Men	200	22.5	80	15.0	120	27.5
Schizophrenia	Women	57	3.5	34	2.9	23	4.3
	Men	103	10.7	58	6.9	45	15.6
Bipolar	Women	62	9.7	45	11.1	17	5.9
	Men	70	20.0	39	17.9	31	22.6
Other psychosis	Women	7	14.3	5	20.0	2	0.0
	Men	22	18.2	11	9.1	11	27.3
Alcohol/drug	Women	71	28.2		*na*		*na*
	Men	134	29.1		*na*		*na*
Personality only	Women	11	27.3		*na*		*na*
	Men	9	22.2		*na*		*na*
Total	Women	401	15.2	218	8.7	112	19.6
	Men	538	21.4	197	13.2	207	24.2

Table 6. Odds Ratios From Logistic Regression Predicting Violence (First 20 Weeks)

	All diagnoses ($n = 939$)		Patients without primary substance abuse diagnosis ($n = 734$)		
Covariates	Model 1	Model 2	Model 3	Model 4	Model 5
Male gender	1.51*	1.53*	1.63*	1.79**	1.53
Primary diagnosis[a]					
Depression	—	2.79**	—	2.85**	2.67**
Bipolar	—	2.12*	—	2.16*	2.25*
Substance disorder		4.57***	—	—	—
Personality only	—	4.12*	—	4.26*	6.41**
Other psychosis	—	2.28	—	2.23	2.23
Co-occurring substance	—	—	—	—	2.36***
Change in chi-square	5.83*	28.14***	5.63*	14.14**	15.56***
Degrees of freedom	1	5	1	4	1

[a]Omitted category: Schizophrenia.
*$p < .05$. **$p < .01$. ***$p < .001$.

and co-occurring substance abuse entered as covariates. As shown in Model 1 of Table 6, gender exhibited a significant bivariate association with violence at the first 20 weeks (odds ratio = 1.5; $\chi^2 = 5.8$, $df = 1$, $p < .05$). Model 2 indicates that the significant gender effect remained after controlling for primary diagnosis. To assess the effects of comorbid substance abuse, subjects with a primary substance abuse disorder were omitted from the sample as these subjects did not possess a primary major mental disorder diagnosis. Models 3 and 4 of Table 6 show once again that the effect of gender was significant controlling for primary diagnosis. Model 5 of Table 6 shows that co-occurring substance abuse disorder was strongly related to violence (odds ratio = 2.4; $\chi^2 = 15.6$, $df = 1$, $p < .001$), holding constant gender and primary diagnosis. In addition, the odds ratio for gender was rendered only marginally significant ($p = .05$) once co-occurring substance abuse was entered into the model. These finding suggests that the effect of gender on violence is in part explained by the increased likelihood of males to possess co-occurring abuse substance disorders, compared to females (see Table 4).

DISCUSSION

Findings from this research that men are no more likely to be violent than women over the course of the 1-year follow-up differ dramatically from results generally found in the criminological literature, but not from findings of other studies of men and women with a mental disorder. In addition, those gender differences that are observed during the first 20 weeks after hospital discharge can be partially explained by the higher prevalence of co-occurring substance diagnosis in patients who are men. As other investigators have averred (Coontz et al., 1994; Lidz et al., 1993; McNiel & Binder, 1995), the underestimation of the likelihood of violence by women patients may be a major factor underlying the lack of validity that plagues clinical violence risk assessment.

Recent research on gender differences in violence risk among adolescent inpatients have observed no difference between males and females (Fehon, Grilo, &

Lipshitz, 2001) but have noted differences in the nature of the violence. And among adults, although the overall prevalence rates are similar for women and men, there are some substantial gender differences in the quality or context of the violence committed (Gelles & Straus, 1988). Men are more likely to have been drinking or using street drugs, and less likely to have been adhering to prescribed psychotropic medication, prior to committing violence. Women are more likely to target family members and to be violent in the home. The violence committed by men is more likely to result in serious injury—requiring treatment by a physician—than the violence committed by women, and perhaps for that reason men are more likely than women to be arrested after committing a violent act. In general, these findings underscore the necessity for clinicians not to underestimate the likelihood of violence committed by women. Although it may be that gender differences are much smaller for recently discharged patients than for the general population, it is equally as likely that the criminological data which depends heavily on arrests and reports from serious injury may miss more of the types of violence we observed with the women. That violence committed by women tends to be less "visible" than violence committed by men—occurring disproportionately against family members, at home, and without response from the police—may help explain why the violence reported for women is often lower and why clinicians tend to underestimate it. Yet accurate risk assessments require accurate estimation of base rates. Because, among people with mental disorder, the base rate for violence by women is substantially the same as the base rate for violence by men, these data indicate that clinicians should be particularly careful to inquire in detail about violence among patients who are women, lest they continue to fall prey to underestimation. Interestingly, recent research by Elbogin, Williams, Kim, Tomkins, and Scalora (2001) found that clinicians who were women were significantly more likely than clinicians who were men to perceive a large gender gap in patients' rates of violence. To the extent that this is the case, it would suggest that women clinicians should pay particular attention to the evidence of near gender parity in violence reported here.

It is clear that the implications of these findings of a lack of differences in rates would highlight the need for clinicians to integrate the gender of the patient in a different way when making discharge decisions: not to discount the propensity of women to commit violence but to consider the possible different situational contexts of the violence that may be committed. These findings and implications become especially noteworthy when taken in the context of noted misperceptions by clinicians that exist when making decisions about the violence, mental disorder, and gender.

ACKNOWLEDGMENTS

The authors gratefully acknowledge the contributions of other members of the Risk Working Group of the MacArthur Network of Mental Health and the Law including Paul S. Appelbaum, Thomas Grisso, Edward P. Mulvey, Loren H. Roth, and Henry J. Steadman, and analytic support of Steven Banks and Roumen Vesselinov.

REFERENCES

Appelbaum, P., Robbins, P., & Monahan, J. (2000). Violence and delusions: Data from the MacArthur Violence Risk Assessment Study. *American Journal of Psychiatry, 157,* 566–572.

Appelbaum, P., Robbins, P., & Roth, L. (1999). A dimensional approach to the assessment of delusions. *American Journal of Psychiatry, 156,* 1938–1943.

Banks, S., Robbins, P., Silver, E., Vesselinov, R., Steadman, H., Monahan, J., et al. (2002). *A multiple models approach to violence risk assessment among people with mental disorder.* Manuscript submitted for publication.

Binder, L., & McNiel, D. (1990). The relationship of gender to violent behavior in acutely disturbed psychiatric patients. *Journal of Clinical Psychiatry, 51,* 110–114.

Brennan, P., Mednick, S., & Hodgins, S. (2000). Major mental disorders and criminal violence in a Danish birth cohort. *Archives of General Psychiatry, 57,* 494–500.

Coontz, P., Lidz, C., & Mulvey, E. (1994). Gender and the assessment of dangerousness in the psychiatric emergency room. *International Journal of Law and Psychiatry, 17,* 369–376.

Elbogin, E., Williams, A., Kim, D., Tomkins, A., & Scalora, M. (2001). Gender and perceptions of dangerousness in civil psychiatric patients. *Legal and Criminological Psychology, 6,* 215–228.

Fehon, D., Grilo, C., & Lipshitz, D. (2001). Gender differences in violence exposure and violence risk among adolescent inpatients. *Journal of Nervous and Mental Disease, 189,* 532–540.

Gelles, R., & Straus, M. (1998). *Intimate violence: The causes and consequences of abuse in the American family.* New York: Simon and Schuster.

Greenfeld, L., & Snell, T. (1999). *Bureau of Justice Statistics special report: Women offenders.* Washington, DC: U.S. Department of Justice.

Grisso, T., Davis, J., Vesselinov, R., Appelbaum, P., & Monahan, J. (2000). Violent thoughts and violent behavior following hospitalization for mental disorder. *Journal of Consulting and Clinical Psychology, 68,* 388–398.

Hiday, V. A., Swartz, M., & Swanson, J. W. (1998). Male–female differences in the setting and construction of violence among people with severe mental illness. *Social Psychiatry and Psychiatric Epidemiology, 33,* 568–574.

Hodgins, S. (1992). Mental disorder, intellectual deficiency and crime: Evidence from a birth cohort. *Archives of General Psychiatry, 49,* 476–483.

Lam, J., McNiel, D., & Binder, D. (2000). The relationship between gender and violence leading to staff injuries. *Psychiatric Services, 51,* 1167–1170.

Lidz, C., Mulvey, E., & Gardner, W. (1993). The accuracy of predictions of violence to others. *JAMA, 269,* 1007–1011.

McNiel, D., & Binder, R. (1995). Correlates of accuracy in the assessment of psychiatric inpatients' risk of violence. *American Journal of Psychiatry, 148,* 1317–1321.

Monahan, J., Steadman, H., Appelbaum, P., Robbins, P., Mulvey, E., Silver, E., et al. (2000). Developing a clinically useful actuarial tool for assessing violence risk. *British Journal of Psychiatry, 176,* 312–319.

Newhill, C., Mulvey, E., & Lidz, C. (1995). Characteristics of violence in the community by female patients seen in a psychiatric emergency service. *Psychiatric Services, 46,* 785–795.

Reiss, A., & Roth, J. (1993). *Understanding and preventing violence.* Washington, DC: National Academy Press.

Sampson, R. J., & Lauritsen, J. L. (1994). Violent victimization and offending: Individual-, situational-, and community-level risk factors. In A. J. Reiss & J. A. Roth (Eds.), *Understanding and preventing violence* (pp. 1–114). Washington, DC: National Academy Press.

Silver, E. (2000). Race, neighborhood disadvantage, and violence among persons with mental disorders: The importance of contextual measurement. *Law and Human Behavior, 24,* 449–456.

Steadman, H., Mulvey, E., Monahan, J., Robbins, P., Appelbaum, P., Grisso, T., et al. (1998). Violence by people discharged from acute psychiatric inpatient facilities and by others in the same neighborhoods. *Archives of General Psychiatry, 55,* 393–401.

Steadman, H., & Silver, E. (2000). Immediate precursors to violence among persons with mental illness: A return to a situational perspective. In S. Hodgins (Ed.), *Effective prevention of crime and violence among the mentally ill* (pp. 35–48). Dordrecht, The Netherlands: Kluwer Academic Publishers.

Steadman, H., Silver, E., Monahan, J., Appelbaum, P., Robbins, P., Mulvey, E., et al. (2000). A classification tree approach to the development of actuarial violence risk assessment tools. *Law and Human Behavior, 24,* 83–100.

Steffensmeier, D., & Allen, E. (1996). Gender and crime: Toward a gendered theory of criminal offending. *Annual Review of Sociology, 22,* 459–487.

Stueve, A., & Link, B. (1998). Gender differences in the relationship between mental illness and violence: Evidence from a community-based epidemiological study in Israel. *Social Psychiatry and Psychiatric Epidemiology, 33,* S61–S67.

Swanson, J., Holzer, C., Ganju, V., & Jono, R. (1990). Violence and psychiatric disorder in the community: Evidence from the epidemiological catchment area surveys. *Hospital and Community Psychiatry, 41,* 761–770.

Wilson, J., & Hernstein, R. (1985). *Crime and human nature.* New York: Simon and Schuster.

[10]

Empirical Limits for the Forensic Assessment of PTSD Litigants[1]

William J. Koch,[2,5] Melanie O'Neill,[3] and Kevin S. Douglas[4]

This paper discusses the limits of expert opinion on posttraumatic stress disorder (PTSD) in personal injury claims. The construct of PTSD is hampered by several empirical limitations. Multiple reliable measures of PTSD exist, but have not been evaluated sufficiently within litigating samples and are infrequently used by forensic assessors. Common methods for trauma screening appear insensitive. Opinions about causation of PTSD and disability are complicated by retrospective memory biases, as well as the failure of most anxiety disorders to be detected within primary medical care. PTSD appears to have a steep spontaneous remission curve during the first year, but at least 10% of trauma-exposed people suffer chronic distress. Little is known about the course beyond 1 year. Efficacious psychological treatments have been developed for PTSD, but are not in common use limiting claimants' access to rehabilitative treatments. Research on functional disability associated with PTSD is in its infancy, but it seems likely that PTSD will account for only a part of the variance in work disability. We provide suggestions for improving forensic practice, advising the courts about the limitations of forensic opinions, and necessary research.

KEY WORDS: posttraumatic stress disorder; forensic assessors; psychological treatments.

> *"There's something happening here/what it is ain't exactly clear."*
>
> Steven Stills, 1969

Steven Stills' classic rock and roll line from the 1960s describes well the current state of our knowledge about the validity of psychological injuries and the best methods

[1]We have omitted any discussion of the assessment of malingering of PTSD in this paper for reasons of space. However, we note that malingering or symptom exaggeration are alternative explanations for PTSD claimants' disability and require appropriate investigation. The interested reader is referred to recent excellent reviews (e.g., Guriel & Fremouw, 2003; Iverson & Lange, in press) of this latter topic.

[2]University of British Columbia, Vancouver, British Columbia, Canada.
[3]Malaspina University College, Nanaimo, British Columbia, Canada.
[4]Simon Fraser University, Burnaby, British Columbia, Canada.
[5]To whom correspondence should be addressed at Department of Psychiatry, University of British Columbia, 2255 Wesbrook Mall, Vancouver, British Columbia, Canada, V6T 2A1; e-mail: willkoch@telus.net.

for assessing and quantifying the losses of psychological injury claimants. Claims of mental injury and work-related disability are a rapidly growing area of personal injury litigation. Both the courts and mental health professionals have recognized the existence of traumatically induced psychological distress since at least the 19th century, particularly in connection with "nervous shock" and "railway mind" stemming from train accidents in Britain (Harrington, 1996), and "irritable heart" developed by Civil War soldiers (Tomb, 1994). More recently, the introduction of the diagnosis of posttraumatic stress disorder (PTSD) into the Diagnostic and Statistical Manual of Mental Disorders (DSM-III) of the American Psychiatric Association (APA, 1980) was "made to order for personal injury and worker compensation claimants because the diagnostic criteria explicitly include an etiological stressor" (Melton, Petrila, Poythress, & Slobogin, 1997, p. 376). PTSD may be a fortuitous diagnosis for personal injury claimants. However, the proof of such a legally compensable injury will depend largely upon expert evidence (e.g., see discussion by Douglas, Huss, Murdoch, Washington, & Koch, 1999), and thus the quality of such expert evidence is important to examine.

We are focusing on the diagnosis of PTSD as a mental health correlate of compensable personal injury, despite our own appreciation that the law does not compensate individuals for specific mental health diagnoses, so much as it compensates claimants for their economic losses and pain and suffering that are only partially described by the symptoms comprising individual mental health diagnoses. Nonetheless, PTSD is commonly referred to in the professional (e.g., Melton et al., 1997; Simon, 2003), and legal (*Johnson v. May* [1992; Ill. App. Ct.]; *Quaglio v. Tomaselli* [1984]) literature concerning personal injury litigation. Thus, we believe our focus on this frequently litigated condition to be timely. We recognize that PTSD is just one of several potential mental injuries that may arise following some negligent trauma. Psychological injuries include diagnosable conditions such as PTSD, depression, other anxiety disorders. They may also include less well-defined states of anxiety, fear or other negative emotions that interfere with mental tranquility and daily functioning. What is important for legal purposes is that these adverse emotional states cause sufficient harm that compensation is appropriate.

Therefore, within this paper, we are focusing on the assessment of a limited subset of psychological injuries. The purpose of this paper is to highlight four issues in forensic assessments of PTSD claims. First, we will review those limited inferences about personal injury claims related to PTSD symptoms that clinicians *can* make based on psychological science; specifically (a) evidence about the validity and diagnosis of PTSD, (b) predisposing factors for the development of PTSD, (c) comorbidity of other disorders with PTSD, (d) short term prognosis of PTSD, and (e) treatment of PTSD. Second, we will review those legal questions that psychological science *cannot* yet address sufficiently, but for which the courts and legal counsel need answers. In particular, difficulties with personal injury claims associated with the diagnosis of PTSD include: (a) difficulties in making reliable estimates of pretrauma status, (b) determining whether Criterion A (the traumatic stressor criterion) has been met in a given case, (c) assessment of functional disability related to individual PTSD claims, and (d) the deficits in our knowledge of the long-term prognosis for PTSD sufferers. These latter areas are those in which forensic assessors often write speculative opinions that have limited empirical bases.

Finally, we will follow-up by discussing how mental health experts can improve PTSD assessments and better inform the court about the limitations of expert opinion. Finally, we will make some suggestions for psychological research in this area.

LEGAL CONTEXT FOR PTSD CLAIMS

Viable claims for psychological damages must satisfy the following requirements. First, the defendant must have some demonstrated responsibility (e.g., through negligence) for the injury suffered by the plaintiff.

Second, the plaintiff must have some documented mental disorder (e.g., PTSD) or other emotional condition that poses objective losses to his/her occupational, social or other important functioning. Such mental or emotional conditions are wide ranging and can encompass (a) gross changes in personality functioning; (b) specific clusters of disabling symptoms characterized by such DSM diagnoses as PTSD, depression, other anxiety disorders; (c) sub-clinical variants of a diagnosable condition (e.g., subsyndromal PTSD) that result in significant functional interference; or (d) specific dysfunctional behaviors that may not necessarily qualify as a common mental disorder diagnosis but cause the claimant both distress and functional disability (e.g., problematic anger that interferes with occupational functioning, specific phobias of automobile travel). Diagnosis and description of mental disorders, personality dysfunction, and description of behavior all fall within the legally acknowledged competencies of psychiatrists and psychologists.

Third, the disorder or condition must have been caused or worsened by the negligent act. This means that the disorder cannot have existed in the plaintiff prior to the negligent act, or if it did exist, it must have been in a less severe and disabling fashion. This "causality" question, despite its paramount importance in tort litigation, poses some striking challenges to mental health professionals, in particular because of the difficulties in reliably estimating pretrauma mental health. Fourth, the injury must have resulted in some loss by the plaintiff. Such losses include reduced occupational or social functioning, and (dependent on statute) may extend to pain and suffering associated with the injury. Damage to, or "loss" of a person's "mental tranquility" typically is considered a compensable injury by the law. Mental health professionals are frequently asked to comment on the extent of a plaintiff's occupational and social disability as they relate to his/her PTSD. Such opinions arguably require the mental health professional to integrate actuarial data (e.g., employment deficits associated with PTSD generally) with the plaintiff's idiosyncratic presentation. Compensation awards may then vary in size dependent on the extent and duration of the plaintiff's distress and disability, as well as the court's determination of the likely prognosis for the plaintiff's recovery. Estimations of prognosis require the assessor to predict a trajectory for the claimant's distress and disability into the future. Such opinions require the assessor to integrate epidemiological data on the course of the disorder with individual characteristics of the plaintiff that make him/her likely to diverge from the modal course. This question has several potential pitfalls for the careless assessor. Part of the general prognosis question involves the prescription of treatment and prediction of disorder course following such treatment. Therefore, forensic assessments of personal injury claims based on PTSD must accomplish four aims. They must describe (a) the existence/nonexistence of PTSD and related disorders or general emotional distress, (b) the temporal/functional relationship of the PTSD or other emotional distress to the negligent act, (c) an opinion about the likely rate of remission of any PTSD symptoms with and without appropriate treatment, and (d) the extent of functional disability associated with the PTSD following from the negligent act. Thus, expert opinions require an integration of our scientific knowledge, epidemiological data, or actuarial data with the plaintiff's idiosyncratic characteristics that predict positive versus negative outcomes.

PTSD AS A MENTAL INJURY

We will presume for the purposes of this paper that the legal status of PTSD in tort litigation generally has been accepted by the courts (see *Johnson v. May,* 1992). Having said that, we must ask the following three questions; (a) is PTSD a valid diagnosis, (b) can health professionals diagnosis PTSD reliably, (c) under what circumstances do they diagnose most reliably, and (d) what are the common threats to validity of PTSD diagnoses?

Is PTSD a Valid Diagnosis?

Space does not permit an historical review of the evolving concept of PTSD. However, we note a number of debates that focus on the validity of PTSD as a psychiatric diagnosis and unitary construct.

Sociopolitical Origins

First, an interesting debate still rages over the sociopolitical origins of the PTSD diagnosis. Critics such as Scott (1990) have suggested that inclusion of PTSD in the modern versions of the DSM was more a consequence of advocacy efforts of psychiatrists involved in the treatment of combat veterans than it was of scientific discovery, per se. That is, the diagnosis grew out of the efforts of advocacy efforts on behalf of a presumed disadvantaged population (Vietnam combat veterans). This early sociopolitical influence, still visible in the comments of many practitioners and researchers, may have held back empirical advances in the field through its emphasis on the importance of the trauma, discouragement of research on personality predictors, and lesser emphasis on posttrauma coping.

Personality Predictors

Second, some authors (e.g., Bowman, 1999) criticize PTSD based on the extensive research literature showing that preexisting personality/mental health histories are better predictors of PTSD status than are objective trauma characteristics, per se. There is very strong evidence from longitudinal and cross-sectional studies (see review by Miller, 2003) that basic personality dimensions such as negative emotionality (NEM, often called neuroticism), positive emotionality (PEM, often called extraversion), and constraint/inhibition play strong predisposing roles in the development of PTSD. This research literature is perhaps most convincing for the reliable contributions of high levels of NEM to the prediction of PTSD status. Data from clinical samples examining the comorbidity personality disorders with PTSD is consistent with this argument. For example, Feeny, O'Neill, and Foa (under review) found that assaulted women who met symptom criteria for PTSD had higher numbers of Axis II diagnoses (39.1%) than women who did not meet symptom criteria for PTSD (19.6%). Thus, it is arguable that PTSD is an extreme state of NEM, composed in various parts of exacerbated levels of NEM as well as diagnostically/situationally unique dysfunctional characteristics such as intrusive memories, nightmares, and specific forms of behavioral and cognitive avoidance.

Other Predictors of PTSD Status

PTSD is not randomly distributed even if one ignores preexisting personality characteristics. Female gender has often been found to predict greater risk of PTSD from MVAs (see reviews by Douglas & Koch, 2000; Koch, Douglas, Nicholls, & O'Neill, in press). However, this may be accounted for in multiple ways. For example, the greater incidence of PTSD in females may be part of the more general phenomenon in which females display more psychological distress independent of exposure to traumatic stressors, and women may be exposed differentially to more frequent nontraumatic stressors (e.g., Almeida & Kessler, 1998). Thus, the utility of female gender as a predictor of PTSD may be mediated by socially mediated characteristics of feminine gender, rather than by gender, per se.

An individual's previous history of traumatic experiences or other psychosocial stressors has been shown in some studies (e.g., Astin, Lawrence, & Foy, 1993; Blanchard, Hickling, Taylor, & Loos, 1995a; Bolstad & Zinbarg, 1997) to predict PTSD subsequent to a later index trauma, but this relationship has not always been replicated. To some extent, the previous development of PTSD may be a better predictor of PTSD following a subsequent index trauma than previous trauma. Ursano et al. (1999), for example, found previous trauma did not predict PTSD following subsequent trauma events, but previous PTSD diagnoses did. Another strong predictor of PTSD is a history of previous episodes of general emotional problems or psychopathology (e.g., Blanchard, Hickling, Taylor, Loos, & Gerardi, 1994; Ehlers, Mayou, & Bryant, 1998).

Unequal Diagnostic Contributions by Different Symptoms

Current diagnostic criteria for PTSD (APA, 2000) require the patient to manifest at least one of five potential reexperiencing symptoms (e.g., nightmares), at least three of seven potential avoidance and numbing symptoms (e.g., loss of interest in usual activities, loss of emotional closeness with loved ones), and at least two of five potential hyperarousal symptoms (e.g., sleep disturbance, irritability), in addition to significant distress or functional impairment. A number of factor analytic studies have tried to confirm this tripartite structure but most have failed to do so. Maes et al. (1998), for instance, found two factors, labeled "depression-avoidance" and "anxiety-arousal," best described the PTSD symptom grouping. They failed to find support in either exploratory principal components analysis or confirmatory factor analysis for the three-factor model of PTSD proposed by the DSM system. They reported that only Criterion C symptoms were able to differentiate trauma victims with and without PTSD. Yet, the prevalence of these symptoms was substantially lower than for Criteria B and D. This led Maes et al., to argue that Criterion C, although largely responsible for PTSD diagnoses, is also too restrictive (or that B and D are too sensitive). Others have made similar arguments (Schützwohl & Maercker, 1999). In an evaluation of MVA survivors and Canadian peacekeepers, Taylor, Kuch, Koch, Crockett, and Passey (1998) reported an "intrusion and avoidance" and a "hyperarousal and numbing" factor, which was later replicated by Buckley, Blanchard, and Hickling (1998). Asmundson et al. (2000), however, reported that a four-factor model best fit the data (reexperiencing, avoidance, numbing, and hyperarousal). Taken as a whole, these findings are less consistent with the tripartite model of PTSD and more consistent with a model of PTSD as superordinate negative affectivity that becomes exacerbated in response to stress (given the prominence of depression and anxiety in the model). This is consistent with Bowman's (1999) and Miller's (2003) arguments that PTSD is better accounted for by individual differences on such factors such as NEM than it is by event characteristics.

These findings that depart from the DSM model of PTSD have led some to criticize PTSD for not reflecting empirical reality (Buckley et al., 1998) but rather expert consensus. Schützwohl and Maercker (1999) reported that certain subthreshold PTSD cases (people who did not meet Criterion C) were more distressed on psychological measures than were some people who met criteria for PTSD. They proposed that "partial PTSD" be recognized as a legitimate classification option for persons who do not meet criteria for PTSD but who clearly are traumatized. Similarly, Buckley, Blanchard, and Hickling (1996) showed that people with a diagnosis of PTSD are not always more distressed than people without such a diagnosis, largely because the latter have many symptoms within a certain cluster but not enough in another.

In summary, few attempts at confirming the tripartite model of PTSD have been able to do so. PTSD may reflect more a general negative affectivity composed of various parts anxious, depressive, avoidant, and mental intrusions symptoms. This debate is especially relevant for forensic assessment. If one adopts a noncategorical approach to defining psychological injuries, then individuals who have a larger number of symptoms, more severe symptoms, or higher scores on continuous measures of psychological distress may be considered to have suffered the greater injury. This supports an assessment model that would call for not only categorical classification (PTSD vs. no PTSD), but comparison of individual claimants' PTSD symptom scores or other dimensional measures of distress to known normative groups.

The Problem of Multiple Comorbidity

The aforesaid perception that PTSD may reflect nothing more than general negative affectivity is bolstered by the high degree of comorbidity with other diagnoses. PTSD has a higher rate of comorbidity with other anxiety and mood diagnoses than any other anxiety disorder. Among treatment seeking outpatients, Brown, Campbell, Lehman, Grisham, and Mancill (2001) found 92% with principal PTSD diagnoses had another active mental health diagnosis, and 100% had at least one other mental health diagnosis in their history. Other treatment-seeking samples (e.g., Blanchard et al., 2003) suggested especially high comorbidity of depression and anxiety disorders with PTSD, with the number of comorbid diagnoses increasing with the severity of PTSD symptoms (Zayfert, Becker, Under, & Shearer, 2002). Within a community sample of women, Boudreaux, Kilpatrick, Resnick, Best, and Saunders (1998) found those with PTSD were more likely to have any Axis I disorder (64 vs. 25%) and some specific Axis I disorders (e.g., major depressive episode) than women without PTSD. Female victims of sexual and nonsexual assault are also more likely to be diagnosed with another Axis I disorder (lifetime and current) than victims without PTSD (Feeny et al., under review).

The difficult task for a forensic assessor in psychological injury claims related to a traumatic stressor is to determine how much comorbid psychopathology predated the subject trauma. Because legally compensable psychological injuries are not limited to specific diagnoses like PTSD, in a case of PTSD that appears to have arisen following the trauma, but is comorbid with (for example) a major depressive disorder, the important questions revolve around (a) the date of onset for the depression, and (b) the relative contributions of these discrete, yet related, disorders to functional disability. To take one potential example, it is theoretically possible for a claimant to suffer a legitimate case of PTSD following a trauma, but to have a major depressive disorder that (a) predated the subject trauma, and (b) makes a more substantial contribution to the claimant's functional disability.

In short, the diagnosis of PTSD appears to be associated with substantially higher rates of depression, other anxiety disorders, and personality disorders; to be strongly predicted by basic personality characteristics of NEM; to have an inconsistent factor structure; and to be excessively influenced by one of three clusters of symptoms (i.e., the avoidance/numbing cluster). Trauma survivors appear to suffer a complex and variable array of mental health symptomms that are not limited to a diagnosis of PTSD, per se. The implications of such comorbidity and personality correlates are four-fold. First, the discussion above suggests that the concept of PTSD is in need of further theoretical refinement and empirical study. Second, psychological assessment of a plaintiff in a personal injury claim should not be limited to PTSD, but should include assessment of other apparently inter-related diagnoses of major depression and other anxiety disorders. Third, forensic assessors should be encouraged to assess across multiple dimensions of psychological distress for evidence of cases of psychological distress that result in significant disability. Fourth, forensic assessors need to differentiate the mere presence of posttrauma high levels of NEM and low levels of PEM or other facets of dysfunctional personality functioning from behaviors more specific to PTSD.

Can Health Professionals Diagnose PTSD Reliably?

With respect to differentiation of PTSD from other mental health conditions, "expert" clinicians can differentiate PTSD from similar disorders (major depressive disorder, generalized anxiety disorder) when given a list of criteria and associated symptoms (Keane, Taylor, & Penk, 1997). Reliable and valid diagnostic tools for the assessment of PTSD are readily available to clinicians. For example, the Clinician Administered PTSD Scale (Blake et al., 1998) has very good inter-rater reliability for PTSD symptoms with correlations between raters ranging from .82 to .99 (Blanchard et al., 1995b), and excellent diagnostic agreement (Kappa = .81; Blanchard et al., 1995a). Other structured diagnostic interviews (e.g., *Anxiety Disorders Interview Schedule for DSM-IV* [ADIS-IV], DiNardo, O'Brien, Barlow, Waddell, & Blanchard, 1982) have adequate levels of reliability as well. The ADIS-IV is particularly relevant for forensic assessment of PTSD because it covers the range of anxiety, mood disorders, as well as some somatoform disorders, reflecting the comorbidity of both emotional and somatic complaints common in PTSD litigants.

Although the CAPS may be the current gold standard for PTSD interviews, a number of self-report inventories are useful and reliable for assessing the severity of PTSD symptoms. For example, Blanchard, Jones-Alexander, Buckley, and Forneris (1996) evaluated the validity of the civilian version of the PTSD Checklist (PCL-C), a 17-item self-report instrument. The overall correlation between the PCL and CAPS was .93. Using the recommended PCL cutoff of 50, prediction parameters (diagnostic efficiency) were good (e.g., .78 for sensitivity, .86 for specificity). The interested reader is referred to Koch et al. (in press) for a more detailed summary of psychometrically adequate structured interviews and self-report instruments for the assessment of PTSD.

The implications for forensic assessment are that although most clinicians have an appreciation of the diagnostic criteria for PTSD, and there are multiple reliable and valid assessment tools to enhance the forensic assessment of PTSD; it is still unclear whether PTSD is a categorical diagnosis so much as the centerpiece of a set of intercorrelated dimensions of psychological distress. Although it is preferable for psychologists and psychiatrists conducting forensic assessments of PTSD to use reliable and valid measures of PTSD status, forensic assessors need to beware of the limitations on the validity (e.g., unclear factor structure, extensive comorbidity) of this diagnosis. Also troubling is that most of the empirical research for PTSD assessment instruments has not accounted adequately for the presence of important variables such as compensation, compensation-seeking, or litigation. We know little about the impact of compensation status or litigation on PTSD-specific measures.

Despite the guardedly optimistic picture concerning reliability of assessment provided above, the clinical assessment of mental disorders has a checkered record.

Clinical assessors often have very low levels of agreement on otherwise straightforward diagnoses (e.g., chance agreement for the diagnosis of Panic Disorder, Steiner, Tebes, Sledge, & Walker, 1995), and their disagreement is too frequently associated with the use of different standards for clinically relevant symptoms or complaints, as well as by variations in the nature of questions and observations during their assessments (Ward, Beck, Mendelson, Mock, & Erbaugh, 1962).

Although similar research has not been conducted with PTSD claimants, it seems likely that the same limitations of unstructured assessments will apply in the forensic arena. Whereas it is possible, using available structured interviews and specific psychological tests, to reliably diagnose PTSD, assessments of PTSD that do not use such empirically supported methods are likely to be of limited reliability. Unfortunately, we have not adequately studied the extent to which forensic assessors use such empirically-supported assessment methods when evaluating PTSD claims. The only study of test utilization by personal injury assessors (Boccaccini & Brodsky, 1999) suggests that there is little consistency among experienced forensic assessors about a standard test battery for the assessment of psychological injuries. Only the MMPI-2 and *Beck Depression Inventory* (BDI; Beck, Steer, & Brown, 1996) are frequently used by forensic assessors in psychological injury cases. This suggests that none of the most reliable and valid PTSD assessment tools are commonly used in personal injury assessments of PTSD litigants

Diagnostic Biases

We emphasize the use of empirically established assessment standards within forensic assessments because, left to their own devices, mental health professionals, like adolescents, too easily express poor judgment. By poor judgment, we refer in this case to a number of biases that may reduce the validity of expert opinions. Illusory correlation refers to the phenomenon in which clinicians observe two events co-occur within a limited sample and draw the conclusion that these two events co-occur more commonly than they would in a more representative sample (see Garb, 1998), e.g., "most MVA survivors I see have driving phobias, so driving phobias must be uniquely related to MVA trauma." Confirmatory bias refers to a cognitive process in which clinicians review patient information in a manner that is more likely to support than refute their hypothesis (Garb & Boyle, 2003). It is clear that patients' ethnicity contributes significantly to clinician diagnoses independent of the clinical presentation (e.g., Loring & Powell, 1988). We do not yet know whether ethnic minority group members receive different diagnoses in psychological injury evaluations. Gender bias also has been shown to occur in clinicians with respect to the diagnosis of mental health conditions (e.g., Becker & Lamb, 1994). In short, the biases described above, among others, adversely impact on the diagnosis of PTSD claimants, either through leading to the over- or under-diagnosis of PTSD or misattribution of causality. Greater adherence to structured assessment procedures and a more detailed understanding of the relevant scientific literature are important for reducing the incidence of such biases.

PROGNOSIS OF PTSD FOLLOWING TRAUMA

The law has a need to know the probability of remission for each individual PTSD claimant. However, there are many gaps in our knowledge and many apparent complexities in describing the emotional recovery of trauma survivors. We have broken our discussion of the current knowledge into four categories; (a) the rate of spontaneous remission of PTSD sufferers, (b) the phenomenon of delayed onset PTSD, (c) cross-sectional evidence of the probability that PTSD can be present for long periods of time posttrauma, and (d) the question of whether PTSD may present as an episodic versus continuous phenomenon.

Spontaneous Remission

PTSD is a unique mental health disorder because it is related to a specific noxious event and thus begs the question of the temporal course of symptoms dating from that event, in contrast with depression where we do not usually date the onset of symptoms to a particular environmental or social stressor. Thus, knowledge of the rate of spontaneous remission of PTSD symptoms following trauma exposure is helpful to forensic assessors. We discuss separately below those studies based on treatment-seeking or nonrandomly recruited samples and those studies based on continuous admission samples as the treatment-seeking samples should arguably have higher rates of PTSD.

Continuous Admission Samples

There are a number of continuous admission or random samples of trauma survivors with follow-ups between 6 months and 2 years in duration that allow us to estimate the rate of spontaneous remission of PTSD. With respect to MVA survivors, initial estimates of PTSD have ranged from 29% (Delahanty et al., 1997) to 34% (Harvey & Bryant, 1999; Ursano et al., 1999). Delahanty et al., and Ursano et al., saw between 50 and 60% of their initial PTSD subjects spontaneously remit at 1 year. On the other hand, Harvey and Bryant's sample showed only a 10% remission at 2 years. La Greca, Silverman, Vernberg, and Prinstein (1996) assessed elementary school children following Hurricane Andrew, and found an initial 39% incidence of PTSD that declined by 54% at 10 months. Rothbaum and Foa (1993), in a prospective study of adult female sexual assault victims, found that 94% of their sample initially met symptomatic criteria for PTSD, but that 55% of these women had remitted at 6 months. In an anomalous study with combat veterans, Wolfe, Erickson, Sharkansky, King, and King (1999) followed a large sample of Persian Gulf veterans for 2 years. The initial incidence of PTSD was estimated at 3%, but a full 8% of the sample were estimated as having PTSD when followed up between 18 and 24 months later. That is, the incidence of PTSD more than doubled as time passed following removal from the combat zone.

Treatment Seeking Samples

Perhaps the most systematic study of the spontaneous remission of PTSD following trauma comes from the large MVA–PTSD studies of Blanchard and his colleagues. In a study of short-term remission, Blanchard et al. (1997) recruited 158 MVA survivors who had sought medical care one to 4 months prior to their assessment. At initial assessment, 40% of their subjects met criteria for PTSD. At 6 month reassessment; 55% of their original PTSD sufferers had remitted. Blanchard et al. (1996), in an expanded sample and extension of previous research, examined remission over the course of 18 months in 158 MVA victims. Over 12 months, the number of persons with PTSD dropped from 30% of the original sample to 10%, resulting in a spontaneous remission rate of about 67%. For the 35 initial people with PTSD who were followed between 12 and 18 months, there was little further remission beyond what occurred in the first 12 months. Halligan, Michael, Clark, and Ehlers (2003) assessed victims of sexual or physical assault. Thirty-five percent of their sample met criteria for PTSD at the initial assessment, reduced to 30% at 6 months for only a 10% rate of spontaneous remission.

In summary, whereas some studies show that approximately one-half to two-thirds of initial PTSD cases remit within the first year, other research suggests a lower rate of spontaneous remission. Some studies (e.g., Wolfe et al., 1999) suggest that PTSD prevalence may grow over the first several months posttrauma. Even the most optimistic of these studies suggests that as many as 10% of initial PTSD sufferers remain symptomatic 1 year posttrauma.

Delayed Onset PTSD

The study above by Wolfe et al. (1999) suggests that cases of PTSD may emerge some months following the traumatic stressor that serves as the putative precipitant. As the critical reader will surmise, the concept of delayed onset PTSD is problematic for PTSD as a diagnostic entity and for arguing PTSD in personal injury claims. According to *DSM-IV* (1994), clinicians should specify delayed onset if 6 months have passed between the trauma and the onset of PTSD symptoms. There are three important issues here: (a) what phenomenon is delayed, (b) at which temporal point do we start timing in the estimation of delayed onset, and (c) how common is such delayed onset PTSD?

What Phenomenon is Delayed?

The concept of delayed onset PTSD hinges to some degree on the categorical system of description. For example, Buckley, Blanchard, and Hickling (1996) found that delayed onset PTSD cases had more PTSD symptoms at initial assessment shortly following their MVAs than did non-PTSD cases. Thus, "delayed onset" may be a misnomer, and reflect no more than an artifact of categorical diagnoses when continuous measures of distress may better describe trauma survivors' posttrauma changes.

When Does the Timer Start?

This is not a trivial question. Does one's exposure to combat exposure begin and end with the first firefight in which one engages? Does one's exposure to MVA-related trauma end when the vehicle stops rolling over? Common sense and our clinical observations suggest not. Nonetheless, discussions of delayed onset PTSD sometimes imply that there is a valid point at which to start the timer. Comparisons of different types of trauma populations illustrate the problems with this presumption. Schnurr, Lunney, Sengupta, and Waelde (2003) examined the PTSD symptom course of 530 Vietnam veterans. According to these authors 31% of combat veterans suffered their first PTSD symptoms the same year they went to Vietnam, another 31% their first symptoms 1 year postentry, 32% had their first symptoms 2–5 years postentry, and 6% between 6 and 22 years later. One can contrast this apparent very high rate of delayed onset PTSD from a form of stressor that has diffuse temporal boundaries with those of Buckley et al. (1996) in which only 10% of MVA-related PTSD patients had delayed onset. The latter study also indicated that one of the predictors of delayed onset PTSD was the greater physical injury quotient for the delayed onset subjects at their later assessment. The implication of the latter finding is that the sense of threat and loss for those subjects with lingering physical injuries had not yet remitted and thus, it was not entirely clear that the trauma was over. The astute reader will note that this has implications for the definition of the Criterion A stressor, which we discuss later in this paper. Just as we presume that the critical threatening events that contributed to PTSD symptoms in Vietnam veterans did not all occur the moment these soldiers walked into a rice paddy for the first time in battle gear, MVA survivors' threatening events are not temporally limited to the collision itself but may include a number of medical events as well as the dawning realization of permanent physical change that are drawn out over a period of months. It is not clear to us that the concept of delayed onset PTSD is helpful other than drawing attention to the potential for different temporal pathways to PTSD.

How Common is Delayed Onset PTSD?

Given the discussion above, this last topic may be of limited importance. It is clear that delayed onset PTSD, using traditional definitions, is either relatively rare (e.g., ≤10% in Buckley et al., 1996; Ehlers et al., 1998) or common (Schnurr et al., 2003).

Chronic PTSD

Most longitudinal studies are of relatively short duration because of the cost and logistical difficulties related to following a large cohort of trauma victims from date of trauma through multiple assessments. For the most part, we are restricted to estimating longer-term prognosis from cross-sectional studies. One exception is that of Zlotnick et al. (1999), who followed 54 PTSD patients over a 5-year period following their initial diagnosis of PTSD. All participants had suffered from PTSD for at least 1 year at the time of their diagnosis for this particular study, and had one or more comorbid anxiety disorders. The most prominent Criterion A stressors to which these participants had been exposed was some form of childhood abuse. Survival analysis based on yearly assessments showed that these PTSD sufferers had only a .18 probability of remitting over the course of 5 years. Childhood abuse and alcohol abuse, but not the concurrent presence of depression, predicted slower or lesser remission of PTSD.

Cross-sectional studies suggest that there is indeed a hard core of trauma survivors who remain symptomatic with PTSD for many years. For example, Schnurr et al. (2000) assessed 363 U.S. military veterans from World War II who had been exposed to mustard gas experiments. The assessment took place in 1996, more than 50 years posttrauma. Thirty-two percent of these veterans met criteria for full PTSD, and 10% met criteria for subsyndromal PTSD as assessed by the PCL. Other studies (e.g., Green, Lindy, Grace, & Leonard, 1992; Kilpatrick & Resnick, 1993) found a sizeable proportion of trauma survivors to suffer from PTSD years following the trauma.

In short, there appears to be a sizeable minority of trauma survivors who suffer from PTSD for many years following the index trauma. Failure of individual PTSD claimants to remit within a year or two following the index trauma should, therefore, not be surprising to forensic assessors or the consumers of psychological evidence.

Episodic Versus Continuous Distress

In a creative study utilizing a Veterans Health Administration database, Ronis et al. (1996) looked at the records of mental health services to PTSD patients to study their use of mental health services, and by implication their functioning over time. Patients with PTSD tended to use fewer mental health services than patients with Schizophrenia, but more than patients with Depression. Of note here, patients with PTSD were relatively chronic users of mental health services but did have episodes when they did not use mental health services (average of 2.2 "nonuse intervals" of 100 days or more in duration). This suggests that individuals with PTSD are highly likely to return for mental health care because of either a full or partial relapse, or are likely to have periods of better functioning even during a prolonged episode of PTSD.

Summary of Treatment Prognosis

We discuss the treatment of PTSD here because (a) PTSD plaintiffs theoretically desire treatment if they suffer this disorder, (b) the costs of returning them to full functioning will be part of the damages, and (c) the availability of efficacious treatment for PTSD has implications for the future remission of this condition and limitations in the plaintiff's losses. The absence of any efficacious treatments therefore is bad for both plaintiff (because of continued suffering) and for the defendant (because of the potential for longer lasting disability and greater damages).

The Good News

The last decade has witnessed the development and validation of a number of efficacious treatments for PTSD. Cognitive-behavioral therapy (CBT) appears to be the main efficacious psychological treatment for chronic PTSD. Four variations of CBT have demonstrated significant efficacy. These include stress inoculation training (SIT; Veronen & Kilpatrick, 1983), prolonged exposure (PE; Foa et al., 1999), cognitive processing therapy (CPT; Resick & Schnicke, 1992), and CBT based on Ehlers's and Clark's (2000) cognitive model of PTSD (e.g., Ehlers et al., 2003). The efficacy of cognitive behavioral interventions for chronic PTSD has been demonstrated in a number of different studies with various different trauma populations. These include sexual assault victims (Foa, Rothbaum, Riggs, & Murdock, 1991; Foa et al., 1999; Resick & Schnicke, 1992; Resick, Nishith, Weaver, Astin, & Feuer, 2002), adult survivors of childhood abuse (Cloitre, Koenen, Cohen, & Han, 2002), MVA survivors (e.g., Blanchard et al., 2003), and veterans (e.g., Keane, Fairbank, Caddell, & Zimering, 1989).

There are also pharmaceutical treatments for PTSD that have some efficacy. Despite earlier pessimistic outcomes, increasing evidence supports the effectiveness of selective serotonin reuptake inhibitors (SSRI's) and monoamine oxidase inhibitors (MAOI's) in reducing PTSD symptomatology. For example, Davidson, Rothbaum, van der Kolk, Sikes, and Farfel (2001) compared sertraline and placebo in a double-blind multicenter trial for moderate to severe PTSD. A 60% versus 38% responder rate for sertraline compared with placebo was found for 208 patients over a 12-week period. Davidson, Landerman, Farfel, and Clary (2002) examined the impact of sertraline on the individual symptoms of PTSD using data from two 12-week placebo-controlled trials. Sertraline outperformed placebo on the vast majority of PTSD symptoms particularly with the numbing and arousal clusters of symptoms.

Overall, it appears that the family of SSRI's demonstrates moderate but clinically significant improvement in PTSD symptomatology and overall functioning across a wide variety of trauma populations (Yehuda, Marshall, Penkower, & Wong, 2002). The International Consensus Group on Depression and Anxiety along with a group of PTSD experts recommend SSRI's as the first-line class of pharmaceutical treatment for PTSD with such treatment recommended for at least 12 months (Ballenger et al., 2000).

The Bad News

First, the most efficacious psychological treatments are seldom applied in clinical practice and thus most PTSD claimants who enter treatment have a relatively low probability of receiving an efficacious treatment. In fact, it is apparent that the vast majority of licensed psychologists do not use prolonged imaginal exposure (perhaps the most important component of CBT for PTSD) on any of their PTSD patients. In a survey of 207 licensed psychologists from the Northeastern United States and Texas, Becker, Zayfert, and Anderson (2004) found that 83% of their sample never used imaginal exposure therapy with their PTSD patients. Therefore, although efficacious psychological treatments exist for PTSD, such treatments are not widely used by health professionals, and thus are for all practical purposes unavailable to PTSD claimants.

Second, even efficacious treatments fail to help a substantial minority of PTSD patients. For example, Blanchard et al. (2003) in their recent large trial of CBT for PTSD following MVAs found that 70% of PTSD patients remitted from full PTSD status following treatment. This is perhaps the most optimistic clinical trial outcome of which we are aware involving PTSD sufferers and fully 30% of people receiving the treatment failed to remit. Therefore, forensic assessors must show caution when making predictions about a claimant's probability of remission following treatment. Access to effective treatment is limited and even the most effective treatment has a high failure rate.

LIMITATIONS IN ASCERTAINING PRETRAUMA MENTAL STATE

Determination of a plaintiff's pretrauma mental state requires extensive historical data collection. Valid inferences from such historical data collection are limited by two phenomena: (a) the relatively low reliability of humans' autobiographical memories, and (b) inadequate mental health screening during usual clinical care.

Retrospective Recall Biases

Social psychological research suggests that individuals "reconstruct" their memories of subjective experiences (e.g., pain, emotional distress) based, at least partially, on personal models they use to explain their experiences. Ross (1989) theorized that when individuals attempt to remember their personal characteristics in the past, they engage in a two-step process. The first step involves self-assessment of their current status on the dimension of interest, under the presumption that present status will be related to past status. Step two involves the application of whatever implicit theory the person has about the personal characteristic (e.g., is this characteristic likely to be stable over time or to vary in a particular manner?).

Arising from this theory, McFarland, Ross, and DeCourville (1989) constructed a very creative study that has significant implications for the forensic assessment of PTSD. These authors based their study on the common North American belief that women suffer significantly more physical and emotional distress during their menstrual period. They demonstrated that young university women substantially overestimated the negative affect, bloating, and pain occurring during their menstrual period when asked to retrospectively estimate the same symptoms, but significantly underestimated their negative affect and pain on days outside their menstrual period when asked to retrospectively estimate. Thus, retrospective recall of subjective symptoms of negative affect and physical discomfort appears to be controlled by stereotypical beliefs about causal factors for such distress.

Does this phenomenon apply to trauma survivors? Unfortunately, this retrospective memory bias does appear to occur with the recall of PTSD symptoms. Harvey and Bryant (2000) interviewed 56 accident victims about their ASD symptoms 1 month and 2 years postaccident. In the follow-up interview, they asked the patients when their symptoms had begun. PTSD symptom severity at 2 year follow-up predicted inaccurate recollection of more symptoms during the first month after the accident than the patients had reported at the 1 month assessment. On the other hand, asymptomatic individuals at the 2-year follow-up tended to under-report ASD symptoms they had reported at 1 month.

The forensic assessor who understands this phenomenon of biased retrospective recall will use assessment methods (e.g., review of past health records;

interviewing of collateral informants) that will reduce his/her reliance on the claimant's retrospective recall and perhaps adjust for the bias described above. However, such nonpatient sources of information have their own limitations.

Limits of Collateral Information

Many PTSD symptoms (e.g., intrusive memories, emotional numbing, and concentration deficits) likely occur under the radar of casual observation by spouses, friends, coworkers, family physicians, and even mental health professionals. These are, after all, subjective symptoms of mental distress.

Within health care settings, it appears that anxiety and mood disorders frequently evade detection. This is a more significant problem than most clinicians might appreciate. A number of studies suggest that anxiety and mood problems are common in patients hospitalized with purely medical disorders. Walker, Novack, and Kaiser (1987) found that 36% of medical inpatients had clinically significant anxiety and depression just prior to discharge. Rincon et al. (2001) found that 24 and 17%, respectively, of discharged critical care patients had anxiety or depressive diagnoses. Clark, Minas, and Stuart (1991) found 30% of medical and surgical inpatients to have depressive and anxiety conditions. Silverstone (1996) found that 27% of medical inpatients had a psychiatric diagnosis. Martucci et al. (1999) found that 26% of general hospital patients met criteria for a psychiatric disorder. Nisenson, Pepper, Schwenk, and Coyne (1998) also found a high prevalence of anxiety disorders in primary care practices.

If hospitalized and primary care medical patients have such a high prevalence of anxiety and depressive conditions, one would expect these to be detected by their treating physicians and recorded in clinical records. This is not the case. Fulop (1990) studied 136,977 discharge summaries, excluding those carrying a principal psychiatric diagnosis. Only .8% of these discharge summaries noted an anxiety disorder diagnosis. Considering conservative prevalence estimates, this suggests at least 90% of anxiety disorders in patients hospitalized for medical reasons are overlooked by their caregivers. Other writers (e.g., Eisenberg, 1992) estimate that as many as 50% of psychiatric disorders are not detected in primary care. In one study, when confederates complained of simulated anxiety-related symptoms to general practitioners, 60% were neither diagnosed with any psychiatric disorder, nor prescribed any pharmaceutical or psychosocial treatment (Shahabudin, Almashoor, Edariah, & Khairuddin, 1994).

Therefore, past health records may well underestimate the historical prevalence and severity of PTSD and related disorders. Forensic assessors must be aware of this limitation of past primary care and hospital health records, and acknowledge this limitation in their historical data concerning the claimant's past status.

ASSESSMENT OF THE TRAUMATIC STRESSOR (CRITERION A)

Forensic assessors must address two issues related to traumatic stressors: (a) was the event that precipitated the litigation and the claimant's initial response to the event of sufficient magnitude and threat to qualify as a Criterion A traumatic stressor, and (b) are the claimant's psychological difficulties better explained by a previous Criterion A stressor? The answers to these questions are critical to forensic assessors' opinions about both diagnosis and causality, but have complex underpinnings.

With respect to determination of Criterion A status for the litigation-related stressor, some authors advocate focusing on the objective severity (e.g., physical injury, amount of property damage) of the traumatic event (e.g., Malmquist, 1996), and there appears to be a general fear in some circles (e.g., the insurance industry) that considering the subjective response during trauma exposure will markedly increase claims for psychological distress. This stems both from natural skepticism and admonitions coming out of the DSM Task Force (Frances, First, & Pincus, 1995). However, Kilpatrick et al. (1998) in the DSM-IV field trials found that restrictions on the definition of Criterion A stressors had only modest effects on PTSD prevalence.

Despite the findings of Kilpatrick et al. (1998), we believe that a thorough forensic assessment of PTSD or other emotional consequences of trauma should include a detailed evaluation of the subject trauma and the claimant's initial emotional response. We briefly review our preferred strategy for such evaluation below.

First, did the claimant suffer a life-threatening injury as a result of the traumatic event? Second, did the claimant suffer a physically disabling injury that could conceivably limit their employment or accomplishment of important life goals (e.g., spinal cord injury)? Third, did the claimant witness a death or severe injury, such as death via homicide, vehicular accidents, or within medical settings (e.g., hospital emergency departments)? Fourth, did the claimant have a realistic fear that their life was in danger despite no obvious traumatic injury (e.g., HIV-infected blood splash or needle puncture, stalking by stranger or ex-romantic partner)? Fifth, did the claimant suffer some threat to their physical integrity (e.g., threatened or actual coercive sexual contact)?

If yes to one or more of these types of events, the examiner must ask for a description of the claimant's emotional state at the time of the traumatic event. DSM-IV specifies intense fear, helplessness, or horror as the requisite emotional states. However, the examiner must use his/her clinical judgment to ascertain whether the claimant was in one or more of these states or some similar form of negative emotional arousal. Thus, the assessor should probe to determine if the claimant feared for his/her life, or that something worse than the actual physical outcome might occur (e.g., "what did you think the stalker would do to you?").

Also relevant are descriptions of intense emotional reactions. For example, there is evidence that panic attacks during the subject trauma predict PTSD status (e.g., Nixon & Bryant, 2003). There is considerable debate about the role of dissociation at the time of the trauma ("peritraumatic dissociation") in the prediction of PTSD (e.g., Mellman, David, Bustamante, Fins, & Esposito, 2001). Sometimes, objective data concerning heightened emotional arousal, such as emergency room vital signs (e.g., heart rate), will be available; however, empirical investigation of heart rates has had mixed results with respect to predicting PTSD (e.g., Blanchard, Hickling, Galovski, & Veazey, 2002; Shalev et al., 1998).

Thus, a careful forensic assessment of the Criterion A status of an index trauma will evaluate systematically the objective and subjective threat experienced by the claimant during the trauma, as well as the presence of negative emotional arousal. Beyond DSM-recommended emotional states, the careful assessor will ask the claimant what he/she anticipated happening to him/her during the trauma (e.g., loss of life, life-altering injury, and threat to personal well-being) and assess for the presence of panic, peritraumatic dissociation, and physiological hyperarousal.

Perhaps the greatest weakness in clinical and forensic assessment of Criterion A stressors is the limited screening for lifetime history of trauma exposure. This is problematic in that inadequate screening increases the potential for the assessor to mis-attribute PTSD symptoms to an index stressor when such symptoms are at least partially precipitated by a previous trauma. At one time, traumatic events sufficient to cause PTSD were thought to be rare. According to the APA in 1987, "The essential feature of (PTSD) is the development of characteristic symptoms following a psychologically distressing *event that is outside the range of usual human experience*.... The stressor producing this syndrome would be markedly distressing to almost anyone...." (APA, 1987, pp. 247). Contrary to the statement above, research during the past decade has shown that traumatic stressors are all too common in everyday life, and that many such common events have a relatively high association with PTSD. In fact, exposure to life-threatening or very frightening trauma appears to be common in the general public (e.g., Goodman, Corcoran, Turner, Yuan, & Green, 1998; Kubany et al., 2000; Norris, 1992).

If the average person, not to mention the average personal injury claimant, is more likely than not to have experienced a traumatic stressor in his/her lifetime, it behooves clinicians and forensic assessors to obtain a detailed trauma history from a patient or plaintiff. Lest the reader believe that trauma victims routinely seek help, various sources suggest that many trauma victims do not freely present for mental health assessment and treatment. For example, Kimerling and Calhoun (1994) found that only 19% of rape survivors initially seen in a hospital emergency room later sought mental health care of any kind. Asking patients or plaintiffs about their history of traumatic experiences may be uncomfortable for clinicians and embarrassing for patients. There are a number of strategies for eliciting more accurate trauma histories including: (a) adding a preface about others' experiences of trauma prior to the inquiry, (b) avoiding legal descriptions in favor of behaviorally specific language to describe acts of sexual victimization, and (c) allowing for reports of multiple traumatic experiences (Resnick, Falsetti, Kilpatrick, & Freedy, 1996).

In a move to improve the detection of traumatic events, general prefatory statements about trauma exposure are now more commonly used in structured interviews for PTSD. However, Weaver (1998), in a sample of 43 women found that behaviorally specific inquires (e.g., about childhood physical and sexual abuse, adult sexual assault) markedly increased the endorsement rate for such events when compared to more general questions, such as "things like major earthquakes or floods, very serious accidents or fires, physical assault or rape, seeing other people killed or dead, being in a war or heavy combat, or some other type of disaster. At any time during your life have any of these kinds of things happened to you?" (Weaver, 1998, p. 182). Close examination of this particular prefatory remark suggests that respondents might understandably not mention exposure to date rape, motor vehicle accidents, sexual harassment, life-threatening medical illness, among other potentially threatening events. In Weaver's sample of battered women, a behaviorally specific question about childhood sexual abuse increased the endorsement rate from 7 to 53%. Within forensic mental health assessments, failure to inquire in such a detailed manner about trauma histories increases the risk of mis-attribution of PTSD symptoms and associated disability.

LIMITATIONS IN RELATING PTSD TO FUNCTIONAL DISABILITY

Posttraumatic stress is correlated with impairment in social, financial, physical, and psychological functioning (e.g., Amaya-Jackson et al., 1999; McCarren et al., 1995; Zatzick et al., 1997). However, this conclusion is taken from specific samples that may not generalize to survivors of other types of trauma. MVAs may be the most common precipitants of PTSD in western society (Norris, 1992), yet we have no empirical data about the overall economic impact of PTSD in MVA survivors. As well, the association of PTSD with underemployment merely indicates that PTSD increases risk for reduced employment. Differences in economic performance between PTSD and non-PTSD samples obscure important differences between PTSD individuals who suffer significant functional disadvantage secondary to their psychological disorder and those who suffer no such functional disadvantage by dint of environmental advantages.

There are only scattered studies within the general disability literature relevant to our current topic. Both PTSD symptoms (Regehr, Goldberg, Clancy, & Knott, 2002) and depression (Kouzis & Eaton, 1994) have been shown to predict work disability. However, Regehr et al. (2002) found that factors such as personality characteristics of suspiciousness, hostility and isolation were stronger predictors of mental health leave than PTSD symptoms, per se. In a sample of PTSD claimants, Emsley, Seedat, and Stein (2003) found that 90% had negative feelings about their previous work and over half believed that changes in the work environment played a substantial role in their emotional discomfort. Two large studies from Finland examined the predictors of disability. Krause et al. (1997) found that psychosocial constructs such as mental strain on the job, job dissatisfaction, limited communication with fellow workers, and less social support from supervisors all contributed to disability, while Appelberg, Romanov, Heikkilae, and Honkasalo (1996) found that life dissatisfaction predicted disability for both genders, interpersonal conflict at work predicted disability in women, and monotonous work, neuroticism, and daily stressors predicted disability in men. Yet another Scandinavian study (Olstad, Sexton, & Sogaard, 2001) found that social support appeared to buffer work-related stress.

Although it appears likely that high levels of PTSD and depressive symptoms place an individual at risk for work disability, social/interpersonal factors such as hostility and social isolation, social support, perceived or actual low support from employers, and work/life dissatisfaction are all variables that may influence the claimant's ability to work productively. Forensic assessors can thus assert with some confidence that PTSD places the sufferer at risk for work-related disability, but must admit that other variables play a role in disability claims. Assessors must then venture into idiographic behavioral analyses of the characteristics of the individual PTSD claimant that make him/her more or less vulnerable to work-related disability.

CONCLUSIONS AND RECOMMENDATIONS

To paraphrase our opening quote from Stephen Stills, *something is definitely happening* when litigants claim damages related to PTSD. However, a number of issues with respect to such claims are unclear. First of all, it is not altogether clear just what PTSD is. The factorial structure of PTSD is still unclear, avoidance and numbing symptoms appear to play a disproportionately large role in determining just which trauma survivors receive the diagnosis, and there is a remarkable amount of comorbidity of PTSD with other mental health diagnoses such as depression, other anxiety disorders, and substance abuse. While reliable assessment tools are available, they are apparently not commonly used in clinical and forensic practice. This is a problem because of the known limitations on the reliability of unstructured clinical interviews and because of the potential for a number of different diagnostic biases to arise in such unstructured assessment.

Forensic assessors also have to predict the course of PTSD in claimants. It is clear that among most representative samples of PTSD sufferers there is as much as 50% spontaneous remission within the first year posttrauma. However, as many as 10% of sufferers may stay chronically distressed. The concept of delayed onset PTSD may reflect both methodological difficulties in specifying the temporal boundaries of the trauma (when does it end?) and insensitive methods for detecting substantial psychological distress than it does a unique clinical entity. We know relatively little about the extent to which PTSD sufferers wax and wane over time in their psychological distress.

Attributions of causality are especially difficult in this area for two reasons: (a) the relatively insensitivity of general health care practice to detecting anxiety disorders more generally, and (b) the low reliability of individual's retrospective memories for their subjective states. Finally, while psychological treatments in particular have evolved over the past decade so that there are efficacious treatments for PTSD, these treatments are seldom applied by practitioners in the field and thus are of limited availability.

How to Structure Assessments to Understand the Individual Case

Keeping with the tradition of the multi-trait, multi-method matrix, we will structure this section on a two dimensional matrix of legal questions and assessment methods as summarized in Table 1. We begin with an attempt to describe the clinical problem(s) or arrive at diagnoses. Given the extensive comorbidity of other stress-related conditions with PTSD, use of a broad-band structured interview, covering the gamut of anxiety disorders as well as mood and somatoform disorders, is helpful. Lifetime interviewing and focus on the waxing and waning of symptoms

Table 1. Elements of a Forensic Assessment of PTSD

Questions	Methods: Interviews	Methods: Tests	Methods: Collateral Sources
Presence of PTSD and/or related conditions	Multi-disorder structured interview	Multi-Scale inventory.	Family members.
	PTSD structured interview	PTSD symptom inventory.	Family physician records
	Clinical interview related to fear and avoidance.	Depressive symptoms inventory.	Mental health records.
		PTSD-related cognitions Measure of behavioral avoidance.	
Relationship to trauma	Historical structured diagnostic interview.	Trauma screening measure	Family members.
	Detailed trauma history.		Family physician records.
			Mental health records.
Prognosis	Interview about anger, pain impact, anxiety tolerance, social support, interference by depressed mood	Depression measures. Trait anger measures. Pain severity and interference measures.	Clinical records indicating failed treatments (presuming that empirically supported treatment was provided).
Functional disability	Interview about how specific symptom clusters affect work attendance, function, and interpersonal relations.		Work records. Interviews with coworkers, employers, family.

both prior to and following the subject event is a necessary part of this interview strategy.

There is a place for clinical interviews in gathering data in the following areas. First, a general psychosocial and trauma exposure history is helpful in determining diverse predisposing factors such as negative family environment during childhood, other traumas, and previous anxiety or mood disorders. An interview concerning the plaintiff's own personal perception of the ways in which his/her symptoms interfere with daily function is also helpful. One important domain of inquiry might include mobility deficits that interfere with work attendance (e.g., fear-motivated avoidance of car travel in MVA–PTSD claimants, or social avoidance related to prior criminal victimization). Other lines of inquiry might involve the impact of PTSD-related anger problems on interpersonal relations in the workplace, or lowered tolerance for work-related stressors secondary to high levels of anxious arousal.

To supplement interviews, we use both multi-scale inventories, to screen for a broader array of clinical problems and impediments to treatment, and an array of single scale inventories to assess the extent of (a) PTSD symptoms, (b) PTSD-related characteristics, and (c) other problems that may complicate the plaintiff's clinical presentation and prognosis. The assessor may understand the plaintiff's particular vulnerabilities more clearly if such strictly PTSD assessment is supplemented both with measures of PTSD-related constructs and other clinical problems that can influence the development and remission of PTSD.

Collateral data are important to thorough investigations of PTSD claims although they are prone to the limitations mentioned earlier. Family members can be interviewed with respect to their general observations of the plaintiff's mental health (what are ___________'s main problems now"). Family members' perception of change in the plaintiff's mental health over time is a critical topic. It is likely better to inquire in a manner that deemphasizes the pre–post trauma distinction and focuses the collateral's attention on general periods of time. The assessor might also interview collaterals about their observations of specific behaviors or complaints by the plaintiff about subjective symptoms that might comprise part of PTSD symptomatic criteria or aspects of other conditions such as depression or other anxiety disorders. It is possible to make up parallel forms of PTSD or depression symptom tests worded in such a manner that one is assessing the degree to which the collateral has observed the plaintiff engaging in particular behaviors or complaining of particular symptoms. Given that there are no normative data on such tests, the assessor must be cautious in interpretation.

Health records have both benefits and limitations within forensic evaluations of PTSD. Because they occur in a different context (help-seeking vs. compensation-seeking) and at least the pretrauma records occur prior to the seeking of compensation, they are theoretically less prone to be influenced by anticipation of compensation. However, given the evidence (discussed above) that most primary medical care and specialist (other than psychiatry) medical care records under-represent anxiety and mood disorders, the forensic assessor cannot confidently rule out anxiety and mood problems from a family physician record devoid of comments about such conditions. This applies, of course, equally to pretrauma and posttrauma medical records. Documentation of such problems in family physician records is more easily interpretable but must still be considered carefully because of the methodological limitations of family physicians assessments of mental health problems. In the end, conservative use of family physician records is probably to use the noted presence of problems to indicate some (nonspecific) psychological distress that *may* be consistent with the presence of a specific mental disorder or problem. It is more logically difficult to conclude that such notations indicate the plaintiff had the same disorder at the same level of severity/disability prior to the subject trauma, unless it is clear that the family physician performed a comprehensive diagnostic assessment. Neither can the forensic assessor take the absence of notations as conclusive evidence that no mental disorder or condition existed at that time.

Finally, although space precludes extensive discussion of this issue, a thorough forensic assessment of a PTSD claimant will use a systematic strategy for assessing symptom exaggeration or malingering.

How to Inform Courts of the Limitations of Expert Opinions

The courts need to understand the following limited points concerning expert evidence about PTSD. First, although PTSD can be reliably diagnosed, adherence to structured, multimethod assessment procedures including structured interviews and tests specific to PTSD is critical to ensure adequate diagnostic reliability. Because reliability is the foundation of validity in psychological assessments, courts should be leery of accepting "expert" evidence based on such unstructured procedures.

Second, the courts need to know that PTSD seldom occurs independently, but is often comorbid with other psychiatric disorders (e.g., depression). Although this comorbidity may reflect problems with the concept of PTSD itself, it also requires those forensic assessors conducting putative PTSD evaluations to cast a wide net for related emotional problems that frequently co-occur with PTSD and are compensable losses in their own right. Expert assessments that address the presence/absence of PTSD in isolation are too narrow in scope to adequately inform the court of plaintiffs' potential losses. Related to this issue, experts must inform the courts that because of PTSD's association more diffuse NEM and given the predictive utility of a history of such personality attributes, careful scrutiny must be given to cases of diffuse negative emotion following trauma to ensure that the claimant's concerns are not primarily a reflection of pre-existing personality characteristics.

Third, experts should inform the court that as many as 50% of initial PTSD cases remit without treatment within 1 year, but that a substantial number of PTSD cases do not remit for many years. Therefore, PTSD claims that are over 1-year old have on average a low probability of remitting without some efficacious treatment. Related to this, experts need to inform the courts that, despite the existence of reasonably efficacious treatments for PTSD, these treatments are not necessarily in common use among clinicians and are thus of limited availability. Even if PTSD claimants receive the best psychosocial treatments for PTSD, they have a one-third chance of not remitting following such treatment. The courts need to know that many distressed individuals can be easily missed in initial screenings that missing such cases is a fault of the DSM categorical diagnostic model, insensitive assessment methods, and our difficulties in defining the temporal boundaries of the subject trauma.

Fourth, the courts should be informed by experts that estimation of pretrauma status is a speculative task because of (a) the marked underestimations of anxiety disorders in general medical settings, and (b) biased retrospective recall of humans in general and trauma survivors in particular. Courts must closely examine experts' methods for arriving at opinions about the pretrauma mental health of PTSD claimants.

Finally, courts need to know that although PTSD is a known correlate of lower economic functioning, our knowledge of how PTSD leads to such lower functioning is rudimentary, and comments on the relationship between a given plaintiff's PTSD and his/her occupational disability is largely speculation. Triers of facts should carefully examine the methods by which causal links are claimed between PTSD status and functional limitations.

Future Research Directions

The research literature on PTSD with respect to its underlying psychopathology, prevalence, course and treatment is expanding exponentially. There are, however, some relatively neglected areas that will be of special benefit to the intersection of law and psychology.

Much of what we know about the course characteristics and economic impact of PTSD comes from veteran and treatment-seeking populations. Although this is an important area, it is of unknown application to those PTSD cases more commonly litigated in the courts (e.g., MVAs). Increased research is needed to examine the longer-term course of PTSD and related conditions following physical injury in vehicular and industrial accidents, as well as assault. Because most of what we know about PTSD comes from diverse samples of convenience, treatment-seeking samples, or samples exposed to one particular type of trauma (e.g., MVAs), further research is necessary to generalize our knowledge base.

We still know far too little about common forensic assessment practice with respect to PTSD claims. The field would benefit from research into common interview practices among forensic assessors, utilization of empirically supported assessment methods, and common biases present in forensic decision-making (e.g., gender biases, confirmatory biases). Despite the enormous economic implications of this area of litigation and expert evidence, we know precious little about how "PTSD experts" conceptualize cases, assess cases, and form expert opinions about PTSD.

Despite the availability of efficacious treatments for PTSD, these treatments have not yet been adequately evaluated in multiproblem, compensation seeking or litigating samples within typical community rehabilitation settings. As well, occupational and social functioning have seldom been targeted as critical dependent variables in the clinical trials for PTSD. Whereas changes in diagnostic status are clinically and scientifically meaningful, return to functioning is the bottom line, both for determining losses secondary to the PTSD and for returning the claimant to a gratifying life. Only a series of such clinical trials will help us to understand whether PTSD claimants can be restored to adequate functioning following their injury with our currently available or enhanced treatments.

Finally, a virtually ignored area is that of the economic consequences of PTSD and related disorders. In particular, some very basic research is necessary to determine what it takes to be an adequate worker in various occupational tracks, and how different forms of psychological dysfunction result in economic impairment. It is not the diagnosis of PTSD that causes sufferers to earn less money and attend work less successfully. Rather, it is the as yet undefined behavioral consequences of maladaptive responses to trauma that lead to such economic consequences.

In summary, despite the proliferation of research on PTSD more generally and the increasing role of psychological injuries within our civil courts, much research remains to be done before we can dispute Steven Still's summary of this area. We do know that *something* (currently named PTSD) is going on in the courtrooms. Similarly, we know that mental health professionals can reliably assess PTSD, but suspect that many forensic assessments of PTSD are themselves somewhat unreliable. Further, we are still not entirely sure what PTSD is, whether it is a unique entity in itself, what psychological damages the courts are compensating, or how forensic assessors develop their expert opinions.

REFERENCES

Allen, A. M. (1992). Effects of race and gender on diagnostic judgments with the DSM-III-R (Doctoral dissertation, University of South Dakota, 1992). *Dissertation Abstracts International, 53/05-A,* 1395.

Almeida, D. M., & Kessler, R. C. (1998). Everyday stressors and gender differences in daily distress. *Journal of Personality and Social Psychology, 75,* 670–680.

Amaya-Jackson, L., Davidson, J. R., Hughes, D. C., Swartz, M., Reynolds, V., George, L. K., et al. (1999). Functional impairment and utilization of services associated with posttraumatic stress in the community. *Journal of Traumatic Stress, 12,* 709–724.

American Psychiatric Association (1980). *Diagnostic and statistical manual of mental disorders* (3rd ed.). Washington, DC: Author.

American Psychiatric Association (1987). *Diagnostic and statistical manual of mental disorders* (Rev. 3rd ed.). Washington, DC: Author.

American Psychiatric Association (1994). *Diagnostic and statistical manual of mental disorders* (4th ed.). Washington, DC: Author.

American Psychiatric Association (2000). *Diagnostic and statistical manual of mental disorders* (Text Rev. 4th ed.). Washington, DC: Author.

Appelberg, K., Romanov, K., Heikkilä, K., & Honkasalo, M. (1996). Interpersonal conflict as a predictor of work disability: A follow-up study of 15,348 Finnish employees. *Journal of Psychosomatic Research, 40,* 157–167.

Asmundson, G. J. G., Frombach, I., McQuaid, J., Pedrelli, P., Lenox, R., & Stein, M. B. (2000). Dimensionality of posttraumatic stress symptoms: A confirmatory factor analysis of DSM-IV symptom clusters and other symptom models. *Behaviour Research and Therapy, 38,* 203–214.

Astin, M. C., Lawrence, K. J., & Foy, D. W. (1993). Posttraumatic stress disorder among battered women: Risk and resiliency factors. *Violence and Victims, 8,* 17–28.

Ballenger, J. C., Davidson, J. R. T., Lecrubier, Y., Nutt, D. J., Foa, E. B., Kessler, R. C., et al. (2000). Consensus statement on posttraumatic stress disorder from the international consensus group on depression and anxiety. *Journal of Clinical Psychiatry, 61,* 60–66.

Beck, A. T., Steer, R. A., & Brown, G. K. (1996). *Beck depression inventory manual* (2nd ed.). San Antonio, TX: Psychological Corporation.

Becker, C. B., Zayfert, C., & Anderson, E. (2004). A survey of psychologists' attitudes towards and utilization of exposure therapy for PTSD. *Behaviour Research and Therapy, 42,* 277–292.

Becker, D., & Lamb, S. (1994). Sex bias in the diagnosis of borderline personality disorder and posttraumatic stress disorder. *Professional Psychology: Research and Practice, 25,* 55–61.

Blake, D. D., Weathers, F., Nagy, L. M., Kaloupek, D. G., Charney, D. S., & Keane, T. M. (1998). *Clinician-administered PTSD scale for DSM-IV.* Boston: National Center for Posttraumatic Stress Disorder.

Blanchard, E. B., Hickling, E. J., Devineni, T., Veazey, C., Galovski, T., Mundy, E., et al. (2003). A controlled evaluation of cognitive behavioral therapy for posttraumatic stress in motor vehicle accident survivors. *Behaviour Research and Therapy, 41,* 79–96.

Blanchard, E. B., Hickling, E. J., Forneris, C. A., Taylor, A. E., Buckley, T. C., Loos, W. R., et al. (1997). Prediction of remission of acute posttraumatic stress disorder in motor vehicle accident victims. *Journal of Traumatic Stress, 10,* 215–234.

Blanchard, E. B., Hickling, E. J., Galovski, T., & Veazey, C. (2002). Emergency room vital signs and PTSD in a treatment seeking sample of motor vehicle accident survivors. *Journal of Traumatic Stress, 15,* 199–204.

Blanchard, E. B., Hickling, E. J., Taylor, A. E., Loos, W. R., & Gerardi, R. J. (1994). Psychological morbidity associated with motor vehicle accidents. *Behaviour Research and Therapy, 32,* 283–290.

Blanchard, E. B., Hickling, E. J., Taylor, A. E., & Loos, W. (1995a). Psychiatric morbidity associated with motor vehicle accidents. *Journal of Nervous and Mental Disease, 183,* 495–504.

Blanchard, E. B., Hickling, E. J., Taylor, A. E., Forneris, C. A., Loos, W., & Jaccard, J. (1995b). Effects of varying scoring rules of the Clinician Administered PTSD (CAPS) for the diagnosis of posttraumatic stress disorder in motor vehicle accident victims. *Behaviour Research and Therapy, 33,* 471–475.

Blanchard, E. B., Jones-Alexander, J., Buckley, T. C., & Forneris, C. A. (1996). Psychometric properties of the PTSD Checklist (PCL). *Behaviour Research and Therapy, 34,* 669–673.

Boccaccini, M. T., & Brodsky, S. L. (1999). Diagnostic test usage by forensic psychologists in emotional injury cases. *Professional Psychology: Research and Practice, 30,* 253–259.

Bolstad, B., & Zinbarg, R. E. (1997). Sexual victimization, generalized perception of control, and posttraumatic stress disorder symptom severity. *Journal of Anxiety Disorders, 11,* 523–540.

Boudreaux, E., Kilpatrick, D. G., Resnick, H. S., Best, C. L., & Saunders, B. E. (1998). Criminal victimization, posttraumatic stress disorder; and comorbid psychopathology among a community sample of women. *Journal of Traumatic Stress, 11,* 665–678.

Bowman, M. L. (1999). Individual differences in posttraumatic distress: Problems with the DSM-IV model. *Canadian Journal of Psychiatry, 44,* 21–33.

Brown, T. A., Campbell, L. A., Lehman, C. L., Grisham, J. R., & Mancill, R. B. (2001). Current and lifetime comorbidity of the DSM-IV anxiety and mood disorders in a large clinical sample. *Journal of Abnormal Psychology, 110,* 585–599.

Buckley, T. C., Blanchard, E. B., & Hickling, E. J. (1996). A prospective examination of delayed onset PTSD secondary to motor vehicle accidents. *Journal of Abnormal Psychology, 105,* 617–625.

Buckley, T. C., Blanchard, E. B., & Hickling, E. J. (1998). A confirmatory factor analysis of posttraumatic stress symptoms. *Behaviour Research and Therapy, 36,* 1091–1099.

Clarke, D. M., Minas, I. H., & Stuart, G. W. (1991). The prevalence of psychiatric morbidity in general hospital inpatients. *Australian and New Zealand Journal of Psychiatry, 25,* 322–329.

Cloitre, M., Koenen, K. C., Cohen, L. R., & Han, H. (2002). Skills training in affective and interpersonal regulation followed by exposure: A phase-based treatment for PTSD related to childhood abuse. *Journal of Consulting and Clinical Psychology, 70,* 1067–1074.

Davidson, J. R. T., Landerman, L. R., Farfel, G. M., & Clary, C. M. (2002). Characterizing the effects of sertraline in posttraumatic stress disorder. *Psychological Medicine, 32,* 661–670.

Davidson, J. R. T., Rothbaum, B. O., van der Kolk, B. A., Sikes, C. R., & Farfel, G. M. (2001). Multicenter, double-blind comparison of sertraline and placebo in the treatment of posttraumtic stress disorder. *Archives of General Psychiatry, 58,* 485–492.

Delahanty, D., Herberman, H. B., Craig, K. J., Hayward, M. C., Fullerton, C. S., Ursano, R. J., et al. (1997). Acute and chronic distress and posttraumatic stress disorder as a function of responsibility for serious motor vehicle accidents. *Journal of Consulting and Clinical Psychology, 65,* 560–567.

Dinardo, P. A., O'Brien, G. T., Barlow, D. H., Waddell, M. T., & Blanchard, E. B. (1982). Reliability of DSM-III anxiety disorders using a new structured interview. *Archives of General Psychiatry, 40,* 1070–1074.

Douglas, K. S., & Koch, W. J. (2000, June). *Posttraumatic Stress Disorder arising from motor vehicle accidents: A critical review of predictive factors* (Working Paper for the Insurance Corporation of British Columbia).

Douglas, K. D., Huss, M., Murdoch, L. L., Washington, D. O., & Koch, W. J. (1999). Posttraumatic stress disorder stemming from motor vehicle accidents: Legal issues in Canada and the United States. In E. Hickling & E. Blanchard (Eds.), *The international handbook of road traffic accidents and psychological trauma: Current understanding, treatment and law* (pp. 271–290). Oxford, England: Pergamon Press.

Ehlers, A., & Clark, D. M. (2000). A cognitive model of posttraumatic stress disorder. *Behaviour research and therapy, 38,* 319–345.

Ehlers, A., Clark, D. M., Hackmann, A., McManus, F., Fennell, M., Herbert, C., et al. (2003). A randomized controlled trial of cognitive therapy, self-help, and repeated assessment as early interventions for PTSD. *Archives of General Psychiatry, 60,* 1024–1032.

Ehlers, A., Mayou, R. A., & Bryant, B. (1998). Psychological predictors of chronic posttraumatic stress disorder after motor vehicle accidents. *Journal of Abnormal Psychology, 107,* 508–519.

Eisenberg, L. (1992). Treating depression and anxiety in primary care: Closing the gap between knowledge and practice. *New England Journal of Medicine, 326,* 1080–1084.

Emsley, R. A., Seedat, S., & Stein, D. J. (2003). Posttraumatic stress disorder and occupational disability in South African Security Force members. *Journal of Nervous and Mental Disease, 191,* 237–241.

Feeny, N. C., O'Neill, M. L., & Foa, E. B. (under review). PTSD and Comorbid Axis I and II Disorders.

Foa, E. B., Dancu, C. V., Hembree, E. A., Jaycox, L. H., Meadows, E. A., & Street, G. P. (1999). A comparison of exposure therapy, stress innoculation training, and their combination for reducing posttraumatic stress disorder in female assault victims. *Journal of Consulting and Clinical Psychology, 67,* 194–200.

Foa, E. B., Rothbaum, B. O., Riggs, D. S., & Murdock, T. B. (1991). Treatment of posttraumatic stress disorder in rape victims: A comparison between cognitive-behavioral procedures and counseling. *Journal of Consulting and Clinical Psychology, 59,* 715–723.

Frances, A., First, M. B., & Pincus, H. A. (1995). *DSM-IV guidebook.* Washington, DC: American Psychiatric Press.

Fulop, G. (1990). Anxiety disorders in the general hospital setting. *Psychiatric Medicine, 8,* 187–195.

Garb, H. N. (1998). *Studying the clinician: Judgment research and psychological assessment.* Washington, DC: American Psychological Association.

Garb, H. N., & Boyle, P. A. (2003). Understanding why some clinicians use pseudoscientific methods: Findings from research on clinical judgment. In S. O. Lilienfeld, S. J. Lynn, & J. M. Lohr (Eds.), *Science and pseudoscience in clinical psychology* (pp. 17–38). New York: Guildford Press.

Goodman, L. A., Corcoran, C., Turner, K., Yuan, N., & Green, B. L. (1998). Assessing traumatic event exposure: General issues and preliminary findings for the Stressful Life Events Screening Questionnaire. *Journal of Traumatic Stress, 11,* 521–542.

Green, B. L., Lindy, J. D., Grace, M. C., & Leonard, A. C. (1992). Chronic posttraumatic stress disorder and diagnostic comorbidity in a disaster sample. *Journal of Nervous and Mental Disease, 180,* 760–766.

Guriel, J., & Fremouw, W. (2003). Assessing malingered posttraumatic stress disorder: A critical review. *Clinical Psychology Review, 23,* 881–904.

Halligan, S. L., Michael, T., Clark, D. M., & Ehlers, A. (2003). Posttraumatic stress disorder following assault: The role of cognitive processing, trauma memory, and appraisals. *Journal of Consulting and Clinical Psychology, 71,* 419–431.

Harrington, R. (1996). The "railway spine" diagnosis and Victorian responses to PTSD. *Journal of Psychosomatic Research, 40*(1), 11–14.

Harvey, A. G., & Bryant, R. A. (1999). The relationship between acute stress disorder and posttraumatic stress disorder: A 2-year prospective evaluation. *Journal of Consulting and Clinical Psychology, 67,* 985–988.

Harvey, A. G., & Bryant, R. A. (2000). Memory for acute stress disorder symptoms: A two-year prospective study. *Journal of Nervous and Mental Disease, 1888,* 602–607.

Iverson, G. L., & Lange, R. T. (in press). Detecting exaggeration & malingering in psychological injury claims. In W. J. Koch, K. S. Douglas, T. L. Nicholls, & M. O'Neill (Eds.), *Psychological injuries: Forensic assessment, treatment, and law.* Oxford University Press.

Johnson v. May, 585 N.E.2d 224 (Ill. App. Ct. 1992)

Keane, T. M., Fairbank, J. A., Caddell, J. M., & Zimering, R. T. (1989). Implosive (flooding) therapy reduced symptoms of PTSD in Vietnam combat veterans. *Behavior Therapy, 20,* 245–260.

Keane, T. M., Taylor, K. L., & Penk, W. E. (1997). Differentiating post-traumatic stress disorder (PTSD) from major depression (MDD) and generalized anxiety disorder (GAD). *Journal of Anxiety Disorders, 11,* 317–238.

Kilpatrick, D. G., & Resnick, H. S. (1993). Posttraumatic stress disorder associated with exposure to criminal victimization in clinical and community populations. In J. R. T. Davidson & E. B. Foa (Eds.), *Posttraumatic stress disorder: DSM-IV and beyond* (pp. 113–143). Washington, DC: American Psychiatric Press.

Kimerling, R. E., & Calhoun, K. S. (1994). Somatic symptoms, social support, and treatment seeking among sexual assault victims. *Journal of Consulting and Clinical Psychology, 62,* 33–340.

Koch, W. J., Douglas, K. S., Nicholls, T. L., & O'Neill, M. (in press). *Psychological injuries: Forensic assessment, treatment, and law.* Oxford, UK: Oxford University Press.

Kouzis, A. C., & Eaton, W. W. (1994). Emotional disability days: Prevalence and predictors. *American Journal of Public Health, 84,* 1304–1307.

Krause, N., Lynch, J., Kaplan, G. A., Cohen, R. D., Goldberg, D. E., & Salonen, J. T. (1997). Predictors of disability retirement. *Scandinavian Journal of Work, Environment and Health, 23,* 403–413.

Kubany, E. S., Haynes, S. N., Leisen, M. B., Owens, J. A., Kaplan, A. S., Watson, S. B., et al. (2000). Development and preliminary validation of a brief broad-spectrum measure of trauma exposure: The Traumatic Life Events Questionnaire. *Psychological Assessment, 12,* 210–224.

La Greca, A. M., Silverman, W. K., Vernberg, E. M., & Prinstein, M. J. (1996). Symptoms of posttraumatic stress in children after Hurricane Andrew: A prospective study. *Journal of Consulting and Clinical Psychology, 64,* 712–723.

Loring, M., & Powell, B. (1988). Gender, race and DSM-III: A study of the objectivity of psychiatric diagnostic behavior. *Journal of Health and Social Behavior, 29,* 1–22.

McCarren, M., Janes, G. R., Goldberg, J., Eisen, S. A., True, W. R., & Henderson, W. G. (1995). A twin study of the association of post-traumatic stress disorder and combat exposure with long-term socioeconomic status in Vietnam Veterans. *Journal of Traumatic Stress, 8,* 111–124.

McFarland, C., Ross, M., & DeCourville, N. (1989). Women's theories of menstruation and biases in recall of menstrual symptoms. *Journal of Personality and Social Psychology, 57,* 522–531.

Maes, M., Delmeire, L., Schotte, C., Janca, A., Creten, T., Mylle, J., et al. (1998). The two-factorial symptom structure of post-traumatic stress disorder: Depression-avoidance and arousal-anxiety. *Psychiatry Research, 81,* 195–210.

Malmquist, C. P. (1996). The use and misuse of psychiatry in sexual harassment cases. *Psychiatric Annals, 26,* 146–156.

Martucci, M., Balestrieri, M., Bisoffi, G., Bonizzato, P., Covre, M. G., Cunico, L., et al. (1999). Evaluating psychiatric morbidity in a general hospital: A two-phase epidemiological survey. *Psychological Medicine, 29,* 823–832.

Mellman, T. A., David, D., Bustamante, V., Fins, A. I., & Esposito, K. (2001). Predictors of posttraumatic stress disorder following severe injury. *Depression and Anxiety, 14,* 226–231.

Melton, G. B., Petrila, J., Poythress, N. G., & Slobogin, C. (1997). *Psychological evaluations for the courts: A handbook for mental health professionals and lawyers* (2nd ed.). New York: Guildford Press.

Miller, M. W. (2003). Personality and the etiology and expression of PTSD: A three-factor model perspective. *Clinical Psychology: Science and Practice, 10,* 373–393.

Nisenson, L. G., Pepper, C. M., Schwenk, T. L., & Coyne, J. C. (1998). The nature and prevalence of anxiety disorders in primary care. *General Hospital Psychiatry, 20,* 21–28.

Nixon, R. D. V., & Bryant, R. A. (2003). Peritraumatic and persistent panic attacks in acute stress disorder. *Behaviour Research and Therapy, 41,* 1237–1242.

Norris, F. H. (1992). Epidemiology of trauma: Frequency and impact of different potentially traumatic events on different demographic groups. *Journal of Consulting and Clinical Psychology, 60,* 409–418.

Olstad, R., Sexton, H., & Sogaard, A. J. (2001). The Finnmark Study. A prospective population study of the social support buffer hypothesis, specific stressors and mental distress. *Social Psychiatry and Psychiatric Epidemiology, 36,* 582–589.

Quaglio v. Tomaselli, 99 A.D.2d 487, 470 N.Y.S.2d 427 (1984).

Regehr, C., Goldberg, G., Glancy, G. D., & Knott, T. (2002). Posttraumatic symptoms and disability in paramedics. *Canadian Journal of Psychiatry, 47,* 953–958.

Resick, P. A., Nishith, P., Weaver, T. L., Astin, M. C., & Feuer, C. A. (2002). A comparison of cognitive-processing therapy with prolonged exposure and a waiting condition for the treatment of chronic posttraumatic stress disorder in female rape victims. *Journal of Consulting and Clinical Psychology, 70,* 867–879.

Resick, P. A., & Schnicke, M. K. (1992). Cognitive processing therapy for sexual assault victims. *Journal of Consulting and Clinical Psychology, 60,* 748–756.

Resnick, H. R., Falsetti S. A., Kilpatrick, D. G., & Freedy, J. R. (1996). Assessment of rape and other civilian trauma-related posttraumatic stress disorder: Emphasis on assessment of potentially traumatic events. In T. W. Miller (Ed.), *Theory and assessment of stressful events* (pp. 235–271). Madison, CT: International Universities Press.

Rincon, H. G., Granados, M., Unutzer, J., Gomez, M., Duran, R., Badiel, M., et al. (2001). Prevalence, detection and treatment of anxiety, depression, and delirium in the adult critical care unit. *Psychosomatics: Journal of Consultation Liaison Psychiatry, 42,* 391–396.

Ronis, D. L., Bates, E. W., Garfein, A. J., Buit, B. K., Falcon, S. P., & Liberzon, I. (1996). Longitudinal patterns of care for patients with posttraumatic stress disorder. *Journal of Traumatic Stress, 9,* 763–781.

Ross, M. (1989). The relation of implicit theories to the construction of personal histories. *Psychological Review, 96,* 341–357.

Rothbaum, B. O., & Foa, E. B. (1993). Subtypes of posttraumatic stress disorder and duration of symptoms. In J. R. T. Davidson & E. B. Foa (Eds.), *Posttraumatic stress disorder: DSM-IV and beyond* (pp. 23–35). Washington, DC: American Psychiatric Press.

Schnurr, P. P., Ford, J. D., Friedman, M. J., Green, B. L., Dain, B. J., & Sengupta, J. (2000). Predictors and outcomes of posttraumatic stress disorder in World War II veterans exposed to mustard gas. *Journal of Consulting and Clinical Psychology, 68,* 258–268.

Schnurr, P. P., Lunney, C. A., Sengupta, A., & Waelde, L. C. (2003). A descriptive analysis of PTSD chronicity in Vietnam veterans. *Journal of Traumatic Stress, 16,* 545–553.

Schützwohl, M., & Maercker, A. (1999). Effects of varying diagnostic criteria for posttraumatic stress disorder are endorsing the concept of partial PTSD. *Journal of Traumatic Stress, 12*(1), 155–165.

Scott, W. J. (1990). PTSD in DSM-III: A case in the politics of diagnosis and disease. *Social Problems, 37*(3), 294–310.

Shahabudin, S. H., Almashoor, S. H., Edariah, A. B., & Khairuddin, Y. (1994). Assessing the competence of general practitioners in diagnosing generalized anxiety disorder using standardized patients. *Medical Education, 28,* 432–440.

Shalev, A. Y., Freedman, A., Peri, T., Brandes, D., Sahara, T., Orr, S., et al. (1998). Prospective study of posttraumatic stress disorder and depression following trauma. *American Journal of Psychiatry, 155,* 630–637.

Silverstone, P. H. (1996). Prevalence of psychiatric disorders in medical inpatients. *Journal of Nervous and Mental Disease, 184,* 43–51.

Simon, R. I. (2003). *Posttraumatic stress disorder in litigation: Guidelines for forensic assessment.* Washington, DC: American Psychiatric Publishing, Inc.

Steiner, J. L., Tebes, J. K., Sledge, W. H., & Walker, M. L. (1995). A comparison of the Structured Clinical Interview for DSM-III-R and clinical diagnoses. *Journal of Nervous and Mental Disease, 183,* 365–369.

Taylor, S., Kuch, K., Koch, W., Crockett, D. J., & Passey, G. (1998). The structure of posttraumatic stress symptoms. *Journal of Abnormal Psychology, 107,* 154–160.

Tomb, D. A. (1994). The phenomenology of post-traumatic stress disorder. *Psychiatric Clinics of North America, 17*(2), 237–250.

Ursano, R. J., Fullerton, C. S., Epstein, R. S., Crowley, B., Kao, T., Vance, K., et al. (1999). Acute and chronic posttraumatic stress disorder in motor vehicle accident victims. *American Journal of Psychiatry, 156,* 589–595.

Veronen, L. J., & Kilpatrick, D. G. (1983). Stress management for rape victims. In D. Meichenbaum & M. E. Jaremko (Eds.), *Stress reduction and prevention* (pp. 341–374). New York: Plenum.

Walker, F. B., Novack, D. H., & Kaiser, D. L. (1987). Anxiety and depression among medical and surgical patients nearing hospital discharge. *Journal of General and Internal Medicine, 2,* 99–101.

Ward, C. H., Beck, A. T., Mendelson, M., Mock, J. E., & Erbaugh, J. K. (1962). The psychiatric nomenclature. *Archives of General Psychiatry, 7,* 198–205.

Weaver, T. L. (1998). Method variance and sensitivity of screening for traumatic stressors. *Journal of Traumatic Stress, 11,* 181–185.

Wolfe, J., Erickson, D. J., Sharkansky, E. J., King, D. W., & King, L. A. (1999). Course and predictors of posttraumatic stress disorder among gulf war veterans: A prospective analysis. *Journal of Consulting and Clinical Psychology, 67,* 520–528.

Yehuda, R., Marshall, R., Penkower, A., & Wong, C. M. (2002). Pharmacological treatment for posttraumatic stress disorder. In P. E. Nathan & J. M. Gorman (Eds.), *A guide to treatments that work* (pp. 411–445). New York: Oxford.

Zatzick, D. F., Weiss, D. S., Marmar, C. R., Metzler, T. J., Wells, K., Golding, J. M., et al. (1997). Posttraumatic stress disorder and functioning and quality of life outcomes in female Vietnam veterans. *Military Medicine, 162,* 661–665.

Zayfert, C., Becker, C. B., Unger, D. L., & Shearer, D. K. (2002). Comorbid anxiety disorders in civilians seeking treatment for posttraumatic stress disorder. *Journal of Traumatic Stress, 15,* 31–38.

Zlotnick, C., Warshaw, M., Shea, M. T., Allsworth, J., Pearlstein, T., & Keller, M. B. (1999). Chronicity in posttraumatic stress disorder (PTSD) and predictors of course of comorbid PTSD in patients with anxiety disorders. *Journal of Traumatic Stress, 12,* 89–100.

[11]

A Critical Assessment of Child Custody Evaluations

Limited Science and a Flawed System

Robert E. Emery,[1] Randy K. Otto,[2] William T. O'Donohue[3]

[1]*University of Virginia,* [2]*University of South Florida, and* [3]*University of Nevada–Reno*

SUMMARY—*Most parents who live apart negotiate custody arrangements on their own or with the help of lawyers, mediators, or other professionals. However, psychologists and other mental health professionals increasingly have become involved in evaluating children and families in custody disputes, because of the large number of separated, divorced, and never-married parents and the substantial conflict that often accompanies the breakup of a family. Theoretically, the law guides and controls child custody evaluations, but the prevailing custody standard (the "best interests of the child" test) is a vague rule that directs judges to make decisions unique to individual cases according to what will be in children's future (and undefined) best interests. Furthermore, state statutes typically offer only vague guidelines as to how judges (and evaluators) are to assess parents and the merits of their cases, and how they should ultimately decide what custody arrangements will be in a child's best interests. In this vacuum, custody evaluators typically administer to parents and children an array of tests and assess them through less formal means including interviews and observation. Sadly, we find that (a) tests specifically developed to assess questions relevant to custody are completely inadequate on scientific grounds; (b) the claims of some anointed experts about their favorite constructs (e.g., "parent alienation syndrome") are equally hollow when subjected to scientific scrutiny; (c) evaluators should question the use even of well-established psychological measures (e.g., measures of intelligence, personality, psychopathology, and academic achievement) because of their often limited relevance to the questions before the court; and (d) little empirical data exist regarding other important and controversial issues (e.g., whether evaluators should solicit children's wishes about custody; whether infants and toddlers are harmed or helped by overnight visits), suggesting a need for further scientific investigation.*

We see the system for resolving custody disputes as deeply flawed, for reasons that go beyond the problem of limited science. The coupling of the vague "best interests of the child" test with the American adversary system of justice puts judges in the position of trying to perform an impossible task, and it exacerbates parental conflict and problems in parenting and coparenting, which psychological science clearly shows to be key factors predicting children's psychological difficulties in response to their parents' separation and divorce.

Our analysis of the flawed system, together with our desire to sharply limit custody disputes and custody evaluations, leads us to propose three reforms. First, we urge continued efforts to encourage parents to reach custody agreements on their own—in divorce mediation, through collaborative law, in good-faith attorney negotiations, in therapy, and in other forums. Some such efforts have been demonstrated to improve parent–parent and parent–child relationships long after divorce, and they embrace the philosophical position that, in the absence of abuse or neglect, parents themselves should determine their children's best interests after separation, just as they do in marriage. Second, we urge state legislatures to move toward adopting more clear and determinative custody rules, a step that would greatly clarify the terms of the marriage contract, limit the need for custody evaluations, and sharply narrow the scope of the evaluation process. We find particular merit in the proposed "approximation rule" (recently embraced by the American Law Institute), in which postdivorce parenting arrangements would approximate parenting involvement in marriage. Third and finally, we recommend that custody evaluators follow the law and only offer opinions for which there is an adequate scientific basis. Related to this, we urge professional bodies to enact more specific standards of practice on this and related issues.

Address correspondence to Robert E. Emery, Department of Psychology, Gilmer Hall, Box 400400, University of Virginia, Charlottesville, VA 22904-4400; e-mail: ree@virginia.edu.

INTRODUCTION

Child custody disputes can entail any number of emotionally wrenching circumstances. The prototypical case involves married parents who separate and, in the heat of divorce, cannot reach an agreement about where and how their children should live. In other cases, a marital or cohabiting relationship dissolves before a child is born and parents must negotiate custody without the benefit of a shared history of parenting. Custody disputes also can surface years after a break-up, for example when a parent relocates, an adolescent wants to change living arrangements, or parents have problems with a difficult child.

Child custody disputes also are not limited to conflicts between biological parents. Grandparents may dispute custody of their grandchildren with their own children, birth parents may contest custody in the context of adoption, or same-sex couples may dispute custody with each other or a biological parent. Finally, infidelity and genetic testing, as well as technological and social innovations in conception and childbearing, can create nightmarish scenarios in which biological and social parents can end up disputing custody (Schwartz, 2003). Our focus here is on child custody disputes between parting parents, whether married or not, but many of the same issues and concerns apply across these different circumstances.

Our initial mission for this monograph was simply to critique the psychological science underpinning child custody evaluations. We make such a critique in the section titled "The (Limited) Science of Custody Evaluations." However, the subject of child custody disputes is complicated by many emotional, practical, and legal issues that are of interest and relevance to psychologists. We therefore have broadened the scope of the report to consider these more general issues, particularly developments in child custody law, alternative dispute resolution, ethics, and societal values about family life. Of course, psychological science is our primary focus, and one of the strongest findings of basic research in this area is that children fare better in separation and divorce if parental conflict is minimal or at least contained and if children maintain a good relationship with at least one, and preferably both, of their parents (Emery, 1982, 1999b, 2004). In other words, the process of family dissolution and the nature of continuing family relationships are more important to children's mental health than is the structure of any particular custody arrangement.

This finding, together with our analysis of the context of custody disputes, leads us to call for three sets of reforms. First, we encourage continued efforts to promote the private settlement of child custody disputes through education, good-faith negotiation, and alternative dispute resolution. Private settlement of custody disputes can reduce conflict; it can encourage more cooperative, ongoing relationships between coparents; and it can facilitate positive relationships between children and both of their parents. Second, we support efforts to make child custody law more clear and determinative, in order to substantially reduce the number of custody disputes. Third, in disputes that remain contested, we would limit mental health expert testimony only to opinions clearly supported by psychological science, a circumstance that unfortunately does not characterize some of today's practice. This final point is not so much a call for a reform as a recommendation that expert witnesses in custody evaluations conform to existing standards for expert testimony.

The Deer-Doe Case

We invite the reader to begin to consider the many emotional, legal, empirical, and value conflicts involved in child custody disputes with a hypothetical case. We revisit this case at points throughout the monograph to illustrate and anchor our discussion.

> Jane and John Deer-Doe, both 39 years old, have two children: Isabella, a 10-year-old girl in the fourth grade, and Carlos, a 3-year-old boy who attends preschool but spends most of the day at home with his mother. Jane continued to work full time as a certified public accountant after Isabella was born, but, with John's reluctant agreement, she quit work after Carlos's birth. John, a moderately successful computer engineer and self-described highly involved father, says that he had expected Jane to return to work after a year or two at home with the children.
>
> Jane and John agreed that they had longstanding conflicts about parenting, finances, and sexuality. John tried repeatedly to get Jane to address their unhappiness by seeing a marriage therapist. Jane was open to therapy but also accepting of an imperfect marriage. Jane's acceptance ended, however, when she learned of John's
> 2-year-long affair with a coworker. She immediately contacted an attorney, and shortly thereafter, John left the house at her request.
>
> In their subsequent negotiations, Jane indicated her desire for a divorce, and John agreed. He hoped to remarry soon and wanted the children with him half of the time. Jane countered that John should have the children no more than every other weekend, consistent with his "minimal" involvement during their marriage, and she further insisted that their children have no contact with his "friend."
>
> In the 3 months after her parents' separated, Isabella refused to see her father except on a couple of occasions. She continued to do well in school but was extremely angry with her father for "cheating on my mother." Carlos asked for his father repeatedly in the days and weeks after the separation but did so less after seeing his father only sporadically during this time. His preschool teachers complained that Carlos had become very aggressive in school and had begun to wet and soil himself again.

How can psychological scientists help families like the Deer-Does? As we will review in this monograph, there is good research to help us better understand children, divorce, and custody conflicts, and there is some reasonably strong evidence on some successful interventions. Unfortunately, very little research has been conducted directly on legal issues in the custody context, including child custody evaluations.

Robert E. Emery, Randy K. Otto, William T. O'Donohue

DEMOGRAPHICS OF FAMILY STRUCTURE, CUSTODY DISPUTES, AND CUSTODY ARRANGEMENTS

The structure of American families changed dramatically in the latter part of the 20th century. As indicated in Figure 1, divorce rates trended upward in the United States throughout the 1900s and, following a rapid rise in the late 1960s, peaked in 1981 before turning downward (Bramlett & Mosher, 2002).

Other key elements of the demographic story include an average risk of divorce of somewhat less than 50%, higher divorce rates for African Americans, lower rates for Asian Americans, and the declining risk for divorce as a function of years in marriage (Bramlett & Mosher, 2001; see Fig. 2). About 60% of divorces involve children (Clarke, 1995), and about half take place in the first 7 years of marriage (see Fig. 2), so that children are likely to be young when marriages end and custody is disputed (Furstenberg, Peterson, Nord, & Zill, 1983). As we discuss later, special concerns arise about custody for infants, toddlers, and, to a lesser extent, preschoolers.

Unmarried Parents

Over 40% of children born to married parents are expected to experience the divorce of their parents (Bumpass, 1984; U.S. Bureau of the Census, 1992), and the qualification "born to married parents" is an important one. In 2002, 34% of all children in the United States were born outside of marriage (Martin et al., 2003). In fact, the apparent decline in divorce since 1981 may be attributable to at-risk individuals and couples self-selecting out of legal marriage and childbearing. Rapid increases in nonmarital childbirth did not stabilize until about 1990, and cohabitation (which is more difficult to track) apparently is continuing to increase in frequency.

The best estimates suggest that about half of children born outside of marriage actually are born to unmarried but cohabiting parents (Sigle-Rushton & McLanahan, 2002), and cohabiting unions are more likely to dissolve than legal marriages are. Forty-nine percent of cohabiting relationships end within 5 years, whereas 20% of first marriages dissolve within 5 years (Bramlett & Mosher, 2002). Although we know of no data regarding how many disrupted cohabitations involve parents and their biological children, the disruption of relationships between unmarried parents clearly is an important and growing area for research on child custody disputes.

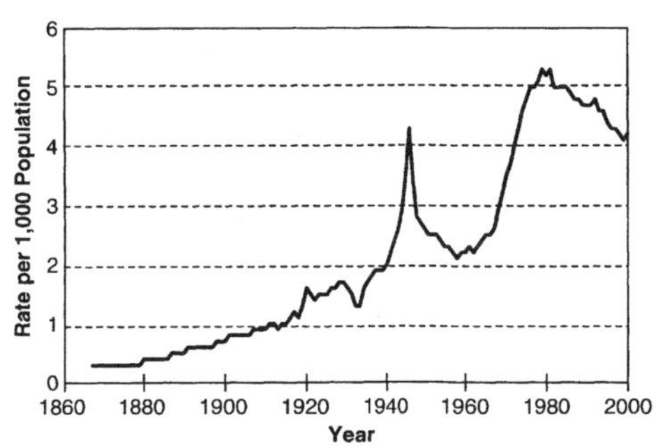

Fig. 1. Annual U.S. divorce rates from 1867 to 2000 (based on Bramlett & Mosher, 2002, and Emery, 1999b).

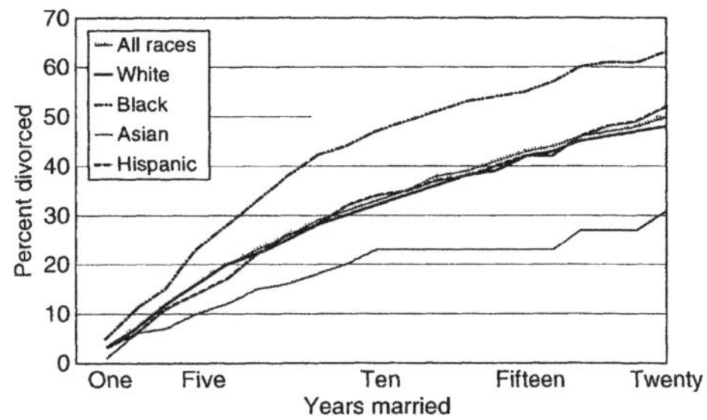

Fig. 2. Risk of divorce over the first 20 years of marriage, by ethnicity (based on Bramlett & Mosher, 2001).

Child Custody Disputes

There is no good national data on how many custody disputes arise when divorcing, cohabiting, or unmarried parents part or on how many such disputes erupt years after the break-up (which may be a more common circumstance). What is clear is that courts are overwhelmed by the huge number of families separating, divorcing, and disputing custody. In 1995, domestic-relations disputes, which include but are not limited to child custody litigation, accounted for one quarter of all legal filings, making this the largest category of court action (Ostrom & Kauder, 1996). Other evidence indicates that custody disputes form the largest percentage of domestic-relations cases (Schepard, 2004).

Child Custody Decisions

The best evidence on how child custody is decided in the context of divorce comes from Maccoby and Mnookin's (1992) study of 1,124 families with children in which the parents filed for divorce in two California counties in the middle 1980s. As illustrated in Figure 3, most of these cases were settled outside of court, as over three quarters of custody arrangements were negotiated either by the parents themselves or through their lawyers. Since 1981, California law has mandated that mediation be attempted before a custody hearing can be held before a judge; an additional 11% of the cases were settled in mediation, while 5% of the cases went the next step up in the hierarchy of legal conflict—a custody evaluation—before reaching a settlement. Only 4% of cases went to

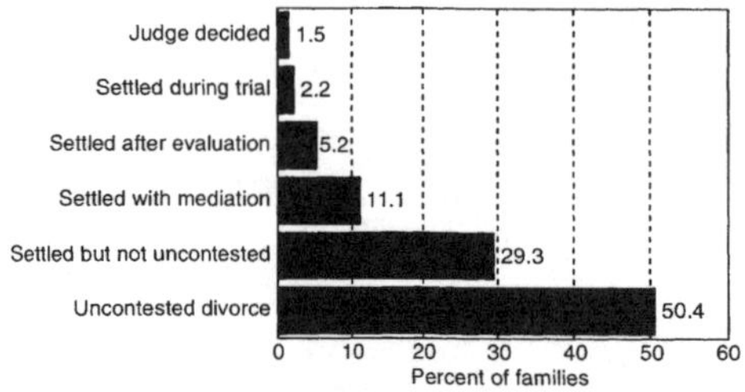

Fig. 3. Percent of 1,124 families in two California counties settling divorce custody using various methods, during the mid-1980s (based on Maccoby & Mnookin, 1992, p. 137).

trial, and most of these were settled during the trial process. A judge decided less than 2% of the cases (Maccoby & Mnookin, 1992).

The generality of these findings is limited by the two-county sampling, as well as by rapidly changing laws and societal expectations. Still, the data highlight several patterns observed across the United States and much of the industrialized world (Emery, 1999b; Pryor & Rodgers, 2001). First, many parents experience at least a mild degree of conflict surrounding child custody, and conflict is substantial in a significant subset of cases. Combining legal indicators and self-reported conflict measures, Maccoby and Mnookin (1992) estimated that 51% of divorces involved negligible conflict over issues related to custody, while 24% had mild conflict, 10% substantial conflict, and 15% intense conflict. Second, as is the case with other litigation, most custody disputes are decided outside of the courtroom. Third, alternative dispute resolution methods such as mediation increasingly are used, often successfully, in an attempt to settle disputed cases. Fourth, mental health professionals often are involved in child custody conflicts as mediators, custody evaluators, or therapists (although the last role is not reflected in these data).

The importance of each of these patterns is multiplied by high rates of separation and divorce, custody disputes between cohabiting and never-married parents, and the potential for conflict throughout the duration of the children's childhood. This means that (a) even if they represent a minority of cases, large numbers of children are exposed to substantial or intense parental and legal conflict in the midst of their parents' separation; (b) judges face the prospect of spending a great deal of their time hearing custody cases; (c) alternative dispute resolution and custody evaluations have become important parts of the process; and (d) mental health professionals are becoming increasingly involved in the child custody arena in a variety of ways.

Child Custody Arrangements Following Separation and Divorce

Although laws, definitions, and terms vary from state to state, most of the key aspects of child custody arrangements are captured by the following concepts:

- *Legal custody* refers to parental authority or decision making. In cases of *sole legal custody*, one parent has the right to make major decisions about the children's lives, especially schooling, elective medical care, and religious training. When *joint legal custody* is in effect, both parents share these major decisions, while each parent makes day-to-day decisions autonomously when the children are with her or him. In some cases, the court will assign more specific decision making over day-to-day matters to one or both parents.
- *Physical custody* refers to the time children actually spend with their parents. In cases of *primary physical custody*, the children spend the majority of their time with one parent and generally "visit" (a term many find pejorative) with the "nonresidential parent" on some agreed-to schedule (e.g., one evening during the week and every other weekend). In cases of *joint physical custody*, children spend close to equal amounts of time with both parents. Although there is no uniform definition of joint physical custody, many consider it to be a minimum of an average of two overnights per week (Maccoby & Mnookin, 1992). This definition is consistent with child-support laws in 28 states that lower support obligations for joint physical custody arrangements and often define joint physical custody at about 100 overnights per year (Elrod & Spector, 2004).
- *Split custody* refers to circumstances in which each parent has sole physical custody of at least one child—that is, when siblings are split up between their parents.

Single Mothers and Single Fathers

The United States Census Bureau generally does not track joint physical custody, but instead lists children as living with two married parents, a single mother, a single father, or in some other arrangement. In 2002, of all children living with a single parent, just over 82% lived with a single mother while approximately 18% lived with a single father (Fields, 2003). This percentage of children living with a single father represents an increase over the historical level of about 10% (Meyer & Garasky, 1993). Interpretation of these census data, however, is clouded by several factors including (a) remarriage, as children who live with remarried parents are counted as living in a two-parent household; (b) cohabitation, as many "single" parents live with a partner, including 11% of single mothers and 33% of single fathers in 2002 (Fields, 2003); and (c) reason for single-parent status, as the category includes separated, divorced, never-married, and widowed parents. Another limitation is that joint physical (or legal) custody is not routinely documented.

Joint Custody

Joint custody (a term that confounds legal and physical custody) has been a much-discussed and much-debated coparenting arrangement since the 1980s (Folberg, 1991). Later, we discuss evidence about the well-being of children living in joint custody. Our present task is to estimate its prevalence.

We know of three national estimates of the frequency of joint custody (Child Trends, 2002; Clarke, 1995; Donnelly & Finkelhor, 1993), the best coming from special supplemental 1998 United States Census data (and also 1994 and 1996 data that provide essentially the same results). In this analysis, 65% of mothers had sole physical and legal custody, 10% had sole physical and joint legal custody, 11% of fathers had sole physical custody (with either joint or sole legal custody), 9% of parents had joint physical and legal custody, and 5% had split custody or some other arrangement (Child Trends, 2002). Thus, about 75% of children not living with both parents lived primarily with their mothers, approximately 10% lived primarily with their fathers, about 10% lived in joint physical custody, and another 5% lived either in split custody or in some other arrangement. Although some people argue that joint physical custody is becoming far more common, no trends for increased prevalence between 1994 and 1998 were found in the census data (Child Trends, 2002).

Historical Trend Evidence and Joint Custody

Historical data from Wisconsin demonstrate the importance of distinguishing legal custody and physical custody, and also make us suspect that joint legal custody is becoming considerably more common than suggested by the census estimates. A review of 9,500 Wisconsin divorce settlements between 1980 and 1992 revealed that sole physical custody to fathers remained stable during these years while sole physical custody to mothers declined (see Fig. 4). Joint physical custody rose from 2% to 14% of the Wisconsin cases, while joint legal custody increased from 18% to 81% (Melli, Brown, & Cancian, 1997). Our experience leads us to believe that this dramatic increase in joint legal custody and more modest increase in joint physical custody have also occurred in many other states. Estimates from 1990 data gathered by the National Center for Health Statistics (Clarke, 1995) also support this suggestion, as different states reported widely varying rates of joint custody (legal and physical custody were not distinguished)—for example, 4% percent in Nebraska compared with 44% in geographically and politically similar Kansas.

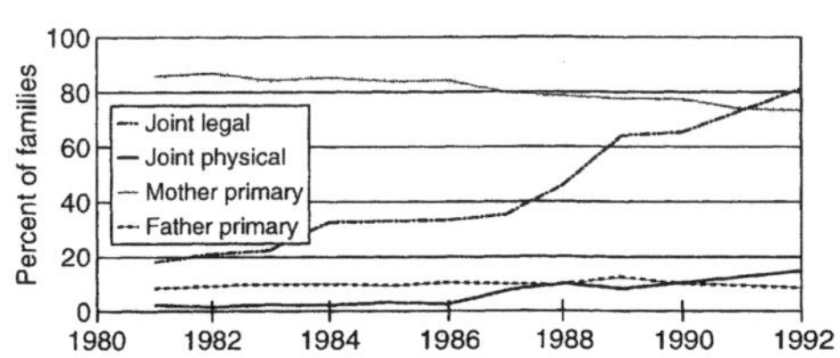

Fig. 4. Percentage of custody arrangements in Wisconsin divorces from 1980 to 1992 (data were collected across calendar years; thus 1982 refers to 1981–82, etc.; based on Melli, Brown, & Cancian, 1997).

Changes in Custody Arrangements

Custody arrangements change over time, and legal agreements often do not correspond to de facto residence. The best evidence on these points also comes from Maccoby and Mnookin's (1992) longitudinal study. For 783 cases where complete data were obtained during the 3-year study, initial legal agreements designated the following custody arrangements in the two California counties: 66% sole mother custody, 9% sole father custody, 21% joint physical custody, and 4% split custody. Shortly after the divorce decree was filed, however, only 52% of the cases with designated joint physical custody actually had a *de facto* joint physical custody. Among the 48% of the joint physical cases in which the living situation was not consistent with the legal agreement, most involved sole mother physical custody. Of cases with designated mother custody, 87% followed that arrangement in practice, as did 82% of father custody agreements, but only 35% of split-custody agreements actually conformed to that arrangement.

Three years later, only 45% of legally designated joint physical custody cases actually conformed to that arrangement, compared to 85% of cases with designated mother custody, 71% of cases of father custody, and 34% of split custody awards (Maccoby & Mnookin, 1992). The absolute percentages of the four types of custody arrangements 3 years after the divorce decree were similar to the initial arrangements, but the longitudinal analysis demonstrated that many families shifted out of their original custody arrangements and into new ones.

CUSTODY LAW AND CHILD CUSTODY EVALUATIONS IN PRACTICE

Later, we consider broad conceptual issues related to child custody law and custody evaluations. We begin, however, with a brief overview of the current legal landscape and a minimal critique.

The "Best Interests of the Child" Standard

Each state legislature in the United States controls its own child custody law, and laws can vary considerably from state to state. Still, every state law indicates that custody decisions are to be made according to "best interests of the child" standard, the principle that judicial determinations should be based on each child's unique future best interests (Elrod & Spector, 2004). Many mental health professionals applaud this "best interests of the child" standard as being responsive to individual children and families. We differ. Individualized decision making is appealing on the surface, but we are deeply concerned that a standard vague enough to be interpreted differently for each family that comes before the court (a) encourages parents to enter into custody disputes (thereby increasing parental conflict), because the outcome of a court hearing is difficult to predict; and (b) allows for bias to intrude in the exercise of judicial discretion.

For reasons we do not fully understand, the law apparently has interpreted children's best interests to be primarily their best psychological interests (as opposed to other possibilities such as their economic, educational, or medical interests). This is evident in the various factors deemed relevant to children's best interests listed in most state laws, which typically are rooted in the Uniform Marriage and Divorce Act (1979), which lists the following:

- The wishes of the children's parent or parents as to their custody
- The wishes of the children regarding their custodian
- The interaction and interrelationship of the children and their parent or parents, their siblings, and any other person who may significantly affect the children's best interests
- The children's adjustment to their home, school, and community
- The mental and physical health of all individuals involved

Because child custody laws differ from state to state, some factors designed to be considered by judges are idiosyncratic to one or only a handful of states. South Carolina, for example, takes into account the religious beliefs and commitment of the parents, while Alabama, Florida, Michigan, North Dakota, and Utah consider parents' "moral character" to be relevant to children's best interests. One of the goals of a child custody evaluation—the overriding goal, according to some—is to assess the child and parents relative to these state-specified best-interest factors.

A Psychological Evaluation for the Deer-Doe Family

After several months of separation and still no custody agreement, Jane's attorney suggested a child custody evaluation as a next step in their negotiations, and, eager for some outside help, John agreed. Several weeks later, a psychologist, Dr. David Hagan, who was mutually agreed upon by both parties, was appointed by the court to assess Jane, John, his girlfriend, and their children.

Over the course of 6 weeks, Dr. Hagan conducted a comprehensive evaluation consisting of interviews and psychological testing with both parents; tests included the Minnesota Multiphasic Personality Inventory-2 (MMPI-2), the Rorschach Inkblot Technique, and the Wechsler Abbreviated Scale of Intelligence. Both children were interviewed, observed interacting with each other, and observed interacting with each parent at Dr. Hagan's office and at the respective parental homes. Dr. Hagan also administered a number of psychological tests to the children including the Achenbach Child Behavior Checklist (with parents and teachers as informants), the Roberts Apperception Test, the Bricklin Perceptual Scales, and the Wechsler Intelligence Scale for Children-IV. In addition, Dr. Hagan obtained collateral information by interviewing the children's teachers and grandparents, reviewing school and medical records, and reading all litigation-related documents. Finally, Dr. Hagan evaluated John's girlfriend by way of extensive interviewing and administration of the psychological tests mentioned earlier.

Dr. Hagan's bill for $7,400 reflected that he spent 37 hours conducting the evaluation, reviewing records, and writing a 35-page report summarizing his observations, findings, and opinions. (We discuss the report later.)

Practices Reported by Custody Evaluators

Given their frequency, high cost, and social and personal importance, we might expect to find a large body of research on custody evaluations and their scientific underpinnings. However, only a few studies of custody evaluations have been completed. One thing these studies show is that, in real life, many evaluators use the instruments employed by our fictional Dr. Hagan. Another thing research shows is that most of these measures are deeply flawed when used in the custody context.

With the exception of one study (Bow & Quinnell, 2002) all research examining child custody evaluation practices has been based on the self-report of examiners. Although these data provide some helpful information, we must keep in mind that professionals' reports of their behavior may not accurately depict their actual practices (Greenberg, Otto, & Long, 2003).

Keilin and Bloom (1986) described the practices reported by 82 custody evaluators (78% psychologists) who responded to an anonymous survey. Respondents devoted an average of 19 hours to each evaluation and almost always reported interviewing each parent and the children. Most used psychological tests with adults (76%) and children (74%); most observed parent–child interactions (69%); half said they observed interactions between the two parents; and about one third reported visiting the children's homes or schools. Approximately one half interviewed third parties (e.g., friends and relatives) in an attempt to gain a better understanding of the children and their parents.

No one particular psychological test was used by a majority of the respondents when assessing children. Intelligence tests were used most frequently, with almost half of the evaluators using them in the majority of their cases. The next most frequently used instruments with children were the Thematic Apperception Test or the Children's Apperception Test (39%), followed by miscellaneous projective drawings, the Rorschach Inkblot Technique, and the Bender-Gestalt Visual Motor Test. In assessments of parents, the MMPI was the most commonly used assessment technique (70%), followed by the Rorschach Inkblot Technique (42%), and the Thematic Apperception Test (38%).

Keilin and Bloom (1986) also asked the evaluators to rank order 21 different factors with respect to their importance when considering custody. In descending order of significance, the ten most important were (1) the stated preferences of a 15-year-old (or older) child, (2) parental attempts at alienation (i.e., attempting to turn a child against the other parent), (3) the nature and quality of the child's emotional relationship with each parent, (4) the emotional or psychological stability of each parent, (5) each parent's parenting skills, (6) each parent's openness towards the child's contact with the other parent, (7) the parents' preseparation caretaking and parenting roles, (8) the parents' expressed anger and bitterness regarding the divorce, (9) the parents' sexual orientation, and (10) the stated preferences of a 5-year-old child.

Ten years later, Ackerman and Ackerman (1997) surveyed 800 doctoral-level psychologists who conducted child custody evaluations and obtained usable responses from 201 (25%). Respondents spent 21 hours per evaluation—similar to the earlier survey—but these respondents reported devoting more time to reviewing collateral materials and report writing. Intelligence tests and projective measures continued to be the instruments most frequently employed with children, and the MMPI/MMPI-2 remained the most frequently used assessment instrument for parents, followed by the Rorschach Inkblot Technique.

Many custody evaluators also reported using assessment instruments with children that were developed specifically for use in custody contexts (Ackerman & Ackerman, 1997). Over one third used the Bricklin Perceptual Scales (Bricklin, 1990a) while 16% used the Perception of Relationships Test (Bricklin, 1989). Fewer respondents (11%) used the Ackerman-Schoendorf Scales for Parent Evaluation of Custody (Ackerman & Schoendorf, 1992), the one custody-assessment measure designed for entire families and adults. Fewer than 10% used other custody-assessment measures, specifically, the Parent Awareness of Skills Survey (Bricklin, 1990b) and the Custody Quotient (Gordon & Peek, 1989). Other investigators (e.g., Bow & Quinnell, 2001; Courley & Stolberg, 2000) have reported findings regarding test usage by custody evaluators similar to those detailed by Keilin and Bloom (1986) and Ackerman and Ackerman.

Like Keilin and Bloom (1986) before them, Ackerman and Ackerman (1997) also asked custody evaluators to rate the importance of various factors to issues of child custody. According to the custody evaluators, the ten most important, in descending order of significance, were (1) the substance abuse status of each parent, (2) the parents' parenting skills, (3) parental attempts at alienation, (4) the nature and quality of the child's emotional relationship with each parent, (5) the emotional or psychological stability of each parent, (6) each parent's openness toward the child's contact with the other parent, (7) the parents' history of compliance with the court during the separation, (8) the parents' preseparation caretaking and parenting roles, (9) the stated preferences of a 15-year-old or older child, and (10) the parents' expressed anger and bitterness regarding the divorce.

THE (LIMITED) SCIENCE OF CUSTODY EVALUATIONS

State statutes regarding children's best interests help us understand at least some of the practices of custody evaluators. We could (and later do) question, for example, whether (or when) a parent's mental health or the wishes of a child should be a central focus in child custody cases. Still, evaluators who assess such factors are following explicit legal guidelines. More difficult to explain and more problematic, however, are other aspects of evaluation practices including the widespread use of well-established measures with no clear relevance to the custody context (e.g., measures of intelligence), attempts to measure constructs created to apply to child custody decision making (e.g., "parent alienation syndrome"), efforts to identify "parent of choice" (e.g., the Bricklin Perceptual Scales), and the use of measures that a significant number of psychologists view with skepticism (e.g., the Rorschach Inkblot Technique).

We are dubious about many child custody evaluation practices, because of the absence of solid psychological science and of clear criteria to be predicted by psychological science. We also hold two much more fundamental questions about child custody evaluations: Why has society and the law placed such importance on a prediction about *psychological* factors in determining custody? And if the goal is to minimize children's psychological risk, might there be better roles for psychologists to play—both as practitioners and as scientists—in custody disputes? For now, however, we focus on the lack of scientific evidence to support many of the instruments and practices of mental health professionals who serve as custody evaluators.

Heilbrun, Rogers, and Otto (2002) described a three-category typology of assessment techniques used in forensic contexts, including custody evaluations. *Clinical assessment instruments* are those developed to assess psychological constructs, typically for intervention purposes (e.g., measures of intelligence, psychopathology, academic achievement). *Forensically relevant instruments* assess constructs that are psychological in nature but may be of particular relevance in forensic contexts (e.g., measures of response style, risk for criminal offending). Finally, *forensic assessment instruments* are specifically designed to assess psycho-legal constructs. Here we review evidence in regard to the third and first categories of assessment techniques. We do not consider forensically relevant instruments because none have been used widely by custody evaluators, although that may change (Posthuma, 2003). We also raise concerns about "parent alienation syndrome" and other constructs that have been created for, and asserted to have scientific standing in, the context of custody evaluations.

Forensic Assessment Instruments: No Scientific Support

In the past 15 years, psychologists have developed a number of forensic assessment instruments purporting to assess children's best interests in custody disputes (see Grisso, 2003). Our bottom-line evaluation of these measures is a harsh one: These measures assess ill-defined constructs, and they do so poorly, leaving no scientific justification for their use in child custody evaluations.

The most widely used forensic assessment instrument (Ackerman & Ackerman, 1997) is the Bricklin Perceptual Scales

(BPS), described as a projective measure of parents' competence, supportiveness, follow-up consistency, and possession of admirable traits (Bricklin, 1990a). Using a stylus and rating card, children rate each parent on 32 different activities considered to be relevant to these four capacities. The parent who receives the greater number of positive ratings is identified as the "Parent of Choice." Bricklin asserts that the nonverbal nature of the task (using a stylus rather than a verbal response) allows for the assessment of the child's "unconscious preferences," which are less likely to be subject to distortion due to social desirability or parental persuasion. However, the BPS has been criticized on numerous grounds: There is no support for claims that it assesses children's unconscious preferences or that responses are not subject to external influence; the developer permits variation from standard test administration; the measure samples a relatively narrow range of parenting domains; the developer has not provided basic norms and psychometric properties of the measure; and data regarding concurrent and predictive validity are either absent or unconvincing (Heinze & Grisso, 1996; Melton, 1995; Melton, Petrila, Poythress, & Slobogin, 1997; Otto & Edens, 2003; Otto, Edens, & Barcus, 2000; Shaffer, 1992).

Another measure used fairly frequently is the Perception of Relationships Test (PORT; Bricklin, 1989), a projective drawing that is described as measuring the "whole organism or gut-level responses a child has toward a parent [that] are much more reflective of what the child's actual interactions or experiences with that parent have been" (Bricklin, 1993, p. 1). Seven drawing tasks completed by the child are scored to identify the "Primary Caretaking Parent." Like the BPS, the PORT has been widely criticized. Objections include the incomplete and confusing manual, unclear administration and scoring guidelines, minimal reliability data, missing norms, and lack of validity data (Carlson, 1995; Conger, 1995; Heinze & Grisso, 1996; Melton et al., 1997; Otto & Edens, 2003; Otto et al., 2000).

Bricklin (1990b) describes another measure, the Parent Awareness Skills Survey (PASS), as a "clinical tool designed to illuminate the strengths and weaknesses in awareness skills a parent accesses in reaction to typical child care situations" (p. 4). The PASS consists of 18 childcare scenarios selected to represent caretaking of children of various ages. The parent's responses are followed up with questioning by the examiner as needed, and scoring is based on guidelines in the test manual. The PASS also has been criticized for basic shortcomings: the absence of norms, reliability and validity data, and clear scoring guidelines (Otto & Edens, 2003; Otto et al., 2000). Of particular concern is the developer's suggestion that "the evaluator, by virtue of appropriate training in psychology and/or child development, can apply his or her own standards in assigning the suggested scores. The PASS allows for wide latitude in scoring since its main purpose is to discover the relative (rather than absolute) strengths and weaknesses any individual or compared set of respondents manifest" (Bricklin, 1990b, p. 11).

The Parent Perception of Child Profile (PPCP; Bricklin & Elliott, 1991) is described as a measure of parents' understanding of a child's development and needs across eight areas: interpersonal relations, daily routine, health history, developmental history, school history, fears, personal hygiene, and communication style. Because parents who more accurately assess their child are assumed to be better parents, the PPCP requires the examiner to assess the accuracy of each parent's report, using vaguely defined criteria that include the examiner's and third-party informants' opinions. According to the manual, data need not be gathered in all eight categories, and the examiner can decide which issues are most critical for a particular child and parent. The PPCP has been criticized for its incomplete manual, lack of scoring directions, and absence of reliability and validity data (Otto et al., 2000; Otto & Edens, 2003).

Another instrument used by evaluators with some frequency, the Ackerman-Schoendorf Scales for Parent Evaluation of Custody (ASPECT), is purported to be "a clinical tool designed to aid mental health professionals in making child custody recommendations" (Ackerman & Schoendorf, 1992, p. 1). The ASPECT is not a test, but an assessment approach that aggregates data from the parent (an open-ended "Parenting Questionnaire," the MMPI-2, the Rorschach Inkblot Technique, and an intelligence test) and from the child (the Rorschach Inkblot Technique, an intelligence test, an academic achievement test, and a projective story). Measures were selected based on the developers' review of the literature, and test scores are used to calculate a "Parental Custody Index" (PCI) for each parent. The PCI is considered to indicate parenting effectiveness, and judgments about the parents are based on their relative PCI values. With rare exceptions (e.g., Brodzinsky, 1993), reviews of the ASPECT have been uniformly negative. Criticisms include the absence of a clear relationship between many of the measures and behavior relevant to custody; the failure to assess factors clearly deemed relevant to custody decisions; and an absence of important data regarding basic psychometric properties, including predictive validity (Arditti, 1995; Heinze & Grisso, 1996; Melton, 1995; Melton et al., 1997; Otto & Edens, 2003; Otto et al., 2000; Wellman, 1994).

In summary, all measures that purport to assess constructs directly relevant to child custody determinations suffer from significant limitations. In fact, no study examining the properties of these measures has ever been published in a peer-reviewed journal—an essential criterion for science and, in theory, for the courts. In our view, the absence of scientific support should preclude the use of any of these forensic assessment instruments for any purpose other than research. We even have doubts about the value of research using these measures, because it is hard to conceive of any psychological test that could measure all the factors that might be relevant to child custody (Shuman, 2002) or that might assess the best custody arrangements for children when the criteria for fulfilling children's best interests are so poorly defined (Emery, 1999b).

Clinical Assessment Instruments: Some Cautions in the Custody Context

Heilbrun et al. (2002) describe measures of intelligence, personality, psychopathology, and academic achievement as clinical assessment instruments. In contrast to forensic assessment instruments, we believe use of many of these measures is warranted in forensic assessment contexts to the degree that they offer reliable and valid assessments of relevant constructs identified in the law. We do, however, wonder about the routine use of measures such as IQ tests, which can add to the time and expense of a custody evaluation without holding a clear relevance to the issue before the court.

A greater concern is the validity of clinical assessment instruments in the custody context, as a number of considerations suggest the need for caution. For one thing, as in other forensic contexts, examinees may be less than candid in their responses, including on psychological tests. Tests that do not include measures of response style are particularly vulnerable to dissimulation, while tests with embedded measures of response style are not necessarily impervious to false reporting.

Whether the constructs assessed by the instrument are, broadly conceived, "states" or "traits" is another important issue. Assessments of characteristics that commonly change over time (e.g., parental depression) provide a weak basis for an evaluator to make claims about how a parent functioned in the past or will function in the future. Because families are evaluated during a period of high stress, moreover, evaluators also must be cautious about drawing inferences about functioning at some later, hopefully less stressful, point in time. Given the very nature of custody disputes and the context in which most custody evaluations occur, it is particularly important that the evaluator not assume that instruments assessing more enduring styles will not change in response to situational factors. The Standards for Educational and Psychological Testing (American Educational Research Association, American Psychological Association, & National Council on Measurement in Education, 1999) direct that "a test taker's score should not be accepted as a reflection of lack of ability with respect to the characteristic being tested for without consideration of alternate explanations for the test taker's inability to perform on that test at that time" (p. 43). The upheaval of divorce constitutes a reasonable "alternative explanation" that should certainly be considered when interpreting a test score.

We do not want to throw out the baby with the bathwater. There may be a role for clinical assessment instruments in some custody evaluation contexts. More specifically, to the degree that there is a psychological construct that is relevant to the issues at the heart of a custody matter and there are valid psychological measures of that construct available, use of such measures can be of some value. Examples of relevant things that may need to be determined in a custody case might include whether a child has a learning disorder that needs special attention, whether a mother suffers from depression that affects her ability to meet her children's emotional needs, or whether a father has a substance-abuse disorder that results in him placing the children in at-risk situations when in his care.

Projective Measures

Our concerns about clinical assessment instruments apply to highly structured, well-validated, and well accepted measures of intelligence, academic achievement, and psychopathology. These issues present the greatest concerns, however, for unstructured, projective measures, given questions that have been raised about even basic psychometric properties of such tests, including their reliability and validity. There is a considerable difference of opinion and ongoing, active debate regarding the general utility of projective measures such as the Rorschach Inkblot Technique (compare Wood, Nezworski, & Stejskal, 1997; Wood, Nezworski, Lilienfeld, & Garb, 2003 and Weiner, 1996; Meyer, 1997, 2001), Draw a Person, and Human Figure Drawings. The very existence of this debate, in combination with some of the specific criticisms and potential dangers in the custody context, lead us to suggest that such measures not be used in child custody evaluation contexts, or any other evaluation contexts for that matter.

We do not have the space, expertise, or the inclination to review the broad and polarized literature on projective tests in this monograph. Thus we only point to the extensive and serious controversy, and note this: Questions about the value of projectives or any other assessment technique need to be debated and answered by psychological scientists outside of the courtroom. It is naive to expect judges to make informed judgments about the psychometric adequacy of projective measures in the context of a custody hearing. We also are concerned about the potential for evaluators to assert that projective measures have scientific authority while the underlying empirical, legal, and values questions remain unanswered, precisely because the "test" is mysterious to lay observers and therefore potentially misleading or difficult to challenge. A nonexpert might feel competent challenging the relevance or the validity of a relatively straightforward measure like an IQ test or an MMPI-2. Yet, despite more significant concerns about its psychometric properties, results of a Rorschach may be more difficult to challenge precisely because of its more obscure source of material and scoring (Shuman, 2002).

Clinical Interviews

The clinical interview is another assessment technique that requires considerable caution when used as a measurement technique in custody evaluations. Interviewers may yield inferences that are reliable or unreliable, valid or invalid, but there are no structured interviews with well-established psychometric properties specifically developed for use in the child custody context, and survey data regarding psychologists' custody evaluation practices indicate that use of any structured interview approach is virtually unheard of (Ackerman & Ackerman, 1997; Keilin & Bloom, 1986). Thus, differences between interviewers may result from variance in the family's responses or from the contrasting structure, content, or interpretation of the interview. We urge psychological scientists to work to develop structured interviews for the custody context. In the meantime, we expect custody evaluators to continue to interview families. Although we are dubious about the psychometrics of unstructured interviews, we find some comfort in the fact that, unlike projective measures, interviews are more straightforward and understandable and hopefully are not presented as providing data as scientific-sounding as that of a test.

Direct Observation

Direct observation of parent–child interactions is another complex and generally unstandardized assessment strategy. Threats to validity include reactivity, unreliable coding systems, unrepresentative samples of behavior, and problematic data compilation and analysis. As with interviews, we urge the development of standardized observation measures for use in the custody context, and urge evaluators to describe their observations clearly and to identify the inferences they draw from observational assessments.

Combining Assessment Results and Drawing Inferences

This last point raises a broader and very important issue. All clinical assessment instruments assess constructs that, at most, are only indirectly relevant to custody; thus their use in custody evaluations typically requires inferences to be made. Once a parent's depression or a child's academic abilities are assessed, for example, the examiner may draw some inference regarding how that factor is relevant to the best interests of a child. The question is: How is the examiner to draw conclusions from a single measure or, even more importantly, combine data from several sources to form a conclusion about the best interests of the child? For example, how does an evaluator weigh the results of a hypothetically accurate (impossible in practice) evaluation where all data indicate that the mother is an effective disciplinarian but not terribly warm and that the father is warmly supportive but not good at setting limits? Thus, our concerns with clinical assessment instruments are not only how to measure relevant constructs reliably and validly in a difficult context, but also how to synthesize multiple measurements in a manner relevant to the ultimate issue of a custody determination. Perhaps ideally, the law would provide a formula for making such decisions, but the factors to be considered in the law are rarely even ranked relative to one another.

Controversial Topics Requiring Further Investigation

Surveys of practicing custody evaluators indicate that, in addition to using clinical assessment instruments and dubious forensic assessment instruments, they also frequently assess certain quite controversial constructs. We illustrate our concerns by focusing on three in particular: (a) parental alienation syndrome (PAS), (b) children's wishes regarding custody, and (c) overnight visitation for very young children.

PAS: Asserting Science Where There Is None

"Parental alienation" is a construct ranked high on the list of factors evaluators consider to be directly relevant to custody decision making. There is no test instrument designed to measure parent alienation. Rather, it is a "diagnosis" reached through clinical interviews. Some experts have testified to making the diagnosis of parental alienation syndrome, and their testimony is claimed to be an important influence on judicial decision making (Gardner, 2004).

"Parental Alienation Syndrome" is a term created by psychiatrist Richard Gardner (2001) based on his clinical experience with custody disputes. Gardner asserts that PAS, which he says develops almost exclusively in the context of custody disputes, is characterized by one parent "programming" a child against the other parent (Gardner, 2001). The assumption is that a child's disdain for one parent is generally unjustified and solely attributable to denigration on the part of the other, alienating parent. Gardner (2004) also claims that PAS can be "diagnosed" reliably and validly by expert evaluators, although he offers no explicit criteria for doing so or objective evidence to support his claim (Emery, 2005).

We recognize that parents often undermine each other's relationships with their children following separation (Emery, 2005; Kelly & Johnston, 2001). We also note that many state statutes include a "friendly parent" rule, a preference for awarding custody to the parent who will be more likely to promote the children's relationship with the other parent (Elrod & Spector, 2004). However, the scientific status of PAS is, to be blunt, nil. As Gardner (2004) himself noted in a recent posthumous publication, only one study of parent alienation ever attempted a statistical analysis: his own. Very recently, Johnston conducted two studies of case records designed to identify the sources of alienation; she found many contributing factors leading to a child aligning with one parent against the other, including high-conflict custody litigation and poor parenting on the part of the "alienated" parent (cited in Johnston & Kelly, 2004).

We believe that it is blatantly misleading to call parental alienation a scientifically based "syndrome" (Emery, 2005). Careful assessments of each parent's willingness to support the other coparent clearly may be relevant to custody, but there is no established way of measuring "alienation." Evaluators therefore must carefully identify the sources of their information concerning a more or less "friendly" parent, as well as the inferences they draw from these assessments. Certainly, these assessments are best conducted by an evaluator who interviews both parents, something Gardner (2001) did not do in many cases.

Children's Wishes

Surveys indicate that custody evaluators place considerable importance on children's stated preferences regarding custody—particularly the preferences of adolescents, but also of children as young as 5 years old (Ackerman & Ackerman, 1997; Keilin & Bloom, 1986). This surely reflects the fact that children's wishes regarding custody typically are included in state laws as a factor to be considered when determining children's best interests. In fact, some statutes explicitly direct that the wishes expressed by a child of a given age—for example, 12 years old—should determine custody if there is no reason why those wishes should not be followed (Elrod & Spector, 2004). Although all agree that the wishes of teenagers can be influenced by unfortunate circumstances (e.g., a parent's greater material resources or permissiveness), laws regarding the expressed wishes of children of a certain age both respect the increasing autonomy of adolescents and recognize the realistic difficulty of trying to keep children in an arrangement to which both they and one parent object.

A policy of acting on the freely expressed wishes of an adolescent is not without problems, but far bigger problems (and controversies) arise in regard to wishes of children who (a) are school aged or even younger and/or (b) do not come forward with a freely expressed preference. Some psychologists have offered that, even in these circumstances, children should be encouraged to express a preference regarding custody as a means of empowering them (see Weithorn, 1987). Others express concern that, instead of giving children the right to have input, such policies give children the responsibility for making adult decisions—decisions that the adults have failed to make themselves (Emery, 2003). Still others say that children's preferences should be assessed only sensitively and indirectly and that this information should be used as feedback to facilitate independent parental decision making (McIntosh, Long, & Moloney, 2004).

One of us has taken a strong position against attempting to assess children's unexpressed wishes (Emery, 2003), but our present concern is more basic. The freely offered preferences of children—particularly older children—are important considerations in custody evaluations for both practical and legal reasons, but there is no direct evidence on how or indeed whether evaluators should assess the wishes of children who, for whatever reason, do not express them.

Overnights With Infants and Toddlers

A final controversy we will discuss is whether or to what extent infants and toddlers should have overnight visits with their nonresidential parents. Children's age in relation to overnights is not a consideration mentioned often in surveys of custody evaluators, but it stands as an example of the sorts of controversial issues that evaluators often are asked to address. Other such issues include the question of whether a residential parent with primary physical custody should be allowed (if there are good reasons) to move with the child away from a nonresidential parent, or under what circumstances parental conflict is so intense that joint physical custody is unworkable.

Using differing interpretations of attachment theory, leading psychological scientists have taken strong and very different positions on the issue of overnights involving young children. A document prepared for the Spokane (Washington) Bar Association, and endorsed by many leading attachment researchers, called attention to the psychological importance of young children's secure attachment with a primary attachment figure. Based on research and theory on the primary attachment, the report recommended against overnight visits with the nonresidential parent until children are 4 years old (Spokane County Bar Association, 1996). In contrast, in a paper published in a major family-court journal, other leading psychological scientists highlighted the importance of children's attachments to multiple caregivers. Focusing on the value of developing multiple attachments, the authors recommended that infants should have regular overnight visits with nonresidential parents in the first year of life (Kelly & Lamb, 2000). Both interpretations offered various caveats about the quality of children's relationship with the nonresidential parent, parental cooperation, and similar issues, but they clearly came to very different substantive conclusions about what psychological science indicates regarding whether, when, or how often infants and toddlers should have overnight visits with nonresidential parents.

There is only meager direct evidence on the harm (Solomon & George, 1999) or absence of harm (Pruett, Williams, Insabella, & Little, 2003) associated with overnight visits for very young children. As with the issue of children's wishes, the psychological scientists debating the question of overnight visits apparently come to logical conclusions based on their own, theoretical premises, yet the limited state of knowledge allows reasonable scientists to come to opposing conclusions. Such differences of opinion are of great value in science, but when translated into policy recommendations, they can confuse and confound judges, lawyers, evaluators, and parents. For example, we have had distraught mothers approach us in shock after being court-ordered to stop breast-feeding their infants to allow for smoother overnight visits, yet we also know of judges who claim to overturn consensual parenting plans if they include overnight visits for children 3 years of age or younger because of worries about disrupting attachments.

One of us has developed a set of guidelines for parents about overnights and other arrangements for young children that represents what we believe to be a balanced position (Emery, 2004). However, our point here is that, whatever conclusion one reaches, it is based on limited evidence. Psychological scientists need to recognize and acknowledge their limited data base.

Our bigger point, to which we turn shortly, is this: Custody decision making and custody evaluations have an impossible task in attempting to determine children's future "best interests" in cases where parents cannot agree. Neither the wisest judge nor the most insightful evaluator has good answers to impossible questions.

The custody report completed by Dr. Hagan in our fictional case illustrates our various concerns with the limited science of custody evaluations and, more importantly, shows the problems that can arise under the regime of vague custody laws and vague professional and ethical standards for custody evaluators.

The Deer-Doe Case: Dr. Hagan's Custody Report

Dr. Hagan wrote a 35-page report summarizing his evaluation of the Deer-Doe family. The report contained precise details of the results of the various standardized tests, but the lawyers were only really interested in the final paragraphs under the heading, *Summary and Recommendations*.

"In summary, substantial evidence points to Ms. Deer-Doe's longstanding depression, her intense, repressed hostility toward Mr. Deer-Doe, and her alienation of the children against their father. In contrast, Mr. Deer-Doe appears to be well adjusted, is eager to promote the children's relationship with their mother, and is able and interested in being a full-time father. It therefore is recommended that, in order to promote his best interests, Carlos Deer-Doe be shifted immediately to his father's custody with regular visits with his mother, provided that she enters into individual psychotherapy.

"Although Isabella's intense anger at her father is largely a product of alienation, no change in custody is recommended for her at this point in time, because she is closely allied with her mother and is likely to continue to reject and rebel against her father's care. Instead, individual psychotherapy and family therapy with her father is recommended for Isabella, with further evaluation in 3 to 6 months depending upon the recommendations of Isabella's therapists and her mother's therapist, if relevant. A key consideration at that time will be whether Isabella's stated wish to live with her mother, if she continues to voice this preference, is a result of alienation."

When he read the evaluation, John Deer-Doe was jubilant. He felt vindicated, eager to be a full-time father again, and excited about the prospect of starting his new family. He vowed he was now going to get remarried "the day after my divorce is final." His lawyer, who also was encouraged by Dr. Hagan's report and recommendations, told John that the evaluation was not only a victory for him but for all fathers. "Sometimes the system really does work," she offered.

Jane Deer-Doe's reactions were understandably quite different. Shocked and panicked, she became emotionally distraught in her lawyer's office. He eventually helped Jane calm down by telling her that he had learned only recently that Dr. Hagan, who used to be fair and evenhanded, had become notoriously biased in favor of fathers as a result of losing custody in his own, bitter divorce. If he had known this a few months ago, Jane's lawyer told her, he never would have agreed to Dr. Hagan as the court-appointed evaluator.

Ms. Deer-Doe's attorney went on to offer that he would postpone the pending hearing in order to get a second evaluation by another mental health professional and have Dr. Hagan's evaluation reviewed by a third professional so as to identify any important limitations or weaknesses. If the court refused to appoint a more objective, neutral evaluator, then he would hire an expert who would do the job right. In any case, the postponement meant that, at a minimum, no changes in custody would take place for 6 to 9 months given the congested court calendar. In the meantime, he urged Ms. Deer-Doe to cheer up, continue to be a wonderful mother, and to be on her very best behavior so as not to give her soon-to-be-ex-husband any ammunition in his campaign against her and motherhood.

A Bigger Problem: The Legal and Emotional Context of Custody Disputes

We could conclude our monograph here with this summary: There is essentially no psychological science to support the measures and constructs designed specifically for the assessment of child custody arrangements for individual children. Moreover, established measures of clinical constructs must be used with caution due to threats to their validity and questions about the relevance in the custody context of the constructs they assess. We also could conclude that the state of psychological science is too limited to reach clear conclusions about controversial issues such as children's wishes, overnight visits, or even PAS, and remind the reader that the burden of proof falls on proponents of a particular hypothesis or recommendation. To these three points, we could add questions about ethics and professional practice—for example, potential concerns about systematic bias on the part of evaluators, questions about whether evaluators should address the "ultimate issue" (i.e., recommend specific custody arrangements), and worries about a battle of experts when each side hires its own evaluator.

However, we believe there are bigger problems in custody evaluations than shoddy science, and we also believe that consideration of these broader issues points the way to some promising solutions for custody evaluations, children, and families. Thus, we turn now to examine the more general literature on children's adjustment to their parents' separation and divorce. After this, we outline three general recommendations that we consider in light of psychological research, legal analysis, and professional responsibilities including various issues we raised about Dr. Hagan's custody evaluation.

AVERAGE EFFECTS AND VARIATION IN THE WELL-BEING OF CHILDREN FROM DIVORCED FAMILIES

There is a large, sophisticated, multidisciplinary research literature on how children are affected by parental separation and divorce. We cannot review many original sources from this literature in this limited space, although we have done so elsewhere (Emery, 1999b). In the following section, we offer an overview of the major conclusions researchers have drawn. After this, we consider what factors predict children's more or less adequate adjustment. For present purposes, research on the average well-being of children from divorced families is of interest primarily as a starting point for examining predictions of individual differences in outcome, one of the main goals of a custody evaluation. Thus, we review this extensive literature only briefly.

On average, parental divorce is associated with an increased risk for a variety of psychological problems among children

(Emery, 1999b; Hetherington & Kelly, 2002; McLanahan & Sandefur, 1994). In a meta-analysis of 92 studies, Amato and Keith (1991) found an average effect size of .14 standard deviation units when comparing children from divorced versus married families across all child outcomes. Another meta-analysis of studies in the 1990s found that the average effect size was somewhat larger than this earlier estimate, ranging from a low of .12 standard deviation units for measures of self-concept to a high of .22 standard deviation units for conduct problems (Amato, 2001).

While the effect sizes suggest a modest, average increase in psychological problems, it is important to underscore the variability in the psychological adjustment of children whose parents separate and divorce. Most children are resilient despite their parents' divorce, as indexed by measures of psychological maladjustment that do not differentiate them from children whose parents remain continuously married (Emery, 1999a; Emery & Forehand, 1994). Still, depending on the outcome, parental separation or divorce is linked with a 25% to 100% (a doubling) increase in the risk for psychological difficulties at the extremes of the distribution (Hetherington & Kelly, 2002; Zill, Morrison, & Coiro, 1993). Given the high prevalence of separation and divorce, even a modest increase in risk translates into an important societal concern.

Nonrandom Selection Into Divorce

Still, at least some of the putative "effects" of parental divorce on children, perhaps as much as 50% of the variance, are due to nonrandom selection into divorce. Many of the problems found among children from divorced families actually are present before the parents separate (Cherlin et al., 1991) and therefore cannot be consequences of parental divorce, although this selection effect seems to be stronger in accounting for the psychological difficulties of children than for those of young adults (Cherlin, Chase-Lansdale, & McRae, 1998). Behavior geneticists have raised the strongest selection argument, suggesting that children's risk in divorce may be fully or partially attributable to the passive gene–environment correlation, because genetic factors influence divorce and may also affect children's behavior (McGue & Lykken, 1992). Despite this important concern, in one adoption study (O'Connor, Caspi, DeFries, & Plomin, 2000) and one twin study (D'Onofrio et al., in press), divorce still was associated with a diminished but increased risk for psychological problems, particularly externalizing problems, among children.

Different Risks for Different Outcomes

Externalizing difficulties are the child emotional problems most strongly linked to parental separation and divorce (Amato, 2001; Amato & Keith, 1991; Emery, 1982, 1999b). Other emotional difficulties less strongly tied to parental marital status include depression; anxiety; poor school behavior and performance; and difficulties in romantic relationships, including an increased risk for divorce among offspring (e.g., McLanahan & Bumpass, 1988). A significantly increased risk for troubled family relationships, especially between children and their fathers, also accompanies divorce. One national study found that fully 65% of young adults between the ages of 18 and 22 whose parents were divorced had poor relationships with their fathers; only 29% of those whose parents were married had poor relationships with their fathers (Zill et al., 1993).

Scientific research notwithstanding, some clinical investigators point to case studies indicating that the adverse consequences of divorce for children are unexpectedly large (e.g., Wallerstein, Lewis, & Blakeslee, 2000). We believe that this conclusion, and much of the debate about it, is due to confusion of psychopathology with what one of us has termed psychological distress or "pain" (Laumann-Billings & Emery, 2000). Even resilient, well-functioning young people whose parents divorce report considerable distress in regard to their memories of their childhood ("I had a harder childhood than most people"), feelings about their current family relationships ("Sometimes I wonder if my father even loves me"), and concern over events where both of their parents will be present ("I worry about big events like graduations or weddings where both of my parents will have to come"; Laumann-Billings & Emery, 2000). Thus, even if resilience—as defined by the absence of mental health problems—is the normative outcome of divorce for children, children's resilience often is colored by painful memories of the past, difficult ongoing feelings about family members, and concerns about future family interactions. There is increasing agreement that making this distress-versus-disorder distinction may help clear up much of the controversy about the consequences of divorce for children (Kelly & Emery, 2003; Wallerstein, 2003).

PREDICTORS OF CHILDREN'S PSYCHOLOGICAL ADJUSTMENT TO DIVORCE

Average outcomes are an important backdrop to our discussion, but the prediction of individual differences in children's psychological well-being is more directly relevant to custody evaluations. In the following sections, we review research on different risk factors, relying primarily on secondary versus original sources because of space limitations and the large number of studies.

Parental Conflict

A large body of research demonstrates that conflict between parents is associated with an increased risk for psychological problems among children in all families, whether the parents are married, separated, or divorced (Ahrons & Miller, 1993; Ahrons & Tanner, 2003; Amato & Keith, 1991; Emery, 1982; Johnston & Roseby, 1997; Otto, Buffington-Vollum, & Edens, 2003). Although nonrandom selection cannot be completely ruled out, many analogue experiments demonstrate that conflict simulated in the laboratory or recorded systematically at home directly causes some adverse reactions among children (Cummings & Davies, 1994; Davies, Harold, Coeke-Morey, & Cummings, 2002).

Parental conflict often precedes a separation or divorce, and various studies demonstrate that children fare better psychologically if they live in a harmonious divorced family than in a conflict-ridden two-parent family (Emery, 1982). Because separation can bring relief from the struggles of living with parents in a conflict-ridden marriage, we therefore must add improved psychological adjustment to the range of variability found in children's psychological outcomes following their parents' divorce. This "relief hypothesis" is supported by research findings that show children's improved adjustment after separation in high-conflict marriages. However, a new and important twist is what happens to children from low-conflict marriages: Several recent studies have found that children fare better following separation from a high-conflict marriage but worse when their low-conflict parents separate (Amato, Loomis, & Booth, 1995; Peris & Emery, in press). In fact, Amato (2001) argues that, in close to half of divorces, the marriage had been "good enough" from the children's perspective. That is, parental conflict had been sufficiently well contained that the children do more poorly following their parents' separation than they would have done had their parents stayed together.

Whether or not more parents could stay together for their children's sake, these data point to the psychological importance of conflict and to the fact that parental separation does not necessarily decrease it. Conflict can, in fact, increase following separation, continue for years, and come to focus more squarely on children who are a point of connection between former partners (Emery, Laumann-Billings, Waldron, Sbarra, & Dillon, 2001; Johnston, 1994).

Parental conflict can affect children directly by creating stress and anxiety (Kelly, 1998) and indirectly by undermining parenting quality and the children's relationship with one or both parents (Otto et al., 2003). As with divorce itself, conflict after divorce is linked with a variety of short- and long-term psychological problems among children, ranging from conduct problems to depression (Emery, 1999b; Schmidtgall, King, Zarski, & Cooper, 2000). However, not all conflict is equally disruptive to children's emotional well-being. The results of systematic analogue studies (Cummings & Davies, 1994), together with field research (Grych & Fincham, 1990) and clinical experience (Emery, 2004), suggest that conflict is least destructive when it (a) is contained between parents; (b) is relatively infrequent; (c) is less intense emotionally or physically; (d) resolves; (e) is not about the children or childrearing; and (f) does not involve the children—which includes not arguing in front of or around the children, not asking children to carry messages between parents, not deriding the other parent to the children, not expecting the children to take sides, not making a child a scapegoat or a mediator, and not asking children to make decisions that the parents themselves cannot make (Emery, 2004). Another brief excerpt from the Deer-Doe case illustrates the sort of conflicts that can be all too familiar in separation and divorce.

Conflict and the Deer-Doe Case

As continued legal maneuvering delayed what he thought would be the speedy implementation of the recommendations made in Dr. Hagan's custody evaluation, John Deer-Doe grew extremely frustrated with his children's mother, with the legal system, and especially with not being able to see his children regularly. As a result of several letters from his lawyer and angry e-mails with Jane, for the first time since the separation, he had the children with him for a long, 3-day holiday weekend. John had a great time with Carlos on his Friday off and on Saturday, but he was deeply disappointed by Isabella's persistent distance and moodiness. His frustration erupted on Saturday evening when he asked Isabella why she didn't spend more time with him and answered his own question by blaming her mother's interference. Before Isabella could even react, he asked, "Wouldn't you like to live with me half of the time?" At this point, Isabella exploded. "I told Mom a hundred times. I want to live with her! I don't want to *see* you! I want to go *home*!"

Hurt and angry, John screamed back, "Fine!" He threw Isabella's things into her backpack, and returned her to her mother's house. They drove in silence, but as Isabella opened the car door, John told her, "You can tell your mother that I'll bring Carlos back tomorrow . . . maybe." Isabella burst into tears, slammed the car door shut, and ran to her mother's front door. John drove away before the door opened, not knowing whether Jane was even home or not.

As this vignette illustrates, hurt, anger, and conflict between separated parents can take many forms, and can erupt even in the absence of the other parent. The vignette also shows how the conflicts that may undermine relationships between separated parents can lead to conflicts between parents and children that undermine crucial parent–child relationships as well.

Parent–Child Relationships

In most studies of children from divorced families, the quality of the relationship between a child and his or her primary residential parent is the strongest predictor of that child's psychological well being (e.g., Buchanan, Maccoby, & Dornbusch, 1996; Hetherington & Kelly, 2002; Martinez & Forgatch, 2002). The most widely accepted classification of parenting groups caretakers into four categories based on the degree of warmth and control they offer to their children (Lamborn, Mounts, Steinberg, & Dornbusch, 1991; Maccoby & Martin, 1983; Novak, 1996; Steinberg, 2001). *Authoritative* parents are warm and involved, and they consistently and democratically enforce developmentally appropriate rules and discipline. *Authoritarian* parents offer their children low warmth and high control, using more frequent and autocratic punishment (Novak, 1996). *Permissive* parents are loving but indulgent, and they offer children little guidance and discipline about controlling their behavior. Finally, *neglectful* parents provide children with little affection or discipline.

Research on two-parent families consistently indicates that children of preschool age through adolescence who are raised by authoritative parents fare best on indicators of psychological and behavioral health, while the children of neglectful parents fare worst (Lamborn et al., 1991; Maccoby & Martin, 1983; Novak, 1996; Steinberg, 2001). Research on children in divorced families also shows that authoritative parenting by the primary residential parent is linked with better postdivorce adjustment (Buchanan et al., 1996; Fauber, Forehand, Thomas, & Wierson, 1990; Hetherington, Cox, & Cox, 1982; Hetherington & Kelly, 2002; Thomson, Hanson, & McLanahan, 1994). We should note, however, that more authoritarian parenting styles are found to be equally or more effective in certain contexts, for example among minority families living in potentially dangerous environments (where increased parental vigilance and authority may be needed; Deater-Deckard, Dodge, & Bates, 1996). Authoritarian parenting also predicts lower levels of substance use among adolescents living with divorced parents (Buchanan et al., 1996).

Mothers Versus Fathers

As noted above, most children live primarily with one parent following separation and divorce—approximately 75% live with their mothers and 10% live with their fathers. Although some early, small-scale studies indicated that children who lived with their same-gender parents were better adjusted than their counterparts living with opposite-sex parents (e.g., Santrock & Warshak, 1979), these findings have not been replicated in more recent research employing large samples (Buchanan et al., 1996; Downey & Powell, 1993). In general, researchers find that children of both genders function equally well living primarily either with their mothers or fathers (Downey, Ainsworth-Darnell, & Dufur, 1998); however, a few investigators have found that children do somewhat better in sole-mother residence than they do in sole-father residence (Buchanan et al., 1996). Still, differences between primary-mother versus primary-father residential arrangements, if they are found at all, are not large in magnitude. Thus, neither parental gender, nor the interaction between parent and child gender, has been found to moderate children's well-being in an important way.

The extent to which children's relationships with their "other" parents predicts their psychological well-being, particularly when there is parental conflict, is one of the most controversial issues in custody law (e.g., favoring or opposing joint physical custody) and in custody evaluations. Data are not conclusive, but there is research relevant to these issues. Given that the issue is so pressing, we believe it is important to draw some clear, if qualified, conclusions from the available research.

Contact Between Children and Nonresident Parents

An important demographic issue that we have not addressed, but that bears in a very important way on parent–child relationships following a separation, is the extent of contact between children and their nonresidential parents. Seltzer's (1991) analysis of the 1987–88 round of the National Survey of Families and Households data provides detailed and high-quality, if somewhat dated, evidence on this issue, especially on the frequency of contact between children and nonresidential fathers. Three broad trends characterized the findings from this national survey. First, contact between nonresident, separated, or divorced fathers and their children was not terribly frequent, even immediately after the separation. For example, only 43% of fathers separated for 2 years or less saw their children on a weekly basis or more frequently, while 30% of fathers separated for less than 2 years saw their children several times a year or less. Second, contact dropped off substantially over time, such that 6 to 10 years following separation, only 19% of nonresident fathers saw their children weekly or more, while 62% had face-to-face contact with their children several times a year or less. Third, higher contact levels were predicted by a variety of factors including less geographic distance between the parents' households, a shorter length of time since separation, absence of remarriages, the child having been born into a legal marriage instead of out of wedlock, and the child being older rather than younger (Seltzer, 1991). Other evidence from national samples shows that nonresidential mothers maintain somewhat more frequent contact with their children than nonresidential fathers do (Zill, 1988).

Some commentators believe that father contact has increased dramatically in the last 15 years, but the relatively modest increases in sole father custody and joint physical custody (reviewed earlier) make us skeptical that there have really been any dramatic changes. In the most recent national data we could locate, an analysis of 1998 U.S. Census data, 40% of nonresident fathers and 22% of nonresident mothers had had no contact with their children in the previous year. Among the 60% of nonresident fathers who had seen their children, contact occurred on an average of 69 days per year. The 78% of nonresident mothers who saw their children did so more often, an average of 86 days per year (Child Trends, 2002). These data were not disaggregated by levels of contact, overnight visits, or time since separation, and they included parents who did not live with their children for a variety of reasons (e.g., divorced, never married). Still, the evidence indicates that, even in a recent cohort, a substantial number of nonresident parents maintain little contact with their children, and contact in the range considered to be joint physical custody (about 100 overnights per year) is not the norm.

Nonresident Fathering and Children's Psychological Well-Being

The normative backdrop is important in considering the question of whether more frequent contact with nonresident parents predicts better psychological adjustment among children. A meta-analysis of 63 studies examining the relationship between children's psychological well-being or academic success and different dimensions of the relationship between a child and his or her nonresident father (i.e., payment of child support, amount of contact, feeling close to the father, and authoritative parenting) indicated that the amount of contact is a poor predictor of children's psychological well-being (Amato & Gilbreth, 1999). As shown in Table 1, the weighted effect sizes (product–moment correlations) between contact levels and three indices of children's psychological well-being were uniformly very small. For externalizing problems and academic success, a fathers' payment of child support was a better predictor of his children's adjustment than was a father's contact with his children. In contrast, authoritative parenting and, to a lesser extent, closeness to the father consistently accounted for a significant if statistically small proportion of variance in all three measured outcomes.

The authors tested for a number of variables that might moderate these relationships, including child gender, age, race, divorce versus nonmarital birth, and remarriage of the parents, but none of these variables moderated the effect sizes in any meaningful way. Although the meta-analysis did not test for the moderating effects of parental conflict, Amato and Gilbreth (1999) discussed the critical role of parental conflict, including research indicating a positive effect of contact when parents cooperate and a negative effect when parents are in conflict (Amato & Rezac, 1994; Hetherington, Cox, & Cox, 1982).

Joint Custody and Children's Psychological Well-Being

Whether joint physical custody is linked with better psychological adjustment among children is an important question in its own right, and if children fare notably better under joint physical custody than in other arrangements, a nonlinear relationship also might explain the weak association between nonresident-father contact and child outcome. Children may benefit from spending more time with their fathers only when contact reaches some high threshold (see, e.g., Cabrera, Tamis-LeMonda, Bradley, Hofferth, & Lamb, 2000; Lamb, 1999; Lewis & Lamb, 2003). Surprisingly, relatively few investigators have examined how joint physical custody is associated with children's well-being. A recent meta-analysis (Bauserman, 2002) located only 11 published studies and 22 unpublished studies (21 of which were unpublished dissertations) with a combined sample size of 814 joint-custody children and 1,846 sole-custody children. Combining the results across measures, Bauserman reported a study-level overall effect size of .23 standard deviation units, slightly above what is traditionally considered to be a small effect. This analysis included both joint physical and joint legal custody, but surprisingly these arrangements did not differ significantly in their effects when compared to sole custody (joint physical, $d = .29$ for 20 studies; joint legal, $d = .22$ for 15 studies).

Importantly, neither presence of past parental conflict (5 studies) nor that of current parental conflict (14 studies) accounted for significant variance in the joint-custody effect sizes; perhaps of more importance, however, joint-custody groups had lower levels of both past and present conflict than sole-custody groups did (Bauserman, 2002). As Bauserman noted, this suggests the very important possibility that self-selection into joint custody may account for part or all of the results. We cannot extrapolate from voluntary joint physical custody to circumstances when joint physical custody is imposed upon parents by laws favoring joint physical custody, by evaluators who recom-

TABLE 1

Meta-Analysis of 63 Studies Showing How Strongly Different Relationships Between Children and Nonresident Fathers Predicted Children's Academic Success and Psychological Well-Being (Adapted From Amato and Gilbreth, 1999)

	Dimension of nonresident father–child relationship			
Child well-being index	Payment of child support by father	Amount of contact between child and father	Child feeling close to father	Authoritative parenting by father
Academic success				
Effect size (weighted *r*)	.09***	.03*	.06*	.15***
Number of effect sizes	17	17	7	11
Sum of sample sizes	7,156	4,918	1,212	1,185
Externalizing problems				
Effect size (weighted *r*)	−.08***	−.02	−.05*	−.11***
Number of effect sizes	8	37	12	26
Sum of sample sizes	2,917	6,808	1,586	2,657
Internalizing problems				
Effect size (weighted *r*)	−.01	−.03*	−.07*	−.12***
Number of effect sizes	8	43	14	13
Sum of sample sizes	1,916	4,841	1,617	545

*$p < .05$. **$p < .01$. ***$p < .001$.

mend that arrangement, or by judges who order it. Finally, it is important to note that, although conflict differences did not account for the advantage of joint over sole custody in the meta-analysis, this analysis does not address the possibility that joint physical custody may be the right solution for the wrong people in contested-custody or other high-conflict situations (Emery, 1999b). At least some research shows that high conflict predicts worse child adjustment within joint-physical-custody groups (Johnston, Kline, & Tschann, 1989).

Thus, our conclusion about the potential benefits of joint physical custody is a cautious one because of (a) the important and unanswered question of whether low-conflict couples self-select into that arrangement; (b) concerns about the potential damage to children caused by likely greater exposure to parental conflict in such an arrangement; (c) the null results for father contact found in a more extensive body of research where self-selection is less of a concern; and (d) the continued low prevalence rates of joint physical custody despite two decades of experimentation. We believe that joint physical custody benefits children when parental conflict is contained. Therefore, more parents who want to attempt joint physical custody (and therefore are likely to be fairly cooperative) should be encouraged to try it. However, joint physical custody seems to be a workable arrangement only for a minority of parents and should not be encouraged as the fair solution for parents who dispute custody or otherwise are in high conflict. Finally, we note that there is no clear line defining when joint physical custody is potentially beneficial or potentially harmful for children. The field would benefit greatly from research on what kinds and levels of parental conflict and cooperation distinguish "good" from "bad" joint physical custody.

Parents' Mental Health

The Uniform Marriage and Divorce Act explicitly indicates that the mental health of all parties should be a consideration in determining children's best interests. Statutes offer little more than this general guidance, however, thereby leaving much room for interpretation. Thus, although mental health professionals can assess mental health with adequate reliability and validity, questions arise about the specific relevance of parents' mental health problems for children, parenting, and custody arrangements.

Emery (1999b) suggested that four mental health problems among parents are of special concern to understanding the potential consequences of divorce for children: (a) depression, (b) antisocial behavior, (c) major mental illness (e.g., schizophrenia and bipolar disorder), and (d) personality disorders. Substance abuse should also be added to this list. Parental depression is associated with negative child outcomes in a number of studies (Otto et al., 2003), but the effects are likely to be mediated through parental conflict and inadequate parenting (Emery, Weintraub, & Neale, 1982). In their review of the literature, Otto and colleagues (Otto et al., 2003) reported that one of the most consistent findings is that parents who engage in antisocial behaviors tend to have children who exhibit a number of behavior problems, particularly aggression, delinquency, and other externalizing problems. Children whose parents suffer from schizophrenia also are at a significantly elevated risk both for schizophrenia and for a range of serious emotional problems, although the increased risk appears to result primarily from genetic effects as opposed to childrearing (Gottesman, 1991). Perhaps the greatest concern in regard to schizophrenia and other major mental illness is whether the parent with the disorder is, with treatment, functioning sufficiently well to care for his or her children. A similar concern arises regarding the well-being of children who have a substance-abusing parent. Evidence shows that both genetic and environmental liabilities contribute to the increased risk for psychological problems among such children (Walden, McGue, Iacono, Burt, & Elkins, 2004), but the most pressing issue is the parent's immediate functioning and whether or not this impairs the parent's ability to care for or protect the safety of his or her children. Finally, little research is available on how children are affected by parental personality disorders, although experts in custody disputes increasingly recognize that personality disorders often are an important concern, particularly in cases characterized by chronic high conflict (Ehrenberg, Hunter, & Elterman, 1996; Johnston & Roseby, 1997).

The literatures on parents' mental health, parent–child relationships, genetic transmission, and children's psychological well-being are too vast and complicated for us to consider in any detail here. Still, several broad conclusions seem clear. First, some evidence shows that children are adversely affected when their parents have emotional, behavioral, or substance-abuse problems, but the children's problems might be caused not by their invariably troubled relationships with their parents but by genetic risk or life hardships associated with their parents' psychological problems (Jenuwine & Cohler, 1999). Second, whether or not a parent is engaged in treatment is a major consideration for serious emotional problems like severe depression, substance abuse, or schizophrenia, since appropriate treatment can do much to mitigate symptoms and improve parents' functioning. Third, although the assessment of parents' mental health is of critical and obvious importance when a parent's emotional difficulties are serious enough to necessitate the involvement of child protective services, in other circumstances (i.e., when a parent's emotional difficulties would not lead to unwanted legal intervention in a two-parent family) such assessment seems to us to be merely a search for a "tie breaker" under a vague custody rule fraught with problems. Once again, our view is that it is better to change an impossible rule than to do one's best to follow it.

In summary we conclude that, as others have suggested (Herman et al., 1997; Otto et al., 2003), a parental diagnosis is not, in and of itself, the primary concern when deciding custody; rather, what is of utmost importance is the impact of parental psychological functioning on the child's development and behavior. When a parent's emotional problems are sufficiently severe that they would warrant legal intervention independent of a custody dispute, we have no doubt that parental mental health should be a central consideration in custody cases. In more ordinary circumstances, however, we see no obvious reason why a history of parental depression, for example, should be a determinative factor in a custody dispute unless it clearly and substantially interferes with parenting.

Economic Well-Being

A family's standard of living falls after separation and divorce, if for no other reason than it is more expensive to live in two households than to live in one. We should note, however, that the average decline is greater for divorced women than for divorced men, as women typically have lower incomes and the extra expense of childrearing (Duncan & Hoffman, 1985). Economic strains can set into motion a number of changes for children, including possibly moving from the family home, changing schools, losing contact with old friends, and spending more time in childcare and having less contact with parents as the parents work to make ends meet. Not surprisingly, research shows that economic stability is an important predictor of postdivorce child functioning (Dunn, 2004; Lamb, Sternberg, & Thompson, 1997). The differences found between the adjustment of children in married and single-parent families are reduced by about half for academic measures like school attainment and by a lesser amount for internalizing and externalizing problems when income is statistically controlled for (Brooks-Gunn & Duncan, 1997; King, 1994; McLanahan, 1997; McLanahan & Sandefur, 1994).

But while family income no doubt is important, much of the variance in children's psychological adjustment in divorced and married families is not explained by economics. Moreover, income may exert its effects indirectly, for example by influencing parenting and other aspects of family functioning, rather than directly, for example by affecting living conditions and opportunities available to children. Results of one study indicated, for example, that divorced working mothers, but not married working mothers, provided less cognitive and social stimulation to their children than married nonworking mothers did (MacKinnon, Brody, & Stoneman, 1982), and other research indicates that parents under economic stress are less likely to be supportive (Thomson et al., 1994).

These findings suggest that caution should be exercised when using parents' incomes as a predictor of children's well-being following divorce; but we particularly call attention to a more basic issue. The suggestion that custody should go to the parent with the higher income sounds outlandish and biased; but we could, if we chose, muster arguments that living with the higher-income parent might be in a child's best interests in terms both of the correlates of greater wealth (e.g., health, well-being) and the direct benefits of greater wealth (e.g., living conditions, opportunities). We would not want to make such arguments too seriously, but we do believe they illustrate an important point: Why should parents' relative mental health, parenting skills, or any other factor determined on a case-by-case basis determine custody? We believe that the essential problem of determining children's "best interests" based on criteria that are only vaguely specified is the same whether evaluators consider children's economic or psychological best interests. In the latter case, the difference is that the core problem is more effectively disguised.

Ranking Predictors

Based on an extensive review of the literature, one of us (Emery, 1999b) concluded that the following four factors were the most consistent predictors of children's positive psychological adjustment following separation and divorce:

- A good relationship with an authoritative residential parent
- Minimal or controlled parental conflict that does not involve the children
- Economic security
- A good relationship with an authoritative nonresidential parent

Our present review is consistent with this earlier conclusion, and also with the suggestion (Emery, 1999b) that the four factors are ranked in their order of importance (defined as proportion of variance explained) for various measures of children's psychological well-being. Given this conclusion, we urge any professional intervening with separating and divorcing families to attempt to promote all four goals. Since this cannot always be accomplished, however, our rank ordering indicates that factors ranked higher should take precedence over factors ranked lower—if, that is, the objective is to minimize children's risk for developing psychological problems. This means, for example, that if parental conflict is high, and if the nature of that conflict is such that it harms children (e.g., revolves around issues of childrearing, involves the children in the parents' disputes) then frequent contact with both parents is likely to be more harmful than beneficial to children. In the face of high conflict, therefore, children would do better living primarily in one household with an authoritative mother or father and having more limited contact with the other parent. Even as we reach this conclusion, we recognize that philosophical or legal considerations might place a higher value on goals other than maximizing children's mental health—for example, the value that children should have frequent contact with both of their parents despite the presence of damaging conflict. We recognize that a degree of conflict between former partners, sometimes intense conflict, can be expected in divorce, but that conflict also can be contained, diminished, and hopefully resolved over time.

A Referral for the Deer-Does

Jane Deer-Doe was frightened and infuriated when she unexpectedly found Isabella knocking on her door a day early, after her father had returned her in a fury. Jane was more angry than worried about Isabella's flood of bitter tears. In the face of Dr. Hagan's adverse custody recommendation, she thought this was her opportunity to turn the tables on John. Secretly, she also hoped for vindication not only for all of her actions since her separation but also for the choices, mistakes, and sacrifices she had made in marriage. Enraged and not wanting to waste a moment—and with Isabella listening in—Jane telephoned her lawyer at his home and tried to tell him about what happened and about her outrage. But he was abrupt with Jane and suggested that she instead come by his office on Monday morning. There was nothing to be done on a Saturday night.

To Jane's surprise, her lawyer did not launch into a case against John, even when she finally related all of the details in his office. He listened patiently, but told Jane he needed to give her a "reality check" about what the courts could and could not do. He talked about the cost of extending the litigation process, delays in hearing dates, legal counter-tactics like bringing up any and all of her vulnerabilities as a parent and as a person (and her husband certainly knew her weak spots), and how children can get caught in the middle of such contests. He pointed out that no court was going to deny John all of his rights as a father, so she was going to have to deal with him one way or another. He also noted that local court rules mandated that parents attempt mediation before a custody hearing could be held.

Jane's lawyer told her that he wanted her to try mediation to see if she and John might work out at least some issues about their children without going to court. He described how mediation works and offered that, even if it failed, her effort would look good if the case did go to court. Jane's lawyer eventually told her that he had, in fact, already spoken with John's lawyer and that she agreed that they should try mediation. John's lawyer had promised she would convince John to try it. After raising a number of objections to the idea, Jane eventually accepted her lawyer's advice—but only with great reluctance and trepidation.

Research shows what the Deer-Does' lawyers intuitively recognized: The process of change, the quality of family relationships, and the management of conflict are more important to children's psychological adjustment to divorce than are the structure of custody arrangements or, indeed, the structure of the family (Ahrons, 1998; Amato & Booth, 1997; Buchanan et al., 1996; Emery, 1999b; Hetherington & Kelly, 2002). This conclusion creates a problem for lawyers in traditional practice, however, because the adversary system on which our legal procedures are based can exacerbate rather than help to contain parental conflict and can further undermine rather than promote coordinated coparenting. The dilemma for lawyers and other professionals who work with custody disputes is particularly vexing under the regime of the vague children's-best-interests standard. We briefly evaluate this custody standard in historical context before turning to our specific recommendations for reform.

CHILDREN'S BEST INTERESTS: A STANDARD WITH NO STANDARDS

In theory, the "best interests of the child" standard gives judges the flexibility to craft custody decisions that are uniquely appropriate for each individual family. In practice, however, the standard has been widely criticized because it (a) encourages litigation by making judges' decisions unpredictable; (b) increases acrimony, because virtually any evidence that makes one parent look bad may be deemed relevant (recall the morality statutes found in some state laws); (c) increases the potential for bias in the exercise of judicial discretion; and (d) limits appellate review, because the guidelines governing judicial decision making are unclear (Garrison, 1996; Mnookin, 1975). In fact, the problems with the best-interests standard have led at least one distinguished legal commentator to propose a fair and simple alternative: Flip a coin (Chambers, 1984). This flip suggestion highlights the extent of the problems that lay hidden underneath the best-interests standard's superficial appeal.

Historical Perspective

Until the middle of the 19th century, custody laws were perfectly clear: Fathers were automatically granted custody of their children, who were viewed, like a wife, as a man's property (Wyer, Gaylord, & Grove, 1987). Laws began to change in the late 1800s with the emergence of the "tender years" doctrine, which held that mothers are uniquely suited to rear children (*Ex Parte Devine*, 1981; Lyman & Roberts, 1985; Mason, 1994; Wyer et al., 1987). The tender-years doctrine came to control custody decision making during much of the 20th century, but in the 1970s the presumption was challenged as sexist (Hall, Pulver, & Cooley, 1996; Mason, 1994). The subsequent decline of the tender-years presumption left courts without clear guidance in following the best-interests standard, a principle that had been place since the beginning of the 20th century (Mnookin, 1975). For decades, children were automatically placed with their mothers in their best interests (unless the mother was "unfit"), but the desire to avoid sexism left courts without a dominant guiding principle.

As we noted earlier, some states today list factors that they deem relevant to children's best interests, at least in general terms, but the ultimate goal is never defined (Mnookin, 1975). This presents judges with an impossible practical, legal, and ethical dilemma. As noted family law professor Robert Mnookin (1975) put it:

> Deciding what is best for a child poses a question no less ultimate than the purposes and values of life itself. Should the judge be primarily concerned with the child's happiness? Or with the child's spiritual and religious training? Should the judge be concerned with the economic "productivity" of the child when he grows up? Are the primary values of life in warm interpersonal relationships, or in discipline and self-sacrifice? Is stability and security for a child more desirable than intellectual stimulation? These questions could be elaborated endlessly. And yet, where is the judge to look for the set of values that should inform the choice of what is best for the child? (pp. 260–261)

Custody Evaluations: A Solution to Judges' Dilemma?

Without clear guidance from the law, judges have turned to mental health professionals and custody evaluations for help in discerning children's best interests (Feller, Davidson, Hardin, & Horowitz, 1992; Mnookin, 1975; Shuman, 2002; Wald, 1976). By doing so, the courts have implicitly embraced the value that children's psychological well-being—their happiness—comes first and foremost on the list of their best interests. Alternative experts the courts instead might employ include accountants who have evaluated each parent's ability to provide for their children economically, educators who can comment on the parents' relative commitment to promoting success in school, religious leaders or philosophers who have assessed the quality of each parent's moral values and training, or perhaps dieticians who have evaluated each parent's preference for healthy versus convenience food. These suggestions may seem outrageous, but so is the idea that custody should be awarded to a parent who has an edge over another parent in promoting children's psychological well-being, particularly when the construct is ill defined or undefined.

We appreciate the terrible dilemma that the vague best-interests standard creates for judges, custody evaluators, and, of course, parents and children. We also believe that a mental health professional or other neutral third party or parties may be in a better position than a judge bound by rules of legal procedure to make recommendations about custody. However, we believe it is legally, morally, and scientifically wrong to make custody evaluators de facto decision makers in custody cases, which is often what happens because judges often accept evaluators' recommendations. As law professor Daniel Shuman (2002) recently summarized, "the role of mental health professionals in custody litigation is being transformed from expert as expert to expert as judge" (p. 160). Shuman went on to point out:

> If society wishes to use mental health practitioners as experts in child custody cases, the law and science demand rigorous threshold scrutiny of their methods and procedures so that courts are informed consumers of this evidence. If society wishes to use mental health practitioners as judges in child custody cases, then social policy demands a public debate and legislative approval of this change . . . (p. 162)

We agree. Establishing panels of mental health professionals who would decide custody disputes would be a major procedural change in the law, perhaps an important one. However, we believe that there are simpler and likely more effective changes in policy that would improve custody decision making for children and divorcing families and simultaneously solve many of the problems faced by custody evaluators, lawyers, judges, and other professionals who now work with custody disputes. Our recommendations include (a) promoting parental self-determination through alternative dispute resolution and other means, (b) working to develop and implement clear custody standards, and (c) altering the practice of current custody evaluations under the best-interests standard.

RECOMMENDATION 1: ENCOURAGE ALTERNATIVE DISPUTE RESOLUTION AND PRIVATE SETTLEMENT

We believe that the best solutions to the problems posed by child custody disputes and unscientific custody evaluations involve changing the system of dispute resolution in ways that encourage parents to reach their own decisions about rearing their children following a separation (Emery, 1999b, 2004). Obviously, there will be fewer custody evaluations, and fewer cases that judges must decide, if more parents resolve their differences by deciding custody arrangements on their own. We also believe that encouraging private settlement is the best way to promote children's mental health in separation and divorce. If the research-based goals are to contain parental conflict, encourage cooperative coparenting, support both parents' authoritative relationships with the children, and preserve economic resources, then it seems reasonable to steer clear of something called "the adversary system," the method of dispute resolution embraced by the American system of justice (Emery & Wyer, 1987b). "Going to war" is not the way to promote peace, certainly not in a divorced family.

Over the last two decades, many legal and mental health professionals, and many divorced parents, have come to this same conclusion. As an alternative, they urge separated parents to determine their own children's best interests by grappling with and working out the difficult issues of residence and childrearing themselves. One important reason to do this from the outset of a separation is that parents ultimately must deal with custody decisions, parenting, and each other on their own. If a degree of cooperation in coparenting is the ultimate goal for promoting children's best interests, then it seems reasonable to hypothesize that a more cooperative approach like mediation, for example, will help parents achieve this outcome better than adversarial negotiations or litigation in the courtroom will.

More cooperative approaches to dispute settlement—those in which parents exercise a greater degree of control over both the process and the outcome than they do in the adversary system—include a range of options such as (a) *pro se* divorce, in which parents manage all legal matters on their own without the use of lawyers; (b) divorce education, usually involving court-mandated classes on parenting in divorce that encourage cooperative coparenting, even during settlement negotiations; (c) more informal, cooperative negotiations between parents and their attorneys, an approach that includes but is not limited to *collaborative law*, a new option invented by family lawyers in which both attorneys agree to represent their clients only so long as they negotiate in good faith and settle their disputes outside of court (Tesler, 2001); (d) family therapy and parent training, which, while not focused on resolving custody disputes, do focus on the importance of authoritative parenting and cooperation in coparenting for separated and divorced parents (Martinez & Forgatch, 2001; Wolchik et al., 2000); (e) divorce mediation, the most firmly established of the new approaches, in which parents negotiate a settlement with the help of a neutral expert, usually a mental health professional or a lawyer (Emery, 1994); and (f) use of family coordinators, for that subset of high-conflict families that cannot participate in or benefit from any of the previous options (e.g., Coates et al., 2003).

The Example of Divorce Mediation

Importantly, research shows that some of these new approaches do help encourage private settlement, cooperative coparenting, and a long-term perspective on childrearing following separation and divorce. The evidence is strongest for divorce mediation, which has been studied more thoroughly than other legal interventions in divorce, although there undoubtedly is a need for more research on all types of custody-dispute-resolution procedures—perhaps especially on the adversary settlement process itself (Beck & Sales, 2001). A few randomized trials and a number of evaluations of large-scale programs have shown the following: Relative to traditional adversary settlement (attorney negotiations and formal courtroom litigation), mediation (a) settles a large percentage of cases otherwise headed for court; (b) possibly speeds the time involved in reaching a settlement, saves money, and increases compliance with agreements; (c) clearly increases party satisfaction with the process of dispute resolution; and, most importantly, (d) leads to improved relationships between nonresidential parents and children, as well as between the separated or divorced parents themselves (Emery, Sbarra, & Grover, 2005).

One of us has conducted a randomized trial of custody mediation and litigation, including a 12-year follow-up of the 71 families in the study (Emery et al., 2001). The study included primarily young, low-income parents, all of whom could be considered high conflict because they failed to reach a settlement on their own and were recruited into the study at the time that they filed a petition for a contested-custody hearing. Participants were randomly assigned at this time to participate either in mediation or in an evaluation by the court (adversary control group), and various tests were conducted to examine self-selection and attrition over time (neither of which proved to bias the study's results in any detectable manner). Among the major findings of an initial study and replication (Emery et al., 2001; Emery, Matthews, & Kitzmann, 1994; Emery, Matthews, & Wyer, 1991; Emery & Wyer, 1987a) were the following:

- Only 11% of cases randomly assigned to mediation appeared in front of a judge, compared with 72% of cases randomly assigned to the adversary-settlement group.
- On average, parents reported greater satisfaction with mediation than with adversary settlement on items assessing both the presumed strengths of mediation (e.g., "your feelings were understood") and the presumed strengths of adversary settlement (e.g., "your rights were protected").
- Reports of greater satisfaction were notably stronger for fathers than for mothers, apparently as a result of a ceiling effect: Mothers almost always won in court and therefore generally were quite satisfied following adversary settlement.
- The pattern of results held not only immediately after the dispute resolutions but also in a 1.5-year follow-up and even 12 years later.
- Nonresidential parents who mediated were far more likely to maintain contact with their children. Thirty percent of nonresidential parents who mediated saw their children once a week or more 12 years after the initial dispute, in comparison to only 9% of parents in the adversary group. In the mediation group, fully 54% of nonresidential parents also spoke to their children on the telephone once a week or more 12 years later, in contrast to 13% in the adversary group.
- The increased contact between parents necessitated by greater nonresidential parent–child contact did not increase parent conflict; rather, conflict was somewhat lower in the mediation group.
- Among parents who mediated rather than continuing with the legal action over the custody dispute, 12 years later the residential parents reported that the nonresidential parents were significantly more likely to discuss problems with them; had a greater influence on childrearing decisions; and were more involved in the children's discipline, grooming, moral training, errands, holidays, significant events, school or church functions, recreational activities, and vacations.

These studies provide strong evidence about the potential for mediation to bring about improved family relationships after separation and divorce, even many years later. Still, while the study's internal validity is strong, its external validity can be questioned. The results of various other evaluations of mediation and adversary settlement help to support the generality of the findings, but an appropriate degree of caution is suggested by variation in the quality of mediation in different settings, the push in some court-based mediation programs to "get agreements" rather than focus on fostering positive postdivorce family relationships, and the general need for more research (Emery, Sbarra, & Grover, 2005).

The limited evidence on other legal and mental health procedures (e.g., divorce education, parent training) also suggests that encouraging parents to take the long view and work together as parents even in the middle of separation and divorce can benefit children, parent–child relationships, and coparents (Emery, Waldron, & Kitzmann, 1999). This is not to suggest that people should not feel hurt, angry, and bitter in the midst of separation and divorce, but instead that, if they have children, former partners who remain parents need to find a way not to act on their understandably painful emotions as they renegotiate their family relationships (Emery, 1994, 2004). Also, despite the proven benefits, it is important to acknowledge that mediation is not a panacea, and there may be a subset of parents for whom mediation is not indicated (e.g., families with a history of significant domestic violence).

The Deer-Does in Mediation

Neither John nor Jane Deer-Doe entered mediation with a sense of optimism, let alone a desire to be in the same room with one another. Their mediator, Dr. Cynthia Barnes, who also was a clinical psychologist and family therapist, was pleasant, calm, and clearly in control of the meeting, but she could not prevent the Deer-Does from erupting into an angry argument after only about 20 minutes. A tense discussion concerning their disagreements about the children exploded when John accused Jane of using the children to meet her own, limitless need for attention. Jane shot back, "It wasn't me who had an affair." In an angry, loud voice, John was retorting, "I never would have had to go outside the marriage if you . . ." when Dr. Barnes interrupted to ask to speak with each parent alone.

At first, Jane fumed during her caucus alone with Dr. Barnes, but she found herself in tears within a few minutes. "I just can't believe I'm losing my marriage," she said, "and now he wants me to lose my kids too." She talked about her feelings of loss, grief, fear, hurt, and anger, not about problems with the custody arrangement. At one point, Jane even confessed that at times she longed to get her marriage back; John had, after all, been a good father and husband. But this revelation quickly led Jane back to John's affair and the pain it caused her; she was becoming angry again when Dr. Barnes interrupted her.

Dr. Barnes offered that she recognized that Jane was in great pain in response to losing so many things, and that she needed to grieve. In fact, Dr. Barnes recommended a therapist for Jane to consult in order to discuss these issues. Yet, Dr. Barnes also pointed out that the goal of mediation was to preserve and protect the best part of Jane's relationship with John—their children. She wanted Jane to think about ways they might be able to try to do that.

John was far less emotional when he met with Dr. Barnes alone. He clearly was very frustrated, but kept saying that all he wanted was to have time with his children and get on with his life. Dr. Barnes acknowledged John's feelings, but suggested that maybe Jane—and maybe Isabella and Carlos too—were not as ready to move on as he was, especially in regard to his new relationship. She also obliquely suggested that John might want to slow down his current romantic relationship a bit for his own sake, as well. Her strong advice to John was to work on taking small but positive steps forward with the kids, and to focus on first rebuilding his relationship with them alone before including his new girlfriend in his time with them.

When the Deer-Does and the mediator got back together toward the end of their two hours, Dr. Barnes again acknowledged everyone's difficult emotions, but pointed out how mediation was focused on trying to solve problems. She repeated her theme about taking small but positive steps, and to the parents' surprise, they took one by arranging a plan for Carlos and Isabella to spend time with John for an overnight during the coming weekend. They agreed on very explicit details, not only for timing and transportation but also on what to tell the children about the plan and what to do if one of them grew distraught.

Jane and John did not work everything out in one mediation session, but they did discover a forum where they could bring their conflicts and try to sort them out. Mediation offered them an environment that accepted their painful emotions but simultaneously encouraged them to put their own feelings on hold and focus on a plan for their children. Jane and John did not realize it, but this is exactly what they needed to do in a much bigger way, in order to move forward as parents and also as people in the coming months and years.

RECOMMENDATION 2: ADOPT A CLEAR CUSTODY STANDARD LIKE THE APPROXIMATION RULE

Our primary recommendation is to continue to develop practices and policies that encourage parents to reach their own, hopefully reasonably amicable decisions about residence and parenting, even when they are in the midst of separation and divorce. We view mediation as only one of a range of options designed to facilitate that goal. Our second recommendation is that state legislatures move to enact clear guidelines for determining custody in cases where the parents cannot reach an agreement. A fair standard that results in more predictable outcomes should reduce the number of contested custody cases, alter the need for and nature of custody evaluations, and as a result, we believe, help to reduce or at least not exacerbate conflict between separating parents. In short, a clear, determinative custody rule is likely to serve the children's best interests in separation and divorce.

There is one proposal for a clear custody guideline whose potential we find particularly hopeful. The "approximation rule" suggests that parenting arrangements after divorce should approximate, as much as is possible, the respective involvement of the parents in childrearing during marriage (Scott, 1992). Parents who had equal or near-equal involvement during the marriage would maintain some form of joint physical custody after separation. Parents who divided their childrearing roles disproportionately during the marriage also would continue that arrangement. Parents who had agreed to change their roles over time, or who wanted a different postdivorce custody arrangement for whatever reason, would be encouraged to negotiate their own arrangements according to the primary, private settlement recommendation of those who have advocated for the approximation rule.

In our view, the most important advantage of the approximation rule is that it is a clear, determinative standard. Parents and their lawyers would know what to expect of the courts, and this knowledge would promote settlement. In custody disputes that are nevertheless litigated, the approximation rule would sharply limit the scope of the legal inquiry, as well as any custody evaluations that might occur. Rather than assessing children's future best interests, under the approximation rule judges and custody evaluators would focus on the far clearer and far narrower question of each parent's past involvement in childrearing.

No state has implemented the proposed approximation rule, so there is no evidence on its effectiveness. We note, however, that the American Law Institute (2002), whose model statutes often become the basis for state law, has endorsed the approximation rule in its proposed reforms of divorce and custody law (along with the principle of parent self-determination, consistent with our first recommendation).

We also should be clear that our support of the approximation rule is motivated more by the problems created by the ill-defined nature of the current best-interests standard than by the approximation rule itself. We would be open to any clear and determinative rule for deciding children's best interests, but favor the approximation rule over its two major rivals: (a) a primary-caretaker parent standard, which would award sole legal and physical custody to the parent who did most of the childrearing; and (b) a presumption in favor of joint physical custody. We view the approximation rule as a pluralistic hybrid of these two alternatives.

We find the approximation rule appealing because it is a clear and determinative alternative but not a "one size fits all" solution. At the same time, we are aware that the approximation rule is not without problems. Parents' involvement changes over time and as children grow older (for example, fathers' involvement in childrearing tends to increase). In addition, parents and their lawyers certainly would debate circumstances like the Deer-Does, in which parents agree that one parent will temporarily become more involved in childrearing. We also would not expect the approximation rule to end strategic maneuvering. For example, an unhappily married parent might quit work or even get fired in order to be home with the children—and have an advantage in a future custody dispute.

We do not propose solutions to these possible difficulties, but again note that the best-interests standard is itself fraught with problems—some similar, and some much bigger, in our view. We believe that the benefits of a clear rule potentially far outweigh the costs and that implementing the rule is a social experiment well worth undertaking. In fact, divorce policy already has witnessed the success of moving from vague to specific guidelines. In the early 1980s, the rules governing child support were unclear, and this uncertainty encouraged conflict and poor enforcement. Federal legislation used financial incentives to encourage states to adopt clear child support guidelines by 1986 (National Institute for Child Support Enforcement, 1986). Despite struggles with initial implementation—and many continuing problems with child support—two decades later, all agree that the clear guidelines are a vast improvement for families, legal professionals, and the child-welfare system. We expect the same outcome when legislatures finally move to adopt a clear child custody rule.

RECOMMENDATION 3: LIMIT EXPERT TESTIMONY AND CLARIFY STANDARDS OF PRACTICE

As long as the best-interests principle remains in place as an ill-defined standard, our third and final recommendation is to utilize existing evidence law, professional ethics codes, and practice standards to limit the expert testimony of mental health professionals in child custody cases to the presentation of scientifically supported evidence. Until far stronger scientific support is forthcoming, this recommendation specifically includes the suggestions (reviewed earlier) to (a) abandon use of all custody-specific "tests" that purport to measure children's best interests directly or indirectly, (b) prohibit testimony about PAS or any other "syndrome" that lacks scientific support, (c) identify the specific nature and sources of inference based on unstructured interview and observational assessments, and (d) apply appropriate caution in interpreting established measures and integrating information across different areas of assessment.

Rules of Evidence

Our recommendation to limit expert testimony may seem radical, but our proposal simply urges the application of established rules for expert testimony to such testimony in custody cases (Shuman, 2002). Expert testimony in all legal proceedings is guided by rules of evidence that identify the circumstances under which such testimony is appropriate (Ewing, 2003; Shuman, 2000; Shuman & Sales, 1998). A key problem for courts and legislatures is determining exactly what makes testimony scientific and expert. Historically, the testimony of experts was admitted if it passed a legal test developed by a United States district court. In *Frye v. United States* (1923) the court wrote that

> Just when a scientific principle or discovery crosses the line between the experimental and demonstrable stages is difficult to determine. Somewhere in this twilight zone the evidential force of the principle must be recognized, and while courts will go a long way in admitting expert testimony deduced from a well recognized scientific principle for discovery, the thing from which the deduction is made must be sufficiently established to have gained general acceptance in the particular field in which it belongs (p. 1014).

The *Frye* test, however, has been criticized on a number of grounds (Shuman, 2000). Some have argued that it is too conservative and may result in exclusion of testimony based on novel-yet-valid techniques and approaches; others say it is too liberal and allows for testimony based on techniques that have gained general acceptance despite being invalid. In *Daubert v. Merrell Dow Pharmaceuticals, Inc.* (1993), the United States Supreme Court ruled that the general-acceptance test developed in *Frye* "is not a necessary precondition to the admissibility of scientific evidence under the Federal Rules of Evidence" (p. 2799). The Court ruled that the trial judge should ensure that the opinion is based on an "inference or assertion . . . derived by the scientific method" and determine "whether the reasoning or methodology underlying the testimony is scientifically valid and . . . whether that reasoning or methodology can be applied to the facts in issue" (p. 2796).

The Court went on to identify four factors that judges could employ when considering specific testimony, including (a) the "testability" of the theoretical basis for the opinion; (b) the error rates associated with the approach, if known; (c) whether the technique or approach on which the opinion is based has been subjected to peer review; and (d) whether the technique or approach is generally accepted in the relevant scientific community.

The guidance provided by *Daubert* could be used to examine whether the expert opinions offered by mental health professionals in custody disputes are science based, but there is no evidence indicating that trial judges have actively done this. Those offering anecdotal accounts or personal impressions, however, are essentially unanimous in their impression that evidence offered by experts in custody cases is rarely objected to and even less frequently excluded (Shuman, 2002). Similarly, a review of appellate cases also suggests that the opinions of mental health experts are rarely excluded on the grounds that the basis for the expert opinions offered does not meet required scientific standards. Our view is that the low scientific standards for expert testimony again can be traced to the vague best-interests principle and the impossible dilemma it creates for judges. For this reason, and because individual trial judges rarely have the time or the expertise to evaluate the scientific status of psychological measures, we believe that it is incumbent upon the mental health professions to develop clear professional standards regarding expert testimony in child custody cases.

Professional Standards and Guidelines

The American Psychological Association (APA; 1994), Association of Family and Conciliation Courts (AFCC; 1995), and American Academy of Child and Adolescent Psychiatry (AACAP; 1997) all have developed guidelines for professionals conducting custody evaluations. All of these guidelines recommend an assessment of childrens' needs, parents' abilities to meet these needs, and parents' abilities to provide for future needs. The APA and AACAP guidelines also identify a number of factors considered to be integral to child custody evaluations, including assessment of parenting abilities, assessment of capacity to provide a stable loving home, identification of inappropriate behavior that negatively influences the child (e.g., substance use/abuse), consideration of parental psychopathology as it affects parenting ability or the child directly, and consideration of the child's wishes.

Despite broad agreement about factors that should be assessed, there is little agreement about how to assess them. For example, the AFCC guidelines (which are currently undergoing revision) do not provide assessment guidelines, while APA and AACAP both generally advocate a multimethod approach combining clinical interviews, direct observation, and psychological tests. Guidelines promulgated by AACAP question the value of psychological testing, while suggesting that collateral information be obtained from school personnel, healthcare providers, childcare providers, family, friends, and other individuals who may provide information germane to child custody placement. The lack of consensus begs the question: What accounts for the variability in recommendations? We conclude that much of the variability is the result of a lack of requisite knowledge. There is not enough scientific evidence (and legal guidance) about how evaluations should be conducted and about what type of evaluation is most helpful. Accordingly, we urge professional organizations to develop very clear guidelines concerning acceptable, scientifically based practices and what inferences can appropriately be drawn from them. We have offered our review of the literature on these measures as a starting point to these discussions and negotiations.

We also urge professional organizations to adopt clear ethical standards for mental health professionals to follow in custody evaluations. For example, professional organizations have failed to take a clear stand on principles of practice that are widely embraced by those with extensive professional experience in the custody context. We suggest three such principles are worthy of becoming standards of practice: Evaluators should

- Show preference for evaluations conducted by mutually agreed-upon or court-appointed experts
- Promote settlement and other steps that will facilitate a degree of parental cooperation in childrearing and authoritative parent–child relationships—for example, by providing concrete, private feedback to the parties about the evaluator's opinion before submitting a final report
- Acknowledge that custody is ultimately a legal decision and thus avoid offering "expert opinion" on legal matters—such as who should enjoy primary legal or physical custody and under what conditions—despite considerable pressure to do so within the legal system

CONCLUDING COMMENT: A QUESTION OF VALUES

A clear custody rule—whether the approximation rule, the primary-caretaker-parent standard, a presumption in favor of joint physical custody, or some other law—would necessarily take a stand on values concerning family life, values that often are contested in our changing, pluralistic society. Custody laws once did take a clear and strong stand favoring fathers as property holders, and later, mothers as nurturers. Today, there is no social consensus about the appropriate family roles for men and women, and we believe this is one reason why legislatures have failed to adopt a clearer and more determinant custody standard. The "children's best interests" standard seems to embrace a laudable value, the well-being of children; yet as we have seen, the standard actually encourages uncertainty and parental conflict that is contrary to children's interests.

No matter what the goals or actual effects of the best-interests standard, it is impossible to sidestep the values issue. Beaber (1982) provides some illustrative examples of key value questions raised by child custody disputes:

1. Should brothers and sisters be in the custody of the same parent?
2. Should an older child, over age 12, have veto power in a custody dispute between two parents?
3. Should boys be placed with fathers and daughters with mothers?
4. Should young children, under age five, be placed with mothers?
5. Should continuity of residence and school district control placement?
6. Should children be placed with the parent who does not work outside the home or who works the fewest hours and/or the most convenient hours?
7. Should children be placed in the home that does not have/ will not have a stepparent? (p. 319)

Science cannot answer such value questions. Philosopher of science Carl Hempel (1965) has argued for the demarcation between factual issues that science in principle can settle and value issues that it cannot, and it is perhaps nowhere more important to make this distinction than in matters of child custody. Hempel makes this point using a thought experiment involving Laplace's demon—a hypothetical entity who knows all scientific laws and all initial conditions and who can perfectly and instantaneously make all relevant calculations needed to make an empirical decision:

> Let us assume, then that faced with a moral decision we are able to call upon the Laplacean demon as a consultant. What help might we get from him? Suppose that we have to choose one of several alternative courses of action to use, and that we want to know which of these we *ought* to follow. The demon would then be able to tell us, for any contemplated choice, what its consequences would be for the future course of the universe, down to the most minute detail, however remote in space and time. But having done this for each of the alternative courses of action under consideration, the demon would have completed his task: he would have given us all the information that an ideal science might provide under the circumstances. And yet he would not have resolved out moral problem, for this requires a decision as to which of the several alternative sets of consequences mapped out by the demon as attainable to us is the best; which of them we ought to bring about. And the burden of this decision would still fall upon our shoulders; it is we who would have to commit ourselves to an unconditional judgment of value by singling out one of the sets of consequences as superior to its alternatives. Even Laplace's demon, or the ideal science he stands for, cannot relieve us of this responsibility. (pp. 88–89)

In short, even if all of the relevant empirical relations regarding various child custody options were known, we would still be left with the value questions of what outcomes are the best. This conclusion gives us a final perspective on our three sets of recommendations. Our recommendation favoring alternative dispute resolution and parent self-determination not only recognizes the psychological importance of renegotiating family relationships for children but embraces the value that, except in cases of abuse or neglect, parents themselves should have the option of determining their children's best interests. Our call for the enactment of a custody standard such as the approximation rule that has the potential to produce more predictable outcomes urges a clear articulation of "family values" as embodied in the law. Finally, our recommendation that mental health professionals limit their role in providing expert testimony in custody cases places the value of science above all others in professional practice.

REFERENCES

Ackerman, M.J., & Ackerman, M.C. (1997). Custody evaluation practice: A survey of experienced professionals (revisited). *Professional Psychology: Research and Practice, 28*, 137–145.

Ackerman, M., & Schoendorf, K. (1992). *ASPECT: Ackerman-Schoendorf Scales for Parent Evaluation of Custody.* Los Angeles, CA: Western Psychological Services.

Ahrons, C. (1998). *The good divorce.* New York: Quill.

Ahrons, C.R., & Miller, R.B. (1993). The effect of postdivorce relationships on parent involvement: A longitudinal analysis. *American Journal of Orthopsychiatry, 63*, 441–450.

Ahrons, C.R., & Tanner, J.L. (2003). Adult children and their fathers: Relationship changes 20 years after parental divorce. *Family Relations: Interdisciplinary Journal of Applied Family Studies, 52*, 340–351.

Amato, P.R. (2001). Children of divorce in the 1990s: An update of the Amato and Keith (1991) meta-analysis. *Journal of Family Psychology, 15*, 355–370.

Amato, P.R., & Booth, A. (1997). *A generation at risk.* Cambridge, MA: Harvard.

Amato, P.R., & Gilbreth, J. (1999). Nonresident fathers and children's well-being: A meta-analysis. *Journal of Marriage and the Family, 61*, 557–573.

Amato, P.R., & Keith, B. (1991). Parental divorce and well-being of children: A meta-analysis. *Psychological Bulletin, 110*, 26–46.

Amato, P.R., Loomis, L.S., & Booth, A. (1995). Parental divorce, marital conflict, and offspring well-being during early adulthood. *Social Forces, 73*, 895–915.

Amato, P.R., & Rezac, S.J. (1994). Contact with nonresident parents, interparental conflict, and children's behavior. *Journal of Family Issues, 15*, 191–207.

American Academy of Child and Adolescent Psychiatry (1997). Practice parameters for child custody evaluation. *Journal of the American Academy of Child and Adolescent Psychiatry, 36*, 57S–68S.

American Educational Research Association, American Psychological Association, & National Council on Measurement in Education (1999). *Standards for educational and psychological testing* (3rd ed.). Washington, DC: American Educational Research Association.

American Law Institute (2002). *Principles of the law of family dissolution: Analysis and recommendations.* Bender: Newark, NJ.

American Psychological Association (1994). Guidelines for child custody evaluations in divorce proceedings. *American Psychologist, 49*, 677–680.

Arditti, J.A. (1995). Ackerman-Schoendorf Scales for Parent Evaluation of Custody. In J.C. Conoley & J.C. Impara (Eds.), *The twelfth mental measurements yearbook* (pp. 20–22). Lincoln, NE: Buros Institute of Mental Measurements.

Association of Family and Conciliation Courts (1995). *Model standards for child custody evaluation*. Madison, WI: Author.

Bauserman, R. (2002). Child adjustment in joint-custody versus sole-custody arrangements: A meta-analytic review. *Journal of Family Psychology, 16*, 91–102.

Beaber, R.J. (1982). Custody quagmire: Some psychological dilemmas. *Journal of Psychiatry & Law, 10*, 309–326.

Beck, C.J.A., & Sales, B.D. (2001). *Family mediation: Facts, myths, and future prospects*. Washington, DC: American Psychological Association.

Bow, J.N., & Quinnell, F.A. (2001). Psychologists' current practices and procedures in child custody evaluations: Five years after American Psychological Association guidelines. *Professional Psychology: Research and Practice, 32*, 261–268.

Bow, J.N., & Quinnell, F.A. (2002). A critical review of child custody evaluation reports. *Family Court Review, 40*, 164–176.

Bramlett, M.D., & Mosher, W.D. (2001). *First marriage dissolution, divorce, and remarriage: United States* (Advance Data From Vital and Health Statistics No. 323). Hyattsville, MD: National Center for Health Statistics.

Bramlett, M.D., & Mosher, W.D. (2002). *Cohabitation, marriage, divorce, and remarriage in the United States* (Vital and Health Statistics, Series 23, No. 22). Hyattsville, MD: National Center for Health Statistics.

Bricklin, B. (1989). *Perception of Relationships Test*. Furlong, PA: Village Publishing.

Bricklin, B. (1990a). *Bricklin Perceptual Scales*. Furlong, PA: Village Publishing.

Bricklin, B. (1990b). *Parent Awareness of Skills Survey*. Furlong, PA: Village Publishing.

Bricklin, B. (1993). *Test Manuals Supplement #9*. Furlong, PA: Village Publishing.

Bricklin, B., & Elliott, G. (1991). *Parent Perception of Child Profile*. Furlong, PA: Village Publishing.

Brodzinsky, D. (1993). On the use and misuse of psychological testing in child custody evaluations. *Professional Psychology: Research and Practice, 24*, 213–219.

Brooks-Gunn, J., & Duncan, G.J. (1997). The effects of poverty on children. *The Future of Children, 7*, 55–71.

Buchanan, C.M., Maccoby, E.E., & Dornbusch, S.M. (1996). *Adolescents after divorce*. Cambridge, MA: Harvard.

Bumpass, L., (1984). Children and marital disruption: A replication and update. *Demography, 21*, 71–82.

Cabrera, N., Tamis-LeMonda, C.S., Bradley, R.H., Hofferth, S., Lamb, M.E. (2000). Fatherhood in the twenty-first century. *Child Development, 71*, 127–136.

Carlson, J.N. (1995). Perception of Relationships Test. In J.C. Conoley & J.C. Impara (Eds.), *The twelfth mental measurements yearbook* (pp. 746–747). Lincoln, NE: Buros Institute of Mental Measurements.

Chambers, D.L. (1984). Rethinking the substantive rules for custody disputes in divorce. *University of Michigan Law Review, 83*, 480–569.

Cherlin, A.J., Chase-Lansdale, P.L., & McRae, C. (1998). Effects of parental divorce on mental health throughout the life course. *American Sociological Review, 63*, 239–249.

Cherlin, A.J., Furstenberg, F.F., Jr., Chase-Lansdale, P.L., Kiernan, K.E., Robines, P.K., Ruane Morrison, D., Teitler, J.O. (1991). Longitudinal studies of effects of divorce on children in Great Britain and the United States. *Science, 252*, 1386–1389.

Child Trends (2002). *Charting parenthood: A statistical portrait of fathers and mothers in America*. Washington, DC: Child Trends.

Clarke, S.C. (1995). *Advance report of final divorce statistics, 1989 and 1990*. (Monthly Vital Statistics Report, Vol. 43, No. 9, Supplement). Hyattsville, MD: National Center for Health Statistics.

Coates, C.A., Jones, W., Bushard, P., Deutsch, R., Hicks, B., Stahl, P., Sullivan, M., Sydlik, B., & Wistner, R. (2003). Parenting coordination: Implementation issues. *Family Court Review, 41*, 533–564.

Conger, J. (1995). Perception-of-Relationships Test. In J.C. Conoley & J.C. Impara (Eds.)., *The twelfth mental measurements yearbook* (pp. 747–748). Lincoln, NE: Buros Institute of Mental Measurements.

Cummings, E.M., & Davies, P. (1994). *Children and marital conflict*. New York: Guilford.

Davies, P.T., Harold, G.T., Goeke-Morey, M.C., & Cummings, E.M. (2002). Child emotional security and interparental conflict. *Monographs of the Society for Research on Child Development, 67*, vii–viii.

Daubert v. Merrell Dow Pharmaceuticals, Inc., 509 U.S. 579, 113 S. Ct. 2786 (1993).

Deater-Deckard, K., Dodge, K.A., & Bates, J.E. (1996). Physical discipline among African American and European American mothers: Links to children's externalizing behaviors. *Developmental Psychology, 32*, 1065–1072.

Donnelly, D., & Finkelhor, D. (1993). Who has joint custody? Class differences in the determination of custody arrangements. *Family Relations, 42*, 57–60.

D'Onofrio, B., Turkheimer, E., Emery, R., Slutske, W., Heath, A., Madden, P., & Martin, N. (in press). A genetically informed study of marital instability and its association with offspring psychopathology. *Journal of Abnormal Psychology*.

Downey, D.B, Ainsworth-Darnell, J.W., & Dufur, M.J. (1998). Sex of parent and children's well-being in single-parent households. *Journal of Marriage and the Family, 60*, 878–893.

Downey, D.B., & Powell, B. (1993). Do children in single-parent households fare better living with same-sex parents? *Journal of Marriage and the Family, 55*, 55–71.

Duncan, G.J., & Hoffman, S.D. (1985). Economic consequences of marital instability. In M. David & T. Smeeding (Eds.), *Horizontal equity, uncertainty and well-being* (pp. 427–469). Chicago: University of Chicago Press.

Dunn, J. (2004). Annotation: Children's relationships with their non-resident fathers. *Journal of Child Psychology and Psychiatry, 45*, 659–671.

Ehrenberg, M.F., Hunter, M.A., & Elterman, M.F. (1996). Shared parenting agreements after marital separation: The roles of empathy and narcissism. *Journal of Consulting and Clinical Psychology, 64*, 808–818.

Elrod, L.D., & Spector, R.G. (2004). A review of the year in family law: Children's issues remain the focus. *Family Law Quarterly, 37*, 527–575.

Emery, R.E. (1982). Interparental conflict and the children of discord and divorce. *Psychological Bulletin, 92*, 310–330.

Emery, R.E. (1994). *Renegotiating family relationships: Divorce, child custody, and mediation*. New York: Guilford.

Emery, R.E. (1999a). Changing the rules for determining child custody in divorce cases. *Clinical Psychology: Science and Practice, 6*, 323–327.

Emery, R.E. (1999b). *Marriage, divorce, and children's adjustment* (2nd ed.). Thousand Oaks, CA: Sage.

Emery, R.E. (2003). Childen's voices: Listening—and deciding—is an adult responsibility. *Arizona Law Review, 45*, 621–627.

Emery, R.E. (2004). *The truth about children and divorce: Dealing with the emotions so you and your children can thrive*. New York: Viking.

Emery, R.E. (2005). Parental alienation syndrome: Proponents bear the burden of proof. *Family Court Review, 43*, 8–13.

Emery, R.E., & Forehand, R. (1994). Parental divorce and children's well-being: A focus on resilience. In R.J. Haggerty, L. Sherrod, N. Garmezy, & M. Rutter (Eds.), *Risk and Resilience in Children* (pp. 64–99). London: Cambridge University Press.

Emery, R.E., Laumann-Billings, L., Waldron, M., Sbarra, D.A., and Dillon, P. (2001). Child custody mediation and litigation: Custody, contact, and co-parenting 12 years after initial dispute resolution. *Journal of Consulting and Clinical Psychology, 69*, 323–332.

Emery, R.E., Matthews, S.G., & Kitzmann, K.M. (1994). Child custody mediation and litigation: Parents' satisfaction and functioning a year after settlement. *Journal of Consulting and Clinical Psychology, 62*, 124–129.

Emery, R.E., Matthews, S., & Wyer, M.M. (1991). Child custody mediation and litigation: Further evidence of the differing views of mothers and fathers. *Journal of Consulting and Clinical Psychology, 59*, 410–418.

Emery, R.E., Sbarra, D., & Grover, T. (2005). Divorce mediation: Research and reflections. *Family Court Review, 43*, 22–37.

Emery, R.E., Waldron, M., & Kitzmann, M. (1999). Delinquent behavior, future divorce or nonmarital childbearing, and externalizing behavior among offspring: A 14-year prospective study. *Journal of Family Psychology, 13*, 568–579.

Emery, R.E., Weintraub, S., & Neale, J.M. (1982). Effects of marital discord on the school behavior of children with schizophrenic, affectively disordered, and normal parents. *Journal of Abnormal Child Psychology, 10*, 215–228.

Emery, R.E., & Wyer, M.M. (1987a). Child custody mediation and litigation: An experimental evaluation of the experience of parents. *Journal of Consulting and Clinical Psychology, 55*, 179–186.

Emery, R.E., & Wyer, M.M. (1987b). Divorce mediation. *American Psychologist, 42*, 472–480.

Ewing, C.P. (2003). Expert testimony: Law and practice. In A. Goldstein (Ed.), *Forensic Psychology* (pp. 55–66). New York: Wiley.

Ex Parte Devine, 398 So.2d 686 (Ala.1981).

Fauber, R.L., Forehand, R., Thomas, A.M., & Wierson, M. (1990). A mediational model of the impact of marital conflict on adolescent adjustment in intact and divorced families: The role of disrupted parenting. *Child Development, 61*, 1112–1123.

Feller, J.N., Davidson, H.A., Hardin, M., & Horowitz, R.M. (1992). *Working with the courts in child protection*. Washington, DC: U.S. Department of Health and Human Services.

Fields, J. (2003). *Children's living arrangements and characteristics: March 2002*. (Current Population Reports, P20–547). Washington, DC: U.S. Census Bureau.

Folberg, J. (1991). *Joint custody and shared parenting*. New York: Guilford.

Frye v. United States, 293 F. 1013 (D.C. Cir. 1923).

Furstenberg, F.F., Peterson, J.L., Nord, C.W., & Zill, N., (1983). The life course of children of divorce: Marital disruption and parental contact. *American Sociological Review, 48*, 656–668.

Gardner, R.A. (2001). Should courts order PAS children to visit/reside with the alienated parent? A follow-up study. *American Journal of Forensic Psychology, 19*, 61–106.

Gardner, R.A. (2004). Commentary on Kelly and Johnston's "The Alienated Child: A Reformulation of Parental Alienation Syndrome." *Family Court Review, 42*, 611–621.

Garrison, M. (1996). How do judges decide divorce cases? An empirical analysis of discretionary decision making. *North Carolina Law Review, 74*, 401–552.

Gordon, R., & Peek, L.A. (1989). *The Custody Quotient: Research manual*. Dallas, TX: Wilmington Institute.

Gottesman, I.I. (1991). *Schizophrenia genesis: The origins of madness*. New York: Freeman.

Gourley, E.V., & Stolberg, A.L. (2000). An empirical investigation of psychologists' custody evaluation practices. *Journal of Divorce and Remarriage, 33*, 1–29.

Greenberg, S., Otto, R.K., & Long, A. (2003). The utility of psychological testing in personal injury evaluation. *Assessment, 10*, 410–419.

Grisso, T. (2003). *Evaluating competencies: Forensic assessments and instruments* (2nd ed). New York: Kluwer/Plenum.

Grych, J.H., & Fincham, F.D. (1990). Marital conflict and children's adjustment: A cognitive-contextual framework. *Psychological Bulletin, 108*, 267–290.

Hall, A.S., Pulver, C.A., & Cooley, M.J. (1996). Psychology of the best interests standard: Fifty state statutes and their theoretical antecedents. *American Journal of Family Therapy, 24*, 171–180.

Heilbrun, K., Rogers, R., & Otto, R.K. (2002). Forensic assessment: Current status and future directions. In J.R.P. Ogloff (Ed.), *Taking psychology and law into the twenty-first century* (pp. 119–146). New York: Kluwer/Plenum.

Heinze, M., & Grisso, T. (1996). Review of instruments assessing parenting competencies used in child custody evaluations. *Behavioral Sciences and the Law, 14*, 293–313.

Hempel, C. (1965). *Aspects of scientific explanation and other essays in the philosophy of science*. New York: Collier-MacMillan Limited.

Herman, S.P., Duanne, J.E., Ayres, W., Arnold, V., Benedek, E., Benson, R.S., Bernet, W., Bernstein, G.A., Bryant, E., Licamele, W., McClellan, J., & Shaw, K. (1997). Practice parameters for child custody evaluation. *Journal of the American Academy of Child & Adolescent Psychiatry, 36*, 57S–68S.

Hetherington, E.M., & Clingempeel, W.G. (1992). Coping with marital transitions: A family systems perspective. *Monographs of the Society for Research in Child Development, 57*(2–3), 1–242.

Hetherington, E.M., Cox, M., & Cox, R. (1982). Effects of divorce on parents and children. In M. Lamb (Ed.), *Nontraditional families* (pp. 233–288). Hillsdale, N.J.: Erlbaum.

Hetherington, E.M., & Kelly, J. (2002). *For better or for worse: Divorce reconsidered*. New York: W.W. Norton.

Jenuwine, M.J., & Cohler, B.J. (1999). Major parental psychopathology and child custody. In R.M. Galatzer-Levy & L. Kraus (Eds.), *The scientific basis of child custody decisions* (pp. 285–318). New York: Wiley.

Johnston, J.R. (1994). High conflict divorces. *The Future of Children, 4*, 165–182.

Johnston, J.R., & Kelly, J.B. (2004). Rejoinder to Gardner's "Commentary on Kelly and Johnston's 'The Alienated Child: A Reformulation of Parental Alienation Syndrome.'" *Family Court Review, 42*, 622–628.

Johnston, J.R., Kline, M., & Tschann, J. (1989). Ongoing postdivorce conflict in families contesting custody: Effects on children of joint custody and frequent access. *American Journal of Orthopsychiatry, 59*, 576–592.

Johnston, J.R., & Roseby, V. (1997). *In the name of the child*. New York: Free Press.

Keilin, W.G., & Bloom, L.J. (1986). Custody evaluation practice: A survey of experienced professionals. *Professional Psychology: Research and Practice, 17*, 338–346.

Kelly, J. (1998). Marital conflict, divorce, and children's adjustment. *Child and Adolescent Psychiatric Clinics of North America, 7*, 259–271.

Kelly, J.B., & Emery, R.E. (2003). Children's adjustment following divorce: Risk and resilience perspectives. *Family Relations: Interdisciplinary Journal of Applied Family Studies, 52*, 352–362.

Kelly, J.B. & Johnston, J.R. (2001). The alienated child: A reformulation of Parental Alienation Syndrome. *Family Court Review, 39*, 249–266.

Kelly, J., & Lamb, M.E. (2000). Using child development research to make appropriate custody and access decisions for young children. *Family and Conciliation Courts Review, 38*, 297–311.

King, V. (1994). Nonresident father involvement and child well-being: Can dads make a difference? *Journal of Family Issues, 15*, 78–96.

Lamb, M.E. (1999). Noncustodial fathers and their impact on the children of divorce. In R.A. Thompson & P.R. Amato (Eds.), *The postdivorce family: Children, parenting, and society* (pp. 105–125). Thousand Oaks, CA: Sage.

Lamb, M.E., Sternberg, K.J., & Thompson, R.A. (1997). The effects of divorce and custody arrangements on children's behavior, development, and adjustment. *Family and Conciliation Courts Review, 35*, 393–404.

Lamborn, S., Mounts, N., Steinberg, L., & Dornbusch, S.M. (1991). Patterns of competence and adjustment among adolescents from authoritative, authoritarian, indulgent, and neglectful homes. *Child Development, 62*, 1049–1065.

Laumann-Billings, L., & Emery, R.E. (2000). Distress among young adults from divorced families. *Journal of Family Psychology, 14*, 671–687.

Lewis, C., & Lamb, M.E. (2003). Fathers' influences on children's development: The evidence from two-parent families. *European Journal of Psychology of Education, 18*, 211–228.

Lyman, R.D., & Roberts, M.C., (1985). Mental health testimony in child custody litigation. *Law & Psychology Review, 9*, 15–34.

Maccoby, E.E., & Martin, J.A. (1983). Socialization in the context of the family: Parent–child interaction. In E.M. Hetherington (Vol. Ed.), *Handbook of child psychology: Vol. 4. Socialization, Personality, and Social Development* (4th. ed, pp. 1–102). New York: Wiley.

Maccoby, E.E., & Mnookin, R.H. (1992). *Dividing the child: Social and legal dilemmas of custody.* Cambridge, MA: Harvard University Press.

MacKinnon, C.E., Brody, G.H., & Stoneman, Z. (1982). The effects of divorce and maternal employment on the home environments of preschool children. *Child Development, 53*, 1392–1399.

Mason, M.A. (1994). *From father's property rights to children's rights: The history of child custody in the United States.* New York: Columbia University Press.

Martin, J.A., Hamilton, B.E., Sutton, P.D., Ventura, S.J., Menacker, F., & Munson, M.L. (2003). *Births: Final data for 2002.* (National Vital Statistics Reports, Vol. 52., No. 10). Hyattsville, MD: National Center for Health Statistics.

Martinez, C.R., & Forgatch, M.S. (2001). Preventing problems with boys' noncompliance: Effects of a parent training intervention for divorcing mothers. *Journal of Consulting & Clinical Psychology, 69*, 416–428.

Martinez, C.R., & Forgatch, M.S. (2002). Adjusting to change: Linking family structure transitions with parenting and boys' adjustment. *Journal of Family Psychology, 16*, 107–117.

McGue, M., & Lykken, D.T. (1992). Genetic influence on risk of divorce. *Psychological Science, 6*, 368–373.

McIntosh, J., Long, C., & Moloney, L. (2004). Child-focused and child-inclusive mediation: A comparative study of outcomes. *Journal of Family Studies, 10*, 87–95.

McLanahan, S.S. (1997). Parent absence or poverty: Which matters more? In G.J. Duncan & J. Brooks-Gunn (Eds.), *Consequences of growing up poor* (pp. 35–48). New York: Russell Sage.

McLanahan, S.S., & Bumpass, L.L. (1988). Intergenerational consequences of family disruption. *American Journal of Sociology, 94*, 130–152.

McLanahan, S., & Sandefur, G. (1994). *Growing up with a single parent: What hurts, what helps.* Cambridge, MA: Harvard University Press.

Melli, M.S., Brown, P.R., & Cancian, M. (1997). Child custody in a changing world: A study of postdivorce arrangements in Wisconsin. *University of Illinois Law Review, 3*, 773–800.

Melton, G.B. (1995). Ackerman-Schoendorf Scales for Parent Evaluation of Custody. In J.C. Conoley & J.C. Impara (Eds.), *The twelfth mental measurements yearbook* (pp. 22–23). Lincoln, NE: Buros Institute of Mental Measurements.

Melton, G.B., Petrila, J., Poythress, N., & Slobogin, C. (1997). *Psychological evaluations of the courts: A handbook for mental health professionals and lawyers* (2nd ed.). New York: Guilford.

Meyer, G. (1997). Thinking clearly about reliability: More critical corrections regarding the Rorschach Comprehensive System. *Psychological Assessment, 9*, 495–498.

Meyer, G. (2001). Introduction to the final special section in the special series on the utility of the Rorschach for clinical assessment. *Psychological Assessment, 13*, 419–422.

Meyer, D.R., & Garasky, S. (1993). Custodial fathers: Myths, realities, and child support policy. *Journal of Marriage and the Family, 55*, 73–89.

Mnookin, R. (1975). Child custody adjudication: Judicial functions in the face of indeterminacy. *Law and Contemporary Problems, 39*, 226–293.

National Institute for Child Support Enforcement (1986). *History and fundamentals of child support enforcement* (2nd ed.). Washington, DC: U.S. Government Printing Office.

Novak, G. (1996). *Developmental psychology: Dynamic systems and behavior analysis.* Reno, NV: Context Press.

O'Connor, T.G., Caspi, A., DeFries, J.C., Plomin, R. (2000). Are associations between parental divorce and children's adjustment genetically mediated? An adoption study. *Developmental Psychology, 36*, 429–437.

Ostrom, B.J., & Kauder, N.B. (1996). *Examining the work of state courts, 1995: A national perspective from the court statistics project.* Williamsburg, VA: National Center for State Courts.

Otto, R.K., Buffington-Vollum, J., & Edens, J.F. (2003). Child custody evaluation: Research and practice. In A. Goldstein (Ed.), *Forensic psychology* (pp. 179–208). New York: Wiley.

Otto, R.K., & Edens, J.F. (2003). Parenting capacity. In T. Grisso (Ed.), *Evaluating competencies: Forensic assessments and instruments* (pp. 229–308). New York: Kluwer/Plenum.

Otto, R.K., Edens, J.F., & Barcus, E. (2000). The use of psychological testing in child custody evaluations. *Family and Conciliation Courts Review, 38*, 312–340.

Peris, T., & Emery, R. (in press). A prospective study of the consequences of marital disruption for adolescents: Pre-disruption family dynamics and post-disruption adolescent adjustment. *Journal of Clinical Child and Adolescent Psychology.*

Posthuma, A. (2003). A new MMPI-2 scale for custody disputes. *American Journal of Forensic Psychology, 21*, 51–64.

Pruett, M.K., Williams, T.Y., Insabella, G., & Little, T.D. (2003). Family and legal indicators of child adjustment to divorce among families with young children. *Journal of Family Psychology, 17*, 169–180.

Pryor, J. & Rodgers, B. (2001). *Children in changing families: Life after parental separation*. Boston, MA: Blackwell Publishers.

Santrock, J.W., & Warshak, R.A. (1979). Father custody and social development in boys and girls. *Journal of Social Issues, 35*, 112–135.

Schepard, A.I. (2004). *Children, courts, and custody: Interdisciplinary models for divorcing families*. New York: Cambridge University Press.

Schmidtgall, K., King, A., Zarski, J.J., & Cooper, J.E. (2000). The effects of parent conflict on later child development. *Journal of Divorce and Remarriage, 33*, 149–157.

Schwartz, L.L. (2003). A nightmare for King Solomon: The new reproductive technologies. *Journal of Family Psychology, 17*, 229–237.

Scott, E. (1992). Pluralism, paternal preferences, and child custody. *California Law Review, 80*, 615–672.

Seltzer, J.A. (1991). Relationship between fathers and children who live apart: The father's role after separation. *Journal of Marriage and the Family, 53*, 79–101.

Shaffer, M.B. (1992). Bricklin Perceptual Scales. In J.C. Conoley & J.C. Impara (Eds.), *The twelfth mental measurements yearbook* (pp. 118–119). Lincoln, NE: Buros Institute of Mental Measurements.

Shuman, D.W. (2000). *Psychiatric and psychological evidence*. Minneapolis: West Group.

Shuman, D.W. (2002). The role of mental health experts in custody decisions: Science, psychological tests, and clinical judgment. *Family Law Quarterly, 36*, 135–162.

Shuman, D.W., & Sales, B. (1998). The impact of Daubert and its progeny on the admissibility of behavioral and social science evidence. *Psychology, Public Policy, and Law, 5*, 3–15.

Sigle-Rushton, W., & McLanahan, S. (2002). The living arrangements of new unmarried mothers. *Demography, 39*, 415–433.

Solomon, J., & George, C. (1999). The effects on attachment of overnight visitation in divorced and separated families. In J. Solomon & C. George (Eds.), *Attachment disorganization* (pp. 243–264). New York: Guilford.

Spokane County Bar Association (1996). *Child-centered residential schedules*. Spokane, WA: Author.

Steinberg, L. (2001). We know some things: Parent-adolescent relationships in retrospect and prospect. *Journal of Research on Adolescence, 11*, 1–19.

Tesler, P.H. (2001). *Collaborative law: Achieving effective resolution in divorce without litigation*. Chicago, IL: American Bar Association.

Thomson, E., Hanson, H.L., & McLanahan, S.S. (1994). Family structure and child well-being: Economic resources vs. parental behaviors. *Social Forces, 73*, 221–242.

Uniform Marriage and Divorce Act, 9A Uniform Laws Annotated, Sec. 316 (1979).

U.S. Bureau of the Census (1992). *Marriage, divorce, and remarriage in the 1990's*. (Current Population Reports, P23–180). Washington, DC: U.S. Government Printing Office.

Wald, M. (1976). State intervention on behalf of "neglected" children: A search for realistic standards. In M. Rosenheim (Ed.), *Pursuing justice for the child* (pp. 246–278). Chicago: University of Chicago Press.

Walden, B., McGue, M., Iacono, W.G., Burt, S.A., & Elkins, I. (2004). Identifying shared environmental contributions to early substance use: The respective roles of peers and parents. *Journal of Abnormal Psychology, 113*, 440–450.

Wallerstein, J.S. (2003). Children of divorce: A society in search of policy. In M.A. Mason, A. Skolnick, & S.D. Sugarman (Eds.), *All our families: New policies for a new century* (2nd ed., pp. 66–95). New York: Oxford University Press.

Wallerstein, J.S., Lewis, J., & Blakeslee, S. (2000). *Unexpected legacy of divorce: The 25 year landmark study*. New York: Hyperion Press.

Weiner, I. (1996). Some observations on the validity of the Rorschach Inkblot Method. *Psychological Assessment, 8*, 206–213.

Wellman, M. (1994). Ackerman-Schoendorf Scales for Parent Evaluation of Custody. In D. Keyser & R. Sweetland (Eds.), *Test critiques* (Vol. 10, pp. 13–19). Austin, TX: Pro-Ed.

Weithorn, L. (1987). *Psychology and child custody evaluations*. Lincoln, NE: University of Nebraska Press.

Wolchik, S.A., West, S.G., Sandler, I.N., Tein, J., Coatsworth, D., Lengua, L., Weiss, L., Anderson, E.R., Greene, S.M., & Griffin, W.A. (2000). An experimental evaluation of theory-based mother and mother-child programs for children of divorce. *Journal of Consulting and Clinical Psychology, 68*, 843–856.

Wood, J.M., Nezworski, M.T., Lilienfeld, S.O., & Garb, H.N. (2003). *What's wrong with the Rorschach?* San Francisco, CA: Jossey-Bass.

Wood, J.M., Nezworski, M.T., & Stejskal, W.J. (1997). The reliability of the Comprehensive System for the Rorschach: A comment on Meyer (1997). *Psychological Assessment, 9*, 490–494.

Wyer, M., Gaylord, S., & Grove, E. (1987). The legal context of child custody evaluations. In L. Weithorn (Ed.), *Psychology and child custody determinations* (pp. 4–22). Lincoln, NE: University of Nebraska Press.

Zill, N.D. (1988). Behavior, achievement, and health problems among children in stepfamilies: Findings from a national survey of child health. In E.M. Hetherington & J.D. Arasteh (Eds.), *Impact of divorce, single parenting, and stepparenting on children* (pp. 325–368). Hillsdale, NJ: Erlbaum.

Zill, N., Morrison, D.R., & Coiro, M.J. (1993). Long-term effects of parental divorce on parent-child relationships, adjustment, and achievement in young adulthood. *Journal of Family Psychology, 7*, 91–103.

Part III
Forensic Treatment

[12]

FROM NOTHING WORKS TO WHAT WORKS: CHANGING PROFESSIONAL IDEOLOGY IN THE 21ST CENTURY

FRANCIS T. CULLEN
University of Cincinnati

PAUL GENDREAU
University of New Brunswick at Saint John

The authors explore changes over time in criminologists' "professional ideology"—a core set of underlying beliefs that focuses academic thinking along certain lines but not others. Until the late 1960s, criminologists believed that the scientific study of the causes of crime would form the basis of individualized treatments that would reduce offender recidivism. By the mid-1970s, this view had collapsed and had been replaced by a professional ideology emphasizing that "nothing works" in corrections, that the causes of criminality are structural, and that crime can only be reduced through social justice. Although not without its merits, the authors suggest that this professional ideology has had the unfortunate consequence of legitimating "knowledge destruction" (showing what does not work) as the core intellectual project of criminology and thus of undermining efforts at "knowledge construction" (showing what does work). A "what works" movement within corrections, however, is advancing an alternative professional ideology that, once again, endorses the use of science to solve crime-related problems. The authors believe that, if embraced, this vision will improve criminology as a discipline and contribute more than "nothing works" scholarship to the commonweal of both offenders and the public order.

A central premise of the sociology of science is that academic thinking, like that of the "common" person in society, is shaped by the prevailing social context (see, e.g., Gould, 1981; Gouldner, 1970). At times, this insight is taken too far. Thus, misguided attempts are made to reduce academic knowledge to "mere" social constructions of reality in which all claims of truth are seen as equally relevant. Or the premise is advanced too deterministically. Observers forget that scientific paradigms are not fully permeable but create their own internal logic—that is, ideas can coalesce and, in a sense, have a life of their own that influences their development apart from outside forces. Still, in a more modest form, the central premise of the sociology of science is surely correct: As a human and thus social undertaking, scientific thinking is not purely a rational exercise in which conclusions are dictated solely by "what the data say."

C. Wright Mills (1942) recognized this fact when he poignantly illuminated the "professional ideology" of the "social pathologists" who studied society's wayward peoples and social problems. A professional ideology is a core set of beliefs—some explicit, some implicit—that focuses academic attention along certain lines of inquiry and away from others. These beliefs may be empirically valid, but they need not be. They may be logically powerful, but this does not mean they are not conditioned by social experiences. In any case, they cause their adherents to resist and reject competing empirical results that are inconsistent with the underlying set of beliefs. For the ideology to be effective, it must be endorsed by enough members within a discipline so that those disputing it will be delegitimated, if not sanctioned. To be *really* effective, the ideology must not be seen as an ideology but as an agreed-on set of beliefs and "background assumptions" that are "obviously true."

In this context, it is our thesis that the academic study of corrections—and the discipline of criminology, more generally—has been dominated by a professional ideology for the past quarter century that is committed to "knowledge destruction" rather than to "knowledge construction." Phrased alternatively, scholars have been "raised" within academic criminology to show what doesn't work as opposed to showing what does work. This professional ideology has been important in the creation of knowledge that reveals the foolishness of numerous correctional interventions. But it has been dysfunctional to the extent that it has inhibited academic criminology's ability to create an evidence-based agenda for how best to correct offenders.

The hegemony of this professional ideology is, fortunately, weakening. Serious efforts are now being initiated to build knowledge on "what works" in corrections (see, e.g., Loeber & Farrington, 1998; MacKenzie, 2000; Pearson & Lipton, 1999; Taxman, 1999). Still, the future of corrections research—and of criminology as a discipline—is hardly settled. It is unclear whether a new professional ideology will emerge that is more diverse in the kinds of research and thinking it will tolerate.

This article is an attempt to call for just such a transformation of what we think our discipline should be about. We start by focusing on the early years of modern American criminology and its views on correctional rehabilitation to show how the prevailing professional ideology was optimistic and open to knowledge construction. We then show how this optimism dissipated into pessimism, with the end result being that criminology became a discipline largely antagonistic to the creation of knowledge that would help the "state" control crime. Finally, we call for the creation of a new sense of what our profession should strive to attain—a professional ideology that takes seriously the opportunity, if not the obligation, it has to build scientific knowledge that contributes to the effectiveness of corrections.

USING SCIENCE TO CHANGE THE LAWBREAKER: THE LOGIC OF CORRECTIONAL TREATMENT

The early years of modern American criminology were informed, if not dominated, by the positivist school of criminology. The biological determinism of positivism—at least that found in Lombroso's work—was eventually forfeited, but the general principles of the positivist criminology paradigm were embraced. These paradigmatic principles structured thinking about crime and, in turn, views on how to control crime. Eventually, these principles became near hegemonic and developed into what we have called a "professional ideology." That is, every "good criminologist" seemed to accept them.

This prevailing professional ideology might be seen as comprising five main principles. First and most important, criminologists believed that crime had definite causes that could be unearthed only through systematic scientific study. The emphasis on science is critical because it meant that the entire framework hinged on the assumption that the study of and fight against crime should be *evidenced-based* and thus constitute a *rational* way of formulating practice and policy. Second, the punishment or infliction of pain on offenders was held to be, at best, of limited effectiveness in reforming offenders and, at worst, counterproductive. Third, because crime had definite causes, interventions should be targeted—as in medicine—on changing these causes. Fourth, using the correctional system in this way to change offenders was challenging but ultimately the only rational approach to crime control. Fifth, because the causes of crime differ for each offender, interventions should be individualized. Notably, this way of thinking had emerged with force by the first part of the 1900s and helped to usher in, during the Progressive Era, a wave of reforms that created probation, parole, indeterminate sentencing, and the juvenile court—innovations based largely on the ideal of individualized treatment (Rothman, 1980).

Arthur Mac Donald's (1893) *Criminology* offers an early illustration of a criminologist expressing this "modern" approach to the study of crime. Mac Donald noted that "whatever the remedy" to crime, "the causes must be studied first" (p. 272). "The method of the scientific study of criminals," he observed, necessitates "a thorough investigation of the criminal himself, both psychologically and physically, so that the underlying and constant cause of crime can be traced out" (p. 272). Although his book is dedicated to Lombroso, he rejected the idea that most offenders are atavistic reversions with little hope of betterment. Rather, he contended that "the greater part of crime arises out of social conditions, and hence is amenable to reformation, by changing these conditions" (p. 272a). An important part of the answer to crime thus rested in developing reformatories for youth and "reformatory prisons" for adults. But Mac Donald also recognized—to use current language—that crime developed over the life course. Many children were allowed "to live the first years of their life in surroundings that almost predestine to crime" (p. 272b). These children required early intervention through the provision of "moral and social education of a home or home-like institution" (p. 272b). "This," Mac Donald concluded, "is the foundation of all prevention of crime" (p. 272b).

As the modern era of criminology developed, these kinds of ideas were endorsed by most of the giants in the field. An exemplar of the professional ideology of positivism is found in the 1939 edition of Edwin Sutherland's *Principles of Criminology*, whose Preface began with the telling sentence: "A science of criminology is greatly needed both for satisfactory understanding [of crime] and for adequate control" (p. v).

Sutherland (1939) recognized that "a large proportion of the offenders under the care of any agency are recidivists" (p. 585). This "persistence of criminals" was important because "a large proportion of crimes can be attributed to recidivists" (p. 585). These observations led to the question of what interventions might be undertaken to reduce reoffending and its concomitant problems. One common answer based on "strictly hedonistic theory," according to Sutherland, was to punish or inflict "suffering" on the offender (p. 591). This approach, however, had "been discarded by psychologists" (p. 591). Although "pain undoubtedly has some value in the control of behavior," he stated, "the value is more or less completely balanced by the antagonism, isolation, and [criminal] group loyalties it produces" (p. 591). Similarly, "isolation" through imprisonment would have little impact on recidivism (p. 594).

Why were these correctional strategies unable to reduce reoffending? In large part, their ineffectiveness stemmed from their failure to target for change the actual causes of crime and, in particular, of recidivism: differential association. "The essential reason why persons become criminals is that they have been isolated from the culture of the law-abiding group . . . or else have been in contact with a rival criminal culture" (Sutherland, 1939, p. 595). It makes sense, therefore, that "criminality, which is the product of this isolation from culture, will not be overcome by more isolation" (p. 595). Similarly, making offenders suffer is ineffective because "the infliction of punishment upon the offender does not change the situation which produced the criminality" (p. 591).

Indeed, for correctional interventions to be effective, they needed to prompt the offender to have more contact with and "assimilation" into conventional culture and relationships. Sutherland (1939) thus favored correctional policies that fostered "more and more provision for contact" (p. 595). These included, for example,

> probation, which permits or assists the offender to come into contact with society instead of isolating him behind prison walls; education and self-government in prison, which are attempts to develop social interaction even while offenders are physically isolated; classification of similar offenders within prisons; parole, which acts in the same way as probation, though it begins after a period of imprisonment; and various other efforts to assist the offender after release from prison to gain or regain contacts with normal groups. (p. 595)

Sutherland (1939) also maintained that a key to the effective delivery of correctional interventions was "individualization." Giving all offenders "fixed sentences" was analogous to the time when medicine did not practice individualization of treatment but rather exposed the sick to "blood-letting... varying in amount with the seriousness of the ailment" (p. 596). Sutherland thus embraced the practice of the "intensive study of the individual offender for the purpose of learning the specific conditions, circumstances, processes, and mechanisms involved in the criminality" (p. 597). Once this investigation was completed, an intervention could be devised that used this "knowledge regarding the offender, in connection with knowledge previously secured regarding the methods of dealing with such cases" (p. 597). Notably, this kind of individualization did not mean that every offender would have a unique treatment, "any more than scientific treatment of diseases means an entirely different policy for each patient" (p. 597). But would not such individualization cause "criminal justice to be discredited in the eyes of the public because of the inequalities of penalties" (p. 599)? He rejected this reasoning because he was persuaded that "real confidence must be based on a belief in the scientific efficiency of the courts" (p. 599).

Sutherland (1939), we should note, did not argue that interventions should be limited to the correctional system; instead, he favored attacking the sources of crime across multiple contexts. As with treatment, he endorsed "policies . . . for the prevention of crime" that were "closely related to the theories of crime causation" (p. 617). He cautioned that some interventions, such as boys clubs, could be criminogenic by "directly or indirectly promoting delinquency, probably through the association of boys who were inclined to delinquency" (p. 625). Still, he advanced a range of possible interventions—from child guidance clinics and "visiting teachers" for at-risk "predelinquents" to attempts to reduce social disorganization through community organization. After all, "prevention is a logical policy to use in dealing with crime. . . . It is futile to take individual after individual out of the situations which produce criminals and permit the situations to remain as they were" (p. 614).

This type of thinking became standard fare in textbooks conveying the accepted wisdom in the field. Take, for example, Donald Taft's (1960) *Criminology* in which he discusses the "apparent principles of effective correctional programs for adults" (p. 727). Taft noted that the best ways to rehabilitate offenders had not been settled and that criminologists continued to differ on whether programs should place "emphasis on dealing with the individual [or] emphasis on working through groups." Regardless, he asked rhetorically, "But can it not be asserted that the neoclassical basis of current correctional practices has been largely discredited?" It is obviously the case that "criminals are not alike. They came to crime by different roads." And punishment is inherently limited, for "it may deter at the moment, but it never socializes and so never protects society in the future" (all quotes from p. 728).

The prevailing professional ideology did not mean that existing correctional and preventative practices were naively assumed to be effective. But if not, their ineffectiveness was defined largely as a problem of science: These practices just were not based on the correct scientific theory of crime. This perspective is seen in the work of another set of criminological giants, Sheldon and Eleanor Glueck. In *Unraveling Juvenile Delinquency*, Glueck and Glueck (1950) presented their empirical analysis of whether a range of factors differentiated one sample of 500 delinquent boys from a second sample of 500 nondelinquent boys. They reported that the roots of maladjustment and criminality often extend to childhood and that across multiple factors, "delinquent boys differ—often markedly so—from non-delinquents" (p. 286). These distinguishing factors are important because they offer "specific targets for clinical and preventative programs." The difficulty, however, is that because "sufficiently exact knowledge of the causes of youth's maladjustment" is not available, correctional interventions—including the juvenile court—"cannot be too successful in curing or even curbing juvenile delinquency" (p. 4). Indeed, they characterized as "naive" the officials dealing with wayward youths:

> How can it reasonably be expected that a brief judicial contact with a delinquent, whether it be entirely sympathetic or accompanied by a threat of punish-

> ment if the boy does not "turn over a new leaf," will change an emotional and conduct pattern that is often deeply anchored? (pp. 3-4)

They called for continued scientific study of the multiple causes of crime that will help reveal "the numerous factors and forces, which, in their dynamic interplay, make for persistent delinquency" (p. 286). This knowledge will then make it possible to "concentrate psychologic, psychiatric, and sociologic activities in those areas in which action gives the highest promise of good results, instead of galloping in all directions at once" (p. 286). Effective intervention will require "specialized training" and the "scientific experiment with therapeutic models based on sound and early diagnosis" (pp. 288, 289). Importantly, they noted the need to move beyond correctional interventions because they often occur when it is "too late for effective results" (p. 287). "Among the forces that count most in whether or not a boy will be conditioned to antisocial behavior," the Gluecks reminded us, "is the home atmosphere, and especially the intimate emotional relationships of the parent and child and their psychologic deposits in the personality and character of the boy" (p. 287). Therefore, good science compelled the conclusion that

> little progress can be expected in the prevention of delinquency until family life is strengthened by a large-scale, continuous, pervasive program designed to bring to bear all the resources of mental hygiene, social work, education, and religious and ethical instruction upon the central issue. (p. 287; see also Laub & Sampson, 1991, pp. 1428-1429)

We will offer one more illustration of the prevailing professional ideology—an essay authored by Donald Cressey (1958). With his penetrating mind, Cressey was quick to see the problems plaguing correctional rehabilitation. He noted, for example, how virtually any activity in an institution—"whatever is done with prisoners to keep them occupied and/or productive and quiet"—can "be called a correctional measure" (p. 763). He revealed how the main goal of those running intervention programs—although seemingly in favor of evaluation research—was to ensure that "research results can be interpreted as 'conclusive' if they favor continued utilization of the technique and as 'inconclusive' if they do not" (p. 759). In the latter regard, any unfavorable finding from an evaluation could be rendered "inconclusive" by subjecting it to a range of spurious methodological critiques, thus ensuring the continued funding of questionable interventions (pp. 761-763). Furthermore, he ended his essay with "the rather obvious conclusion that most of the 'techniques' used in 'correcting' criminals have not been shown to be either effective or ineffective and only vaguely related to any reputable theory of behavior or of criminality" (p. 770).

Still, despite this skepticism, Cressey (1958) did not favor abandoning rehabilitation (see also Cressey, 1978, 1982); science still held answers for him. "If correctional work were scientific," he claimed, "each correctional technique would be established on a rational basis" (p. 764). As the paradigm suggests, "we would be reasonably sure that men commit crime in certain describable circumstances and not in others, and then we would set out to modify their crime-producing circumstances." As the caretaker of Sutherland's differential association theory, Cressey proposed that interventions would be more effective if they focused less on personality traits and more on a "group-relations" approach in which the goal is to modify the group or social relations of offenders. He then deduced that many prison programs—such as education, vocational training, and prison labor—will be effective only to the extent that they serve as a conduit through which "the offender's postinstitutional group relationships" are changed (p. 767).

In short, the positivist professional ideology could accommodate a diverse lot—sociologists and psychologists, skeptics and supporters of rehabilitation. Program failures were not a reason to reconsider the whole enterprise but occasions to point out how treatment might be done better—that is, more scientifically. Indeed, the ideological hegemony was sufficiently tight that, as described by Gibbons (1999),

> it seemed to many criminologists that they were about to become "scholar princes" who would lead a social movement away from punitive responses to criminals and delinquents and toward a society in which treatment, rehabilitation, and reintegration of deviants and lawbreakers would be the dominant cultural motif. (p. 272)

In Toby's (1964) words, the authors of criminology textbooks felt comfortable suggesting, implicitly if not explicitly, that "punishment is a vestigial carryover of a barbaric past and will disappear as humanitarianism and rationality spread" (p. 332).

At least on the surface, the "real world" was not inconsistent with this academic vision. Although the rehabilitative idea was never implemented as intended (Rothman, 1980), the language of "corrections" became commonplace. In 1954, for example, the American Prison Association changed its name to the American Correctional Association. Prisons became known as "correctional institutions" (Irwin, 1980; Rotman, 1995). But real programmatic changes also ensued. Prison labor, industrial/vocational training, and basic education—long the staple of prison rehabilitation—were increasingly supplemented with psychological classification systems, therapeutic milieus, token economies, work release and furloughs, and college education. "During the 1960s," observes Keve (1991), "many of the country's correctional systems instituted special treatment programs, in an optimistic hope that the behavioral sciences could diagnose individual criminal cases and devise corrective strategies. It was a time of widespread creative experimenting in rehabilitation" (p. 216). It was also a time when calls were being made to explore community-based treatment programs, spurred on by theories such as differential association that stressed the curative benefits of prosocial reintegration into local neighborhoods.

Reflecting the tenor of the times, the Task Force on Corrections (1967)—part of the President's Commission on Law Enforcement and Administration of Justice—officially sanctioned the professional ideology of criminologists. "Excessively harsh penalties," warned the task force, "may simply backfire by fostering hostility and despair." The challenge is to achieve community safety "by reducing the incidence of crime." And the "rehabilitation of offenders to prevent their return to crime is in general the most promising way to achieve this goal" (all quotes from p. 16).

"NOTHING WORKS" AS A PROFESSIONAL IDEOLOGY

In 1974, Robert Martinson published his celebrated assessment of the effectiveness of correctional treatment, "What Works? Questions and Answers About Prison Reform"—an article that would have both substantive and symbolic significance. Distilled from a larger coauthored report published a year later (see Lipton, Martinson, & Wilks, 1975), Martinson (1974a) presented the results of an analysis of 231 program evaluation studies conducted between 1945 and 1967. "With few and isolated exceptions," he pessimistically concluded, "the rehabilitative efforts that have been reported so far have had no appreciable effect on recidivism" (p. 25). Importantly, Martinson then went on to pose a provocative question. "Do all of these studies," he asked, "lead irrevocably to the conclusion that *nothing works* [italics added], that we haven't the faintest clue about how to rehabilitate offenders and reduce recidivism?" (p. 48). He refrained from answering in the affirmative, but it was clear what he was suggesting. Soon after, it became a criminological wisdom that "nothing works" in the correctional system to change offenders.

Instead of the ready acceptance of the "nothing works doctrine," we might have expected a more detached appraisal of this strongly put finding (for an exception, see Sechrest, White, & Brown, 1979). As Merton (1973) points out, a core norm of the scientific enterprise is "organized skepticism" in which the community of scholars subjects claims of truth to withering scrutiny. If criminologists had adhered to this normative prescription, they might have noticed that the Martinson review covered only 138 measures of recidivism—not 231—and that in these studies, fewer than 75 of the evaluated interventions could be called "treatments" (Cullen & Gendreau, 2000, p. 127). They also might not have chosen to ignore Martinson's (1974b, p. 5) admission that his review did not include a category for behaviorally oriented programs—even though readily available literature at this time showed that this treatment modality had achieved promising results with other problem populations and had demonstrated successes in some correctional settings (see Gendreau & Ross, 1979; Milan & McKee, 1974).

If the traditional positivist professional ideology had been reigning undisturbed, Martinson's (1974a) report would have received such scrutiny—such organized skepticism—and warnings would have been forthcoming not to read too much into it. The technical finding of "no appreciable effects" would have been treated as regrettable and then used as evidence that correctional treatment was still based on faulty theories of crime, was using scientifically inappropriate intervention technique, and/or lacked quality in its implementation. A call for more research and experimentation would have been made. The idea that "nothing works" would not have been broached or, if put forward, accepted.

But the traditional paradigm was not left undisturbed. It had been shattered, and thus a very different response to Martinson's (1974a) study was forthcoming. Indeed, a profound transformation in criminologists' professional ideology was well under way when the "nothing works" essay appeared. Between the late 1960s and mid-1970s, the paradigm organizing how criminologists thought had been increasingly abandoned, and "new criminologies" were now flourishing (Cressey, 1978). Michael Gottfredson (1979) captured how this paradigmatic shift changed views on rehabilitation in his amusing but poignant essay, "Treatment Destruction Techniques."

Writing 5 years after Martinson, Gottfredson (1979) introduced his essay with the observation that "the conventional wisdom in criminology is that rehabilitation has been found to be ineffective" (p. 39). In fact, this view was so widespread that "the lack of demonstrated effectiveness is agreed upon by criminologists of nearly every persuasion and theoretical orientation" (p. 39). This consensus, however, rested on shaky empirical ground. As Gottfredson pointed out, about half of the studies with the most rigorous methodological designs in the Martinson report showed *positive* treatment results (see also Palmer, 1975). But criminologists were no longer interested in defending rehabilitation but rather were ideologically predisposed to prove that "nothing works." Accordingly, in the face of promising results, they used "treatment destruction techniques"—biased methodological critiques and ex post facto arguments—to show why promising evaluation results were, in fact, inconclusive, if not misleading (see also Gendreau, 1996a). He characterized these techniques and their use in defense of the new professional ideology in this way:

> There is a variety of general principles (or, more accurately, pseudoscientific criteria) that may be invoked to fend off any attack on our conventional wisdom regarding the effectiveness of treatment. In fact, there are at least five distinguishable methods that may be used to demonstrate the ineffectiveness of any and all treatment modalities in the criminal justice system. Individually (but, most effectively, in combination), these methods are capable of destroying any positive results that might appear in the literature. Perhaps more important, each can be used to show that continuing research in the area would be a mistake. . . . Because no study or research proposal can withstand an assault from a carefully chosen arsenal of these destruction techniques, their value is obvious. (p. 40)

A number of factors had coalesced in a short period of time to prompt criminologists to relinquish one professional ideology for another. Like others in the United States, criminologists experienced the social and political upheaval of the decade spanning the middle parts of the 1960s and 1970s. Civil rights marches, urban unrest, the Vietnam War, Kent State, Attica, and Watergate—these events and more created a "confidence gap" between the public and the government (Lipset & Schneider, 1987). This rapidly declining trust in the government had direct implications for how scholars came to view the so-called "welfare state," of which corrections and, more generally, the "therapeutic state" were a part (see Kittrie, 1971).

Previously, the expansion of government interventions into the lives of the poor and deviant had been portrayed as benevolent paternalism—as well-intended efforts to address problems in people's lives. But the events of the day fostered the view that the state wielded its power not benevolently but abusively. It was now possible to see welfare programs for mothers and children not as assistance but as an attempt to "regulate the poor" (Piven & Cloward, 1971) or to see "hospitals" for the mentally ill and mentally retarded as a means both to inhumanely incapacitate them and to make them undergo "enforced therapy" (Kittrie, 1971). Vulnerable Americans did not need help from the state but protection from it.

As Rothman (1980) points out, the issue of the discretionary power of the state was integral to the correctional paradigm first initiated in the Progressive Era. Indeterminate sentencing, community supervision, and parole release gave correctional officials unfettered discretion to individualize treatment. The bargain was that this discretion was to be exercised responsibly and according to scientific criminological knowledge. In the prevailing context of the state waging an unpopular war, shooting down college students and inmates, and plotting illegal political schemes, such a bargain seemed strangely and naively trusting.

Indeed, with minorities crowding the courts and prisons, criminologists now worried about whether the unfettered discretion accorded criminal justice officials was an invitation for race and class discrimination—that is, for "extra-legal" factors to shape decision making. They worried as well that release from prison was not earned through true rehabilitation but linked to effective playacting before the parole board (i.e., to "prove" one was cured) and to coerced compliance to institutional rules while locked up (i.e., unless one obeyed, there would be no release). Academic studies, media exposés, and inmate accounts seemed to show that, in fact, benevolence had been corrupted (Irwin, 1974; Rothman, 1980). For many criminologists, offenders needed legal rights to protect them from a powerful state that had its own, not their, interests in mind. In this context, the idea that "nothing works" in correctional treatment was awfully appealing and not grounds for "organized skepticism" (Cullen & Gilbert, 1982).

Within criminology, exciting intellectual developments—"new criminologies" that challenged old ways of thinking—were reinforcing this rejection of rehabilitation. Starting in the first part of the 1960s, labeling theorists warned that stigmatizing "societal reaction" triggered a "self-fulfilling prophecy" that would trap offenders in criminal roles and amplify their offending (Becker, 1963). The logical extension of this thinking was Schur's (1975) call for "radical nonintervention"—a call to keep juvenile offenders out of the justice system whenever possible.

Critical criminology, with its roots in Marxism, offered an even harsher portrayal of rehabilitation as its adherents unmasked the "good intentions" of correctional "reformers" as efforts to reinforce existing privileges and structural inequalities. For example, the "child savers" who created the juvenile court were now portrayed as embarking on a moral crusade that legitimated their class values and extended control over the lives of poor children (Platt, 1969). From Foucault (1977), we learned that penitentiaries and youth reformatories were not civilized advances over public whippings and hangings but insidious, covert means to discipline the disadvantaged. More broadly, rehabilitation was seen as an effort to adjust offenders to a society that was, at its core, unjust and criminogenic. The solution to crime was not fixing people but fixing social injustices.

These intellectual and social influences combined to create a new set of interrelated principles or shared understandings that were now the lens through which criminologists viewed their world and subject matter. The traditional positivist model did not lose all its adherents, but the emergent professional ideology dominated scholarly discourse and publication. Indeed, even today this ideology shapes academic criminology, as succeeding cohorts of criminologists have been socialized, to varying degrees, into it. On the broadest level, the core feature of this ideology is the rejection of science as a means of building correctional knowledge and, instead, the use of science—and, if need be, rhetoric—to show that virtually nothing related to the correctional system reduces crime. More specifically, this professional ideology of "knowledge destruction" rests on five main principles.

First, nothing works to rehabilitate offenders. Martinson's (1974a) study is seen as providing final and definitive proof that correctional rehabilitation is a failure. It is not, of course, necessary to actually read this study—only to cite it and perhaps one or two more (e.g., Whitehead & Lab, 1989). The wealth of contrary evidence is to be systematically ignored, especially the empirical studies of Canadian psychologists (see, e.g., Andrews & Bonta, 1998; see also Gendreau, 1996a). When discussing rehabilitation, it is essential to unmask its hypocrisy by noting that "good intentions have bad results" and that "benevolence is corrupted"; ignore as well the possibility that the policy results are even worse when the intentions are simply nakedly "bad." Whenever possible, refer to probation officers, correctional counselors, and the like as "state agents of social control" and refer to rehabilitation as "state-enforced therapy"; this will ensure that their coerciveness will not be missed (Binder & Geis, 1984). In contrast, when studies report that fortuitous events—such as job stability or marriage—cause persistent offenders to change and desist from crime (Sampson & Laub, 1993), cite this research uncritically and repeatedly. Meanwhile, retain the assumption that *planned* interventions—even well-designed, high-dosage, targeted treatment programs—are incapable of changing offenders.

Second and closely related, nothing that the state does in the criminal justice system will reduce crime. This is the corrections "nothing works" criticism writ large. There is no need to conduct more research to verify this principle empirically, but studies are always welcome that show the ineffectiveness of new "get-tough" laws, diversion programs, drug crackdowns, policing patrol strategies, and so on. There are two exceptions to this generic nothing works principle: White-collar offenders, especially corporate executives, and perpetrators of domestic violence are good candidates for deterrence, apparently because they are exquisitely sensitive to criminal sanctions.

Third, prisons have virtually no effect on the crime rate and should only be used for serious violent offenders—of which there are few. This principle is important because it is prima facie evidence that the United States overincarcerates its citizens. After all, if prisons have "no effect" and few people inside them are dangerous, why are we locking up so many folks? Relatedly, it is always better to place an offender in the community than behind bars. Even though "nothing works" that we do in the community either, at least this intervention "does less harm" than incarceration. Meanwhile, do not discuss the risks to public safety posed by placing felony offenders into local neighborhoods (see Petersilia, Turner, Kahan, & Peterson, 1985). If pressed on this issue, defend community corrections by saying that it is more "cost-effective."

Fourth, engaging in "penal science" is a bad thing for criminologists to do. Using criminological knowledge to show how to make control exercised by the criminal justice system more effective is to become a "tool of the state." Especially if paid by the state to do this work, the criminologist is suspect ethically. The real danger is not so much that penal science will be effective but that it will lend an air of legitimacy or academic respectability to the repressive measures of the state.

Fifth, crime is caused by structural factors, especially forms of social and economic inequality. This principle has several functions. Thus, it explains why rehabilitation and other types of state control are ineffective: They cannot change the structural "root causes" of crime. It also explains why individual theories of crime are wrong and can be safely ignored. In fact, because these astructural theories divert attention to individual pathology, they run the risk of acquitting the social structure of its complicity in crime. As such, individual differences theories are likely to blame the victim and foster repressive crime control policies.

CRIMINOLOGISTS AND THE PUNITIVE STATE

To select a somewhat arbitrary line, the "nothing works" professional ideology was fairly entrenched by 1980. Although this ideology arose largely as a critique of the "therapeutic state," it was clear by this time that rehabilitation—although still seen as ineffective—was the least of criminologists' problems. Until the early 1970s, the rate of incarceration in the United States had remained relatively stable for half a century (Blumstein & Cohen, 1973). But by the time the Reagan era arrived, the steep increase in prison populations was the major concern of criminologists studying corrections and broader issues of social control. The policies and practices of the 1980s ensured a full transformation from a "therapeutic state" to a "punitive state." Worries about the use of rehabilitation to mask coercion were replaced by worries about policies explicitly formulated to deliver, as Clear (1994) aptly puts it, "penal harm."

Of course, most attention was given to the inordinate numbers of offenders behind bars. Then there was the attempt to transform community "corrections" into community "control," with an emphasis on intensive supervision, drug testing, electronic monitoring, and home confinement (Cullen, Wright, & Applegate, 1996). But equally disquieting was the sheer punitiveness of the rhetoric surrounding crime policy and, at times, the gratuitous attempts to inflict suffering on offenders (e.g., eliminate access to college courses, reimplement chain gangs). Corrections had entered a "mean season," and criminologists could not simply sit by as the human toll mounted. In response, criminologists did what they knew best: They wrote books and articles showing the foolhardiness of the punitive state (see, e.g., Beckett, 1997; Clear, 1994; Currie, 1985, 1998; Irwin & Austin, 1994; Mauer, 1999; Petersilia, 1992; Tonry, 1995; Welch, 1999).

Most of these works carted out a laundry list of familiar criticisms as to why prisons and harsh penalties "don't work." These arguments varied in their scholarly merit—some convincing, some questionable—but they functioned, in essence, as "punishment destruction techniques." It was often argued, for example, that America had engaged in a two- or three-decade "punishment experiment" that had proved to be a failure; that prison populations had to be doubled to achieve even a small percentage reduction in the crime rate; that other nations imprisoned less and had less crime; and that community sanctions were more "cost-effective" than building and operating an endless flow of new institutions (cf. Bennett, DiIulio, & Walters, 1996).

Although a worthy battle to have fought, the downside of the attack on the punitive state was that criminologists continued to spend enormous amounts of time showing what did not work. Knowledge destruction, not construction, remained the dominant theme of these writings. To be sure, exceptions existed (see, e.g., Currie, 1985, 1998), but most works that had offered splendid critiques of punitively oriented correctional policies and practices ended with half-baked or vacuous recommendations for an *alternative way of doing things*. Mostly, there was a call for using prisons less and communities more as places where less harmful punishments might be exacted. Meanwhile, most criminologists declined to build a *science of corrections*, based on criminological knowledge on the causes of criminality, that might show what worked to reduce recidivism, improve the lives of offenders, and foster public safety (Gendreau, Goggin, Cullen, & Paparozzi, in press).

THE "WHAT WORKS" MOVEMENT IN CORRECTIONS

Any attempt to characterize the professional ideology of an entire discipline, such as criminology, or a group within a discipline, such as corrections scholars, is open to the charge of ignoring intellectual richness and nuance of opinion. Although admitting that we undoubtedly underplay the diversity of viewpoints among criminologists, the portrayal of the "nothing works" professional ideology captures, we believe, assumptions that are pervasively held and that tend to "load on the same factor." Again, core features of this professional ideology are not without merit or empirical support. Still, belief in this ideology is typically not a rational choice that follows a careful assessment of competing empirical realities. Instead, this way of thinking is socially transmitted in graduate school, in texts, and in journals. At professional meetings, the ideology is reinforced. Here, we learn which criminological statements are disciplinarily "correct" (e.g., "structural reform is needed to reduce crime") and which are "incorrect" (e.g., "prisons reduce crime").

Take, for example, the reception given to the writings of Wilson and Herrnstein's (1985) *Crime and Human Nature* and Gottfredson and Hirschi's (1990) *A General Theory of Crime*. Because these works were provocative in tone, they brought some criticisms onto themselves. Nonetheless, their preference to explain crime by individual differences, not structural circumstances, earned them a disproportionate level of harsh written and unwritten criticism. In contrast, we can point to the warm reception accorded Sampson and Laub's (1993) *Crime in the Making*. Although truly a wonderful book—a contemporary classic—this work is now uncritically cited as definitive proof that persistent individual differences in criminal propensity can be changed when offenders, virtually by chance, acquire quality jobs and marriages. It is accepted that the delivery of "social capital" and "informal social control"—whose conceptual components are broadly defined and measured indirectly— are integral to crime causation. Sampson and Laub's findings certainly are plausible, but we suspect that criminologists' ready embrace of their interpretations is because they are consistent with conventional disciplinary wisdom. Even better, Sampson and Laub's views have the special benefit of rebutting central claims of Gottfredson and Hirschi's "general theory"—a perspective that antagonizes the field's conventional wisdom (see Sampson & Laub, 1995).

In this context, it is perhaps not surprising that the challenge to Martinson's (1974a) "nothing works" doctrine came disproportionately, if not primarily, from scholars from outside criminology and often from outside the United States—that is, from Canadian psychologists (see, e.g., Andrews, 1995; Andrews & Bonta, 1998; Andrews et al., 1990; Gendreau, 1996b; Gendreau & Ross, 1979, 1987; see also Lipsey, 1992; Lipsey & Wilson, 1998; Palmer, 1975, 1992). Note that the collateral movement to discover what works in early interventions with children and adolescents at risk for crime also is rooted largely outside traditional criminology (see, e.g., Catalano, Arthur, Hawkins, Berglund, & Olson, 1998; Henggeler, 1997; Yoshikawa, 1994; see also Farrington, 1994).

As social scientists embracing the norm of organized skepticism, psychologists engage in a fair amount of knowledge destruction, falsifying commonsense myths and academic nonsense. It is a discipline, however, that also is devoted to constructing knowledge about what works to change people. In part, of course, this is because they have an economic interest in doing so: If no one could be helped through psychological treatment, much legitimacy and many jobs might be threatened. In any case, the discipline of psychology—especially its clinical component—largely believes that behavioral change among troubled individuals is possible and that interventions can bring this about. The data, it appears, are supportive of this assumption (Lipsey & Wilson, 1993).

How psychologists view corrections also differs from how mainstream criminologists, especially those with a sociological orientation, view corrections. Criminologists see prisons as a "society of captives" that is characterized by power relationships, racial conflict, violence and victimization, inmate insurgency, and subcultural formation. The study of corrections thus is the study of social problems writ small; the task is to take the social domain of corrections, especially the prison, and to detail what is wrong with it. In contrast, although not unmindful of these phenomena (Haney & Zimbardo, 1998), clinically oriented psychologists tend to focus on the *individual* within the prison or other correctional settings. An important reality for them is "the program" or "intervention" through which psychological treatment is delivered. It is the quality of this intervention that counteracts the offender's criminality and that, implicitly, outweighs the effects of what else is going on in the correctional setting. Individual change of the offender, not structural change of prison dynamics, is their concern.

Given these considerations, we can perhaps understand why Canadian (and other) psychologists, especially those working in correctional agencies, did not jump on Martinson's (1974a) "nothing works" bandwagon. Coming from a different discipline and society, Martinson's results did not resonate with them as being "obviously true" but as "obviously false." And providing treatment to offenders did not strike them as a form of "repression" but as a genuine attempt to help these individuals overcome behavioral patterns damaging to themselves and others.

Indeed, the findings reported by Martinson (1974a) were anomalies within the psychologists' disciplinary paradigm and inconsistent with their professional ideology; they "couldn't be true." In response, they published reviews of the extant empirical literature revealing the effectiveness of treatment, which they then hoped would provide "bibliotherapy for cynics" (Gendreau & Ross, 1979; see also Gendreau & Ross, 1987). They also developed "principles of effective intervention" that, if followed, promised to achieve meaningful reductions in recidivism. For the most part, however, these empirical reviews and theoretical insights changed few minds, again because the message being conveyed was incompatible with the "conventional wisdom" of criminologists' prevailing professional ideology.

In the latter part of the 1990s, however, the "what works" view within corrections seemed to capture more adherents and to be accepted as "possibly true" by criminology in general. Why this is so, we do not really know, but we can speculate about two factors that may have played a role. First, with a Democratic administration in the White House and heading the National Institute of Justice, doing research—especially funded research—aimed at reducing crime became more acceptable. Scholars now might be seen as "chasing money," but at least they were less likely to be stigmatized as "tools of the state."

Second and more consequential, the data from meta-analyses of tens, if not hundreds, of studies confirmed that the Canadians might, in the end, be right. With rather consistent results drawn from meta-analyses conducted in North America and Europe, it appeared that across all types of treatments, rehabilitation programs worked to reduce recidivism. However, the key finding from these analyses was that treatment effects were *heterogeneous*. Some interventions—especially those that were punitively oriented (e.g., boot camps)—did not work, but others—especially those reflecting the principles of effective treatment—did work to cut recidivism meaningfully (Cullen, in press; Cullen & Gendreau, 2000). Scholars might interpret these findings with a different degree of optimism (cf. Cullen & Gendreau, 2000, with Losel, 1999, and Gaes, Flanagan, Motiuk, & Stewart, 1999), but the case against the "nothing works" doctrine has become pretty convincing (see also Lurigio, 2000; MacKenzie, 1997; Pearson & Lipton, 1999; Pearson, Lipton, Cleland, & Yee, 2000; Prendergast, Anglin, & Wellisch, 1995; Redondo, Sanchez-Meca, & Garrido, 1999; Taxman, 1999).

In many ways, the professional ideology underlying the "what works" approach overlaps with that of the earlier days of modern American criminology. The key theme is that science is a way of knowing the world and changing it for the better. More specifically, the "what works" professional ideology encompasses five principles or core beliefs—ideas that inform, explicitly or implicitly, the scholarship of those now working in this approach (see, e.g., Andrews & Bonta, 1998; Cullen & Gendreau, 2000).

First, scientific criminology is the basis for effective correctional intervention. As early criminologists understood, interventions can only be effective if they target for change the causes or known predictors of recidivism. Understanding what causes persistent criminal involvement, however, requires research into the factors that place offenders at risk of recidivism. Theory plays an important role in this enterprise by directing research into potentially salient risk factors.

Second, scientific criminology should be used to "destroy" knowledge that is not evidence based. Many correctional interventions are based on faulty theories and employ treatment techniques that are inconsistent with decades of social psychological research on behavioral change (e.g., "boot camps," "Scared Straight" programs). Resources should not be allocated to these interventions. Furthermore, if such ill-advised programs are initiated, evaluation research should be undertaken to test the claims being made. In all likelihood, such studies will show that these programs are hopelessly ineffective (see, e.g., Gendreau, Goggin, Cullen, & Andrews, 2000).

Third, scientific criminology should be used to "construct" knowledge about what does work. This is the central premise of the "what works" ideology. There is a belief that offenders are not trapped for life in their criminality but can change. There is a belief that such change is more effectively accomplished by interventions that use treatment modalities (e.g., cognitive-behavioral treatment) that are capable of reducing the known predictors of recidivism. And there is the belief that sustained research and the systematic accumulation of knowledge will improve our ability to discern how best to deliver effective treatments in correctional settings. Indeed, knowledge construction is every bit as important as knowledge destruction. More generally, this approach assumes that scientific criminology is capable of producing knowledge about "what works" in others areas, such as in policing and in situational crime prevention.

Fourth, although pure research is a noble activity, it is equally legitimate for criminologists to produce knowledge that can reduce crime. The failure to make correctional policies and practices "evidence based" merely ensures that ineffective interventions will abound, as they now do. Unless criminologists can provide a persuasive blueprint for what should be done in corrections, we will be saddled with programs—such as boot camps—that potentially damage offenders and harm public safety. Furthermore, criminologists who help to develop effective interventions are not "tools of the state" but servers of the commonweal. The exercise of state control is not an inherent evil but a resource that should be used to foster effective and humane interventions. This task is daunting, but it is precisely why criminologists should not leave it exclusively to other people.

Fifth, "what works" scientific criminology is not limited, a priori, to any one level of analysis or theoretical perspective. The project is to use science to build criminological knowledge that is the basis of more effective interventions. The "nothing works" professional ideology assumed a priori that theories focusing on offenders' individual differences were incorrect and thus incapable of forming the basis for effective interventions. In contrast, the "what works" paradigm believes that there is heterogeneity in individual propensities to engage in crime—propensities that reflect both traits and differential exposure to social circumstances. At present, the research is strongest in showing that proximate causes of crime—such as antisocial attitudes and relations, faulty cognitions, low self-control, and dysfunctional family relations—are more amenable to intervention than are causes that are more distal (e.g., concentrated disadvantage in neighborhoods, society inequality) (Andrews & Bonta, 1998). This state of affairs, however, may reflect the failure of criminologists to investigate systematically and empirically how interventions targeted at social arrangements beyond the level of the individual offender might affect criminal involvement (e.g., specific housing, welfare, or employment policies) (but see Currie, 1998). There is no inherent reason, though, why a "what works" approach could not operate at, or across, different levels of analysis.

Sixth, scientific criminology will result in more "good" in the world than a criminology that ignores what really works. The "nothing works" doctrine is a fiction that is not based on science. The "cost of ignoring success," to use Van Voorhis's (1987) words, is that we are consigned either to inaction—doing nothing—or to supporting faulty actions—doing the wrong thing. It is particularly disquieting that criminologists would prefer to call for more social justice—to "preach to the choir" and receive accolades from their professional colleagues—even when such statements do not materially change the lives of offenders now in the correctional system. In contrast, constructing knowledge about what does work can foster programming that can "do good" in the real world and in real people's lives.

CONCLUSION: CHOOSING THE FUTURE

What set of beliefs—what "professional ideology"—should guide criminology and the study of corrections in the 21st century? We have suggested that in the late 1960s and early 1970s, criminology experienced a paradigm shift in its underlying set of operating assumptions. The professional ideology of positivist criminology, which hoped to use knowledge to improve the correctional system, was replaced by a criminology that sought to show that "nothing works" when "state control" is exercised and to argue that larger social justice is the solution to crime. This paradigm shift was made possible, at least in part, by the inability of the older criminological paradigm to "deliver the goods"—to make matters better. But it also was a product of events outside and inside the discipline that shaped how a new generation—and subsequent generations—of scholars saw their work.

The new professional ideology was attractive. It seemed ennobling because it placed criminologists on the side of the casualties of social injustice and lined us up against the entrenched powers of capitalism. It implored us to become collective deconstructionists devoted to unmasking the hypocrisy of good intentions that justified repression, to showing how inequities flourished under the cover of claims of equal justice, and to deflating the many myths in society that legitimated inane "get-tough" policies. We were in a fight with powerful forces, and knowledge destruction was our weapon.

The limits of this professional ideology, however, are now clear: It was a recipe for never being able to provide a positive agenda for corrections—of never being able to tell anyone of consequence "what really works." We largely became a discipline of naysayers—people who could tell what not to do but not what to do. Indeed, in the absence of knowledge construction—knowledge whose persuasiveness comes from data and not from mere ideology—we have been able to offer only value-laden opinions about the need to "do less harm" to offenders. In short, we have been largely bereft of any scientifically based answers as to how we can reduce crime effectively and humanely.

The professional ideology of the past quarter century is hardly diminished, never mind dead. It continues to inform how nearly all of us approach correctional issues. In part, this is a good thing. Knowledge destruction is part of criminologists' role. Even so, we believe that the hegemony of this professional ideology has outlived its utility and has become counterproductive. The challenge that lies ahead is to use science to develop "evidence-based" corrections that not only tells us what not to do but also what to do (Cullen & Gendreau, 2000; MacKenzie, 2000). At its core, this challenge involves using what is unique to our field—our capacity to undertake scientific criminology—to construct knowledge both about the nature of crime and about "what works" to change offenders.

We are not unmindful of the criticisms of "logical positivism" or of the assumption that cumulative scientific knowledge ineluctably produces social progress. Any choice regarding what criminology should be about, however, has its costs and benefits, its dangers and its possibilities. Even so, if we are to experiment with one choice or the other, we will cast our lot with those who believe that criminology is a discipline that should use scientific knowledge to improve our world. Already within corrections, we can see that the efforts of a rather small cadre of researchers have produced a "what works" knowledge base about the "principles of effective treatment" that is shaping how correctional officials in a variety of jurisdictions view and implement interventions. We are convinced that a large-scale "what works" movement would increasingly construct powerful sets of knowledge about controlling crime that would meaningfully influence policy debates and actual practice. Not to make this choice is to consign criminologists to irrelevance and to forfeit crime policy and practice to those whose knowledge—and often whose motives—are suspect.

REFERENCES

Andrews, D. A. (1995). The psychology of criminal conduct and effective treatment. In J. Maguire (Ed.), *What works: Reducing reoffending—Guidelines from research and practice* (pp. 35-62). New York: John Wiley.

Andrews, D. A., & Bonta, J. (1998). *The psychology of criminal conduct* (2nd ed.). Cincinnati, OH: Anderson.

Andrews, D. A., Zinger, I., Hoge, R. D., Bonta, J., Gendreau, P., & Cullen, F. T. (1990). Does correctional treatment work? A clinically-relevant and psychologically-informed meta-analysis. *Criminology, 28*, 369-404.

Becker, H. S. (1963). *Outsiders: Studies in the sociology of deviance.* New York: Free Press.

Beckett, K. (1997). *Making crime pay: Law and order in contemporary politics.* New York: Oxford University Press.

Bennett, W. J., DiIulio, J. J., Jr., & Walters, J. P. (1996). *Body count: Moral poverty . . . and how to win America's war against crime and drugs.* New York: Simon & Schuster.

Binder, A., & Geis, G. (1984). *Ad populum* argumentation in criminology: Juvenile diversion and rhetoric. *Crime & Delinquency, 30*, 624-647.

Blumstein, A., & Cohen, J. (1973). A theory of the stability of punishment. *Journal of Criminal Law and Criminology, 64*, 198-206.

Catalano, R. F., Arthur, M. W., Hawkins, J. D., Berglund, L., & Olson, J. J. (1998). Comprehensive community- and school-based interventions to prevent antisocial behavior. In R. Loeber & D. P. Farrington (Eds.), *Serious and violent juvenile offenders: Risk factors and successful interventions* (pp. 248-283). Thousand Oaks, CA: Sage.

Clear, T. R. (1994). *Harm in American penology: Offenders, victims, and their communities.* Albany: State University of New York Press.

Cressey, D. R. (1958). The nature and effectiveness of correctional techniques. *Law and Contemporary Problems, 23*, 754-771.

Cressey, D. R. (1978). Criminological theory, social science, and the repression of crime. *Criminology, 16*, 171-191.

Cressey, D. R. (1982). Foreword. In F. T. Cullen & K. E. Gilbert (Eds.), *Reaffirming rehabilitation* (pp. xi-xxiii). Cincinnati, OH: Anderson.

Cullen, F. T. (in press). Rehabilitation and treatment programs. In J. Q. Wilson & J. Petersilia (Eds.), *Crime: Public policies for crime control* (2nd ed.). San Francisco: ICS Press.

Cullen, F. T., & Gendreau, P. (2000). Assessing correctional rehabilitation: Policy, practice, and prospects. In J. Horney (Ed.), *Criminal justice 2000: Vol. 4. Policies, processes, and decisions of the criminal justice system* (pp. 109-175). Washington, DC: National Institute of Justice, U.S. Department of Justice.

Cullen, F. T., & Gilbert, K. E. (1982). *Reaffirming rehabilitation.* Cincinnati, OH: Anderson.

Cullen, F. T., Wright, J. P., & Applegate, B. K. (1996). Control in the community: The limits of reform? In A. T. Harland (Ed.), *Choosing correctional interventions that work: Defining the demand and evaluating the supply* (pp. 69-116). Thousand Oaks, CA: Sage.

Currie, E. (1985). *Confronting crime: An American dilemma.* New York: Pantheon.

Currie, E. (1998). *Crime and punishment in America.* New York: Metropolitan.

Farrington, D. P. (1994). Early developmental prevention of juvenile delinquency. *Criminal Behaviour and Mental Health, 4*, 209-227.

Foucault, M. (1977). *Discipline and punish: The birth of the prison.* New York: Plenum.

Gaes, G. G., Flanagan, T. J., Motiuk, L. L., & Stewart, L. (1999). Adult correctional treatment. In M. Tonry & J. Petersilia (Eds.), *Prisons: Crime and justice—A review of research* (Vol. 26, pp. 361-426). Chicago: University of Chicago Press.

Gendreau, P. (1996a). Offender rehabilitation: What we know and what needs to be done. *Criminal Justice and Behavior, 23*, 144-161.

Gendreau, P. (1996b). The principles of effective intervention with offenders. In A. T. Harland (Ed.), *Choosing correctional interventions that work: Defining the demand and evaluating the supply* (pp. 117-130). Thousand Oaks, CA: Sage.

Gendreau, P., Goggin, C., Cullen, F. T., & Andrews, D. A. (2000). The effects of community sanctions and incarceration on recidivism. *Forum on Corrections Research, 12*, 10-13.

Gendreau, P., Goggin, C., Cullen, F. T., & Paparozzi, M. (in press). The common sense revolution and correctional policy. In J. McGuire (Ed.), *Offender rehabilitation and treatment: Effective programs and policies to reduce re-offending.* Chichester, UK: Wiley.

Gendreau, P., & Ross, R. R. (1979). Effective correctional treatment: Bibliotherapy for cynics. *Crime & Delinquency, 25*, 463-489.

Gendreau, P., & Ross, R. R. (1987). Revivification of rehabilitation: Evidence from the 1980s. *Justice Quarterly, 4*, 349-407.

Gibbons, D. C. (1999). Review essay: Changing lawbreakers—What have we learned since the 1950s. *Crime & Delinquency, 45*, 272-293.

Glueck, S., & Glueck, E. (1950). *Unraveling juvenile delinquency.* Cambridge, MA: Harvard University Press.

Gottfredson, M. R. (1979). Treatment destruction techniques. *Journal of Research in Crime and Delinquency, 16*, 39-54.

Gottfredson, M. R., & Hirschi, T. (1990). *A general theory of crime.* Stanford, CA: Stanford University Press.

Gould, S. J. (1981). *The mismeasure of man.* New York: Norton.

Gouldner, A. W. (1970). *The coming crisis of Western sociology.* New York: Avon.

Haney, C., & Zimbardo, P. (1998). The past and future of U.S. prison policy: Twenty-five years after the Stanford prison experiment. *American Psychologist, 53*, 709-727.

Henggeler, S. W. (1997). *Treating serious anti-social behavior in youth: The MST approach.* Washington, DC: Office of Juvenile Justice and Delinquency Prevention, U.S. Department of Justice.

Irwin, J. (1974). Adaptation to being corrected: Corrections from the convict's perspective. In D. Glaser (Ed.), *Handbook of criminology* (pp. 971-993). Chicago: Rand McNally.

Irwin, J. (1980). *Prisons in turmoil.* Boston: Little, Brown.

Irwin, J., & Austin, J. (1994). *It's about time: America's imprisonment binge.* Belmont, CA: Wadsworth.

Keve, P. W. (1991). *Prisons and the American conscience: A history of U.S. federal corrections.* Carbondale: Southern Illinois University Press.

Kittrie, N. N. (1971). *The right to be different: Deviance and enforced therapy.* Baltimore: Penguin.

Laub, J. H., & Sampson, R. J. (1991). The Sutherland-Glueck debate: On the sociology of criminological knowledge. *American Journal of Sociology, 96*, 1402-1440.

Lipset, S. M., & Schneider, W. (1987). *The confidence gap: Business, labor, and government in the public mind* (Rev. ed.). Baltimore: Johns Hopkins University Press.

Lipsey, M. W. (1992). Juvenile delinquency treatment: A meta-analytic inquiry into the variability of effects. In T. D. Cook, H. Cooper, D. S. Cordray, H. Hartmann, L. V. Hedges, R. J. Light, T. A. Lewis, & F. Mosteller (Eds.), *Meta-analysis for explanation: A casebook* (pp. 83-127). New York: Russell Sage.

Lipsey, M. W., & Wilson, D. B. (1993). The efficacy of psychological, educational, and behavioral treatment. *American Psychologist, 48*, 1181-1209.

Lipsey, M. W., & Wilson, D. B. (1998). Effective intervention for serious juvenile offenders: A synthesis of the research. In R. Loeber & D. P. Farrington (Eds.), *Serious and violent and juvenile offenders: Risk factors and successful interventions* (pp. 313-345). Thousand Oaks, CA: Sage.

Lipton, D., Martinson, R., & Wilks, J. (1975). *The effectiveness of correctional treatment: A survey of treatment evaluation studies.* New York: Praeger.

Loeber, R., & Farrington, D. P. (Eds.). (1998). *Serious and violent juvenile offenders: Risk factors and successful interventions.* Thousand Oaks, CA: Sage.

Losel, F. (1995). The efficacy of correctional treatment: A review and synthesis of meta-evaluations. In J. Maguire (Ed.), *What works? Reducing reoffending—Guidelines from research and practice* (pp. 79-111). New York: John Wiley.

Lurigio, A. (2000). Drug treatment availability and effectiveness: Studies of the general and criminal justice populations. *Criminal Justice and Behavior, 27*, 495-528.

Mac Donald, A. (1893). *Criminology.* New York: Funk and Wagnalls.

MacKenzie, D. L. (1997). Criminal justice and crime prevention. In L. W. Sherman, D. Gottfredson, D. MacKenzie, J. Eck, P. Reuter, & S. Bushway (Eds.), *Preventing crime: What works, what doesn't, what's promising* (pp. 9.1-9.76). Washington, DC: National Institute of Justice.

MacKenzie, D. L. (2000). Evidence-based corrections: Identifying what works. *Crime & Delinquency, 46*, 457-471.

Martinson, R. (1974a). What works? Questions and answers about prison reform. *The Public Interest, 35*, 22-54.

Martinson, R. (1974b). Viewpoint. *Criminal Justice Newsletter, 5*, 4-5.

Mauer, M. (1999). *The race to incarcerate*. New York: New Press.

Merton, R. K. (1973). *The sociology of science: Theoretical and empirical investigations*. Chicago: University of Chicago Press.

Milan, M. A., & McKee, J. M. (1974). Behavior modification: Principles and applications in corrections. In D. Glaser (Ed.), *Handbook of criminology* (pp. 745-776). Chicago: Rand McNally.

Mills, C. W. (1942). The professional ideology of social pathologists. *American Journal of Sociology, 49*, 165-180.

Palmer, T. (1975). Martinson revisited. *Journal of Research in Crime and Delinquency, 12*, 133-152.

Palmer, T. (1992). *The re-emergence of correctional intervention*. Newbury Park, CA: Sage.

Pearson, F. S., & Lipton, D. S. (1999). A meta-analytic review of the effectiveness of corrections-based treatment for drug abuse. *The Prison Journal, 79*, 384-410.

Pearson, F. S., Lipton, D. S., Cleland, C. M., & Yee, D. S. (2000). *The effects of behavioral/cognitive behavioral programs on recidivism*. Unpublished paper, National Development and Research Institutes, New York.

Petersilia, J. (1992). California's prison policy: Causes, costs, and consequences. *The Prison Journal, 72*, 8-36.

Petersilia, J., Turner, S., Kahan, J., & Peterson, J. (1985). *Granting felons probation: Public risks and alternatives*. Santa Monica, CA: RAND.

Piven, F. F., & Cloward, R. A. (1971). *Regulating the poor: The functions of public welfare*. New York: Pantheon.

Platt, A. M. (1969). *The child savers: The invention of delinquency*. Chicago: University of Chicago Press.

Prendergast, M. L., Anglin, M. D., & Wellisch, J. (1995). Treatment for drug-abusing offenders under community supervision. *Federal Probation, 59*, 66-75.

Redondo, S., Sanchez-Meca, J., & Garrido, V. (1999). The influence of treatment programs on the recidivism of juvenile and adult offenders: An European meta-analytic review. *Psychology, Crime and Law, 5*, 251-278.

Rothman, D. J. (1980). *Conscience and convenience: The asylum and its alternatives in Progressive America*. Boston: Little, Brown.

Rotman, E. (1995). The failure of reform: United States, 1865-1965. In N. Morris & D. J. Rothman (Eds.), *The Oxford history of the prison: The practice of punishment in Western society* (pp. 169-197). New York: Oxford University Press.

Sampson, R. J., & Laub, J. H. (1993). *Crime in the making: Pathways and turning points through life*. Cambridge, MA: Harvard University Press.

Sampson, R. J., & Laub, J. H. (1995). Understanding variability in lives through time: Contributions of life-course criminology. *Studies in Crime and Crime Prevention, 4*, 143-158.

Schur, E. M. (1973). *Radical nonintervention: Rethinking the delinquency problem*. Englewood Cliffs, NJ: Prentice Hall.

Sechrest, L., White, S. O., & Brown, E. D. (Eds.). (1979). *The rehabilitation of criminal offenders: Problems and prospects*. Washington, DC: National Academy of Sciences.

Sutherland, E. H. (1939). *Principles of criminology* (3rd ed.). Chicago: J. B. Lippincott.

Taft, D. R. (1960). *Criminology* (3rd ed.). New York: Macmillan.

Task Force on Corrections, President's Commission on Law Enforcement and Administration of Justice. (1967). *Task force report: Corrections.* Washington, DC: Government Printing Office.

Taxman, F. S. (1999). Unraveling "what works" for offenders in substance abuse treatment services. *National Drug Court Institute Review, 2,* 93-134.

Toby, J. (1964). Is punishment necessary? *Journal of Criminal Law, Criminology, and Police Science, 55,* 332-337.

Tonry, M. (1995). *Malign neglect: Race, crime, and punishment in America.* New York: Oxford University Press.

Van Voorhis, P. (1987). Correctional effectiveness: The high cost of ignoring success. *Federal Probation, 51,* 59-62.

Welch, M. (1999). *Punishment in America: Social control and the ironies of imprisonment.* Thousand Oaks, CA: Sage.

Whitehead, J. T., & Lab, S. P. (1989). A meta-analysis of juvenile correctional treatment. *Journal of Research in Crime and Delinquency, 26,* 276-295.

Wilson, J. Q., & Herrnstein, R. J. (1985). *Crime and human nature.* New York: Simon & Schuster.

Yoshikawa, H. (1994). Prevention as cumulative protection: Effects of early family support and education on chronic delinquency and its risks. *Psychological Bulletin, 115,* 28-54.

[13]

Psychopathy and therapeutic pessimism Clinical lore or clinical reality?

Randall T. Salekin*

Department of Psychology, University of Alabama, P.O. Box 870348, Tuscaloosa, AL 35487-0348, USA

Received 4 June 1999; received in revised form 6 January 2000; accepted 7 December 2000

Abstract

It is a widely held belief that psychopathic individuals are extremely difficult to treat, if not immune to treatment. This therapeutic pessimism is pervasive and undermines motivation to search for effective modes of intervention for psychopathic individuals. A review of 42 treatment studies on psychopathy revealed that there is little scientific basis for the belief that psychopathy is an untreatable disorder. Three significant problems with regard to the research on the psychopathy–treatment relation cast doubt on strident conclusions that deem the disorder untreatable. First, there is considerable disagreement as to the defining characteristics of psychopathy. Second, the etiology of psychopathy is not well understood. Third, there are relatively few empirical investigations of the psychopathy–treatment relationship and even fewer efforts that follow up psychopathic individuals after treatment. Psychologists are encouraged to investigate the psychopathy–treatment relation from multiple perspectives as well as to conduct long-term follow-up studies to establish a modern view of the psychopathy–treatment relation.

Keywords: Psychopathy; Treatment; Meta-analysis

1. Perspective on psychopathy and treatment: a need for further integration of science and practice?

Clinical lore has led clinicians and researchers to believe that psychopathy is, essentially, an untreatable syndrome. This view is echoed by prominent theorists' claims that the disorder is difficult, if not impossible, to treat (e.g., Cleckley, 1941; Hare, 1991; McCord & McCord,

* Tel.: +1-205-348-6619; fax: +1-205-348-8648.

E-mail address: rsalekin@bama.ua.edu (R.T. Salekin).

1964; Suedfeld & Landon, 1978). In his more recent writings on psychopathy, Cleckley (1981, p. 275) stated that he was "profoundly impressed by two difficulties that stood in the way of dealing effectively with the psychopath. One of these was his apparent immunity, or relative immunity, from control by the law. The other was his lack of response to psychiatric treatment of any kind."

There is no doubt that psychopathy brings a considerable amount of therapeutic frustration, confusion, and pessimism to researchers and clinicians alike (e.g., Greenwald, 1967; Losel, 1998; Ogloff, Wong, & Greenwood, 1990; Rice, 1997). This frustration, however, may have blurred psychologists' perception of important clinical realities and stalled enthusiasm for research pursuits that would have produced and enhanced interventions for this complex clinical problem.

Social policy considerations make the search for effective treatments for psychopathic individuals even more pressing. For instance, continued problems with adult and juvenile offending indicate that untreated offenders will continue to create serious problems for society in both the short and long run. These problems are likely to include violent crimes given that violence, in part, stems from individuals who lack important human characteristics such as empathy and remorse (Hare & Hart, 1993). In fact, recent research efforts have shown that there is a relationship between psychopathy and both general and violent crimes (e.g., Salekin, Rogers, & Sewell, 1996), further emphasizing the need for preventative measures and treatment programs for those most at risk of committing future violent acts.

The purpose of the present article is to identify and characterize the current status of research that exists on psychopathy and treatment, to prompt and guide investigations in this area of investigation, and to encourage future research into the etiology of psychopathy. In order to address these purposes, I (a) briefly discuss problems that exist with classification of psychopathy specifically dealing with terminology and heterogeneity that make work in this area particularly difficult, (b) examine the developmental and etiological theories of psychopathy as they relate to treatment, and (c) present empirical evidence on the treatability of psychopathy in the form of a meta-analysis.

2. Classification of psychopathy

Abundant theoretical and empirical attention has been directed toward understanding the psychopathic personality since Phillippe Pinel first introduced the concept approximately 200 years ago. Most contemporary conceptualizations are linked, at least in part, to the work of Cleckley (1941) and his book *The Mask of Sanity*. Cleckley provided extensive clinical descriptions of the characteristics of psychopathy, which have now received widespread acceptance as typifying the concept of psychopathy.

Although Cleckley's definition of psychopathy was included in the DSM-II, subsequent revisions consisted largely of behavioral-based descriptions such as antisocial personality disorder (APD), conduct disorder (CD), and oppositional defiant disorder (ODD). Changes from primarily personality-based conceptualizations of the disorder to primarily behaviorally based ones were predicated on the notion that behavioral characteristics (e.g., truancy) were more reliably assessed than were personality traits (e.g., empathy) (Cloninger, 1978; Robins,

1978). Over the last two decades, however, researchers and clinicians have stressed that behavioral classifications alone are too narrow (Lilienfeld, 1994) and have emphasized the importance of a personality component to the assessment of psychopathy. As such, many researchers and clinicians have continued to make a distinction between psychopathy and DSM-IV classifications of ODD and CD in children and APD in adults (Frick, 1998; Hare & Hart, 1993).

An important development since Cleckley has been the Psychopathy Checklist (PCL; Hare, 1991). Hare's work on psychopathy with adult offenders has shown that two factors emerge: F_1 indicates the "selfish, callous, and remorseless use of others" and F_2 the "chronically unstable, antisocial, and socially deviant lifestyle." Forth, Kosson, and Hare (1994) have extended this construct to adolescents and Frick and Hare (in press) have extended the construct even further to include children with F_1 representing impulsive/conduct problems and F_2 representing callous/unemotional (CU) traits.

Wide-range utilization of psychopathy as a critical clinical construct for adults as well as the development of adolescent and childhood measures of psychopathy (Forth et al., 1994; Frick & Hare, in press) underscore the importance of reevaluating the clinical belief that psychopathy is an untreatable disorder. There are at least three issues related to classification and its implication for treatment that require highlighting here. First, while psychopathy has received increasing attention from both clinicians and scientists over the last two decades, it is important to note that the definitions of the disorder have drifted from earlier conceptualizations provided by Cleckley and theorists before him (Rogers, 1995). To address this important point more thoroughly, Rogers (1995) has shown that when examining the 16 Cleckley criteria only 7 (approximately half) are similar to the items on Hare's more contemporary classification system for psychopathy. Moreover, only one-third of the PCL-R items represent Cleckley criteria of psychopathy. In other words, although intended to assess the Cleckley psychopath, this more recent conceptualization of psychopathy may not capture important Cleckley criteria, some of which could have a direct impact on the degree to which psychopathy is treatable. For instance, the presence of anxiety at the initiation of therapy has been noted as a positive prognostic sign with adult patients (see Garfield, 1994). Thus, "absence of nervousness," a hallmark of earlier psychopathy definitions may fuel hypotheses that psychopathy is difficult to treat. However, psychopathy definitions not incorporating this item may identify individuals who are more amenable to treatment given that they are capable of experiencing some anxiety prior to, and at the initiation of, psychotherapy.

Second, current measures of psychopathy are polythetic in nature with numerous possible variations. Assessment, therefore, rests on the assumption that the criteria should be accorded equal weight and that any combination of the criteria that exceeds a predetermined cutoff score is sufficient to warrant the diagnosis of psychopathy and presumably a conclusion that the individual is unamenable to treatment. However, it may be that different constellations of psychopathy directly impact amenability to treatment. Frick (1998) has foreshadowed this point by suggesting that children with CU traits may be more difficult to treat than children displaying conduct problems alone although this supposition needs to be empirically investigated.

Third, deviations from traditional theory-based diagnosis (e.g., Cleckley, 1941) to contemporary conceptualizations (e.g., Hare, 1991) may have direct consequences with regard to psychologists' expectations as to the treatability of psychopathy. For example, if psychologists operate from a traditional psychoanalytic orientation, then viewing psychopathy as a treatable disorder may fall outside the set of assumptions that guide that particular paradigm. However, with more contemporary conceptualizations (e.g., Frick, 1998; Newman, 1998) psychologists are less bound by traditional theory and may view the disorder as amenable to intervention.

In summary, given that the concept of psychopathy rests upon the assumption that certain individuals have in common a particular set of behaviors and personality traits, the evolution of the disorder as well as the polythetic nature of many recent assessment measures complicate the thesis that psychopathy is an untreatable disorder. In addition, psychologists' paradigmatic perspective may affect their expectations of the likelihood of successful treatment, which in turn, may affect the degree to which clients see themselves as capable of change.

3. Developmental and etiological theories of psychopathy

Remarkably, theory has often been absent when considering treatment programs for psychological disorders (Kazdin, 1999). In order to shed light on why psychopathy is thought to be recalcitrant to efforts at rehabilitation, etiological literature of psychopathy is briefly reviewed. Developmental and etiological theories of psychopathy will likely provide psychologists with important information as to the treatability of psychopathic individuals.[1]

In this article, 12 developmental theories of psychopathy are briefly reviewed: (a) psychodynamic (Aichorn, 1966; Cleckley, 1941; Draughon, 1977; Redl & Wineman, 1951, 1952), (b) learning and cognitive theories (Eron, 1997; Templeman & Wollersheim, 1979), (c) role-playing (Gough, 1948), (d) sensation-seeking (Quay, 1965), (e) extraversion (Eysenck, 1975, 1981), (f) attachment-based (Bowlby, 1969), (g) Hare's neurological models (Hare, 1970, 1998), (h) response modulation (Newman, 1998), (i) low-fear model (Lykken, 1995), (j) somatic marker (Damasio, 1994), (k) CU temperament (Frick, 1998), and (l) psychopathy constraint (Lynam, 1996, 1997) (see Table 1). The purpose of this section is not to present a detailed review of each of the developmental/etiological theories, but rather to present a brief review of the theory and to (a) evaluate whether the theory is comprehensive (e.g., does the theory account for all the symptoms of psychopathy?), (b) examine whether these theories elucidate treatment difficulties that psychologists experience with psychopathic individuals, and (c) if possible, provide suggestions for where psychologists might best focus their treatment efforts.

3.1. Psychodynamic theory of psychopathy

Psychodynamic theories generally state that psychopathy is a function of poor ego and superego development (e.g., Aichorn, 1966; Draughon, 1977). According to Freud (1961),

[1] Because there are numerous theories of psychopathy, it is beyond the scope of this paper to cover comprehensively all etiological theories. Psychologists investigating the etiology and/or treatment of psychopathy should also investigate the utility of other developmental theories of psychopathy not covered in this review (e.g., Millon, 1990; Patrick, 1994; Schmauk, 1970; Zuckerman, 1995).

the superego, originally part of the ego, breaks off into a separate structure when the Oedipus or Electra complex is resolved. The functions of the superego include self-observation, conscience, and maintenance of the ideal. When the ego does not meet the demands of the superego, guilt is experienced by the individual. The crux of this theory is that psychopathic behavior is the result of childhood problems stemming from adverse child–parent interactions that stunt proper development of the superego. The underdevelopment of the superego is reflected in the child's lack of conscience and an inability to experience guilt (Greenacre, 1945; Johnson & Szurek, 1954).

The notion that psychopathy is untreatable may originate from psychoanalytic theory (Draughon, 1977), which suggests that personality is laid down in the first 5 to 6 years of life with relatively few changes made thereafter. However, more recent theories contend that personality is more malleable than previously believed. For instance, Draughon (1977) has found that an expanded view of the ego and superego allows for their development over a longer period of time and has also suggested that the ego can perform many functions of the superego including regulating emotion, delaying gratification, and reality testing.

Kohut (1982) argued for a movement away from the traditional psychoanalytic personality constructs of id, ego, and superego when conceptualizing psychopathology. Instead of focusing on Freud's structural model of the mind, he contended that dysfunction could be conceptualized as stemming from developmental disruptions in the self-structure. The self-structure is thought to consist of the self and internal representations of significant others. Building on Kohut's reformulations of psychoanalytic theory, Noshpitz (1984) argued that aggression stems from a child's need to protect an overly expansive self-system from harm. One hypothesized pathological variant, the "ruthless–psychopath," is characterized by a need to exploit and intimidate others and to use aggression and violence in an attempt to maintain an inflated sense of self, an illusion of control, and the perception of invulnerability.

The symptoms of psychopathy are accounted for in this theory by poor superego development (e.g., criminal activity, disregard for others) and defense mechanisms (e.g., grandiosity, superficial charm). With regard to treatment, whether utilizing an expanded view of the ego and superego (Draughon, 1977) or Kohut's reformulations of psychoanalytic theory, contemporary theories indicate that psychopathy is a treatable disorder. Strengthening ego or superego functions or improving object relations might be the target of intervention depending upon the psychoanalytic theory utilized. More traditional theories would espouse having the interventions occur within the first 5 years of life. One problem with traditional psychoanalytic theory, if inaccurate, is that it may result in withholding treatment from those beyond the age of 5 or 6 years who might benefit from intervention. An additional concern is that it may inappropriately place blame on the parents of psychopathic youth.

3.2. Learning and cognitive theories of psychopathy

Learning theories of psychopathy purport that the syndrome develops through modeling and conditioning (Bandura, 1973; Eron, 1997; Patterson, Dishion, & Chamberlain, 1993). Eron (1997), as well as Ullman and Krasner (1969), theorized that psychopaths are those who

Table 1
Developmental pathways to psychopathy

Theorist	Developmental pathways to psychopathy								
Damasio (1994)	deficiency in somatic markers	→	inability to form or utilize affective associations	→	psychopathy				
Draughon (1977)	poor ego development	→	infantile emotional level	→	egocentricity	→	poor empathy impulsivity, poor tolerance, poor planning, low self-esteem	→	psychopathy
Eysenck (1975)	cortical underarousal (high extraversion, neuroticism, and psychoticism)	→	impairment in ability to condition to environmental stimuli, especially in learning appropriate fear reactions to punishment	→	poorly conditioned moral and social responses, poorly developed conscience	→	a poorly socialized, neurotic, extravert	→	psychopathy
Frick (1998)	unique temperamental style	→	low behavioral inhibition	→	CU traits	→	conduct problems	→	psychopathy
Gough (1958)	deficiency in role-playing ability	→	poor anticipation comprehension of the role of others	→	lack of empathy, lack of remorse	→	psychopathy		
Hare (1970)	brain lesions	→	loss of inhibitory mechanisms	→	diminished capacity to inhibit and a tendency for perseveratory responses	→	psychopathy		

Hare (1998)	subtle neurological problems	→ increased activation in occipital lobe	→ other neurological difficulties	→ psychopathy		
Lykken (1995)	low fearfulness	→ child insufficiently motivated to avoid punishment	→ difficult to socialize using typical parenting	→ psychopathy		
Lynam (1997)	deficient "psychopathy constraint"	→ difficulty incorporating feedback from the environment and using information to modulate responses while pursuing rewards	→ show signs of HIA complex: exhibit more exploratory behaviors and motor restlessness, does not respond to admonitions, and responds impulsively to rewards	→ mild conduct problems oppositional defiant symptoms. Unable to control temper, arguing, lying, and blaming others for own actions	→ increases in structure (school) result in an appearance of heightened HIA and conduct problems including aggression and disregard for others	→ psychopathy
Newman (1998)	information-processing deficiency	→ failure to accommodate meaning of contextual cues	→ failure of self-regulation	→ psychopathy		
Quay (1965)	hyperactive nervous system	→ stimulation-seeking child	→ behavior aversive to parents/others	→ parental retreat, inconsistency rejection, and hostile detachment	→ fewer effective socializing experiences	→ psychopathy
	hyperactive nervous system	→ poor anticipatory responses to pain	→ early excessive punishment	→ increased resistance to effects of treatment	→ reduced level of stimulus input	→ psychopathy
Ullman and Krasner (1969)	reinforced at the wrong time for wrong things	→ psychopathy				

are reinforced at the wrong time and thus have developed a selective inattention to various social stimuli. In this sense, the lack of emotion in the psychopath is traceable to an early history of desensitization to emotional stimuli. More recently, researchers have introduced learning models based on current thinking in cognitive psychology (e.g., Berkowitz, 1990; Dodge, 1980; Guerra & Slaby, 1990). For example, Dodge (1980) emphasizes the importance of attributional biases. Antisocial children are viewed as having defective cognitive processes for the interpretation of others' behavior and the selection of their own behavior from a previously learned repertoire. Huesmann (1988), on the other hand, views the child as a processor of information who develops programs or scripts to guide their (social) behavior. The antisocial child is one who has developed many aggressive and antisocial scripts and few prosocial ones.

While learning theories are relatively comprehensive, it has not been easy to identify a reinforcement schedule that would consistently result in psychopathy. That is, children under similar conditioning environments often develop along very different pathways. Moreover, the various learning theories have differed in terms of exactly what is learned. Specifically, whether certain behaviors, cue–behavior connections, response biases, beliefs, or scripts are learned. In all cases, however, learning is hypothesized to occur both as a result of one's own behaviors and as a result of viewing others behave. With this perspective, researchers (e.g., Lochman, 1990; Rotenberg, 1975; Templeman & Wollersheim, 1979) have viewed behavioral aspects of psychopathy as treatable. Techniques such as counterconditioning, cognitive restructuring, and modeling may affect change.

3.3. Deficiency in role-playing theory of psychopathy

Gough (1948) formulated a sociological theory of psychopathy that described psychopaths as suffering from a deficiency in role-playing ability. As a result, psychopathic individuals are not able to adequately anticipate the reaction or comprehend the role of others. Because of this lack of understanding for others, the symptoms of psychopathy were purported to result. However, research investigating the role-playing abilities of psychopaths has been equivocal (e.g., Doren, 1987; Smith, 1978; Widom, 1976).

Even if psychopathic individuals are assumed to be deficient in role-playing abilities, Gough's (1948) theory lacks comprehensiveness and clarity. One problem with the theory is that it does not delineate underlying factors that would lead to defective role-playing in psychopaths. Another problem is that commonly listed psychopathic personality features, such as guiltlessness, superficial charm, manipulation, and sensation seeking, are difficult to explicate using Gough's theory. In fact, references in the literature (e.g., Cleckley, 1941) to the psychopath's manipulation, adeptness at telling others what they want to hear, and ability to make a positive impression suggest that psychopathic individuals may have a considerable talent at role-taking as opposed to a serious deficit (Doren, 1987). Any link between psychopathy and resistance to treatment is not apparent from this theory. Psychologists developing treatment programs from this etiological perspective may want to enhance these individuals' ability to take on different roles through in-session role-playing and the use of behavioral rehearsal. However, some psychologists may be concerned about the potential risk of increased manipulation by improving this skill with psychopaths.

3.4. Sensation-seeking theory of psychopathy

Quay (1965) described the psychopathic disorder as a manifestation of excessive sensation-seeking behavior. Quay's theory consists of two facets: (a) psychopaths are characterized by an abnormality in their physiological reaction to sensory input, which requires a higher degree of sensory stimulation in order to obtain satisfaction and (b) because of psychopaths higher optimal level of stimulation, an extremely high degree of motivation is required in order to compensate for their underarousal.

Quay (1977) expanded on this theory to include environmental factors in the development of adult psychopathy. This formulation again stated that the psychopath began life with a hyperactive nervous system that resulted in one of two developmental pathways. The first developmental pathway suggests that children's sensation-seeking behavior becomes aversive to parents resulting in parent–child interactions that are hostile, inconsistent, and rejecting. These negative reactions, in turn, result in an increase in their deviancy, which then leads to more inconsistency and hostility on the part of the parent. According to Quay, an endless cycle of poor interpersonal patterns results in the eventual distancing of parents from their children and this decreases the likelihood that the child will experience any form of positive socialization.

The second developmental pathway suggests that psychopathic children are less able to anticipate physical pain due to an underactive nervous system. Thus, punishment by parents must be at a high level to produce avoidance. However, because of habituation, the child's ability to resist the effects of punishment tends to increase. At the same time, parents withdraw from the child who seems beyond their control. The net result is an undersocialized, sensation-seeking child developing along a pathway to adult psychopathy.

Using Quay's formulation alone, it is unclear why psychopaths would (a) be guiltless, (b) be unable to form meaningful relationships, (c) lack morality, (d) lack insight, and (e) possess superficial charm. In short, Quay's theory focuses on sensation-seeking at the exclusion of other aspects of psychopathy. With regard to treatment, Quay did not view psychopathy as untreatable. In fact, Quay offered two types of treatment for psychopaths based on his theoretical notions. The first suggestion was to utilize psychopharmacology to "increase basal reactivity" or decrease their "rapidity of adaptation to stimuli." The second was to use strong, unconditioned stimuli to condition avoidance reactions in psychopaths, and use strong, unconditioned stimuli coupled with reinforcement to condition appropriate approach reactions from persons exhibiting the psychopathic disorder. Parent training may also benefit children with psychopathy because parents would be able to deal more effectively with this unique temperamental style.

3.5. Extraversion theory of psychopathy

Eysenck (1977) based his theory of psychopathy on his three-dimensional model of personality that included: (a) extraversion, (b) neuroticism, and (c) psychoticism. Eysenck's definition of psychoticism differed from more traditional views of psychosis in that he placed psychopathy on a continuum between normality and psychosis. In this theory, the neuroticism factor was viewed as one that dealt with the strength of emotional reactions. Extraversion was hypothesized to be related to the low baseline arousal state of an individual. Eysenck believed that psychopaths had an underaroused state because of an impairment in their ability to condition to environmental stimuli. According to Eysenck, this impairment is especially relevant to the learning of appropriate fear reactions to environmentally punishing contingencies.

More recently, Eysenck (1981) revised his theory of psychopathy. According to his new model, genetic factors contribute to individual differences in physiological processes (e.g., ascending reticular activating system). These differences in physiological processes drive fundamental psychological processes (e.g., motivation, learning) that result in stable differences in personality (e.g., extraversion–introversion), which ultimately influence a person's social behavior and risk for APD. Within Eysenck's model, the relation between personality and antisocial behavior is mediated by psychosocial processes such as perception, cognition, motivation, and emotion. These processes, in turn, influence learning and social adjustment. Thus, according to this theory, antisocial behavior must be understood in light of a myriad of person by situation interactions that shape an individual's response to the environment.

Similar to the aforementioned theories, Eysenck's theory, does not clearly articulate why psychopaths would (a) be manipulative, (b) be guiltless, (c) lack morality, and (d) possess superficial charm. With regard to treatability, Eysenck's theory suggests that treatment might be hampered by learning and motivational deficits. The extent to which these problems would hamper treatment beyond other psychological disorders (e.g., motivational problems in depressed patients and learning deficits in patients with attention deficit–hyperactivity disorder (ADHD)) is unclear. Because this model of psychopathy is interactional with individuals having a predisposition that is effected by the environment, early intervention from the learning paradigm (e.g., counterconditioning, modeling) may be most effective. In addition, parent training would likely augment treatment.

3.6. Attachment-based theory of psychopathy

Several areas of research suggest that psychopathy may be related to neglect or a particular type of insecure attachment. One of the most compelling sources of evidence comes from the vast research on family histories of youth with psychopathy (e.g., McCord & McCord, 1964). Two bodies of research are relevant in this regard. First, numerous studies have consistently shown that family adversity, most notably low socioeconomic standing, single parenthood, parental psychopathology, and exposure to family violence and aggression is related to the development of psychopathy or the related disorder of CD in youth (Megargee & Golden, 1973; Morretti, Holland, & Peterson, 1994; Schuster, 1976). Second, studies (e.g., Patterson & Yoerger, 1993) have shown a robust relationship between punitive and inconsistent parenting practices and the development of psychopathy and related disorders. Family adversity and punitive and inadequate parenting practices commonly occur together (Rutter, Tizard, & Whitmore, 1970; Webster-Stratton, 1990), giving an overall impression that psychopathy may develop in the context of an impoverished and typically abusive primary socialization experience. As such, these individuals lack the attachment experiences that (a) lead to the development of mental representation that guide behavior and affect over time, (b) function to integrate experience, and (c) increase the likelihood of continuity over the life span.

The attachment-based theory of psychopathy is relatively comprehensive but clearer connections between the poor attachment and why psychopaths tend to be manipulative and possess superficial charm, need to be delineated. With regard to treatability, clearly, if this etiological theory is accurate, then treatment of psychopathic individuals may be possible. Treatment efforts that involve extensive training with parents and children and have an emphasis on reconnecting youth with the community may very well be beneficial to children displaying psychopathic traits.

3.7. Hare's neurological theory of psychopathy

Hare (1970) delineated a perspective on psychopathy, which he termed response perseveration. In this early theory, psychopaths are viewed as having lesions in the limbic system of the brain which affect their ability to inhibit or disrupt ongoing behavior. One hypothesized effect of these lesions was a learning deficiency which made it difficult to inhibit an action that was known to lead to punishment. Hare employed this theory to explain why psychopaths seem unable to learn from punishment and appear to be controlled by their immediate needs. Later, however, Hart, Forth, and Hare (1990) concluded that there exists no demonstrable evidence to support the notion that psychopaths have brain damage. Gale (1973) stated that EEG research, which purportedly demonstrated brain abnormalities in psychopaths, has been ambiguous and, if anything, leans against rather than in favor of the contention that psychopaths have brain lesions.

More recently, Hare (1998) suggested that there may be a more subtle neurological basis for psychopathy. In a neurological imaging study of psychopathic individuals with substance abuse disorders, psychopaths exhibited less anterior activation during processing of the neutral and emotional tasks than did nonpsychopaths (Intrator, Hare, Stritzke, Brichstwein, et al., 1997). Moreover, activation was less widespread in psychopaths than nonpsychopaths. For psychopaths, the greatest activation was in the occipital cortex. However, these findings are tempered by the fact that psychopaths differed less from other patient groups than controls suggesting that at least part of the pattern of activation of psychopaths was related to substance abuse.

Hare's early theory of psychopathy fails to account for some of the hallmarks of this syndrome such as superficial charm and manipulation. Given the lack of clarity with regard to psychopathy, brain organization, and neurochemistry it is difficult to critically evaluate Hare's more recent theory for two reasons: (a) it is exploratory and (b) it is incomplete. However, one criticism of Hare's theory is that it may be too reductionistic and fail to explain the intricacies of psychopathy. From a treatment perspective, it is important to note that with the advances in pharmacotherapy, irregularities in neurotransmission can be altered. Moreover, although tentative, Vaughan (1997) has suggested that there may be some evidence for the notion that neurochemistry and brain organization can be altered via psychotherapy. In this regard, both pharmacotherapy and psychotherapy may be worthy of further investigation with this syndrome.

3.8. Response modulation model of psychopathy

Newman and his colleagues have conducted a series of rigorous laboratory studies that indicate that psychopathic individuals may have a form of disinhibitory psychopathology that includes difficulty in passive avoidance learning (Newman & Kosson, 1986; Newman,

Patterson, Howland, & Nichols, 1990; Newman, Widom, & Nathan, 1985), inhibition of well-established dominant responses (Howland, Kosson, Patterson, & Newman, 1993), and poor response modulation (Newman, Patterson, & Kosson, 1987). According to Newman (1998), children at risk for psychopathy suffer from an information-processing deficit that interferes with effective self-regulation. Parental and societal failure to appreciate the existence of this problem and our consequent reactions to the child's behavior compound the risk of psychopathy. Newman's work has been fueled by earlier work on disinhibition conducted by Fowles (1980) and Gray (1987).

The response modulation hypothesis of psychopathy, although intriguing, does not readily account for some practitioners and researchers beliefs about psychopaths ability to plot, manipulate, take on different roles, and display superficial charm to meet their needs. In this way, the theory is not yet comprehensive. If Newman's theory is accurate, then treatment may be hampered by psychopathic individuals' information-processing deficit. It is important to note, however, that Newman has not suggested that a diagnosis of psychopathy would equate to the disorder being unamenable to treatment. In fact, he has suggested that informing psychopaths of their deficit may be the first step toward change. While Newman's theory would indicate that there would be challenges to the treatment of psychopathy it does not lead to the conclusion that psychopathy is treatment refractory.

3.9. Low-fear model of psychopathy

Lykken (1995) posits that the psychopath has an attenuated experience of anxiety and fear. Because of this below average endowment of innate fearfulness, psychopaths are more difficult to socialize using typical parenting methods that rely on a child being motivated to avoid punishment. Lykken's (1957) classic investigation of psychopathy and anxiety used a measure of passive avoidance learning to evaluate the low fearfulness hypothesis. He found that, in general, psychopaths were less fearful of receiving a shock than were nonpsychopaths.

Lykken's theory of psychopathy is relatively comprehensive but clearer connections among low fearfulness and manipulation and superficial charm require delineation. Overall, Lykken's theory is compelling given that most symptoms of psychopathy (Cleckley, 1941; Hare, 1991) can be accounted for with this hypothesis. While Lykken has suggested that there is a genotype for psychopathy, he also sees the development of psychopathy as being highly dependent upon socialization and parenting. Thus, according to Lykken, if parental competence is high, the development of psychopathy is avoidable. Extrapolating from this conclusion, psychotherapy might very well help augment and facilitate parental attempts to socialize children.

3.10. Somatic marker model of psychopathy

A recent theoretical perspective for psychopathy is Damasio's (1994) somatic marker hypothesis. The concept of somatic markers refers to affect-related associations that come to be related with particular stimuli and responses. According to Damasio, somatic markers are created in our brains during the process of socialization and education by connecting specific classes of stimuli with specific classes of somatic state. Once formed, somatic markers facilitate decision-making and behavioral regulation by calling to mind the positively or negatively valenced outcomes that have been associated with particular situations or followed particular responses. Referring to their role in avoidance learning, Damasio stated that a somatic marker functions as an "automated alarm signal" that warns individuals of danger. According to Damasio, whereas normal individuals have a nonconscious process formulating future events or outcomes for a given situation, psychopaths are unable to use punishment or reward to contribute to the automated marking for prediction of future outcomes. Thus, psychopaths have a generalized deficit in the formation and/or utilization of affective associations.

While Damasio's (1994) formulation offers some interesting new theoretical insights into the etiology of psychopathy, it does not adequately account for why psychopaths would (a) con others, (b) be grandiose, and (c) possess superficial charm. Also, this etiological perspective does not explain the belief that psychopathy is an untreatable disorder. For instance other disorders, such as major depression and schizophrenia could also be explained by this theory but are not considered unamenable to treatment. Efforts at enhancing psychopathic individuals' associations between specific classes of stimuli with specific classes of somatic state would be the first step in treating psychopathy from Damasio's etiological perspective.

3.11. Callous/unemotional temperament in children

Frick (1998) has proposed that psychopathy (a) is more etiologically homogeneous than CD and (b) has one causal pathway to conduct problems. CU traits (e.g., absence of empathy, a lack of guilt) are considered to develop as a function of a unique temperamental style and low behavioral inhibition that make a child more difficult to socialize (Frick & Jackson, 1993; Kochanska, 1993). Once they develop, CU traits make a child more likely to act against parental and societal norms and to violate the rights of others. Frick's theory is intriguing and helps to integrate diverse findings from previous research on the etiology of psychopathy. Importantly, the theory addresses directionality suggesting that parents may be reacting to children who are problematic and difficult to satisfy based on a genetic predisposition. Although Frick has suggested that CU traits may be more resistant to treatment than conduct problems, his theory also suggests that there is an important interaction between parents and children that can facilitate prosocial behavior. Frick's theory is relatively comprehensive and suggests that parental training and child psychotherapy in combination may be warranted to prevent the development of psychopathy.

3.12. Psychopathy constraint model

According to Lynam (1996), "fledgling psychopaths" are found to have a combination of hyperactivity–impulsivity–attention (HIA) and conduct problems from an early age. He has suggested that youth show similar deficits on similar laboratory, psychophysiological, and performance measures to that of adults. For example, Lynam suggests that poor passive avoidance seen in adult psychopaths (Lykken, 1995) is common in children with HIA. In addition, Lynam has drawn similarities between cortical underarousal, frontal lobe deficits, and response modulation in adult psychopaths to that of children with HIA.

Lynam (1996) suggests that psychopathic individuals begin life with a deficiency in constraint (he calls this psychopathic constraint), which hampers their ability to incorporate feedback from the environment and to use this information to modulate responses while pursuing rewards. Because of this lack in "psychopathic constraint," they show signs of HIA. As these individuals age and become more mobile and verbal, and as goal-directed behavior is frequently frustrated by parents, the deficit in constraint leads to mild CD or ODD symptoms. Lynam suggests that this deficit in psychopathic constraint leads to an inability to pause and empathize with others or to feel remorse and guilt and that ultimately these deficits result in psychopathy.

Lynam's theory of psychopathy is compelling but has similar shortcomings to theories previously mentioned when it comes to accounting for the symptomology of psychopathy. Symptom such as superficial charm and manipulation would suggest that psychopathic individuals might be extremely effective at emotion regulation as opposed to having symptoms of hyperactivity and inattention. If, however, this theory for psychopathy is accurate, then approaches designed to treat ADHD in children may be indicated as a first step in the treatment of psychopathic youth. Then, behavioral and parent training may have a beneficial effect on CD or ODD symptoms.

4. General comments on the etiology of psychopathy

As with many psychological disorders, the etiology of psychopathy is not well known. Developmental and etiological theories of psychopathy provide some information as to why psychopathy may be viewed as untreatable (e.g., deficit in their ability to condition); they do not, however, provide strong support for clinical lore that contends psychopaths are unamenable to treatment. In fact, recent compelling theories by Frick (1998), Lykken (1995), Lynam (1997), and Newman (1998) suggest that the better we understand the etiology of psychopathy, the higher the likelihood of developing effective treatments become.

Nine of the twelve theories reviewed in the foregoing suggest that there is a predisposition for psychopathy whether it be a unique temperamental style (Frick, 1998), a deficiency in somatic markers (Damasio, 1994), low fearfulness (Lykken, 1995), a deficiency in psychopathy constraint (Lynam, 1997), or some other deficit. The three remaining theories (psychodynamic, cognitive–behavioral, and attachment based) suggest that psychopathy develops in children through a specific set of environmental conditions (e.g., poor attachment due to maltreatment). It is possible that psychopathy develops in different ways for different individuals with some individuals having a predisposition, others developing the condition through harsh environments, and still others through the interaction between temperament and environment. In fact, Lykken (1995) has suggested that this is the case and that the prevalence of "sociopathy" is increasing among the group that develops this condition primarily from the environment.

An important point from the aforementioned research is that a style in temperament (or a deficit in learning) does not necessitate that the disorder is untreatable. In fact, of the theorists who suggest there may be a temperamental style to psychopathy, none have purported that the disorder is untreatable (Frick, 1998; Lykken, 1995, Lynam, 1997; Newman, 1998). The theories proposed in the foregoing suggest that even individuals with a particular temperamental style interact with parents, peers, and society in ways that can either foster detachment and aggression or attachment and prosocial behavior in such youth. It may be that considerably more treatment effort is needed for those individuals highest at risk.

To this point in the article, two problems (classification and etiology of psychopathy) have been reviewed, which suggest that the clinical belief that psychopathy is untreatable or extremely difficult to treat is either complicated or not well supported by the available evidence. The next logical step is to examine the treatment studies of psychopathy to determine whether or not interventions attempted in the past have been successful. In the following section, I present research that specifically examines the treatability of psychopathy.

5. Review of studies investigating the psychopathy–treatment relation

Previous researchers have rendered conclusions about the treatability of psychopathy based on clinical lore or their readings of the literature (e.g., Gacono, Nieberding, Owen, Rubel & Bodholt, 2001; Losel, 1998; Suedfeld & Landon, 1978). Unfortunately, this type of summary does not provide an overall comparison between theoretical orientations/techniques nor does it report quantitatively the magnitude of the outcome. The present investigation provides an integration of existing research on the relation between psychopathy and treatment. To this end, meta-analysis was employed to estimate the magnitude of the relationship between treatment and outcome. Also examined were the various theoretical orientations and their approach to the treatment of psychopathy and their reported outcome. An important aspect of the study was to evaluate whether treatment studies were aligned with developmental theories of psychopathy. This meta-analytic review of the effectiveness of intervention methods for psychopathy is unique in that no previous review has summarized quantitatively such a comprehensive database for the psychopathy–treatment relation.

5.1. Compilation of psychopathy and treatment studies

A computerized search was performed to locate all studies that examined the psychopathy–treatment relationship. Articles that examined treatment outcome of psychopathy were of interest. The search was limited to psychopathy and not related disorders (e.g., APD, CD, ODD). Search procedures included use of the PsychLIT database, an examination of previous reviews of the literature, and the reference sections of individual studies and chapters. The last year of specialized journals that might address the issue of psychopathy and treatment that were too recent to be included in computer databases were also reviewed (i.e., *American Journal of Psychotherapy, American Psychologist, Clinical Psychology: Science and Practice, Clinical Psychology Review, International Journal of Offender Therapy, Journal of Clinical Psychology, Journal of the American Academy of Psychiatry and the Law, Journal of Consulting and Clinical Psychology, Journal of Forensic Psychiatry, Law and Human Behavior, Psychological Bulletin, Psychotherapy: Theory, Research, and Practice*). These search procedures yielded 42 published investigations with 44 samples and 43 effect sizes on treatment outcome.

5.2. Calculation of effect sizes

Meta-analytic studies employ different, although closely related, quantitative procedures. Because few studies have been conducted on psychopathy and treatment, the current study did not restrict the review to designs utilizing only control groups nor did it exclude case studies. One limitation of the current study was that not all studies utilized control groups. According to Hunter (1990), this limitation in individual studies can be circumvented in a meta-analysis because the control group for one intervention study can serve as a control group for other intervention studies that do not have control groups. Control groups are used to estimate the success rate without any treatment. Thus, the "treatment" is the same across all studies (i.e., no treatment), and findings for studies that include control groups can be generalized to studies that do not. The control group figure used should represent the average across all studies with control groups. Meta-analysts (e.g., Hunter, 1990; Hunter & Schmidt, 1990) state that a meta-analysis of the results from all available control groups provides a better benchmark to evaluate any intervention than does the control group from any one particular study because the idiosyncracies of the individual control groups are averaged out. Therefore, in the current meta-analysis, eight control group samples were meta-analyzed together to obtain a more robust and reliable estimate of the average reduction in psychopathic traits/behavior without any intervention. The resulting mean was then compared to the mean success rates for different interventions for psychopathy, thereby allowing estimates of "net" success rates.

In the present study, proportions of treatment success were cumulated. Available from each study were the sample sizes (n_i) used and the proportion who improved from psychotherapy (P_i). The mean success rate ($\bar{p}$) was computed as $\sum n_i P_i / \sum n_i$ and the observed variance is given as $\sum n_i (P_i - \bar{p})^2 / \sum n_i$. Thus, for each intervention method, the sample size-weighted mean and the sample size-weighted variance of success rates were obtained. The formula for sampling error variance of proportions was obtained from standard statistical textbooks as $P_i Q_i / n_i$, where $Q_i = 1 - P_i$. A sample-weighted mean of the sampling error variance of proportions to be cumulated was then obtained as $(\sum n_i P_i Q_i / \sum n_i) / \sum n_i = \sum P_i Q_i / \sum n_i$. This sample-weighted mean sampling error variance was then subtracted from the observed variance, yielding an estimate of the true variance plus variance due to other artifacts, such as unreliability (Hunter & Schmidt, 1990), that could not be corrected for. Lacking any information about other artifacts, it can be assumed that the true variance estimate is an upper bound value on the real variability of the effectiveness of an intervention method. Also calculated were effect sizes based on the formula from Rosenthal (1991) for proportions: $d' = P_{tx} - P_c$ where P_{tx} is the proportion of patient who benefited from psychotherapy and P_c is the proportion of patients who benefited without any formal treatment.

5.3. "File-drawer" analysis

Rosenthal's (1991) prescription for estimate of the number of unreported nonsignificant studies needed to reduce the current meta-analytic results to a significance of $P=.05$ or higher was utilized. This estimate is referred to as the "file-drawer" statistic, as these results languish unreported in various academic file-drawers. The following formula was used: $X = K(KZ_P^2 - 2.706)/2.706$ where K is the number of studies included in the analysis, Z_P is the mean of standard normal deviates of P for the studies analyzed, and X is the number of unpublished null studies needed to reduce the overall significance to $P = .05$ or less. The algebraic derivation of this formula results in the use of 2.706, the square of 1.645, the Z for $P = .05$.

6. Results

A total of 42 studies on the treatment of psychopathy were compiled and yielded information about outcome for those who were treated for a psychopathic condition. The results from individual studies are presented in Table 2. The overall proportion of successful intervention for all treatment studies was .62 ($P < .01$). This number remained virtually the same when case studies were dropped from the analysis (.60). File-drawer analyses for the overall sample determined that 160 studies (almost four times the amount of studies reported in this review) with null results would be required to reduce the significance level of this finding to $P = .05$.

Most studies presented in this meta-analysis approached the treatment of psychopathy from a psychoanalytic orientation. Many of the studies (52%) conceptualized psychopathy from a Clecklian perspective and only four studies (9%) utilized the more contemporary conceptualization put forth by Hare (1991). Four other studies (9%) used Craft's conceptualization and two studies (4%) utilized Partridge's conceptualization. For 11 studies (26%), the conceptualization of psychopathy was not specified or was the only study that utilized a particular conceptualization (e.g., So scale of the California Personality Inventory; Gough, 1997). Although some studies did not specify the conceptualization utilized, most studies had hallmark psychopathic traits of psychopathy as described by Cleckley (1941). The average age of psychopathic individuals being treated was 22.38 and most were males (91%).

As can been seen in Table 2, a variety of treatment methods have been employed for psychopathic individuals ranging from electroconvulsive therapy (ECT; Cleckley & Beard, 1942) to psychodrama (Corsini, 1958) to traditional psychoanalysis (Schmideberg, 1978). Interestingly, when group psychotherapy was combined with individual psychotherapy the proportion of patients that improved was relatively high (81%). Also, the inclusion of family members in treatment programs appeared to increase the proportion of patients who improved (75%). Intensive individual psychotherapy (on average four sessions per week for 1 year or longer) had a highly successful treatment rate (91%). The success rates in column 10 of Table 2 provide a basis for comparing across the individual studies. Studies for which proportions could not be obtained were also included in Table 2 and provide descriptive information about the effectiveness of a given approach to the treatment of psychopathy.

6.1. Average success rates

In addition to providing information across individual studies, the mean success rates in column 4 of Table 3 provide a basis for comparison across the intervention methods. Values

Table 2
Effects of treatment for psychopathic personalities for 42 studies

Author	Orientation	Psychopathy conceptualization	*n*	Age	Gender	Frequency/ duration	Parent/ group	Outcome	*p*	*d'*
Beacher (1962)	psychoanalytic	Cleckley	1	29.0	m	2/18 mo	G	less hostile, more social, improved internalized value system, less grandiose, improved communication skills	1.00	.80
Berman (1964)	psychoanalytic	Cleckley	1	18.0	m	3/26 mo	P[m]	warmer to family members, more productive (started working), court reports that patients behavior has been good and was released from probation, improved relationships, long-term follow-up found patient to be in graduate school	1.00	.80
Borriello (1979)	psychoanalytic	Cleckley	4	a	m	–	G[o]	gained insight, less manipulative, internalized new value system, decreased acting out behaviors, improved perspective taking	1.00	.80
Butterworth (1951)	psychoanalytic	Cleckley	1	28.0	m	5/12 mo	N	improved ability to provide economic support for self (started work), improved planning abilities	1.00	.80
Chrzanowski (1965)	psychoanalytic	Cleckley	2	–	m	–	F	one terminated prematurely with having made no progress, a second case reported to be making progress	.50	.30
Chwast (1961)	psychoanalytic	Cleckley	10	20.5	8m/2 f	1/6 mo	N	five dropped prematurely, five improved social relations	.50	.30

Cleckley & Beard (1942)	ECT	Cleckley	6	–	–	3/0.5 mo	N	three patients no change, three limited data	.00	−.20
Copas, O'Brien, Roberts, and Whiteley (1984)	therapeutic community	Cleckley	37	26.5	m/f	7/>0.5 mo	G	reduction in subsequent criminal convictions and psychiatric hospitalizations	.60	.40
Copas and Whiteley (1976)	therapeutic community	Cleckley	87	a	m	–	G°	did not reoffend	.47	.27
Corsini (1958)	psychodrama	Cleckley	1	15.0	m	?/8 mo	G	less destructive, respectful of others, significant drop in reprimands, adopted social norms, school work improved, respectful	1.00	.80
Craft (1968)	cognitive–behavioral	Craft	94	19.2	m	3/11.1 mo	G	success in treatment was based on offense rates	.63	.43
	cognitive–behavioral	Craft	92	18.3	m	2/9.1 mo	G	success in treatment was based on offense rates	.43	.23
Craft, Stephenson, and Granger (1964)	cognitive–behavioral	Craft	23	19.0	m	7/12 mo	G	clinical improvement improved work records	.83	.63
	therapeutic community	Craft	21	19.0	m	3/12 mo	G	clinical improvement improved work records	.67	.47
Darling (1945)	ECT	Cleckley	3	20.7	m	–	N	drop in violent behavior, less hostility, increased stability	.66	.46
Ellis (1961)	rational therapy	Cleckley	1	25.0	m	1/12 mo	N	stopped antisocial behavior	1.00	.80
Glaus (1968)	cognitive–behavioral	Cleckley	3	a	m	–/>12 mo	–	increased stability	1.00	.80
Heaver (1943)	psychoanalytic	Cheney	40	28.7	m	7/3.85 mo	G	conformed with societies expectations	.40	.20
Henderson (1972)	psychoanalytic	DSM-II/Cleckley	3	–	m	1/–	G	not reported	–	–
Humphreys (1940)	psychoanalytic	Hendersen	3	30.7	m	–	N	no improvement	.00	−.20
Ingram, Gerard, Quay, and Levinson (1970)	action-oriented	Quay	20	y	m	7/6 mo	G	decrease in institutional aggressive behavior	.75	.55
								overall improved adjustment in community	1.00	.80

Table 2 *(continued)*

Author	Orientation	Psychopathy conceptualization	*n*	Age	Gender	Frequency/ duration	Parent/ group	Outcome	*p*	*d*
Kiger (1967)	therapeutic community	Cleckley	100	–	m/f	5/3 mo	G	better able to handle feelings about authority, less impulsive, more giving, increased self-respect, responsible, less need to control, less blaming	–	–
Korey (1944)	pharmacotherapy, Benzedrine sulfate	Cleckley	6	16.0	m	20 mg qd/1 mo	N	increased work effort/efficacy, accelerated school performance, increased sociability, decreased number of misconducts, more temperate	.57	.37
Kristiansson (1995)	pharmacotherapy (lithium or SSRI) and cognitive behavioral	Hare-PCL-R	4	41.5	m	–	N	improved socially and behaviorally	1.00	.80
Maas (1966)	personal construct	Gough	46	25.0	f	2/3.3 mo	G	significant decrease in sociopathy scores	.63	.43
Miles (1969)	therapeutic community	Cleckley	40	21.7	m	7/12 mo	G	improvement in ability to communicate and solve problems, improved empathy more social	.65	.45
Noshpitz (1984)	psychoanalytic	Cleckley	5	14.0	2m/3f	3/6–16 mo	G	patients were able to experience guilt and anxiety, decrease in aggressive behavior	1.00	.80
Ogloff et al. (1990)	therapeutic community	Hare-PCL-R	21	26.9	m	5/3.3 mo	N	"slight" improvement in treatment and "slight" no motivation for treatment	.16	−.04
Partridge (1928)	not specified	Partridge	6	29.7	3m/3f	–	–	more productive, more cooperative	.17	−.03
Persons (1965)	eclectic	Applezweig	12	22.0	m	2/2.5 mo	N	lower sociopathy scores on two measures, significant decrease in disciplinary reports issued by correctional officers	.92	.72

Reiss, Grubin, and Meux (1996)	eclectic	Legal	40	19.2	m	5/4.6 years	G	improvement in social activity/relations	.89	.69
		Hare-PCL-R						did not offend, PCL-R scores were not related to offending	.80	.69
Rice, Harris, and Cormier (1992)	therapeutic community	Hare-PCL-R	46	23.4	m	7/ ≥ 24 mo	G°	did not recidivate violently, treatment group had a 78% violent recidivism rate while the control group had only a 55% violent recidivism rate indicating a reverse effect	.22	.02
Sandhu (1970)	therapeutic community	Cleckley	18	a	m	7/9 mo	G°	improved attitude to work, improved conduct in prison	.72	.52
Savitt (1940)	psychoanalytic	Cheney	2	15.0	m	7/0.75 mo	P^{mf}	moderate improvement	1.00	.80
Schmideberg (1947)	psychoanalytic	not specified	2	–	m	–	N	unclear	–	–
Schmideberg (1978)	psychoanalytic	Cleckley	1	16.5	m	5/10 mo	N	increase in ability to experience guilt, started work, began to develop career plans, increase in social relations with meaningful relationships	1.00	.80
Skolnick and Zuckerman (1979)	therapeutic community	MMPI-Pd	59	–	m	5/7 mo	G	no change in Pd scores, decrease in sensation-seeking	.00	−.20
Sturup (1948)	psychotherapy castration (for sex offenders)	not specified	300	–	m	–	–	normal life in the community	.55	.35
Szurek (1942)	psychoanalytic	Partridge	1	8.0	m	7/6 mo	P^{m}	increase in concern for others, progressive increase in attention span, interest in school work, decrease in destructive behavior, hyperactivity, and erratic behaviors, more consistent concern about the rights of others	1.00	.80
Thorne (1959)	psychoanalytic	Thorne/Cleckley	7	–	m	–/1–10 years	N	less sociopathic/more honest	1.00	.80

Table 2 *(continued)*

Author	Orientation	Psychopathy conceptualization	*n*	Age	Gender	Frequency/ duration	Parent/ group	Outcome	*p*	*d*'
Vaillant (1975)	psychoanalytic	Cleckley	4	27.5	2m/2f	1/12 mo	P	less sociopathic	1.00	.80
Whitaker and Burdy (1969)	psychoanalytic	not specified	1	–	f	1/6 mo	P	no improvement	.00	–.20
Whiteley (1970)	therapeutic community	Whiteley	122	25.0	m	7/4 mo	G	high drop-out rate (87%), did not offend	.65	.45
Woody, McLellen, Rubersky, and O'Brien (1985)	cognitive–behavioral/ supportive–expressive	RDC	30	a	m	25 sessions	N	improvement in employment, less drug and alcohol use, drop in legal problems	.80	.60
	Psychodynamic	Cleckley	1308	22.3	m	4/12.3 mo	G	less sociopathic	.62	.48

RDC = Research Diagnostic Criteria for APD; m = male; mo = months; Parent/group = either the parent or the psychopathic individual was receiving treatment in a group signified by P = parent received psychotherapy along with the youth; G = patient also participated in group psychotherapy; Go = group therapy only usually in the form of a therapeutic community; N = neither the parents were treated nor did the youth participate in group psychotherapy. ES = effect size that is signified by the proportion of patients who benefited from psychotherapy. – = not reported. Where age was not provided we used "y" for children and adolescents and "a" for adults.

ranged from .22 for ECT to 1.00 for rational therapy, psychodrama, and personal construct therapy. ECT had no therapeutic effect on psychopathic individuals; the average success rate was approximately equal to that of the control sample (.20). Although rational therapy, psychodrama, and personal construct therapy were found to be effective modes of treatment for psychopathy, any optimism is tempered by the fact that these findings were based on single case studies.

A surprising finding was that psychoanalytic therapy appeared to be effective in the treatment of psychopathy. The average success rate was 59% based on 17 studies and 88 psychopathic individuals. These studies (e.g., Beacher, 1962; Berman, 1964; Chwast, 1961; Henderson, 1972; Humphreys, 1940; Noshpitz, 1984; Schmideberg, 1947, 1978; Szurek, 1942; Thorne, 1959; Vaillant, 1975) found that following psychoanalytic psychotherapy psychopathic individuals ranging widely in age (8 to 55 years) and across genders improved. This finding was surprising given that many early psychoanalytic therapists believed that personality remained relatively stable after the first 5–6 years of life. This finding indicates that insight-oriented therapies may decrease psychopathic traits and that psychopathic individuals gained some awareness of their general approach to life through this therapeutic approach.

Cognitive–behavioral therapies had a success rate of 62% suggesting that this approach might be slightly more effective than psychoanalytic therapies although the difference between the two perspectives is minuscule (3%). The average success rate for cognitive–behavioral therapies was a robust finding given that it was based on 5 studies and 246 psychopathic individuals. Cognitive–behavioral therapies may have been effective because they often addressed patients' thoughts about themselves, others, and society. Thus, they tended to directly treat some psychopathic traits. Eclectic therapies that often included a combination of both cognitive–behavioral techniques and insight-oriented approaches were also highly effective. The average success rate based on this method of psychotherapy was 86% suggesting that augmenting cognitive–behavioral therapies with insight therapies and other psychotherapeutic techniques may be optimal for the treatment of psychopathic individuals.

Therapeutic communities were the least effective methods for treating psychopathy with an average success rate of 25%. This success rate was based on 8 studies and 372 psychopathic individuals. Again, this rate of success was only slightly greater than that of the control group (20%). This finding is not particularly surprising. Although therapeutic communities have often been utilized for the treatment of psychopathic individuals the programs are not designed to target psychopathic symptomatology. Therapeutic community programs tended to have little psychologist–patient contact. This factor may have had a direct impact on the effectiveness of these programs. In fact, this issue was raised by Warren (1994) to explain the variance across therapeutic community treatment outcome studies.

A treatment program specifically designed by Ingram et al. (1970) to address psychopathic symptomatology in youth demonstrated a high success rate (88%). Unlike therapeutic communities, the Ingram et al. treatment program was designed specifically for psychopathic youth and they selected staff based on their training and ability to deal with psychopathic youth. The program was based on the sensation-seeking model and as such kept youth interested in treatment. These two factors may, in part, account for the success of this treatment program.

Two very small-scaled studies utilized pharmacotherapy to target psychopathic traits and behaviors. The average success rate for these studies was 70%. However, it should be noted that one study (Kristiansson, 1995) combined cognitive–behavioral therapy with pharmacotherapy (either the use of lithium or an SSRI). This study had an average success rate of 100% but this was found for a small sample of only four psychopathic individuals. The second study (Korey, 1944), consisted of six adolescents who received Benzedrine sulfate. The average success rate for this group was 57%. Because of the very small sample sizes utilized in these two studies and the use of cognitive–behavioral therapy in one study, the effectiveness of pharmacotherapy for the treatment of psychopathy requires further study.

Several other approaches were reviewed but many consist of only a single study and sometimes these involved only a single psychopathic individual. While these studies are important to include in a review such as this, the conclusions that can be drawn from them are minimal. At best, they may be utilized to spur further research in that area. These studies (e.g., rational emotive therapy; Ellis, 1961) are depicted in Tables 2 and 3.

The success rate of the control group indicates the percentage of psychopathic individuals who had a decrease in psychopathic traits/behaviors without any intervention. The present analysis included eight control groups, with a total sample of 287, indicated that 19.8% of psychopathic individuals showed improvement over time without any intervention. To determine the net effectiveness of the intervention methods in Tables 2 and 3, 20 percentage points must be subtracted from each success rate. Adjustments produce larger percentage reductions for some interventions than others. For example, the for the cognitive–behavioral interventions, the adjustment is $.62-.20=.42$, a 32% reduction, whereas for therapeutic communities, the adjustment is $.23-.20=.03$, an 87% reduction. Thus, the control group adjustment changes the ratios of success rates. For example, the net effectiveness of cognitive–behavioral interventions is 14 times greater than that of therapeutic communities. But for unadjusted success rates, cognitive–behavioral therapies would be found to be only 2.7 times greater than that of therapeutic communities. Therefore, in comparing relative success rates, the control group adjustment is very important. Moreover, as can be seen for therapeutic communities, such an adjustment has important implications for the absolute value of the intervention; the net effectiveness of therapeutic communities is nearly zero. Table 2 provides d' effect sizes for all treatment studies that calculates the aforementioned adjustments.

6.2. *Tests of possible moderator effects*

In order to test for the presence of moderator effects, the classification of psychopathy (e.g., Cleckley, Hare-PCL-R), patient age, and treatment duration were examined to determine if they had an impact on treatment outcome results. Table 4 summarizes the effect size estimates for all analyses reported below. Cautious interpretation of moderator effects are warranted given that the number of samples is small. Future research will be needed to conclusively clarify these differences.

Table 3
Meta-analysis results for psychopathy intervention studies

Type of psychotherapy	Number of studies	Total sample	Mean p (success rate)	Observed variance	Sampling error variance	Percent variance accounted for	Corrected S.D.[a]	80% credibility interval[b]
1. Psychoanalytic	17	88	0.59	.0879	.0089	10.1	.17	.34–.84
2. Cognitive–behavioral	5	246	0.62	.0238	.0026	10.9	.03	.58–.66
3. Therapeutic communities	8	371	0.25	.1768	.0035	1.9	.06	.17–.33
4. Actional procedures	1	20	0.88	–	.0053	–	–	–
5. Eclectic	2	62	0.86	.0024	.0036	100.0	.01	.85–.87
6. Pharmacotherapy (2)[c]	2	10	0.70	.0461	.0245	53.1	.10	.55–.85
7. ECT	2	9	0.22	.1789	.0242	13.5	.17	–.03–.47
8. Personal construct	1	46	1.00	–	–	–	–	–
9. Rational therapy	1	1	1.00	–	–	–	–	–
10. Psychodrama	1	1	1.00	–	–	–	–	–
11. Not specified	1	6	0.17	–	.0235	–	–	–
12. Control	8	287	0.20	.0428	.0038	8.8	.04	.18–.29

– = unable to calculate because statistics are based on a single or few cases.

[a] Standard deviation of success rates after the effects of sampling error have been eliminated.

[b] The 80th credibility interval values indicate the range of proportions after the extreme 10% of values on either side of the mean have been eliminated from the distribution.

[c] Meta-analysis results when studies in those categories are combined.

Table 4
Examination of potential moderators of effect

Moderator	Proportion	Number of samples
Classification		
Cleckley	$.88_a$	19
Hare-PCL-R	$.57_b$	4
Craft	$.64_b$	4
Partridge	$.59_b$	2
Other	$.56_b$	11
Age of psychopath		
Youth	$.96_a$	8
Adult	$.63_b$	33
Duration of psychotherapy		
<6 months	$.61_a$	10
≥ 6 months	$.77_a$	23
>12 months	$.91_b$	12

Proportions with different subscripts differ significantly from each other within categories. These differences are based on small sample sizes and replication will be necessary in the future.

6.2.1. *Classification of psychopathy*

All samples were grouped according to classification type: Cleckley ($n=22$), Hare-PCL-R ($n=4$), Craft ($n=4$), Partridge ($n=2$), and other ($n=11$). Treatment outcome studies showed that psychotherapy was more effective with psychopaths defined by Cleckley criteria (.88) than those individuals meeting Hare-PCL-R (.57), Craft (.64), or Partridge (.59) criteria. Craft psychopaths also benefited from treatment to a greater degree than any of the other conceptualizations with the exception of Cleckley (1941). Differences in the types of treatment provided for the differing conceptualizations limit these findings and suggest that further research is needed in this area. Interestingly, no matter which way psychopathy was defined all classifications showed some benefit from treatment.

6.2.2. *Age of psychopathic individual*

Studies were also coded for subject age: youth ($n=8$), and adults ($n=22$). The results revealed that a greater proportion of psychopathic youth benefited from psychotherapy than did adults. The proportion of youth (.96) that benefited from treatment was substantially higher than the proportion of adults (.63) that benefited from treatment. Yet, treatment appeared to be effective for both.

6.2.3. *Duration of psychotherapy*

Studies were classified based on the duration of psychotherapy: short term (<6 months) and long term (≥ 6 months). If treatment lasted less than 6 months, then psychopathic individuals were less likely to benefit from treatment than if they participated in treatment that lasted longer than 6 months. If the treatment lasted for a year or longer, 91% of the psychopathic individuals were found to have benefited from treatment (on average these individuals met four times a week with a mental health professional).

7. General discussion

In many clinical circles, psychopaths are seen as untreatable although there is little scientific support for this belief. In the current review, cognitive–behavioral, psychodynamic, and eclectic intervention methods for psychopathy were shown to be effective. Moreover, psychopathic individuals were shown to have improved following rational therapy, personal construct psychotherapy, and other more specific psychotherapy programs. The most notable benefits included a reduction in psychopathic traits and characteristics (e.g., a decrease in lying, an increase in remorse and empathy, improved relations with others) and a reduction in recidivism. These findings indicate that contrary to clinical lore, the syndrome of psychopathy does not appear to be completely recalcitrant to treatment. Because of the high cost these individuals pose to society and themselves, the findings from the present review are encouraging and have important implications for future development and implementation of treatment programs for psychopathy.

The most successful interventions (e.g., cognitive–behavioral and psychoanalytic) tended to be intensive including an average of four sessions of individual psychotherapy per week for at least 1 year. Individual psychotherapy when augmented with group psychotherapy, at least preliminarily appears to be beneficial. In addition, treatment programs that incorporate family members appears to be beneficial. These results indicate, at least preliminarily, that for complex problems such as psychopathy, more elaborate and intensive intervention programs involving individual psychotherapy, treatment of family members, and input from groups (other patients/inmates) are beneficial and may enhance their overall effectiveness. Thus, based on the current review, the scope, intensity, and duration of treatment for psychopathy may have been key in the overall adjustment of these individuals.

Not unexpectedly, the review revealed that intervention programs with little professional psychological input and little-to-no one-to-one patient–psychologist contact resulted in poor treatment outcomes. This was most notable with therapeutic communities where mental health professionals had little or no contact with patients and essentially allowed inmates to "treat" other inmates often with very different symptom patterns. In the case of therapeutic communities, 25% of the patients benefited from treatment. Of the ones that did not benefit, significant costs to the community resulted in terms of violent recidivism (see Rice et al., 1992). These results suggest that when mental health professionals are not directly involved in treatment programs for serious forms of psychopathology then, clinically, patients exhibit little or no change and "interventions" possibly allow psychopathic conditions to worsen (Rice et al., 1992).

Several specific psychotherapy techniques were found to decrease psychopathic traits/characteristics. Specifically, four techniques/approaches that appeared to reduce psychopathic traits and characteristics included rational therapy, action-oriented therapies, interventions that involved fixed-role therapy, and psychodrama. The action-oriented program that involved intensive treatment of psychopathic youth was highly successful (75% of the sample decreased institutional infractions and the entire group (100%) made positive adjustments to the community). Maas (1966) found that fixed-role psychotherapy and role-playing in general with a group of psychopathic women was beneficial and significantly reduced psychopathic traits. Ellis (1961) found that one individual improved after the use of rational therapy. Finally, Corsini (1958) found that a youth improved after the use of psychodrama.

There is little question that from a purely scientific perspective that many of the studies reviewed in this review and meta-analysis, including some of the experimentally designed studies, could have been improved in terms of their internal, external, construct, and statistical conclusion validity. However, dismissing this early research as well as clinical opinions and treatment experience with psychopathic individuals written in case study form when reviewing a first generation of research on psychopathy would, in my opinion, be neglectful. In fact, Strupp (1996) has stressed the importance of looking at previous literature on treatment outcome and using it to inform current treatment outcome studies. Though the studies in the current review may be less than optimal in scientific rigor, their inclusion is considered to be both necessary and important given our current state of knowledge on psychopathy.

Although the current article's primary purpose was to clarify our current state of knowledge on the psychopathy–treatment relation, an equally important goal of this article was to spur a second generation of research on this important topic area. In order to address the problems experienced with the first generation of research it is necessary to underscore the limitations in past research that psychologists should attempt to rectify in the future. This process involves first asking what problems exist and where we as psychologists should go with regard to treatment outcome studies for psychopathy. Both the current problems and suggested future directions are highlighted in the next several paragraphs.

Three problem areas are clear from the present review. First, classification is a critical issue with regard to treatment. Further clarity regarding the features of the disorder are necessary with regard to the treatment amenability query. This clarity can, in part, be gained by specifying the conceptualization of psychopathy utilized in treatment outcome studies as well as the specific constellation of symptomatology that the psychopathic individual(s) have. Relatedly, use of polythetic models of psychopathy will likely mean that researchers will have to investigate the relative effect of various constellations of psychopathic traits on treatment amenability.

Related to this problem and possibly more problematic to the conclusions about the treatability of psychopathy in this article is that there are few studies that examine the psychopathy–treatment relation from the contemporary conceptualization of the disorder. A finding of the current meta-analysis was that the Cleckley psychopath was the most frequently investigated conception of the syndrome in treatment outcome studies. Yet, many researchers and clinicians utilize Hare's conceptualization of psychopathy. Given that his definition differs from Cleckley, treatment outcome studies that employ this definition are necessary, particularly if psychologists are to make statements about treatment amenability based on the PCL-R.

Second, etiological theories of psychopathy require refinement. If effective treatment programs are to be developed for psychopathy then it will be necessary for psychologists to determine the specific causes of the disorder. Furthermore, there was only a low-to-moderate degree of correspondence between treatment programs and current etiological/developmental theories. More specifically, while psychodynamic, cognitive–behavioral, and sensation-seeking theories tended to be incorporated into the treatment programs investigated in this review, several developmental theories have not been formally tested. Specifically, no studies had treatment programs that focused on deficits in learning, few studies emphasized the need for improving role-playing abilities of psychopaths, and there have been few programs developed from attachment-based theories. Expectedly, more recent theories of psychopathy (Frick, 1998; Hare, 1998; Lykken, 1995; Lynam, 1997; Newman, 1998) have not yet been implemented in treatment studies. In the future, such theories may furnish psychologists with the necessary therapeutic guidelines for treatment programs. Rudderless treatment investigations are likely to be less successful.

Third, to better understand the psychopathy–treatment relationship, several issues should be addressed in future treatment studies. Treatment programs should be developed with specific aims and experimental research is needed to systematically determine the effects of different treatment modalities with psychopathic individuals in well-controlled experimental designs. For example, researchers should utilize psychopathy instruments pre- and posttreatment in order to examine changes in symptomatology. Such ratings should be made by masked raters. Third, external criteria such as recidivism and conduct problems should be systematically investigated. This type of information would inform psychologists as to whether there is evidence that psychological change implies reduced risk of reoffending. In addition, research needs to make some attempt to determine whether clients are "faking good" in treatment studies or whether the changes are genuine.

Finally, prevention of psychopathy requires study. Because many of the developmental theories suggest that there is a predisposition (temperamental style) to this syndrome, early intervention may be particularly important. Lykken has shed light on this issue by suggesting that with competent parenting and "skillful help" children can in fact be socialized, albeit this effort is considerable. Nevertheless, given the high cost of this disorder on society, early intervention seems worthy. Moreover, withholding treatment from youth thought to develop psychopathy because of beliefs that the disorder is refractory to treatment would be unethical.

It seems clear from the current review that the widely held clinical belief that psychopathy is an untreatable disorder is unwarranted and that conclusions either way for this first generation of research are premature. At best, what we can glean scientifically suggests that psychopathy may be treatable. Further research on the psychopathy–treatment relation will help to increase the accountability of the profession for the treatment of those individuals who are psychopathic. Collaborative efforts between clinicians and researchers will enhance the richness and complexity of the psychotherapeutic process with psychopathic individuals as it unfolds over time. Considering the present state of our knowledge, the current review suggests that therapeutic pessimism with regard to the psychopathy–treatment relation is not warranted and efforts to develop and advance treatment technology in this area should be initiated.

Acknowledgments

The author would like to thank Alan E. Kazdin and George H. Davis of Yale University for their helpful comments on an earlier draft of this article.

References

Aichorn, A. (1966). *Wayward youth.* New York: Viking Press.

Bandura, A. (1973). *Aggression: a social learning analysis.* Englewood Cliffs, NJ: Prentice-Hall.

* Beacher, A. I. (1962). Psychoanalytic treatment of a sociopath in a group situation. *American Journal of Psychotherapy, 16,* 278–288.

Berkowitz, L. (1990). On the formation and regulation of anger and aggression: a neo-associationistic analysis. *American Psychologist, 45,* 497–503.

* Berman, S. (1964). Techniques of treatment of a form of juvenile delinquency, the antisocial character disorder. *Journal of the American Academy of Child Psychiatry, 3,* 24–52.

* Borriello, J. F. (1979). Group psychotherapy with acting-out patients: specific problems and techniques. *American Journal of Psychotherapy, 33,* 521–530.

Bowlby, J. (1969). *Attachment and loss, vol. 1. Attachment* (2nd ed.). New York: Basic Books.

* Butterworth, A. T. (1951). Psychopathic personality in treatment. *New Orleans Medical Journal, 104,* 197–200.

* Chrzanowski, G. (1965). The psychotherapeutic management of sociopathy. *American Journal of Psychotherapy, 19,* 372–381.

* Chwast, J. (1961). Reversibility–irreversibility: problems in the treatment of offenders. *American Journal of Psychotherapy, 15,* 221–232.

Cleckley, H. (1941). *The mask of sanity.* St. Louis, MO: Mosby.

Cleckley, H. (1981). *The mask of sanity* (4th ed.). St. Louis, MO: Mosby.

* Cleckley, H., & Beard, B. (1942). Electric shock therapy in personality disorders. *Journal of the Medical Association of Georgia, 31,* 303–308.

Cloninger, C. R. (1978). The antisocial personality. *Hospital Practice, 13,* 97–106.

* Copas, J. B., & Whiteley, J. S. (1976). Predicting success in the treatment of psychopaths. *British Journal of Psychiatry, 129,* 388–392.

* Copas, J. V., O'Brien, M., Roberts, J., & Whiteley, J. S. (1984). Treatment outcome in personality disorder: the effects of social, psychological and behavioral variables. *Personality and Individual Differences, 5,* 565–573.

* Corsini, R. J. (1958). Psychodrama with a psychopath. *Group Psychotherapy, 11,* 33–39.

* Craft, M. (1968). Psychopathic disorder: a second trial of treatment. *British Journal of Psychiatry, 114,* 812–820.

* Craft, M., Stephenson, G., & Granger, C. (1964). A controlled trial of authoritarian and self-governing regimes with adolescent psychopaths. *American Journal of Orthopsychiatry, 34,* 543–554.

Damasio, A. R. (1994). *Descartes' error: emotion, reason and the human brain.* New York: Putnam.

* Darling, H. F. (1945). Electric shock treatment in psychopathic personality. *Journal of Nervous and Mental Disease, 101,* 247–250.

Dodge, K. A. (1980). Social cognition and children's aggressive behavior. *Child Development, 53,* 620–635.

Doren, D. M. (1987). *Understanding and treating the psychopath.* New York: Wiley.

Draughon, M. (1977). Ego-building: an aspect of the treatment of psychopaths. *Psychological Reports, 40,* 615–626.

Ellis, A. (1961). The treatment of a psychopath with rational psychotherapy. *Journal of Psychology, 51,* 141–150.

Eron, L. D. (1997). The development of antisocial behavior from a learning perspective. In: D. M. Stoff, J. Breiling, & J. D. Maser (Eds.), *Handbook of antisocial behavior* (pp. 140–147). New York: Wiley.

Eysenck, H. J. (1975). Genetic factors in personality development. In: A. R. Kaplan (Ed.), *Human behavior genetics.* Springfield, IL: Thomas.

Eysenck, H. J. (1977). *Crime and personality* (3rd ed.). London: Routledge & Kegan Paul.

Eysenck, H. J. (1981). General features of the model. In: H. J. Eysenck (Ed.), *A model for personality* (pp. 1–37). New York: Springer-Verlag.

Forth, A. E., Kosson, D., & Hare, R. D. (1994). *Psychopathy Checklist — Youth Version.* Toronto, ON: Multi-Health Systems.

Fowles, D. C. (1980). The three arousal model: implications of Gray's two factor learning theory for heart rate, electrodermal activity, and psychopathy. *Psychophysiology, 17,* 87–104.

Freud, S. (1961). The ego and the id. In: J. Strachey (Ed.), *The standard edition of the complete psychological works of Sigmund Freud, vol. 19* (pp. 3–56). London: Hogarth.

Frick, P. J. (1998). Callous-unemotional traits and conduct problems: a two factor model of psychopathy in children. In: D. J. Cooke, A. E. Forth, & R. D. Hare (Eds.), *Psychopathy: theory, research, and implication for society* (pp. 161–188). Dordrecht, Netherlands: Kluwer Academic Publishing.

Frick, P. J., & Hare, R. D. (in press). *The psychopathy screening device.* Toronto, ON: Multi-Health Systems.

Frick, P. J., & Jackson, Y. K. (1993). Family functioning and childhood antisocial behavior: yet another reinterpretation. *Journal of Clinical Child Psychology, 22*, 410–419.

Gacono, C .B., Nieberding, R. J., Owen, A., Rubel, J., & Bodholt, K. (2001). Treating conduct disorder, antisocial, and psychopatic personalities. In J. B. Ashford, B. D. Sales, & W. H. Reid (Eds.), *Treating adult and juvenile offenders with special needs.* Washington, DC: American Psychological Association.

Gale, A. (1973). The physiology of individual differences: studies on extraversion and the EEG. In: P. Kline (Ed.), *New approaches to physiological measurement.* Chichester, England: Wiley.

Garfield, S. L. (1994). Research on client variables in psychotherapy. In: S. L. Garfield, & A. E. Bergin (Eds.), *Handbook of psychotherapy and behavior change* (3rd ed.) (pp. 190–228). New York: Wiley.

* Glaus, A. (1968). The handling of criminal psychopaths in Switzerland. *International Journal of Offender Therapy, 12*, 29–36.

Gough, H. G. (1948). A sociological theory of psychopathy. *American Journal of Sociology, 53*, 359–366.

Gough, H. G. (1958). *California Psychological Inventory.* Palo Alto, CA: Consulting Psychologists Press.

Gough, G. H. (1997). *California Psychological Inventory (revised).* Palo Alto, CA: Consulting Psychologists Press.

Gray, J. A. (1987). *The psychology of fear and stress* (2nd ed.). Cambridge: Cambridge Univ. Press.

Greenacre, P. (1945). Conscience in the psychopath. *American Journal of Orthopsychiatry, 15*, 495–509.

Greenwald, H. (1967). Treatment of the psychopath. *Voices, 3*, 50–60.

Guerra, N. G., & Slaby, R. G. (1990). Evaluative factors in social problem solving by aggressive boys. *Journal of Abnormal Child Psychology, 17*, 277–289.

Hare, R. D. (1970). *Psychopathy: theory and research.* New York: Wiley.

Hare, R. D. (1991). *Manual for the revised Psychopathy Checklist.* Toronto, ON: Multi-Health Systems.

Hare, R. D. (1998). Psychopathy, affect, and behavior. In: D. J. Cooke, A. E. Forth, & R. D. Hare (Eds.), *Psychopathy: theory, research, and implications for society* (pp. 105–138). Dordrecht, Netherlands: Kluwer Academic Publishing.

Hare, R. D., & Hart, R. D. (1993). Psychopathy, mental disorder, and crime. In: S. Hodgins (Ed.), *Mental disorder and crime* (pp. 104–115). Newbury Park, CA: Sage.

Hart, S. D., Forth, A. E., & Hare, R. D. (1990). Performance of criminal psychopaths on selected neuropsychological tests. *Journal of Abnormal Psychology, 99*, 374–379.

Howland, E. W., Kosson, P. S., Patterson, C. M. & Newman, J. P. (1993). Altering a dominant response: performance of psychopaths and low socialization college students.

* Heaver, W. L. (1943). A study of forty male psychopathic personalities before, during and after hospitalization. *American Journal of Psychiatry, 100*, 342–346.

* Henderson, J. M. (1972). The doing character. *Adolescence, 7*, 309–326.

* Humphreys, E. J. (1940). Psychopathic personality among the mentally defective. *Psychiatric Quarterly, 14*, 231–247.

Hunter, J. E. (1990). *The control group and meta-analysis.* Unpublished manuscript, Department of Psychology, Michigan State University (May).

Hunter, J. E., & Schmidt, F. L. (1990). *Methods of meta-analysis: correcting error and bias in research findings.* Newbury Park, CA: Sage.

* Ingram, G. L., Gerard, R. E., Quay, H. C., & Levison, R. B. (1970). An experimental program for the psychopathic delinquent: looking in the "correctional wastebasket". *Journal of Research in Crime and Delinquency, 7*, 24–30.

Intrator, J., Hare, R. D., Stritzke, P., Brichstwein, K., Dorfman, D., Harper, T., Bernstein, D., Handelsman, L., Keilp, J., Rosen, J., & Machac, J. (1997). A brain imaging (SPECT) study of semantic and affective processing in psychopaths. *Biological Psychiatry, 42*, 96–103.

Johnson, A. M., & Szurek, S. A. (1954). Etiology of antisocial behavior in delinquents and psychopaths. *Journal of the American Medical Association*, *154*, 814–817.

Kazdin, A. E. (1999). Current (lack of) status of theory in child and adolescent psychotherapy research. *Journal of Clinical Child Psychology*, *28*, 533–543.

* Kiger, R. S. (1967). Treating the psychopathic patient in a therapeutic community. *Hospital and Community Psychiatry*, *18*, 191–196.

Kochanska, G. (1993). Toward a synthesis of parental socialization and child temperament in early development of conscience. *Child Development*, *64*, 325–347.

Kohut, H. (1982). Introspection, empathy, and the semi-circle of mental health. *International Journal of Psychoanalysis*, *63*, 395–407.

* Korey, S. R. (1944). The effects of Benzedrine sulfate on the behavior of psychopathic and neurotic juvenile delinquents. *Psychiatric Quarterly*, *18*, 127–137.

* Kristiansson, M. (1995). Incurable psychopaths? *Bulletin of the American Academy of Psychiatry and the Law*, *23*, 555–562.

Lilienfeld, S. O. (1994). Conceptual problems in the assessment of psychopathy. *Clinical Psychology Review*, *14*, 17–38.

Lochman, J. E. (1990). Modification of childhood aggression. In: A. M. Hersen, R. Ersler, & P. Miller (Eds.), *Progress in behavior modification* (p. 23). New York: Academic Press.

Losel, F. (1998). Treatment and management of psychopaths. In: D. J. Cooke, A. E. Forth, & R. D. Hare (Eds.), *Psychopathy: theory, research, and implications for society* (pp. 105–138). Dordrecht, Netherlands: Kluwer Academic Publishing.

Lykken, D. T. (1957). A study of anxiety in the sociopathic personality. *Journal of Abnormal and Social Psychology*, *55*, 6–10.

Lykken, D. T. (1995). *The antisocial personalities*. Hillsdale, NJ: Erlbaum.

Lynam, D. R. (1996). The early identification of chronic offenders: who is the fledgling psychopath? *Psychological Bulletin*, *120*, 209–234.

Lynam, D. R. (1997). Pursuing the psychopath: capturing the fledgling psychopath in a nomological net. *Journal of Abnormal Psychology*, *106*, 425–438.

* Maas, J. (1966). The use of actional procedures in group psychotherapy with sociopathic women. *International Journal of Group Psychotherapy*, *16*, 190–197.

McCord, W., & McCord, J. (1964). *The psychopath: an essay on the criminal mind*. New York: Van Nostrand-Reinhold.

Megargee, E. I., & Golden, R. E. (1973). Parental attitudes of psychopathic and subcultural delinquents. *Criminology*, *35*, 427–439.

* Miles, A. E. (1969). The effects of therapeutic community on the interpersonal relationships of a group of psychopaths. *British Journal of Criminology*, *9*, 22–38.

Millon, T. (1990). *Toward a new personology: an evolutionary model*. New York: Wiley.

Morretti, M. M., Holland, R., & Peterson, S. (1994). Long term outcome of an attachment-based program for conduct disorder. *Canadian Journal of Psychiatry*, *39*, 360–370.

Newman, J. P. (1998). Psychopathic behavior: an information processing perspective. In: R. D. Hare, D. J. Cooke, & A. E. Forth (Eds.), *Psychopathy: theory, research, and implication for society* (pp. 81–104). Dordrecht, Netherlands: Kluwer Academic Publishing.

Newman, J. P., & Kosson, D. S. (1986). Passive avoidance learning in psychopathic and nonpsychopathic offenders. *Journal of Abnormal Psychology*, *95*, 252–256.

Newman, J. P., Patterson, C. M., Howland, E. W., & Nichols, S. L. (1990). Passive avoidance in psychopaths: the effects of reward. *Personality and Individual Differences*, *11*, 1101–1114.

Newman, J. P., Patterson, C. M., & Kosson, D. S. (1987). Response perseveration in psychopaths. *Journal of Abnormal Psychology*, *96*, 145–148.

Newman, J. P., Widom, C. S., & Nathan, S. (1985). Passive–avoidance in syndromes of disinhibition: psychopathy and extraversion. *Journal of Personality and Social Psychology*, *48*, 1316–1327.

* Noshpitz, J. D. (1984). Opening phase in the psychotherapy of adolescents with character disorders. *Bulletin of the Menninger Clinic*, *21*, 153–164.

* Ogloff, J. R. P., Wong, S., & Greenwood, A. (1990). Treating criminal psychopaths in a therapeutic community program. *Behavioral Sciences and the Law, 8*, 181–190.

* Partridge, G. E. (1928). A study of 50 cases of psychopathic personality. *American Journal of Psychiatry, 7*, 953–973.

Patrick, C. J. (1994). Emotion and psychopathy: startling new insights. *Psychophysiology, 31*, 319–330.

Patterson, G. R., Dishion, T. J., & Chamberlain, P. (1993). Outcomes and methodological issues relating to the treatment of antisocial children. In: T. R. Giles (Ed.), *Effective psychotherapy: a handbook of comparative research* (pp. 43–88). New York: Plenum.

Patterson, G. R., & Yoerger, K. (1993). Developmental models for delinquent behavior. In: S. Hodgins (Ed.), *Mental disorder and crime* (pp. 140–172). London: Sage.

* Persons, R. W. (1965). Psychotherapy with sociopathic offenders: an empirical evaluation. *Journal of Clinical Psychology, 21*, 205–207.

Quay, H. C. (1965). Psychopathic personality as pathological sensation-seeking. *American Journal of Psychiatry, 122*, 180–183.

Quay, H. C. (1977). Psychopathic behavior: reflections on its nature, origins, and treatment. In: I. Uzgiris, & F. Weizmann (Eds.), *The structuring of experience*. New York: Plenum.

Redl, F., & Wineman, D. (1951). *Children who hate*. New York: Free Press.

Redl, F., & Wineman, D. (1952). *Controls from within: techniques for the treatment of the aggressive child*. New York: Free Press.

* Reiss, D., Grubin, D., & Meux, C. (1996). Young "psychopaths" in special hospital: treatment and outcome. *British Journal of Psychiatry, 168*, 99–104.

Rice, M. E. (1997). Violent offender research and implications for the criminal justice system. *American Psychologist, 52*, 414–432.

* Rice, M. E., Harris, G. T., & Cormier, C. A. (1992). An evaluation of a maximum security therapeutic community for psychopaths and other mentally disordered offenders. *Law and Human Behavior, 16*, 399–412.

Robins, L. N. (1978). Etiological implications in childhood histories relating to antisocial personality. In: R. D. Hare, & D. Schalling (Eds.), *Psychopathic behavior: approaches to research* (pp. 255–272).

Rogers, R. (1995). *Diagnostic and structured interviewing: a handbook for psychologists*. Odessa, FL: Psychological Assessment Resources.

Rosenthal, R. (1991). *Meta-analytic procedures for social research* (2nd ed.). Beverly Hills, CA: Sage.

Rotenberg, M. (1975). Psychopathy, insensitivity, and socialization. *Professional Psychology, 6*, 283–292.

Rutter, M., Tizard, J., & Whitmore, K. (1970). *Education, health, and behavior*. London: Longman.

Salekin, R. T., Rogers, R., & Sewell, K. W. (1996). A review and meta-analysis of the Psychopathy Checklist and Psychopathy Checklist — Revised. *Clinical Psychology: Science and Practice, 3*, 203–215.

* Sandhu, H. S. (1970). Therapy with violent psychopaths in an Indian prison community. *International Journal of Offender Therapy, 14*, 138–144.

* Savitt, R. A. (1940). An approach to the problem of psychopathic personality. *Psychiatric Quarterly, 14*, 255–263.

Schmauk, F. J. (1970). Punishment, arousal, and avoidance learning in sociopaths. *Journal of Abnormal Psychology, 76*, 325–335.

* Schmideberg, M. (1947). The treatment of psychopaths and borderline patients. *American Journal of Psychotherapy, 1*, 45–70.

* Schmideberg, M. (1978). The treatment of a juvenile "psychopath". *International Journal of Offender Therapy and Comparative Criminology, 22*, 21–28.

Schuster, R. (1976). Trust: its implication in the etiology and treatment of psychopathic youth. *International Journal of Offender Therapy, 20*, 128–133.

Skolnick, N. J., & Zuckerman, M. (1979). Personality change in drug abusers: a comparison of therapeutic community and prison groups. *Journal of Consulting and Clinical Psychology, 47*, 768–770.

Smith, R. J. (1978). *The psychopath in society*. New York: Academic Press.

Strupp, H. H. (1996). The tripartite model and the consumer reports study. *American Psychologist, 51*, 1017–1024.

* Sturup, G. K. (1948). The management and treatment of psychopaths in a special institution in Denmark. *Proceedings of the Royal Society of Medicine, 41*, 765–768.

Suedfeld, P., & Landon, P. B. (1978). Approaches to treatment. In: R. D. Hare, & D. Schalling (Eds.), *Psychopathic behavior: approaches to research* (pp. 347–378). New York: Wiley.

* Szurek, S. A. (1942). Notes on the genesis of psychopathic personality trends. *Psychiatry, 5*, 1–6.

Templeman, T. L., & Wollersheim, J. P. (1979). A cognitive–behavioral approach to the treatment of psychopathy. *Psychotherapy: Research and Practice, 16*, 132–139.

* Thorne, F. C. (1959). The etiology of sociopathic reactions. *American Journal of Psychotherapy, 13*, 319–330.

Ullman, L. P., & Krasner, L. (1969). *A psychological approach to abnormal behavior.* New York: Prentice-Hall.

* Vaillant, G. E. (1975). Sociopathy as a human process: a viewpoint. *Archives of General Psychiatry, 32*, 178–183.

Vaughan, S. C. (1997). *The talking cure: the science behind psychotherapy.* New York: G.P. Putnam and Sons.

Warren, F. (1994). What do we mean by a "therapeutic community" for offenders? Commentary on papers by Harris et al. and Cullen. *Therapeutic Communities: International Journal of Therapeutic and Supportive Organizations, 15*, 312–318.

Webster-Stratton, C. (1990). A potential disrupter of parent perceptions and family interactions. *Journal of Clinical Child Psychology, 19*, 302–312.

* Whitaker, C. A., & Burdy, J. (1969). Family psychotherapy of a psychopathic personality: must every member change? *Comprehensive Psychiatry, 10*, 361–364.

* Whiteley, J. S. (1970). The response of psychopaths to a therapeutic community. *British Journal of Psychiatry, 116*, 517–529.

Widom, C. S. (1976). Interpersonal conflict and cooperation in psychopaths. *Journal of Abnormal Psychology, 85*, 330–334.

* Woody, G. E., McLellan, A. T., Luborsky, L., & O'Brien, C. P. (1985). Sociopathy and psychotherapy outcome. *Archives of General Psychiatry, 42*, 1081–1086.

Zuckerman, M. (1995). Good and bad humors: biochemical bases of personality and its disorders. *Psychological Science, 6*, 325–332.

[14]

Evaluation of a National Prison-Based Treatment Program for Sexual Offenders in England and Wales

CAROLINE FRIENDSHIP
RUTH E. MANN
Her Majesty's Prison Service, London, United Kingdom
ANTHONY R. BEECH
University of Birmingham, United Kingdom

Treatment efficacy is described for a sample of sexual offenders who had undertaken treatment in United Kingdom prisons (N = *647) and for a retrospectively selected comparison group* (N = *1,910). The outcomes under observation in this study were sexual, sexual and/or violent, and general reconviction. Treatment impact was also examined in relation to offenders' risk of reconviction. The treatment group had slightly lower 2-year sexual reconviction rates than the comparison group, but these differences were not statistically significant. Significant differences were found between the treatment and comparison group for sexual and/or violent reconviction. Further analysis suggested that treatment produced a reduction in the probability of sexual and/or violent reconviction* ($p < .05$) *when other relevant variables were controlled for. General reconviction rates were consistently lower in the treatment group, but these differences were not significant.*

Keywords: *sexual offenders; prison; static risk; sexual offender treatment; reconviction; recidivism*

Sexual offenses represent less than 1% of all crimes recorded by the police in England and Wales (Povey, 2001). But this minority behavior is known to have a significant negative impact on its victims (Beitchman et al., 1991; Finkelhor & Browne, 1985), and this provides a compelling argument for constructive intervention with sexual offenders.

Authors' Note: The authors would like to thank David Thornton, the founder of this program, and Matthew Erikson for assisting in the analysis of the criminal conviction data.

Over the past decade, as a direct result of meta-analytic studies of treatment effectiveness, there has been a shift in the management of offenders, from a punitive approach to offending to a treatment/rehabilitative approach (McGuire, 1995). The development of cognitive behavioral approaches in the treatment of sexual offenders has been well documented, and treatment outcomes for cognitive behavioral programs have been comprehensively reviewed (Marshall, Anderson, & Fernandez, 1999). The authors summarized both positive and negative treatment outcomes in the literature, but concluded that on balance, the empirical evidence supported the view that the treatment of sexual offenders has a positive impact on reducing recidivism.

Whether treatment works remains a debated issue, not least because few studies have achieved the ideal research design, a randomized experiment. Many studies have matched a suitable comparison group to treatment offenders on relevant criminal history variables. In such studies, a reduction in recidivism for treatment offenders may be attributed to differences in offender characteristics between the treatment and comparison groups rather than to the treatment per se. The most rigorous study to date (Marques, 1999) did not show a reduction in the rates of sexual recidivism for treated offenders.

In England and Wales, the 1980s saw an increase in the public and political profile of sexual offending. The *Woolf Report* (1991), published in the aftermath of a number of serious prison riots, and the *Criminal Justice Act: England and Wales* (1991) made specific recommendations for the management of imprisoned sexual offenders. In June 1991, the United Kingdom government announced a strategy for the containment and treatment of sexual offenders in England and Wales. This involved holding sexual offenders in fewer prison establishments to provide a safe and supportive environment for the consistent delivery of treatment programs. In 1992, a national Sex Offender Treatment Program (SOTP) was established. It was centrally designed, adhering to research evidence regarding treatment efficacy for sexual offenders (i.e., it adopted a cognitive behavioral approach). Program monitoring and evaluation were an integral part of the program. The development and implementation of the SOTP have been described in detail (Beech, Fisher, & Beckett, 1999; Grubin & Thornton, 1994; Mann & Thornton, 1998; Thornton & Hogue, 1993).

The aim of the current study is to evaluate the effectiveness of the SOTP in terms of recidivism using reconviction as an outcome measure. The number of offenders in this study is higher than in the studies reported by Marshall et al. (1999) and probably forms the largest study of sexual offenders who have participated in the same program. This study is unique in that it examines the relationship between risk of reconviction, treatment, and reconviction rates (see Beech, Friendship, Erikson, & Hanson, 2002).

METHOD

Participants

The treatment group consisted of 647 adult male offenders who had been sentenced to prison for at least 4 years for a sexual offense and had voluntarily participated in and completed the SOTP between 1992 and 1994. All of these offenders had subsequently been discharged from prison and had spent at least 2 years in the community. During this time period, the SOTP was only available for offenders serving a custodial sentence for 4 years or more. This was due to the limited number of places available for treatment, and sentence length was used as part of the criteria for prioritizing offenders for treatment. Procedures for program data collection at this time varied from prison to prison. For some prisons, the data returned centrally included treatment drop-outs, although drop-out cases were not specifically identified. In other prisons, treatment dropouts were not included in the program data returned. For this reason, not all drop-out cases are included in the treatment sample, and drop-out offenders cannot be identified as a separate group.

The comparison group consisted of 1,910 adult male offenders serving a prison sentence of 4 years or more for a sexual offense. They were matched to the treatment sample by year of discharge. As mentioned above, there was no complete record of treatment dropouts collected for the program during this period. There was a very small possibility that some treatment dropouts would appear in the comparison group, but it was not possible to identify these offenders.

Criminal conviction data for England and Wales do not routinely record victim information (i.e., the age and gender of the victim of the offense). For this reason, it was not possible to give a detailed breakdown of the sample according to these characteristics. The sexual conviction for which the offenders in the sample were originally sentenced to prison differed between the treatment and comparison groups. Comparison group offenders were not matched to the treatment offenders according to the original sexual conviction.

Table 1 describes the treatment and comparison group samples in terms of offender criminal history. Independent *t* tests were used to assess the differences between the treatment and comparison group samples on these vari-

TABLE 1: Mean Values for Selected Variables

Variable	*Treatment Group M (N = 647)*	*Comparison Group M (N = 1,910)*	*95% Confidence Interval for the Difference Between the Ms*	t *Value*
Risk or raw score for Static-99	2.35	1.75	0.43, 0.76	6.98***
Sentence length	6.13	7.52	0.47, 2.32	2.96**
Age at first conviction	27.66	25.68	0.77, 3.18	–3.16***
Age at discharge	41.23	39.83	0.38, 2.52	–2.65**
Number of previous sentencing occasions for any type of offense	4.72	5.69	0.5, 1.44	4.02***
Number of previous sentencing occasions for sexual offenses	1.49	1.42	–0.17, 0.42	–1.19
Number of previous sentencing occasions for violent offenses	1.65	2.10	0.24, 0.65	4.23***

NOTE: Sentencing occasions counted the number of times an offender had been sentenced before the courts for any number of offenses.
$^{**}p < .01$. $^{***}p < .001$.

ables. If equal variance could not be assumed (Levine's test for equality of variance), the nonequal variance *t* test was used. It can be seen from Table 1 that there were significant differences between all the selected variables, except for the number of previous sentencing occasions for sexual offenses (Table 1).

Both treatment and comparison group samples excluded life sentence prisoners who are subject to unique community supervision on discharge from prison, a supervision license for life. Re-offending in this group may not proceed through the criminal courts but lead to direct recall to prison. A small minority of the treatment and comparison groups may have engaged in a variety of group and/or one-on-one offense-related interventions, but these were unlikely to fulfill principles of evidence-based practice.

Design and Analysis

This study compared a group of treated offenders and a retrospective comparison group who shared the same broad characteristics as the treatment group. The treatment and comparison groups were equated by risk of reconviction using an existing risk assessment schedule, Static-99 (Hanson & Thornton, 2000), developed for use with sexual offenders. The offenders were placed in one of four risk groups based on this assessment of their demographic details and criminal history. Reconviction rates were compared between groups using chi-square analysis. The factors theoretically demonstrated to be predictive of sexual reconviction in the literature (e.g., age at current offense, age at conviction, number of previous sexual appearances, and length of sentence) were controlled for in post hoc analysis using logistic regression. A forward selection stepwise model was used. Variables were accepted into the model on the basis of significant change in the –2 log likelihood statistic. Predictor variables were also entered into a hierarchical logistic regression analysis with reconviction as the outcome. Significant variables were forced first, and then treatment was entered last to see if it produced a significant improvement to the prediction of reconviction.

Description of Treatment

Two versions of a United Kingdom treatment program are included in this evaluation. Both versions were based on a cognitive behavioral model. For both versions, group facilitators were drawn from a variety of professional disciplines, principally psychologists, probation officers (from a social work background), and prison officers (Mann & Thornton, 1998). All staff attended 2 weeks of nationally organized residential training.

The first version of the Core Program was composed of about 29 two-hour sessions. The program started by getting the offender to provide a simple offense account, based on the Finkelhor (1984) model. The offense account was then repeated with cognitive distortions (Murphy, 1990) being challenged to produce an active account where the offender took more responsibility for his offending. Following this, 4 sessions were devoted to developing victim empathy. Methods used included group discussion, based on group members' own childhood experiences, and exposure to video or audio accounts presented by victims of sexual abuse. A decision matrix session followed, where each offender examined the costs and gains of his offending to increase motivation to avoid further offending. Offenders then examined their offending patterns using the cycles of offending model (Wolf, 1988). The course finished with 2 to 4 sessions looking at relapse prevention, where the concept of a lapse was introduced and group members discussed ways of coping with their own high-risk situations. The emphasis was on "escape" as the most appropriate strategy. By today's standards (e.g., Fisher & Beech, 2002; Marshall, Fernandez, Hudson, & Ward, 1998), this program would be seen as simplistic and short.

The second version of the Core Program was a considerable expansion in terms of length, depth, and style. This version took 70 to 75 sessions to deliver. The time allocated for active accounts was expanded. Group facilitators used questioning rather than confrontation to "unpick" cognitive distortions. The victim empathy sessions became more sophisticated and incorporated victim empathy role-plays, a method adopted from Pithers's (1994) sex offender program in Vermont. Individual cognitive-behavioral chains (Nelson & Jackson, 1989) replaced offense cycles. Finally, the relapse prevention sessions were expanded so that group members identified their individual risk factors with recognition cues and planned coping strategies. Although better than the first version of the United Kingdom program, by today's standards this program also lacked sophistication. In particular, there was little or no emphasis on therapeutic style or group process (Beech & Fordham, 1997), and facilitators worked with no formal supervision or monitoring of their practice.

Selection Criteria

Offenders were selected for the program if they were serving a prison sentence for a sexual offense of 4 years or more. Offenders with an IQ of less than 80 were excluded from the program. Offenders were also excluded from the SOTP if they totally denied their offense. When the program first started in the prison service, only a few prisons ran it. The offenders who were selected for treatment tended to be offenders who were highly motivated and eager to enter into the treatment process.

Risk Assessment Measure

Static-99 (Hanson & Thornton, 2000) is a 10-item instrument that assesses offenders' past criminal conviction and demographic details to predict sexual recidivism in sexual offenders. It contains the following items: prior sex offenses, prior sentencing dates, noncontact offenses, index of nonsexual violence, prior nonsexual offenses, unrelated victim, stranger victim, male victim, young, and single. The raw item score can range from 0 to 12. The raw score can also be grouped into one of four categories or risk groups: low, medium-low, medium-high, and high.

Procedure

Criminal conviction histories were obtained from official records for both offender groups using the Offenders Index, a United Kingdom conviction database. Reconviction outcomes were derived from this data.

The reconviction outcomes were defined using legal offense categories for the United Kingdom. Sexual reconviction was defined as the conviction of another sexual offense during a specified follow-up period. Furby,

Weinrott, and Blackshaw (1989) described this as the most commonly used definition of sexual reconviction, and this definition has been extensively adopted in studies in the United Kingdom. This study excluded sexual offenses that were considered to be consensual or victimless (i.e., gross indecency between males, soliciting by a man, bigamy, and living off immoral earnings). The reasons for this were twofold. First, it is rare to receive a custodial sentence for these types of offenses. Second, the offenders convicted of such offenses were not considered to possess the criminogenic needs targeted by the program.

Violent reconviction was defined as the conviction of another violent offense (excluding sexual violence) during a specified follow-up period. Violent offenses were composed of the following: murder, manslaughter, wounding, assault, cruelty, blackmail, kidnapping, rioting, violent disorder, and firearm offenses. General reconviction was defined as the conviction for any offense during follow up.

A static risk procedure for sexual offenders, Static-99 (Hanson & Thornton, 2000) was scored for the whole sample, based on criminal conviction history and basic demographic data. It was not possible to score three items of Static-99 due to lack of information. Criminal conviction data in England and Wales do not include factors such as the perpetrator's relationship to the victim or the perpetrator's marital status. The excluded items were any unrelated victims, any stranger victims, and single. The impact of scoring Static-99 with missing items is explored in the discussion.

RESULTS

The distribution of the treatment and comparison group samples is presented by Static-99 risk category (Hanson & Thornton, 2000) in Table 2. Only a quarter of the sample had completed the revised program. When the sample was broken down by program type and risk level, this left too few offenders in the high-risk groups for robust analysis. In addition, the reconviction rates for the original and revised programs followed a similar pattern. For this reason, the analysis conducted combined offenders who had completed the original program with offenders who had completed the revised.

Two-year sexual reconviction rates were calculated for the treatment and comparison groups (see Table 3). The 2-year rates examined reconviction within a fixed time period (i.e., whether the offender was reconvicted within the first 2 years postdischarge from prison). All the offenders in this study had short follow-up periods. Standardization of the follow-up period allowed

TABLE 2: Sample by Risk Category (Static-99)

	Treatment Group (N = 647)		*Comparison Group (N = 1,910)*	
Risk Category	n	%	n	%
Low	263	41	969	50
Medium-low	225	35	655	34
Medium-high	109	17	229	12
High	50	7	57	4

TABLE 3: Two-Year Sexual Reconviction Rates for Treatment (*N* = 647) and Comparison (*N* = 1,910) Groups by Static-99 Risk Category

	Treatment Group		*Comparison Group*	
Risk Category	%	n	%	n
Low	1.1	3	1.2	12
Medium-low	1.3	3	3.4	22
Medium-high	2.8	3	5.2	12
High	16.0	8	14.0	8
Overall	2.6	17	2.8	54

direct comparison with other United Kingdom studies where this convention is commonly used. The 2-year rates of sexual reconviction were low in both the treatment and comparison groups, although the rate was elevated for high-risk offenders. Differences between the treatment and comparison groups' sexual reconviction rates were assessed using chi-square statistic. There were no significant differences.

Table 4 reports 2-year sexual and/or violent reconviction rates. This combined sexual and violent outcome raises the base rate of reconviction. Differences between sexual and/or violent reconviction rates were assessed using chi-square statistic. There was a significant difference overall between the treatment and comparison groups for 2-year sexual and/or violent reconviction rates. In terms of risk level, significant differences were also present in the medium-low and medium-high offender groups. For low and high-risk offenders there was a trend in the expected direction with treatment group offenders showing a slightly lower rate of reconviction.

Two-year reconviction rates for any type of offense (general reconviction) are shown in Table 5. The differences between comparison and treatment

TABLE 4: Two-Year Sexual and/or Violent Reconviction Rates for Treatment (N = 647) and Comparison (N = 1,910) Groups by Static-99 Risk Category

	Treatment Group		*Comparison Group*			
Risk Category	%	n	%	n	df	χ^2 *Value*
Low	1.9	5	2.6	25	1	0.40
Medium-low	2.7	6	12.7	83	1	18.44**
Medium-high	5.5	6	13.5	31	1	4.88*
High	26.0	13	28.1	16	1	0.06
Overall	4.6	30	8.1	155	3	8.71**

*$p < .05$. **$p < .01$.

TABLE 5: Two-Year General Reconviction Rates for Treatment (N = 647) and Comparison (N = 1,910) Groups by Static-99 Risk Category

	Treatment Group		*Comparison Group*	
Risk Category	%	n	%	n
Low	5.7	15	6.7	65
Medium-low	13.3	30	25.3	166
Medium-high	21.1	23	27.1	229
High	36.0	18	38.6	22
Overall	13.3	86	16.5	315

groups were also assessed using chi-square statistic, and no significant differences were found. General 2-year reconviction rates were, however, consistently lower in the treatment group.

Logistic regression analysis was used to assess the respective influence of treatment and other empirically related variables on reconviction. A forward stepwise method was used. Variables were accepted into the model on the basis of significant change in the –2 log likelihood statistic. The dependent variables were sexual reconviction, sexual and/or violent reconviction, and general reconviction. The independent variables were the following: age at first conviction, age at discharge from prison, number of previous sentencing occasions for any offense, number of previous sentencing occasions for a sexual offense, number of previous sentencing occasions for a violent offense, sentence length (years), Static-99 risk score, Static-99 risk category, and treatment status.

TABLE 6: Logistic Regression Model to Predict Reconviction Within 2 Years of Discharge From Prison

Variable	B	SE	df	*Significance*	*Exponential(β)*
Risk category					
Low[a]			3	.000	
Medium-low	0.295	0.441	1	.503	1.344
Medium-high	0.181	0.488	1	.711	1.198
High	1.623	0.506	1	.001	5.068
Number of previous sentencing occasions (all types)	0.051	0.018	1	.004	1.053
Age at discharge	–0.070	0.014	1	.000	0.933
Number of previous sentencing occasions (violence)	0.142	0.065	1	.029	1.153
Treatment status	–0.860	0.339	1	.011	0.423
Constant	–0.620	0.600	1	.302	0.538

a. Low is the reference category.

Treatment was *only* significant in the final regression model for the dependent variable sexual and/or violent reconviction. Here, the model also included the variables risk category, number of previous sentencing occasions for violent offenses, number of previous sentencing occasions for all types of offenses, and offender age at discharge from prison (see Table 6). Static-99 risk score was not accepted into the model.

The last column in Table 6, Exponential(ß), represents an odds ratio that describes the relationship of the independent variable to the dependent variable. With logistic regression, Exponential(ß) allows us to describe the unique effect of an independent variable when all other variables in the model have been controlled for. If a variable has an Exponential(ß) less than 1, it can be considered to be reducing the odds of reconviction, and if it is greater than 1, then it can be considered to be increasing the odds of reconviction.

In the logistic regression model (Table 6), both treatment and age at discharge from prison are reducing the odds of reconviction. Treatment produced a robust reduction in the probability of reconviction ($p < .05$) and can be seen to reduce reconviction by a factor of 0.42. This translates into a 58% reduction in the chances of being reconvicted within 2 years for a sexual and/or violent offense. Age at discharge produced only a slight reduction (7%) in the odds of reconviction. Offender risk level, number of previous sentencing occasions for any type of offense, and number of previous sentencing occasions for violence all increase the odds of reconviction. For risk category, it is the high-risk category as compared to the low-risk category that substantially increases the odds of reconviction. High-risk offenders are 5 times more likely to be reconvicted within 2 years for a sexual and/or violent offense than are low-risk offenders.

Hierarchical logistic regression analysis was conducted with treatment only allowed to enter the regression after the forced entry of the other variables. Treatment did produce a significant improvement in the prediction of reconviction ($\chi^2 = 5.56$, $df = 1$, $p < .05$).

In this study, the risk predictor Static-99's performance accuracy was good. Receiver operating characteristic (ROC) analysis was used to evaluate the predictive accuracy of Static-99. The area under the ROC curve statistic was 0.70 for sexual reconviction and 0.70 in terms of predicting sexual and/or violent reconviction.

DISCUSSION

The 2-year sexual reconviction rates for both treatment and comparison group offenders are low, but the treatment group sample had slightly lower reconviction rates than the comparison group sample. There were no significant differences between these rates. Friendship and Thornton (2001) have discussed the possible absence of statistical significance for evaluation studies in England and Wales. They suggested that as the rate of sexual reconviction is already low for untreated sexual offenders (i.e., 5% within 2 years of release), any reduction in this rate as a result of treatment would be so small that it would be difficult to statistically demonstrate that it was due to the effect of treatment rather than chance factors. Marques (1999) reported nonsignificant differences between treatment offenders and controls in the preliminary evaluation of a California sexual offender treatment program but stated that this was not unexpected as the evaluation was a longitudinal evaluation and the final results would be 5 years hence.

The reliance on official sexual reconviction rates to evaluate the effectiveness of SOTP is unrealistic in light of the low base rate of sexual reconviction (Friendship & Thornton, 2001). In England and Wales, official recording of crime relates only to criminal conviction variables and a small number of demographic details. Supplementing sexual reconviction data with nonofficial data has been recommended and adopted by various studies (Allam, 1998; Marques, Day, Nelson, & West, 1994; Marshall & Barbaree, 1988) and should be the aim of future evaluative research.

A combined outcome measure of sexual and/or violent reconviction demonstrated that there were overall significant differences between the treatment and comparison groups in the rate of reconviction (Table 4). In terms of risk group, for low- and high-risk offenders, there was a trend in the expected direction, with the treatment group showing a slightly lower rate of reconviction. Significant differences were found between medium-low and medium-high risk offenders. The mechanism behind this may simply be that the combination of both sexual and violent outcomes serves to raise the reconviction base rate.

A further explanation for this could be that a proportion of the violent reconvictions were in fact sexually motivated offenses. A recent United Kingdom study assessed the violent reconvictions of a sample of sexual offenders discharged from prison (who had not been reconvicted of a sexual offense). The study concluded that 12% of the violent reconvictions had a sexual motivation (Corbett, Patel, Erikson, & Friendship, in press). Research has also demonstrated that some sexual offenses result in a conviction for a nonsexual offense (e.g., Marshall, 1994), and this results from the legal processes that may include plea-bargaining.

Finally, these results could be due to the known differences between the treatment and offender samples, particularly in terms of their previous history of violence (see Table 1). This notion was examined in further logistic regression analysis where these differences were controlled for. The results of this suggested that when other relevant factors were controlled for, the effect of treatment was maintained ($p < .05$). Hierarchical logistic regression also confirmed this result.

Although there were no significant differences between the treatment and comparison groups in terms of general reconviction, treated offenders did consistently have lower rates of general reconviction as compared to untreated offenders.

The performance accuracy of the risk predictor Static-99 was shown, in this study, to be good. Using only seven items of Static-99 was not ideal and would to some degree influence risk group categorization and the accuracy of the predictor. However, despite this limitation, the predictive accuracy of Static-99 was maintained to a level reported in other studies (e.g., Hanson & Thornton, 2000). Interestingly, in the logistic regression analysis, Static-99 risk score was not accepted into the model to predict reconviction, whereas Static-99 risk category was accepted.

Research Design

In the absence of a randomized experimental design, the most difficult thing to achieve is comparability between treatment and offender groups. Within Her Majesty's Prison Service, comparison group matching is limited by a number of factors.

First, this study used a comparison group that broadly matched the demographic and criminal conviction characteristics of the treatment group. It could be argued that a more detailed matched comparison group would be superior. The absence of victim-perpetrator information for the comparison group, however, compromises the ability to provide a well-matched group. There are also relatively small numbers of sexual offenders in prison in England and Wales (Marshall, 1994), and as the number of sexual offenders participating in treatment increases, the numbers available for comparison group matching decrease. In a recent United Kingdom study, Erikson and Friendship (2003), revealed that finding an adequate comparison group for sexual offenders is difficult as the SOTP inadvertently selects offenders that are fundamentally different to untreated counterparts in terms of criminal history. In North America, the problem of comparison group matching has been discussed in the recent treatment literature (e.g., Hanson & Nicholaichuk, 2000; Looman, Abracen, & Nicholaichuk, 2000; Nicholaichuk, Gordon, Gu, & Wong, 2000).

Second, this study retrospectively constructed a comparison group. This has limitations as researchers often have to rely on a small number of static factors for matching. Typically, there are far more available data for the treatment sample than the comparison group (e.g., selection for treatment interview and assessment test battery data). As mentioned above, the United Kingdom criminal conviction database does not systematically record victim details, so this level of detail is missing for comparison group cases.

Third, offenders in the treatment group have volunteered to participate in treatment, and because of this, it is argued that they are different from untreated offenders on motivational factors. Sexual offenders who totally deny their offense are excluded from treatment, and so denial may also account for differences between the two groups.

Finally, in this study, the dropouts were not recorded in a systematic way and were not identifiable as a discrete group. Some dropouts appeared within the treatment group, and others did not. This fundamental recording problem has been identified and rectified in current data recording practices for the SOTP.

Future Direction of Evaluative Research

The way forward is a prospective matching of comparison group offenders to treatment counterparts. This could attempt to collect fuller information on the untreated offenders including factors such as victims of offending, motivational factors, and denial and other psychological characteristics. This study would involve systematic data collection for comparison group offenders as the treatment group goes through the treatment process. In a prospective design, offenders could also be matched by treatment center to examine quality of program delivery.

The approach of the traditional reconviction or recidivism study in evaluating treatment efficacy makes the assumption that participation in treatment has the same effect on all offenders. In reality, the success of treatment can be dependent on factors such as the treatment climate, the implementation of the program, and how the individual sex offender responds to treatment. This concept has been explored in detail (Beech et al., 1999). In a study of child abusers who participated in the SOTP, the authors examined change attributable to treatment in four main areas. These were denial or admittance of deviant sexual interests and level of offending behavior, pro-offending attitudes, predisposing personality factors, and relapse prevention skills. A sophisticated analysis then assessed whether individual offenders met a "treated profile" on these four domains. Future research needs to further develop this work to examine the relationship between treatment change and reconviction. This type of approach to evaluation examines the treatment of offenders only and to some extent avoids the issues surrounding comparison group matching.

REFERENCES

Allam, J. (1998). *Effective practice in work with sex offenders: A reconviction study comparing treated and untreated offenders*. Birmingham, UK: West Midlands Probation Service Sex Offender Unit.

Beech, A. R., Fisher, D., & Beckett, R. C. (1999). *STEP 3: An evaluation of the prison sex offender treatment programme*. London: HMSO.

Beech, A. R., & Fordham, A. (1997). Therapeutic climate of sexual offender treatment programs. *Sexual Abuse: A Journal of Research and Treatment, 9*, 219-237.

Beech, A. R., Friendship, C., Erikson, M., & Hanson, R. K. (2002). The relationship between static and dynamic risk factors and reconviction in a sample of UK child abusers. *Sexual Abuse: A Journal of Research and Treatment, 14*, 155-167.

Beitchman, J. H., Zucker, K. J., Hood, J. E., DaCosta, G. A., Ackman, D., & Cassavia, E. (1991). A review of the long-term effects of child abuse. *Child Abuse and Neglect, 16*, 101-118.

Corbett, C., Patel, V., Erikson, M., & Friendship, C. (in press). The violent reconvictions of sexual offenders. *Journal of Sexual Aggression.*

Criminal Justice Act: England and Wales. (1991). London: HMSO.

Erikson, M., & Friendship, C. (2003). *Sexual offenders selected for prison-based treatment: Implications for comparison group matching*. Manuscript submitted for publication.

Finkelhor, D. (1984). *Child sexual abuse: New theory and research*. New York: Free Press.

Finkelhor, D., & Browne, A. (1985). The traumatic impact of child sexual abuse: A conceptualization. *American Journal of Orthopsychiatry, 59*, 238-245.

Fisher, D., & Beech, A. R. (2002). Treating adult sexual offenders. In K. Browne, H. Hanks, P. Stratton, & C. Hamilton (Eds.), *The prediction and prevention of child abuse: A handbook* (pp. 337-353). Chichester, UK: Wiley.

Friendship, C., & Thornton, D. (2001). Sexual reconviction for sexual offenders discharged from prison in England and Wales: Implications for evaluating treatment. *British Journal of Criminology, 41*, 285-292.

Furby, L., Weinrott, M. R., & Blackshaw, L. (1989). Sex offender recidivism: A review. *Psychological Bulletin, 105*, 3-30.

Grubin, D., & Thornton, D. (1994). A national programme for the assessment and treatment of sex offenders in the English prison system. *Criminal Justice and Behavior, 21*, 55-71.

Hanson, R. K., & Nicholaichuk, T. (2000). A cautionary note regarding Nicholaichuk et al. (2000). *Sexual Abuse: A Journal of Research and Treatment, 12*, 189-293.

Hanson, R. K., & Thornton, D. (2000). Improving risk assessments for sexual offenders: A comparison of three actuarial scales. *Law and Human Behavior, 24*, 119-136.

Looman, J., Abracen, J., & Nicholaichuk, T. R. (2000). Recidivism among treated sexual offenders and matched controls. *Journal of Interpersonal Violence, 15*, 279-290.

Mann, R. E., & Thornton, D. (1998). The Evolution of a multisite sexual offender program. In W. L. Marshall, Y. M. Fernandez, S. M. Hudson, & T. Ward (Eds.)., *Sourcebook of treatment programs for sexual offenders* (pp. 47-57). New York: Plenum.

Marques, J. K. (1999). How to answer the question "does sex offender treatment work?" *Journal of Interpersonal Violence, 14*, 437-541.

Marques, J. K., Day, D. M., Nelson, C., & West, M. A. (1994). Effects of cognitive-behavioral treatment on sex offender recidivism: Preliminary results of a longitudinal study. *Criminal Justice and Behavior, 21*, 10-27.

Marshall, P. (1994). Reconviction of imprisoned sexual offenders. *Research Bulletin, 36*, 23-29. (Available from Home Office, London)

Marshall, W. L., Anderson, D., & Fernandez, Y. (1999). *Cognitive behavioural treatment of sexual offenders*. Chichester, UK: Wiley.

Marshall, W. L., & Barbaree, H. E. (1988). The long-term evaluation of a behavioral treatment program for child molesters. *Behavior Research and Therapy, 6*, 499-511.

Marshall, W. L., Fernandez, Y. M., Hudson, S. M., & Ward, T. (Eds.). (1998). *Sourcebook of treatment programs for sexual offenders*. New York: Plenum.

McGuire, J. (Ed.). (1995). *What works: Reducing re-offending—Guidelines from research and practice*. Chichester, UK: Wiley.

Murphy, W. D. (1990). Assessment and modification of cognitive distortions in sex offenders. In W. L. Marshall, D. R. Laws, & H. E. Barbaree (Eds.), *Handbook of sexual assault: Issues, theories and treatment of the offender* (pp. 331-342). New York: Plenum.

Nelson, C., & Jackson, P. (1989). High-risk recognition: The cognitive-behavioral chain. In D. R. Laws (Ed.), *Relapse prevention with sex offenders* (pp. 167-177). New York: Guilford.

Nicholaichuk, T., Gordon, A., Gu, D., & Wong, S. (2000). Outcome of an institutional sexual offender treatment program: A comparison between treated and matched untreated offenders. *Sexual Abuse: A Journal of Research and Treatment, 12*, 139-153.

Pithers, W. D. (1994). Process evaluation of a group therapy component designed to enhance offenders' empathy for sexual abuse survivors. *Behavior Research and Therapy, 5*, 565-570.

Povey, D. (2001). *Recorded crime: England and Wales, 12 Months to September 2000* (Home Office statistical bulletin, national statistics, No. 1/01, pp. 1-34). London: Home Office.

Thornton, D., & Hogue, T. (1993). The large-scale provision of programs for imprisoned sex offenders: Issues, dilemmas and progress. *Criminal Behaviour and Mental Health, 3*, 371-380.

Wolf, S. C. (1988). A model of sexual aggression/addiction. *Journal of Social Work and Human Sexuality, 7*, 131-147.

Woolf report. (1991). *Prison disturbances 1990, report by the Rt Hon. Lord Justice Woolf and his Honour Judge Stephen Tumin.* London: HMSO.

Caroline Friendship, MSc., is a chartered forensic psychologist with Her Majesty's Prison Service, and her main role is evaluating the effectiveness of prison-based programs for offenders in terms of reconviction. She is currently working toward a Ph.D. at the University of Birmingham.

Ruth E. Mann, MSc., is a chartered forensic psychologist with Her Majesty's Prison Service and is the head of the Sex Offender Treatment Program. She is responsible for program implementation, development, and staff training; clinical support monitoring, and clinical evaluation. She is currently engaged in a doctoral research program studying the role of cognition in sexual offending.

Anthony R. Beech, Ph.D., is a senior lecturer at the University of Birmingham and has published more than 30 articles on assessment and treatment of sexual offenders.

[15]

Treatment Effects on Forensic Psychiatric Patients Measured With the HCR-20 Violence Risk Assessment Scheme

Henrik Belfrage and Kevin S. Douglas

This study focuses on the foundational issue of change in violence risk factors in forensic psychiatric patients across multiple assessment periods using the HCR-20 scheme. HCR-20 assessments performed on 150 forensic psychiatric patients at two special (forensic) hospitals in Sweden were studied in relation to the patients' time at institution, with the aim to investigate a possible relation between level of risk and time at institution. A sub-group was followed across an 18-month period of institutionalization to investigate possible changes in risk factors over time. The latter patients were assessed with the HCR-20 three times, with six months between the assessments. Patients with longer treatment times had lower scores on the HCR-20 Clinical and Risk Management sub-scales, compared to patients who had been admitted to the hospitals for a shorter period of time. This finding was particularly evident on the cross-sectional analyses with respect to the R scale. The clinical risk factors in the C scale also dropped overall in connection with treatment time across both cross-sectional and prospective analyses, although not as substantially as the R scale. The results are consistent with and provide support for the HCR-20 system's proposition that the C and R scales are dynamic, or prone to change.

One of the most important issues in the area of correctional and forensic psychiatric treatment is the question of its crime prevention effectiveness. Politicians, media, and the public frequently discuss the issue, and clinicians and researchers in the field are often asked for answers. There have been important developments in terms of the accuracy of assessments of risk for violence among persons with mental disorders (Douglas, Ogloff, Nicholls, & Grant, 1999; McNiel & Binder, 1994; Monahan et al., 2000, 2001; Quinsey, Harris, Rice, & Cormier, 1998; Steadman et al., 2000). In recent years, the field of violence risk assessment has, however, appropriately started to turn its focus to questions of violence prevention rather than merely violence prediction (Hart, 1998, 2001). This shift in attention has, to date, been more conceptual and theoretical than empirical (though see Skeem, Mulvey, & Lidz, 2000), although it represents a needed aspect of a comprehensive model of violence risk assessment.

This concern with violence prevention among risk assessment researchers and commentators is embodied primarily in mounting recognition of risk management as an integral component of risk assessment. For instance, Heilbrun (1997) proposed that there are two major ways in which risk assessment is carried out—prediction versus management. In the management model, the goal is the reduction of risk through ongoing assessments of primarily dynamic (changeable) risk factors. Steadman et al. (1993; see also Monahan, 1988) discussed the reconceptualization of risk assessment to consist of "ongoing, day-to-day decisions about the management and treatment of mentally disordered persons" (p. 41), rather than a one-time prediction. Steadman (2000) similarly has noted that the risk assessment paradigm that has emerged in recent years is sensitive to the likelihood that violence risk may change over time (and hence need re-assessment), and that questions of the intensity of community supervision are as important to the risk assessment task as are decisions related to confinement. The clinical task often calls for the specification of (dynamic) conditions that may aggravate or mitigate risk, rather than an "on-off, context-free prediction of dangerousness based on a consistent algorithm" (Mulvey & Lidz, 1995, p. 136).

Henrik Belfrage is at the Forensic Psychiatric Centre, Sundsvall. Kevin S. Douglas is at the Department of Mental Health Law and Policy, Florida Mental Health Institute, University of South Florida. The authors are grateful to Research Assistant Susanne Strand for her statistical assistance. Address all correspondence to Henrik Belfrage, Box 880, 851 24 Sundsvall, Sweden. (E-mail: henrik.belfrage@lvn.se).

Dvoskin and Heilbrun (2001) noted that most forensic systems use a risk management approach that entails as an important element ongoing evaluations of dynamic risk factors. Under such a model, progress of patients or prisoners on potentially changeable risk factors should be monitored, as mitigation or aggravation of such risk factors has implications for supervision and intervention. As stated by Dvoskin and Heilbrun (2001), "An individual's risk may be seen as changing over time and in response to interventions, as contrasted with the single, unchanging risk estimate yielded under the prediction model by actuarial tools that use static (unchangeable through planned intervention) risk factors" (p. 8).

They went on to state that "the next challenge for the medical and behavioral sciences is to develop an accurate way of measuring those aspects of violence risk that change" (p. 8). They cited the Level of Service Inventory—Revised (LSI-R; Andrews & Bonta, 1995) and the HCR-20 violence risk assessment scheme (Webster, Douglas, Eaves, & Hart, 1997) as two risk assessment instruments that contain putatively dynamic risk factors, and hence as potentially useful vehicles for indexing the change of violence risk. The current research, as described below, focuses on the latter of these two instruments—the HCR-20. As explained in the manual (Webster et al., 1997) and elsewhere (Douglas, Cox, & Webster, 1999; Webster, Douglas, Belfrage, & Link, 2000), the HCR-20 lends itself to use within the emerging management/prevention model of risk assessment because of its inclusion of dynamic risk factors that can serve as intervention targets.

The growing recognition of violence risk management and prevention as the primary purpose to many, if not most, risk assessments has led to the necessity of conceptualizing means by which such management and prevention can be effected. Of course, there exists a fairly large research literature on the effectiveness of correctional treatment of both adult and adolescent offenders. However, there are drastically fewer crime and violence prevention research studies that focus upon forensic and civil psychiatric patients. Further, the field of violence risk assessment has, for the most part, yet to integrate its newfound interest in risk management with existing correctional treatment principles and concepts.

One principle that has found its way into the risk assessment field, however, is the classification of risk factors according to their potential responsiveness to treatment interventions. As has been described in the correctional treatment literature (Andrews & Bonta, 1998), and as alluded to above, risk factors can be *static* or *dynamic*. Static risk factors are those that are highly unlikely to change, and, hence, cannot be considered promising treatment targets. Dynamic factors, on the other hand, are theoretically prone to change, either spontaneously or through intervention, and hence are good candidates for violence prevention interventions.[1] Hanson and Harris (2000) further divided dynamic risk factors into *stable* and *acute* dynamic factors. Stable dynamic factors are unlikely to change over short periods of time, but can change gradually. Acute dynamic factors, however, could in principle change daily or even by the minute. This concern with static and dynamic violence risk factors is foundational to future attempts to mitigate violence risk among forensic and civil psychiatric patients, as it has been to models of crime reduction in the correctional field. As a concept, it is a necessary addition to the emerging risk management and violence prevention focus within the field of risk assessment.

Further, commentators have typically described the risk management model as entailing repeated re-evaluations of risk over time (Douglas et al., 1999; Dvoskin & Heilbrun, 2001; Hart, 1998, 2001; Steadman et al., 1993; Webster et al., 2000). The traditional approach when evaluating both violence prediction and forensic treatment is to focus on two points in time—when the prediction was made or

[1] We would like to point out that the terms *static* and *actuarial* are not synonymous, as is sometimes assumed in the literature. The term *actuarial* refers to the process of combining variables to reach a decision (i.e., in an algorithmic manner according to fixed and explicit rules), not to the nature of risk factors being used (Grove & Meehl, 1996; Meehl, 1954). The term also does not refer to variables that have a good deal of empirical support. A variable that has absolutely no empirical support could be used in an actuarial fashion. Similarly, a variable with a vast amount of empirical support, even if static, could be used in a non-actuarial manner (i.e., in a way that is not algorithmic, explicit, and fixed—typically called clinical decision-making or prediction). Further, dynamic or changeable variables, with or without empirical support, can in theory be used in either actuarial or clinical means.

the intervention started, and when follow-up data were obtained. This approach characterizes most published risk assessment research. What happens between these two points often is excluded, and thus remains unknown (Webster et al., 2000). Chances are, of course, that behavioral and attitudinal changes that occurred never will be captured—changes that might provide important feed-back for people involved in ongoing assessment regimes or various treatment programs.

This traditional method by which to understand risk assessment and treatment outcome is inconsistent with the emerging risk management model that calls for ongoing re-evaluation of risk and attendant adjustment of interventions. The importance and utility of dynamic risk factors to violence prevention and risk management is diminished by a conceptual model that fails to account for the possibility of change in the status of these risk factors. That is, the traditional research study that uses a simple two-point prediction-outcome model, while serving the important role of validating the relationship between predictions/predictors and violence, cannot be of much service to forwarding the scientific basis of a risk management/violence prevention model of risk assessment.

In addition to calls for more attention to risk management by those in the field of risk assessment, there have been some attempts to lay the groundwork for an empirically-grounded approach that integrates risk assessment and risk management and prevention. The HCR-20 violence risk assessment scheme (Webster et al., 1997), the focus of the data presented in this article, is a risk assessment tool that offers the potential of conducting repeated re-evaluations of risk rather than making one-time predictions. As displayed in Figure 1, the instrument contains not only 10 historical, static risk factors such as history of violence and substance misuse, but also 10 potentially changeable, dynamic risk factors. Five of these concern current mental and clinical status (the Clinical scale), and five concern future situational risk factors (the Risk Management scale). This makes it possible to use the HCR-20 to perform repeated evaluations of changeable risk factors over time, and to modify treatment and management strategies accordingly. The questions in focus become: Have we managed to change some important risk factors among patients prior to their release? Are risk factors still under control while patients are being supervised in the community? rather than: How many patients have, after their discharge, relapsed into new criminality according to file information?

Figure 1
The HCR-20 Items (Webster, Douglas, Eaves & Hart, 1997)

Historical (Past)	Clinical (Present)	Risk Management (Future)
H1. Previous Violence	C1. Lack of Insight	R1. Plans Lack Feasibility
H2. Young Age at First Violent Incident	C2. Negative Attitudes	R2. Exposure to Destabilizers
H3. Relationship Instability	C3. Active Symptoms of Major Mental Illness	R3. Lack of Personal Support
H4. Employment Problems	C4. Impulsivity	R4. Noncompliance with Remediation Attempts
H5. Substance Use Problems	C5. Unresponsive to Treatment	R5. Stress
H6. Major Mental Illness		
H7. Psychopathy		
H8. Early Maladjustment		
H9. Personality Disorder		
H10. Prior Supervision Failure		

Note. Adapted with permission from Webster et al. (1997).

There is also a new companion publication to the HCR-20 risk assessment scheme that suggests intervention and management strategies that flow from the 10 potentially changeable or dynamic risk factors. This *HCR-20 Violence Risk Management Companion Guide* (Douglas, Webster, Hart, Eaves, & Ogloff, 2001) provides a small chapter for each of the 5 Clinical and 5 Risk Management items outlining several intervention or management ideas that could be of assistance to clinicians, case workers, or probation/parole officers who are charged with either reducing or monitoring risk. Together, the two manuals are intended to provide one option for an integrated assessment/management system. Doubtless there are many other systems that do or could exist.

This study focuses on the small though foundational issue of change in violence risk factors across multiple assessment periods. This question, as discussed above, is integral to the emerging risk management model of risk assessment, in that changeable risk factors provide the greatest promise for violence risk reduction and, ultimately, violence prevention. However, there have been few investigations in the risk assessment field of change in risk factors across time.

Research on the HCR-20 violence risk assessment scheme has tended to show good validity when used with a traditional "predictive" approach. That is, effect sizes between the HCR-20 scales and various measures of violence have mainly been moderate to large across different populations (i.e., forensic psychiatric; civil psychiatric; correctional; mentally disordered offenders) and different settings (i.e., institutional; community) (for reviews and commentaries, see Beech, 2000; Dolan & Doyle, 2000; Douglas, 2001; Douglas et al., 1999; Douglas & Webster, 1999; Edens & Otto, 2001; Mossman, 2000; Otto, 2000; Witt, 2000). Interrater reliability also has been demonstrated to be acceptable (e.g., Belfrage, 1998; Dernevik, 1998; Douglas, 2001; Douglas & Webster, 1999). It has been officially implemented into practice in forensic psychiatric settings in Germany, Canada, the Netherlands, and the United States (California and New York), and both forensic psychiatric and correctional settings in Sweden (e.g., Belfrage, 1998; Belfrage, Fransson, & Strand, 2000). It has been used among both male patients and female patients (see Nicholls, Ogloff, & Douglas, 2001, and Strand & Belfrage, 2001, for data on female patients). Recent studies have shown, both in violence risk assessments of institutional violence, and in risk assessments of community violence, that the dynamic risk factors on the HCR-20 have a strong link to future aggression and violence (Belfrage, Fransson, & Strand, 1999; Ross, Hart, & Webster, 1998; Strand, Belfrage, Fransson, & Levander, 1999).

Few studies have investigated the utility of dynamic violence risk factors. Hanson and Harris (2000) did report that these variables were related to violence among a sample of sex offenders. Skeem et al. (2000), however, reported that while clinicians were able to predict violence at above-chance levels among a large sample of civil psychiatric patients, they were unable to make "conditional" predictions at above-chance levels. That is, they were unable to forecast the alcohol-related violence of patients.

Only one study has focused on changes in HCR-20 scores *over time*. Douglas and Belfrage (2001; see also Webster et al., 2000) analyzed changes in HCR-20 items across two time periods in civil- and forensic psychiatric patients in Canada and Sweden. Overall, the scores on the risk factors declined over time, albeit differently in various samples. Civil psychiatric patients had a large drop in scores. Among 193 Canadian civil psychiatric patients, the Clinical Scale was coded at both admission and discharge. The mean total Clinical Scale score dropped from approximately 7 (out of 10), to roughly 4, a large change as indexed by Cohen's *d*. The proportion of patients who scored in the 8-10 range dropped from 48% to 3%. Drops on individual risk factors were commensurate with the drop on the overall scale. In two forensic samples—one Canadian and one Swedish—there also were drops on C and R Scale scores and items, although they were more moderate in size.

In the current study, 219 HCR-20 assessments performed on 150 forensic psychiatric patients at two special (forensic) hospitals in Sweden were studied. The HCR-20 assessments were analyzed in relation to the patients' time at institution, with the aim to investigate a possible relation between level of risk and time at institution. The expectation was that there would be a decrease in the scores of HCR-20 violence risk factors over time, owing to intervention efforts.

Additionally, a sub-group of the study group was followed across an 18-month period of institutionalization. These patients were assessed with the HCR-20 three times, with six months between assessments. Since several of the clinical and risk management items incorporated in the HCR-20 may demand a certain amount of time to influence and adjust (e.g., feasible plans for discharge), the aim was to investigate possible changes in scores for certain patients on the dynamic HCR-20 risk factors over a longer period of time than had been done previously.

METHOD

Participants

The sample comprised all forensic psychiatric patients admitted at two maximum-security forensic psychiatric hospitals in Sweden (Sundsvall and Växjö) between 1997–2001 (*N* = 150). Many of these patients had been assessed on more than one occasion, given the length of time they had been institutionalized. In total, there were 219 HCR-20 assessments completed on these 150 participants. Participants were all sentenced to forensic psychiatric care according to the Swedish Penal Code, meaning that they were all convicted for one or more crimes, and it was determined by a judge that mental disorder was a causal factor in the crime, and could be in future crimes as well. The sample was all male, with a mean age at the time of the first assessment of 39 (*SD* = 10). Seventy patients (47%) were diagnosed with psychotic disorders, and eighty (53%) with personality (and "other") disorders. The diagnoses were made by psychiatrists according to the *Diagnostic and Statistical Manual of Mental Disorders, Fourth Edition* (DSM-IV; American Psychiatric Association, 1994).

A majority of the patients (94%) had committed violent crimes. Thirty (20%) had committed homicide/manslaughter, 38 (25%) were sentenced for assault, 38 (25%) had committed a violent sexual crime, and 35 (23%) were sentenced for other violent crimes. At the time of the first assessment, the patients had been admitted to the hospital for an average of 37 months (*SD* = 44), with a range from 1 to 186 months. (If a person started a month, it counted as a month, e.g., 3 months and 4 days, was scored as 4 months.)

Measures

All patients were subjected to real-life assessments (*in vivo*) with the HCR-20 risk assessment scheme, Version 2 (Webster, et al, 1997), including the Psychopathy Checklist: Screening Version (Hart, Cox & Hare, 1995). All items in the HCR-20, which are labeled in Figure 1, are scored as 0 (No), 1 (Possibly) or 2 (Yes). The scale divides items according to past (H), present (C), and future (R) time. The authorized Swedish versions of the HCR-20 (Belfrage & Fransson, 1997) and the PCL:SV (Belfrage, 1997) were used. These are literal translations, worked out in close collaboration with the Canadian authors, and hence findings in this study should be interpretable to the original schemes. The HCR-20 has since 1997 been fully implemented into clinical practice at both hospitals, a process which is described in detail in Belfrage (1998).

Procedure

Every six months, patients appear before a Criminal Review Board seeking conditional or absolute discharge. In addition to these reviews, a team consisting of psychiatrists, psychologists, social workers, and other members of the staff assesses the patients. In the first part of this study, containing cross-sectional between-groups analyses, only complete HCR-20 "Out-assessments" were used (i.e., HCR-20 assessments in which the R items are coded for community release). Thus, no "In-assessments," where the R-scale in the HCR-20 is focused on risk for violence *inside* the institution, were used for these analyses. The reason for this is that the R- scale turned out to have been used slightly differently by different assessment teams. Some always performed both In- and Out- assessments, as was instructed, while some had performed either In- or Out-assessments, depending on where in the treatment phase the patients have been. Some treatment teams, for instance, experienced difficulties assessing a long-term patient with the Out- scale, simply because there were not any plans made for the patient's return into the community since he would be expected to stay for at least 10-15 more years at the hospital. However, in the second part of this study, the prospective, within-group analyses, data on In-assessments will be reported, but with varying sub-group sample number regarding R-assessments.

Cross-sectional, between-groups analyses. The sample was divided into three groups as a function of the amount of time that individuals had spent in the institution. The first group contained those who had been at the institution up to a year, the second group contained those who had been admitted between one and two years, and the last group contained all patients who had been admitted for more than two years. In cases where patients had been subject to more than one HCR-20 assessment, they were included in respective study groups (i.e., a patient who had been assessed at 9 months and 15 months would have their respective scores included in both Group 1 and 2). Thus, one patient can be represented at a minimum once, and at a maximum three times in total. However, no patients are more than once represented in one group (i.e., within each group, there is only one HCR-20 rating per patient). The reason for having some patients appearing in different groups, in a between-group comparison, is that our approach in this first part of the study is directed at the amount of institutional time in relation to HCR-20 risk factors. In the second part of the study, however, change in risk factors over time on the same patients is studied.

From Table 1 it can be seen that the three groups were quite equivalent in size, background factors (age, index crimes, principal psychiatric diagnoses), H-10 scores (i.e., the aspect of the HCR-20 that measures, *inter alia*, historical and static risk factors such as early maladjustment, substance misuse, and previous criminality), and PCL:SV scores. Thus, the only difference between the groups on the measures we have used in this study was time at institution (i.e. length of treatment). Some of this homogeneity in background factors could be explained by the fact that some patients are displayed in more than one group; this represents a minority, however.

The statistics used for these analyses were the non-parametric Mann-Whitney U and the Kruskal-Wallis H tests. The reason for using non-parametric tests in this section, despite that they are less sensitive compared to parametric tests, is the slightly different praxis and routines that had evolved at the two clinics during the study period. Thus, this was an "assurance" from getting results more powerful than they are. (However, we also analyzed the data using the parametric t test, which overall yielded the same results.)

Prospective, within-group analyses. A sub-group consisting of all patients (n = 70) who had been assessed three times, with approximately 6 months between the assessments, was also analyzed. Data regarding two of these three assessment points has previously been reported for 33 patients (47%) in this sub-group (Douglas & Belfrage, 2001; Webster et al., 2000).

The statistics used in this sub-group was the dependent t test, which is a parametric statistical test commonly used to measure differences in mean scores. The reason for using parametric tests in this section was that we here are interested in changes within the the same persons. However, analyses were also made using the non-parametric Wilcoxon's test, which yielded the same results as for the t test. Only the results from the t test analyses are therefore presented in the following.

Table 1
Certain background factors for 219 assessments on 150 mentally disordered offenders divided into three sub-groups depending on institutional time

	Group 1 (0-12 months) N = 81	Group 2 (13-24 months) N = 57	Group 3 (25-186 months) N = 81
Institutional time, *Md*	4.7 months	16.4 months	57.2 months
Age in years, *M (SD)*	36.6 (10.0)	38.0 (9.6)	40.4 (10.0)
H-scale, *M (SD)*	13.4 (4.5)	13.2 (4.3)	13.3 (3.8)
PCL:SV, *M (SD)*	13.4 (5.5)	12.5 (5.9)	12.4 (5.5)
Violent crimes, *N (%)*	75 (93%)	53 (93%)	76 (94%)
Psychosis diagnoses, *N (%)*	41 (51%)	27 (47%)	41 (51%)
Personality (and other) disorders, *N (%)*	40 (49%)	30 (53%)	40 (49%)

Table 2
Distribution of HCR-20 dynamic risk factors in 219 HCR-20 assessments on 150 mentally disordered offenders divided into three sub-groups depending on institutional time

HCR-20 Scale and Item	Group 1	Group 2	Group 3	Kruskal Wallis	Mann-Whitney		
				H-test	U-test		
	0-12 mos. $N = 81$ M (SD)	13-24 mos. $N = 57$ M (SD)	25-186 mos. $N = 81$ M (SD)	1,2,3 p value	1-2 p value	2-3 p value	1-3 p value
H-Scale							
Total	13.4 (4.5)	13.2 (4.3)	13.3 (3.8)	0.931	0.738	0.912	0.768
C Scale							
C1	1.5 (0.5)	1.3 (0.6)	1.3 (0.6)	0.040	0.035	0.996	0.026
C2	1.3 (0.7)	1.2 (0.7)	1.1 (0.7)	0.164	0.251	0.563	0.064
C3	0.6 (0.8)	0.5 (0.7)	0.5 (0.8)	0.657	0.558	0.784	0.379
C4	0.9 (0.7)	0.8 (0.5)	0.8 (0.6)	0.381	0.305	0.830	0.205
C5	1.3 (0.7)	1.1 (0.6)	1.1 (0.7)	0.154	0.179	0.658	0.070
Total	5.7 (2.3)	5.0 (2.1)	4.8 (2.3)	0.074	0.077	0.768	0.038
R Scale (Out)							
R1	1.7 (0.5)	1.4 (0.6)	1.3 (0.8)	0.000	0.003	0.277	0.000
R2	1.8 (0.5)	1.7 (0.5)	1.5 (0.5)	0.003	0.179	0.075	0.001
R3	1.5 (0.6)	1.2 (0.7)	1.2 (0.7)	0.009	0.037	0.503	0.003
R4	1.6 (0.7)	1.2 (0.7)	1.0 (0.8)	0.000	0.004	0.140	0.000
R5	1.8 (0.5)	1.6 (0.6)	1.4 (0.6)	0.000	0.066	0.019	0.000
Total	8.3 (2.1)	7.2 (2.5)	6.4 (2.7)	0.000	0.010	0.068	0.000
HCR-20	27.4 (7.4)	25.4 (7.4)	24.6 (7.2)	0.033	0.081	0.543	0.012
PCL:SV	13.4 (5.4)	12.5 (5.9)	12.4 (5.5)	0.496	0.465	0.780	0.240

RESULTS

Cross-Sectional, Between-Groups Analyses

The distribution of the risk factors that comprise the HCR-20 C and R scales across the three groups is shown in Table 2. The data in Table 2 show that the mean scores for the C and R total scores are significantly lower the longer that patients have been hospitalized. That is, while the total scores for the C and R scales do not change between Groups 1 (0-12 months) and 2 (13-24 months), or 2 and 3 (25+ months), both declined significantly between Groups 1 and 3. It should be pointed out that some of the individual R scale items changed between Groups 1 and 2, and between 2 and 3, and all changed between Groups 1 and 3. As is evident, there was a greater degree of change for the R scale and its items compared to the C scale, both in terms of magnitude and number of individual factors that changed. We calculated Cohen's d based on the means and standard deviations presented in Table 2. For the significant C scale total score change (between Groups 1 and 3), it was .40 (small to moderate in size).[2] The significant changes for the R scale total score were larger ($d = .48$ [moderate in size] for the Group 1-2 comparison, and .79 [large in size] for the Group 1-3 comparison). It thus seems, as was one of our hypotheses, that those who had longer treatment times had a more feasible planning regarding their discharge into the community (which is reflected in the decline of their R scale scores).

[2] Cohen (1988, 1992) defines the size or magnitude of d, which is the standardized difference between means, as follows: small = .30, moderate = .50, large = .80+.

It might be viewed as somewhat surprising that there was no improvement at all between Groups 2 and 3 on the C scale. When analyzed closer, however, it turned out that there was a group of long-term patients in Group 3 with very high scores on the C and R scales as well as on the complete HCR-20. When those 5% of the patients with the longest treatment times in group 3 were deleted, there was, in fact, a significant change in the R scale between Groups 2 and 3 ($p < 0.03$). Under these conditions, then, the R scale total score differed significantly between each group. No improvement, however, appeared on the C scale.

It is noteworthy that there were differences on the HCR-20 total score between groups, albeit they were not highly significant. These could be attributed to the changes in the R and, to a lesser extent, the C scale, given that there were no changes on the H scale, as was expected (it is defined in part by the static nature of its items). Thus, it is important in studies using the HCR-20 to carefully analyze all parts of this instrument and not just the HCR-20 total score. Significant changes might be hidden in the sub-scales.

Within-Groups, Prospective Analyses

The analysis of this sub-group of patients from the study group was performed with the aim to study possible changes in risk factors over time for the same patients ($n = 70$). The analysis above concerned different patients, with different treatment times. The current sub-group of 70 patients differed from the whole study group in an important aspect—the treatment times were significant longer. At the time of the first assessment, the patients in this sub-group had been admitted to the hospital for an average of 3 years (*MDN* 1.35 years, $SD = 3.37$), with a range from 1 to 15 years.

The scores on the HCR-20 C and R items for this sub-group across three assessment times are shown in Table 3. From Table 3 it can be seen that the mean scores on the C scale total dropped significantly over time, in a manner similar to the result from the whole study group (between-groups analyses), albeit somewhat less significantly and substantially ($d = .15$ and .26, or small, for time 1-2 and 1-3 comparisons). However, the scores on the R scale (Out) did not drop at all, which differs from the findings for the whole study group, where changes in these risk factors were significant. An explanation could well be, that much of the improvement in these patients already had taken place, due to their comparatively long treatment times. Their mean score on the R scale (Out), for example, is considerably lower at the time for their first assessment, compared to those who had been subject to treatment for a period of up to one year in the whole study group (Group 1 in Table 2). This probably reflects that, given their longer treatment times at the time of their first assessment, either much improvement concerning their discharge plans already had been done, or that these patients have substantially long treatment periods still in front of them, and consequently not much planning for their discharge seems to have been done. This is reflected by their very high scores on the R scale Total (Out).

Concerning the ratings for the R scale (In), there were significant drops across time for the total score and some of the individual risk factors. This suggests that while there had not yet been significant change in terms of planning for community release (the R scale "Out" assessment), there seems to have been some progress made in terms of institutional risk management planning ($d = .46$ and .45, respectively, for time 1-2 and 1-3 comparisons).

Additionally, considering these patients' comparatively longer treatment times, they must be regarded as a high-risk group of violent offenders, where any possible changes of dynamic risk factors for violence are well known to take a certain amount of time, if it is possible at all.

DISCUSSION

The basic logic underlying dynamic violence risk factors is that they are prone to change, particularly if they are targeted for violence-reducing treatment strategies. The overall finding of this study is that this basically is the case. Patients with longer treatment times had lower scores on the HCR-20 Clinical and Risk management subscales, compared to patients who had been admitted to the hospitals for a shorter period of time. This finding was particularly evident on the cross-sectional analyses with respect to the R scale (which used the "Out" scoring version). Using a prospective, within-groups

Table 3
Changes in HCR-20 C and R items across three assessment times in a forensic psychiatric sample (N = 70)

HCR-20 Scale and Item	Time 1 M (SD)	Time 2 M (SD)	Time 3 M (SD)	Difference Score (SD) Time 1-2	t	Difference Score (SD) Time 1-3	t
C Scale				N = 70		N = 70	
C1	1.44 (0.55)	1.40 (0.60)	1.32 (0.61)	0.04 (0.40)	0.90	0.11 (0.53)	1.82
C2	1.29 (0.68)	1.20 (0.69)	1.09 (0.72)	0.09 (0.41)	1.76	0.20 (0.55)	3.02**
C3	0.64 (0.82)	0.54 (0.77)	0.54 (0.76)	0.10 (0.49)	1.72	0.10 (0.64)	1.30
C4	0.89 (0.65)	0.81 (0.57)	0.81 (0.60)	0.07 (0.62)	0.96	0.07 (0.57)	1.04
C5	1.20 (0.69)	1.14 (0.73)	1.03 (0.66)	0.06 (0.66)	0.73	0.17 (0.68)	2.11*
Total	5.46 (2.48)	5.10 (2.36)	4.80 (2.51)	0.36 (1.44)	2.07*	0.66 (1.86)	2.96**
R Scale (In)				N = 40		N = 36	
R1	0.85 (0.74)	0.54 (0.74)	0.47 (0.61)	0.10 (0.74)	0.85	0.28 (0.66)	2.53*
R2	0.63 (0.63)	0.38 (0.49)	0.42 (0.55)	0.20 (0.61)	2.01*	0.14 (0.72)	1.15
R3	1.25 (0.74)	1.08 (0.79)	1.08 (0.81)	0.03 (0.62)	0.26	0.08 (0.55)	0.90
R4	1.30 (0.65)	1.00 (0.62)	1.00 (0.68)	0.30 (0.72)	2.62*	0.22 (0.68)	1.96
R5	0.98 (0.58)	1.02 (0.60)	1.03 (0.61)	0.00 (0.64)	0.00	-0.08 (0.69)	-0.72
Total	5.00 (2.16)	4.02 (2.13)	4.00 (2.24)	0.63 (1.89)	2.09*	0.64 (1.77)	2.16*
R Scale (Out)				N = 53		N = 52	
R1	1.42 (0.72)	1.43 (0.69)	1.37 (0.79)	0.02 (0.57)	0.24	0.04 (0.71)	0.39
R2	1.60 (0.53)	1.59 (0.49)	1.54 (0.54)	0.38 (0.48)	0.57	0.06 (0.50)	0.83
R3	1.13 (0.71)	1.20 (0.74)	1.10 (0.75)	0.04 (0.55)	0.49	0.02 (0.61)	0.23
R4	1.15 (0.84)	1.19 (0.73)	1.08 (0.79)	-0.06 (0.54)	-0.78	0.06 (0.64)	0.65
R5	1.51 (0.64)	1.58 (0.58)	1.52 (0.64)	-0.57 (0.50)	-0.83	-0.02 (0.54)	-0.26
Total	6.81 (2.79)	7.00 (2.57)	6.60 (2.88)	-0.02 (1.80)	-0.08	0.15 (2.10)	0.53

Notes. *$p < 0.05$; **$p < 0.01$, ***$p < 0.001$. The difference score in this table refers simply to the differences between means, and not to Cohen's *d*.

approach on a subsample of 70 patients produced similar findings, although observed significant effects for the R scale for the "In" assessment only, not for the "Out" assessment.

The clinical risk factors in the C scale also dropped overall in connection to treatment time across both cross-sectional and prospective analyses, although not as substantially as the R scale. Nonetheless, this can be seen as a reasonably promising result, since some clinical risk factors (insight, attitudes), as mentioned above, can take a long time to change, if it is possible at all. The scores on some items, such as C1, C3 and C4 (lack of insight, active symptoms, and impulsivity) might have reached their "barrier," since there were no changes at all on these items between the second and the third assessments.

Overall, the results are consistent with and provide support for the HCR-20 system's proposition that the C and R scales are dynamic, or prone to change. It is important to point out, as well, that the groups that were compared were very similar regarding certain background variables such as age, criminality, psychiatric diagnoses, psychopathic traits, and so forth.

In the sub-sample of 70 high-risk patients undergoing long-term treatment, the HCR-20 dynamic risk factors did change, but more moderately. While the C scale and R scale (for "In" ratings of institutional risk management planning) changed moderately, there were no changes for the R scale "Out" rating (for community-based release ratings of the Risk Management factors). One can speculate about why these changes were relatively moderate in this subsample, or, in the case of R-Out, non-existent. On the one hand, the sample is a high-risk group of mentally disordered offenders where changes in such factors as insight, attitudes, and so forth, are well known to be hard to accomplish. It also could be that, as pointed out by Webster et al. (2000), that the C variables are too broadly conceived to detect precise changes in attitudes and behavior in samples such as the present one. Further, it could well be that the treatment programs for this high-risk group deserve review or contrived alteration.

Whatever is the most probable scenario, this study stresses the importance of a careful analysis of the study groups. Different groups can, as in this study, yield different results. If we, for example, had analyzed only the group that had been subject to three assessments over time, we would have concluded that the R scale (Out) had not changed at all, pointing to a very disappointing treatment effect. However, the changes on the "In" R scale ratings suggests that, even in this high risk group, some changes had been accomplished. If, on the other hand, we only had analyzed the total study group, without analyzing the high-risk sub-group, we might have arrived at different conclusions, perhaps being somewhat more positive about the forensic psychiatric treatment provided in the two special hospitals in this study. None of the above scenarios is of course quite correct.

Undoubtedly, data from assessments using the HCR-20, and similar tools, can help not only researchers, but also clinicians, administrators, politicians, and others, in thinking about program planning and intervention in a more fruitful way than has been almost standard for a number of years (i.e., merely in terms of "relapse in new criminality after a certain number of years after discharge"). That is, the field is undergoing a change of paradigm in evaluation research in the area of mental disorder and crime. Modern risk assessment places more emphasis on prevention than in previous years (Dvoskin & Heilbrun, 2001). The consequences of this model are that the field is less focused *solely* on forecasting possible crimes in the future, and is placing resources into the careful monitoring and following up of patients during their treatment and after-care periods. Instruments such as the HCR-20 (Webster et al., 1997), the SARA (Kropp et al., 1999), and the SVR-20 (Boer et al., 1997) can inform this prevention-based model in that they promote the repeated re-assessment of potentially dynamic risk factors, changes of which would be important for constructing and revising risk management and violence prevention plans. These instruments can all be described as structured professional judgment guidelines, rather than exact instruments where the interest is focused on a single total score. They promote comprehensive, thorough evaluations of risk based on empirically-supported risk factors that also can adapt to changing circumstances and be used to inform risk management. Hart (1996, 1998, 1999) has pointed out that using instruments with focus on static risk factors with fixed scores, can sometimes lead to curious conclusions. The instrument becomes "more than the assessor," which is not the idea behind the professional guidelines mentioned above. These instruments, when used in clinical practice, should be an aid, and an "anchor," for the assessor.

Having said this, it becomes more important that contemporary risk assessment instruments are carefully and properly incorporated into clinical practice, and that standards for training are established and maintained. In this study, slightly different assessment techniques were used on the R-scale across the hospitals, and across different assessors, despite the fact that the HCR-20 was implemented into clinical practice at both institutions in the same way (Belfrage, 1998). Some teams had scored both In- and Out- assessments for the R scale, while others had scored either In- or Out- assessments. Some had even varied In- and Out-assessments over time, for the same patients. Thus, practice has a tendency to slightly change over time, and if not monitored and evaluated repeatedly, it could well be that the instrument eventually is used in a way in which it was never intended.

The use of professional guidelines is demanding for professionals who use them, and implies undoubtedly a great responsibility. Used in improper ways, they can be unethical and counter-productive. The "professional guidelines" manual HCR-20, for example, can be used as a strict statistical and quantitative risk assessment research tool, where only the total score is in focus. But it could also be used in clinical practice as a check-list of important risk factors from which the assessor has to consider the quality of the risk factors that apply. In practice, risk may never be as easy as a linear function of a certain number of risk factors (Hart, 2001).

One strategy to prevent misuse and misunderstanding of how the professional guidelines instruments are to be used in practice has been tested with good results in Sweden. In the Swedish HCR-20 manual, an additional score sheet has been added. One score sheet is for research use, where risk factors are scored with numbers (0, 1, 2), while the other score sheet is for clinical use, where risk factors are noted with letters (No, Partly, Present). This strategy helps clinicians, and others, to focus on the HCR-20 basically as a checklist of important risk factors when used in clinical practice, instead of focusing on a single total score, which unfortunately sometimes has been the case, despite the absence in the manual for any basis to do so.

Future studies in this field will undoubtedly focus considerably on dynamic risk factors for violence. How to index and define these risk factors in various offender and patient populations, and how to manage and improve them, will be of great importance. Instruments such as the HCR-20 might play an important role in this work.

REFERENCES

American Psychiatric Association. (1994). *Diagnostic and statistical manual of mental disorders* (4th ed.). Washington, DC: Author.

Andrews, D. A., & Bonta, J. (1995). *The Level of Service Inventory-Revised (LSI-R)*. Toronto: Multi-Health Systems.

Andrews, D. A., & Bonta, J. (1998). *The psychology of criminal conduct* (2nd ed.). Cincinnati, OH: Anderson.

Beech, A. R. (2000). Case material and interview. In C. R. Hollin (Ed.), *Handbook of offender assessment and treatment* (pp. 123-136). Chichester, UK: Wiley.

Belfrage, H. (1997). The interrater reliability of the HCR-20 scheme for risk assessment: A study of 6 clinicians assessments of the same 43 patients. *Nordic Forensic Medicine, 3*, 79-81.

Belfrage, H. (1997). The Hare PCL:SV. Swedish Manual Supplement. Multi-Health Systems, Ontario, Canada. Svensk översättning av Hart SD, Cox DN & Hare RD: *The Hare PCL:SV (The Psychopathy Checklist: Screening Version)*. Svensk distribution av Psykologiförlaget, Stockholm (Swedish).

Belfrage, H. & Fransson, G. (1997). *HCR-20. Bedömning av risk för framtida våld.* Manual med instruktioner och kommentarer. Växjö: Forskningsenheten, Regionpsykiatriskt centrum (Swedish).

Belfrage, H. (1998). Implementing the HCR-20 scheme for risk assessment in a forensic psychiatric hospital: Integrating research and clinical practice. *Journal of Forensic Psychiatry, 9*, 328-338.

Belfrage H., & Fransson G. (2000). *HCR-20. Bedömning av risk för framtida våld.* Manual med instruktioner och kommentarer. Andra reviderade upplagan. Växjö: Forskningsenheten, Regionpsykiatriskt centrum (Swedish).

Belfrage, H., Fransson, G., & Strand, S. (2000). Prediction of violence using the HCR-20: A prospective study in two maximum security correctional institutions. *Journal of Forensic Psychiatry, 11*, 167-175.

Boer, D. P., Hart, S. D., Kropp, P. R., & Webster, C. D. (1997). *Manual for the Sexual Violence Risk—20: Professional guidelines for assessing risk of sexual violence.* Vancouver, BC: British Columbia Institute Against Family Violence.

Cohen, J. (1988). *Statistical power analysis for the behavioral sciences* (2nd ed.). Hillsdale, NJ: Erlbaum.

Cohen, J. (1992). A power primer. *Psychological Bulletin, 112*, 155-159.

Dernevik, M. (1998). Preliminary findings on reliability and validity of the Historical-Clinical-Risk Assessment in a forensic psychiatric setting. *Psychology, Crime, and Law, 4*, 127-137.

Dolan, M., & Doyle, M. (2000). Violence risk prediction: Clinical and actuarial measures and the role of the Psychopathy Checklist. *British Journal of Psychiatry, 177*, 303-311.

Douglas, K. S. (2001). *HCR-20 violence risk assessment scheme: Overview and annotated bibliography* [On-line]. Available: http://www.sfu.ca/psychology/groups/faculty/ hart.violink.

Douglas, K. S., & Belfrage, H. (2001). Use of the HCR-20 in violence risk management: Implementation and clinical practice. In K. S. Douglas, C. D. Webster, D. Eaves, S. D. Hart & J. R. P. Ogloff (Eds.), *The HCR-20 violence risk management companion manual.* Burnaby, BC: Mental Health, Law, and Policy Institute, Simon Fraser University.

Douglas, K. S., Cox, D. N., & Webster, C. D. (1999). Violence risk assessment: Science and practice. *Legal and Criminological Psychology, 4*, 149-184.

Douglas, K. S., Ogloff, J. R. P., Nicholls, T. L. & Grant, I. (1999). Assessing risk for violence among psychiatric patients: The HCR-20 violence risk assessment scheme and the Psychopathy Checklist: Screening Version. *Journal of Consulting and Clinical Psychology, 67*, 917-930.

Douglas, K. S., & Webster, C. D. (1999). Predicting violence in mentally and personality disordered individuals. In R. Roesch, S. D. Hart, & J. R. P. Ogloff (Eds.), *Psychology and law: The state of the discipline* (pp. 175-239). New York: Plenum.

Douglas, K.S., Webster, C.D., Hart, S.D., Eaves, D., & Ogloff, J.R.P. (Eds.) (in press). *HCR-20: Violence risk management companion guide.* Burnaby, BC: Mental Health, Law, and Policy Institute, Simon Fraser University.

Dvoskin, J. A., & Heilbrun, K. (2001). Risk assessment and release decision-making: Toward resolving the great debate. *Journal of the American Academy of Psychiatry and the Law, 29*, 6-10.

Edens, J. F., & Otto, R. K. (2001). Release decision making and planning. In J. B. Ashford, B. D. Sales, & W. H. Reid (Eds.), *Treating adult and juvenile offenders with special needs* (pp. 335-371). Washington, DC: American Psychological Association.

Grann M., Belfrage, H. & Tengström, A. (2000). Actuarial assessment of risk for violence: Predictive validity of the VRAG and the historical part of the HCR-20. *Criminal Justice and Behavior, 27*, 97-114.

Hanson, R. K., & Harris, A. J. R. (2000). Where should we intervene? Dynamic predictors of sexual offense recidivism. *Criminal Justice & Behavior, 27*, 6-35.

Hart, S. D. (1996). *Conceptual issues in predicting violence: Some unasked and unanswered questions about risk assessment.* Paper presented at the Biennial Meeting of the American Psychology-Law Society (APA Div. 41), Hilton Head, South Carolina.

Hart, S. D. (1998). The role of psychopathy in assessing risk for violence: Conceptual and methodological issues. *Legal and Criminological Psychology, 3*, 121-137.

Hart, S. D. (1999). Assessing violence risk: Thoughts and second thoughts. [Review of the book *Violent offenders: Appraising and managing risk*]. *Contemporary Psychology, 44*, 486-488.

Hart, S. D. (2001). *Complexity, uncertainty, and the reconceptualization of violence risk assessment* [On-line]. Available: http://www.sfu.ca/psychology/groups/faculty/hart.

Hart, S. D., Cox, D., & Hare, R. D. (1995). *The Hare Psychopathy Checklist: Screening Version (PCL:SV).* Toronto, ON: Multi-Health Systems.

Heilbrun, K. (1997). Prediction versus management models relevant to risk assessment: The importance of legal decision-making context. *Law and Human Behavior, 21*, 347-359.

Kropp, P. R., Hart, S. D., Webster, C. D., & Eaves, D. (1999). *Manual for the Spousal Assault Risk Assessment Guide* (3rd ed.). Toronto, ON: Multi-Health Systems.

McNiel, D. E., & Binder, R. L. (1994). Screening for risk of inpatient violence: Validation of an actuarial tool. *Law and Human Behavior, 18*, 579-586.

Monahan, J., Steadman, H. J., Appelbaum, P. S., Robbins, P. C., Mulvey, E. P., Silver, E., Roth, L. H., & Grisso, T. (2000). Developing a clinically useful actuarial tool for assessing violence risk. *British Journal of Psychiatry, 176*, 312-319.

Monahan, J., Steadman, H. J., Silver, E., Appelbaum, P. S., Robbins, P. C., Mulvey, E. P., Roth, L. H., Grisso, T., & Banks, S. (2001). *Rethinking risk assessment: The MacArthur study of mental disorder and violence.* New York: Oxford University Press.

Mossman, D. (2000). Evaluating violence risk 'by the book': A review of HCR-20: Assessing risk for violence, Version 2 and The manual for the Sexual Violence Risk—20. *Behavioral Sciences and the Law, 18*, 781-789.

Mulvey, E. P., & Lidz, C. W. (1995). Conditional prediction: A model for research on dangerousness to others in a new era. *International Journal of Law and Psychiatry, 18*, 129-143.

Monahan, J. (1988). Risk assessment of violence among the mentally disordered: Generating useful knowledge. *International Journal of Law and Psychiatry, 11*, 249-257.

Nicholls, T. L., Ogloff, J. R. P., & Douglas, K. S. (2001). *Assessing risk for violence among female and male psychiatric patients: The HCR-20, PCL:SV, and McNiel & Binder's Screening Measure.* Manuscript submitted for publication.

Otto, R. K. (2000). Assessing and managing violence risk in outpatient settings. *Journal of Clinical Psychology, 56*, 1239-1262.

Quinsey, V. L., Harris, G. T., Rice, G. T., & Cormier, C. A. (1998). *Violent offenders: Appraising and managing risk.* Washington, DC: American Psychological Association.

Ross, D. J., Hart, S. D., & Webster, C. D. (1998). *Aggression in psychiatric patients: Using the HCR-20 to assess risk for violence in hospital and in the community.* Unpublished manuscript.

Skeem, J. L., Mulvey, E. P., & Lidz, C. W. (2000). Building mental health professionals' decisional models into tests of predictive validity: The accuracy of contextualized predictions of violence. *Law and Human Behavior, 24*, 607-628.

Steadman, H. J. (2000). From dangerousness to risk assessment of community violence: Taking stock at the turn of the century. *Journal of the American Academy of Psychiatry and the Law, 28*, 265-271.

Steadman, H. J., Monahan, J., Robbins, P. C., Appelbaum, P., Grisso, T., Klassen, D., Mulvey, E. P., & Roth, L. (1993). From dangerousness to risk assessment: Implications for appropriate research strategies. In S. Hodgins (Ed.), *Mental disorder and crime* (pp. 39-62). London: Sage.

Steadman, H. J., Silver, E., Monahan, J., Appelbaum, P. S., Robbins, P. C., Mulvey, E. P., Grisso, T., Roth, L. H., & Banks, S. (2000). A classification tree approach to the development of actuarial violence risk assessment tools. *Law and Human Behavior, 24*, 83-100.

Strand, S., & Belfrage, H. (2001). Comparison of HCR-20 scores in violent mentally disordered men and women: Gender differences and similarities. *Psychology, Crime & Law, 7*, 71-79.

Strand, S., Belfrage, H., Fransson, G., & Levander, S. (1999). Clinical and risk management factors in risk prediction of mentally disordered offenders—more important than historical data? A retrospective study of 40 mentally disordered offenders assessed with the HCR-20 violence risk assessment scheme. *Legal and Criminological Psychology, 4*, 67-76.

Webster, C. D., Douglas, K. S., Belfrage, H., & Link, B. (2000). Capturing change: An approach to managing violence and improving mental health. In S. Hodgins & R. Müller-Isberner (Eds.), *Violence among the mentally ill: Effective treatment and management strategies* (pp. 119-144). Dordrecht, Netherlands: Kluwer/Academic.

Webster, C. D., Douglas, K. S., Eaves, D., & Hart, S. D. (1997). *HCR-20: Assessing risk for violence* (version 2). Burnaby, BC: Mental Health, Law, and Policy Institute, Simon Fraser University.

Witt, P. H. (2000). A practitioner's view of risk assessment: The HCR-20 and SVR-20. *Behavioral Sciences and the Law, 18*, 791-798.

[16]

Evaluation of a Mental Health Treatment Court with Assertive Community Treatment

Merith Cosden, Ph.D.,* Jeffrey K. Ellens, M.A., Jeffrey L. Schnell, M.A., Yasmeen Yamini-Diouf, M.A., and Maren M. Wolfe, M.A.

Without active engagement, many adults with serious mental illnesses remain untreated in the community and commit criminal offenses, resulting in their placement in the jails rather than mental health facilities. A mental health treatment court (MHTC) with an assertive community treatment (ACT) model of case management was developed through the cooperative efforts of the criminal justice and mental health systems. Participants were 235 adults with a serious mental illness who were booked into the county jail, and who volunteered for the study. An experimental design was used, with participants randomly assigned to MHTC or treatment as usual (TAU), consisting of adversarial criminal processing and less intensive mental health treatment. Results were reported for 6 and 12 month follow-up periods. Clients in both conditions improved in life satisfaction, distress, and independent living, while participants in the MHTC also showed reductions in substance abuse and new criminal activity. Outcomes are interpreted within the context of changes brought about in the community subsequent to implementation of the MHTC.

Many adults with serious mental illnesses remain untreated in the community and engage in illegal activities. The disproportionate number of adults with mental illnesses in the nation's jails suggests that jails have become the largest *de facto* institution for the seriously mentally ill (Turnbo & Murray, 1997).

People with serious mental illness require stabilization, including medication maintenance, as well as treatment that addresses their practical psychosocial needs for housing, job training, and safety (Heilbrun & Griffin, 1998). Without treatment,

*Correspondence to: Dr Merith Cosden, Counseling/Clinical/School Psychology, Gevirtz Graduate School of Education, University of California, Santa Barbara, CA 93106, U.S.A.
E-mail: cosden@education.ucsb.edu
This research was sponsored by a grant from the California State Board of Corrections, the Mentally Ill Offender Crime Reduction Grant (MIOCRG) Program.

Contract/grant sponsor: California State Board of Corrections.

the individual with a serious mental illness is likely to continue to commit offenses, enter jail, become released to the community, and soon enter jail again. Efforts to break this cycle have to balance the individual's right to accept or refuse treatment with the need to maintain community safety.

Stein and Test (1980) developed a model of intensive case management commonly referred to as "assertive community treatment" (ACT), which has become a popular method for trying to meet the needs of this population. ACT has many elements, however, and the fidelity of its implementation across sites has been questioned (see, e.g., McGrew & Bond, 1995). McGrew and Bond surveyed experts to develop a consensus on critical characteristics of the model. They identified a number of key factors, including use of a team approach with a small case manager–client ratio; treatment provided where the client lives, with a focus on helping the client obtain their basic needs; and assertive, persistent engagement of weakly motivated clients.

Despite the recent proliferation of ACT programs, studies on its effectiveness have been mixed. In an early review, Bond, McGrew, and Fekete (1995) reported that ACT resulted in greater retention, fewer hospitalizations, and improved GAF scores relative to other treatments. Recent studies have also reported positive outcomes. Marshall and Lockwood (2001) compared standard community care without case management, typical case management, and more intensive ACT. They found that clients receiving either case management or ACT were more likely to remain in treatment than clients receiving less intensive services. Clients with ACT were also less likely to be admitted to a psychiatric hospital or to be arrested or homeless. However, no differences were noted for clients' mental state or social functioning. In other studies (e.g., Clarke et al., 2000; Hamernick & Pakenham, 1999) both ACT and comparison treatment groups demonstrated similar improvements in outcomes such as improved life skills and reductions in hospitalizations.

A more recent treatment model for adults with mental illness who commit criminal offences has been the mental health treatment court. This follows a broader movement within the criminal justice system toward "therapeutic jurisprudence," in which the courts have become more involved in the treatment as well as punishment of offenders (Wexler, 2001). Drug courts have been the major form of specialty court to emerge from this movement, and have shown considerable promise (Belenko, 2001). Typically, these courts involve cooperative agreements within the criminal justice system and between the courts and treatment providers. These agreements allow decisions to be made that can serve the client therapeutically while also protecting public safety. Mental health courts have similarly arisen to provide offenders with mental illnesses with the opportunity for treatment instead of jail time, with the hope of decreasing the recidivism of this population. As a relatively new form of specialty court, mental health courts lack the structure of drug courts (Steadman, Davidson, & Brown, 2001). Early studies of mental health courts cite problems with finding comparison groups and describe the complexity of examining outcomes for this population (McGaha, Boothroyd, Poythress, Petrila, & Ort, 2002).

Both mental health courts and ACT contain elements that may be perceived by clients as coercive. Assertive Community Treatment has been called "paternalistic" because of the intrusive nature of its case management (McGrew & Bond, 1995), while mental health courts require the client to comply with court requirements or face consequences that in some mental health courts may include jail time.

Nevertheless, both programs can also be viewed as giving the clients a greater role than is traditional in their own treatment. For example, ACT often involves the client in a group decision-making process, while mental health courts allow clients to talk directly to the judge in a non-adversarial atmosphere, In combination, these treatments provide a coordinated effort to retain clients in treatment while the clients retain autonomy to effect, and refuse, treatment.

In an effort to reduce recidivism among offenders with mental illnesses, California passed the Mentally Ill Offender Criminal Reduction Act (MIOCR) funded by California Senate Bill 1485 ('Rosenthal' Bill, S.B. 1485, Section 1(g), 1998). This Act funds innovative programs that would provide and evaluate services to non-violent, seriously mentally ill offenders. This study focuses on one such program designed to improve the quality of life and reduce recidivism within this population.

The purpose of this study was to evaluate the impact of a mental health treatment court (MHTC) with intensive case management, relative to "treatment as usual" (TAU), consisting of less intensive case management, and adversarial criminal processing. This study is part of a 4 year funded project, which will evaluate client outcomes over a 24 month period. Client outcomes during their first 12 months of treatment are presented in this paper.

The following hypotheses were tested: (i) clients participating in the MHTC would report more improvement in their baseline life satisfaction after 6 and 12 months in treatment than would clients receiving TAU; (ii) clients participating in the MHTC would report a greater reduction in their initial psychological distress after 6 and 12 months in treatment than would clients receiving TAU; (iii) clients participating in the MHTC would demonstrate a more extensive change in their global independent functioning after 6 and 12 months in treatment than would clients receiving TAU; (iv) clients participating in the MHTC would show more improvement in their alcohol and drug problems after 6 and 12 months in treatment than would clients receiving TAU; and (v) clients participating in the MHTC would show a greater reduction in criminal activity after 6 and 12 months in treatment than would clients receiving TAU.

METHOD

Sample Selection

This experimental program was open to adults who were charged with either a felony or misdemeanor, had at least one prior booking, were diagnosed with a serious and pervasive mental illness, and were residents of Santa Barbara County. Diagnosis was determined by a psychiatrist or psychologist working with county inmates, and was developed on the basis of a clinical interview and observations. Potential clients who were already part of the county mental health care system were re-evaluated for the purpose of this program to ascertain whether or not they still met the diagnostic criteria. In addition, substance abuse problems were assessed via administration of the Addiction Severity Index (ASI; McLellan, Kushner, Metzger, & Peters, 1992).

Offenders could enter the program either pre-plea or post-adjudication. Pre-plea participants could have no prior offenses that involved serious acts of violence. Post-conviction participants could have some violence in their past, if they were seen as no longer posing a threat of danger to others as determined by the District Attorney and other MHTC team members.

All offenders who were booked into the county jail and who met the eligibility criteria for the program over a two-year period were offered the opportunity to enroll. Potential participants came to the attention of the program either because they had a record of prior contact with mental health services, or by a referral from someone processing the offender, a family member, or the offender. Participation was voluntary and could be terminated by the client at any time. While, at least in some instances, the decision facing the client was jail or "treatment," recent studies (e.g. Poythress, Petrila, McGaha, & Boothroyd, 2002) report that mental health court defendants do not perceive their court process as being as coercive as other types of criminal processing. Premature termination from the program resulted in the client being faced with the same legal charges they had on entry to the program. For pre-plea clients, graduation from the program resulted in their charge being dropped, while post-conviction clients typically had a reduction in their terms of probation. The program could also terminate the client's participation, and did so primarily when clients committed new crimes that sent them to prison and made them ineligible for the program.

Participants

There were 235 participants in this study, 137 enrolled in the MHTC, and 98 in "treatment as usual" (TAU). Of this initial sample, 12 month follow-up assessments were available on 150 participants, 85 in the MHTC and 65 in TAU. There were three reasons that initial participants did not have follow-up data: 59 (32 MHTC, 27 TAU) could not be located for follow-up, 2 (1 MHTC, 1 TAU) died, and 24 (19 MHTC, 5 TAU) had not reached their 12 month follow-up period at the time of the analysis. A larger number of MHTC than TAU clients had not reached follow-up because a decision was made to randomly assign participants to the MHTC and TAU on a 2–1 ratio toward the end of the project in order to provide the more intensive service to a larger number of clients.

Demographic characteristics of the initial and 12 month samples are shown in Table 1. While there were small, chance differences in the characteristics of clients between conditions, a series of chi-square analyses determined that these differences were not significant at intake or 12 months. Overall, the population contained more women, and fewer Latinos, than would be expected from a local, jail-based population. The most likely explanation for the over-representation of women in the sample is that there are more men who have convictions for violent activity that precluded their participation in the study. Discrepancies in the ethnic composition of the sample is a function of the program requirement that clients be citizens of the US, as some people of Latino descent in the local area are not legal citizens. A majority of clients had a drug or alcohol problem in addition to their primary mental illness.

Program Description

Enhanced treatment consisted of a mental health treatment court (MHTC) and intensive case management that followed an assertive community treatment (ACT)

Table 1. Number of participants with specific demographic characteristics at intake and 12 month follow-up

Variable	MHTC		TAU	
	Intake	12 month	Intake	12 month
Gender				
Male	67	41	51	36
Female	70	45	47	33
Ethnicity				
European–American	97	66	69	49
Hispanic/Latino	24	9	17	9
African–American	10	7	8	7
Other	6	4	4	4
Diagnosis				
Mood disorder	51	34	32	24
Schizophrenia	38	27	38	29
Bipolar disorder	32	16	20	11
Other	16	9	8	5
Dual diagnosis	114	68	81	51

model of service delivery. The mental health treatment court was developed by a policy council composed of key members of the criminal justice system, including judges, the district attorney, public defender, probation officer, and sheriff, and chief administrators for alcohol, drug, and mental health services. It was adapted from the drug court model of non-adversarial criminal processing and intensive court supervision. Once clients entered the program decisions regarding their disposition were made by the treatment team, which met before each court session to discuss the client's progress. Clients were scheduled for weekly, or bi-weekly, court supervision. The Judge spoke with the client and gave the client feedback in the form of praise for good progress, or sanctions, often in the form of jail days, when the client was not following the program.

Clients were also assigned a case manager within the intensive care team. Following the ACT model of intervention, case managers had frequent contact with their clients and helped them obtain resources, including transportation to meetings, Section 8 housing vouchers, horticulture vocational training, and group skills training in community re-entry and substance abuse management maintenance. Unlike traditional ACT models that have no time limit, however, this program could only serve each client for 18 months in order to comply with the grant's requirements. Clients who completed the program were transferred, if necessary, to the long-term care team to receive ongoing treatment available from the county.

Treatment as usual (TAU) consisted of traditional, adversarial court proceedings and a referral to the long-term care team at county mental health services. That is, after leaving jail, clients were admitted to county mental health care services, where they received case management for the duration of the project. Clients were also eligible for housing vouchers and had access to Department of Rehabilitation vocational services. There was considerable variability in services received by clients, as any community resource not funded by the MIOCR grant was available to them. Clients remained with the long-term care team for at least 18 months, after which they could be terminated or continue to receive care as long as needed.

Table 2. Differences between mental health treatment court and usual mental health services

Mental health treatment court	Treatment as usual
Non-adversarial court proceedings	*Adversarial court proceedings*
Decisions made by team	Decisions made by judge
Intensive court supervision and drug testing	Regular court supervision
Charges dropped with program completion or conditions of probation reduced	Regular sentencing
	Same judge as in MHTC
Assertive community treatment	*Long-term care team*
Case manager with 1:15 client ratio	Case manager with 1:50 client ratio
Section 8 housing	Waitlist for Section 8 housing
Horticulture vocational program	Department of Rehabilitation programs
Transportation	Other county programs available
Group skills training on substance abuse treatment and community re-entry	

Differences between the MHTC and TAU conditions are delineated in Table 2. Primary variations between the two programs were the adversarial versus non-adversarial method of criminal processing, the intensity of care management, opportunities for housing, specialized vocational training, and the availability of groups to help with substance abuse and community integration. However, as noted in Table 2, the same Judges and other court personnel processed both groups of clients.

Measures

Four assessments were administered to clients at each time interval. Two were self-assessments: the *Behavior and Symptom Identification Scale-32* (Eisen, 1996), and the *Lehman Quality of Life Scale—Short Form* (QOL-SF, Lehman, 1988). In addition, the *Addiction Severity Index* (ASI, McLellan et al., 1992) was used to obtain a measure of the need for drug and alcohol services, and a clinician rating of client skills, the *Global Assessment of Functioning* (GAF), was used. Finally, criminal data, including arrests, convictions, and jail days, were obtained from a review of county records by a deputy probation officer.

The BASIS-32 is a self-report scale designed to assess the client's perception of difficulty in five areas: depression/anxiety, psychotic symptoms, relation to self/others, daily living skills, and impulsive/addictive behaviors. Investigators have found acceptable to high internal consistency estimates for the subscales (Chow, Snowden, & McConnell, 2001; Hoffman, Capelli, & Mastrianni, 1997) with full-scale internal consistency estimates as high as 0.95 (Eisen, Wilcox, Leff, Schaefer, & Cuhlane, 1999). Test–retest reliability coefficients have ranged from 0.65 to 0.85 (Eisen, Dill, & Grob, 1994). Chow et al. (2001) replicated a consistent factor structure across different ethnic groups. Researchers have found evidence of criterion validity (Eisen et al., 1994), and discriminant validity (Eisen et al., 1999).

The Lehman QL-SF measures the client's perception of quality of life in seven domains: general living, daily activities, family and social, finances, work/school, legal problems, and personal safety. Psychometric investigations have demonstrated a replicable factor structure and high internal consistency, with subscale reliability ranging from 0.80 to 0.92 (Russo et al., 1997). Evidence of construct validity (Lehman, 1988) and discriminant validity (Russo et al., 1997) are also noted. The measure of general life satisfaction was used in this study.

The ASI is a structured interview, designed to evaluate client problems across seven domains. Severity ratings, based on the interviewer's perception of the client's need for additional treatment and composite scores, derived from client responses, are obtained in each domain. Analyses have demonstrated high reliability, including concurrent reliability estimates ranging from 0.94 to 0.99 across subscales (McLellan et al., 1985), internal consistency estimates ranging from 0.65 to 0.89 (Leonhard, Mulvey, Gastfriend, & Schwartz, 2000), and good to excellent test–retest reliability of lifetime items (Cacciola, Koppenhaver, McKay, & Alterman, 1999). Good reliability and validity have also been obtained for specific populations including homeless substance abusers (Joyner, Wright, & Devine, 1996; Zanis, McLellan, Cnaan, & Randall, 1994).

The Global Assessment of Functioning (GAF) is often used as part of a clinical assessment. Researchers note that it has adequate reliability (Hall, 1995; Roy-Byrne, Dagadakis, Unutzer, & Ries, 1996). The Kennedy-Axis Approach was used to calculate the GAF in this study. This method distinguishes the components of the GAF (psychological impairment, social skills, violence, activities of daily living/ occupational skills) and calculates client functioning in each area separately, averaging them to obtain a total score.

Design and Procedures

This study followed a true experimental design, with qualifying clients randomly assigned to one of the two treatment conditions: MHTC or TAU. Given the likelihood that not all clients would continue through the 18 month enhanced treatment, the MHTC group was assigned clients on a two to one basis relative to TAU for a six month period, but still using a random number table. Eligibility for the program was determined after a review of each case by the team probation officer, district attorney (for pre-plea cases), public defender, and jail-based mental health practitioner. The project was described to the offender by either the mental health practitioner or the public defender. If interested, offenders were asked to sign a consent to participate in the study, with the understanding that they would be randomly assigned to either MHTC or TAU. Clients assigned to the MHTC signed an additional contract outlining their rights and responsibilities as a client in the enhanced program.

All clients were assessed at intake and at 6 month intervals over a 24 month period of time; the first three assessments (intake, 6 months, 12 months) will be examined in this study. Assessments were conducted by a full time employee of the mental health system who used a variety of techniques to locate clients, including traveling with homeless outreach organizations. Clients were interviewed in a range of locations, from the mental health offices, to local parks or the jail. Participants were paid $15 at the completion of each follow-up interview.

RESULTS

The first four hypotheses were tested using a repeated measure ANOVA to examine changes in client perceptions and behaviors over time. As 59 clients (25% of the original sample) could not be located at follow-up, an analysis was conducted to assess the nature of the differences between the missing clients and those on whom follow-up data were available. A 2 (MHTC, TAU) × 2 (with follow-up, missing follow-up) MANOVA was conducted with intake Lehman, BASIS-32, and GAF scores as the outcome measures. No significant differences were found on these measures between those who were located for follow-up and those who were not, Wilks's $\Lambda = 0.97, F(3, 229) = 1.61$, NS. Thus, while it is likely that clients who could not be found differed from other participants in some ways, their initial assessments were similar.

To test the first hypothesis, a 2 × 3 repeated measures ANOVA was conducted between clients in the MHTC and TAU conditions over three periods of time (intake, 6 month follow-up, 12 month follow-up) examining differences on client ratings of life satisfaction on the Lehman QOL-SF. There was a main effect for time, Wilks's $\Lambda = 0.79, F(2, 148) = 19.72, p < 0.001, \eta^2 = 0.21$. Statisticians indicate that an η^2 of 0.01 represents a small effect size, 0.06 a medium effect size, and 0.14 a large effect size (Green, Salkind, & Akey, 2000, p. 190). Thus, the changes that occurred were significant and represented a relatively large effect size. Client in both groups improved in life satisfaction from intake to 6 months in treatment, with gains maintained at the 12 month follow-up (see Table 3). There was no treatment × time interaction, indicating that both groups had similar gains over time.

Hypothesis 2 was that clients in the MHTC would report a greater reduction in distress over time than would clients in TAU. A repeated measure ANOVA was conducted using the averaged subscale scores on the BASIS-32. There was a significant interaction of condition and time, Wilks's $\Lambda = 0.96$, $F(2, 147) = 3.38$, $p < 0.05$, $\eta^2 = 0.04$, reflecting a significant but relatively small effect size. This interaction was a function of chance higher scores (greater problems) for MHTC clients relative to TAU clients at intake, resulting in greater gains over time, as both groups had similar scores at 6 and 12 month assessments. There was also a significant main effect of time, Wilks's $\Lambda = 0.73$, $F(2, 147) = 27.43$, $p < 0.001$,

Table 3. Changes on the Lehman QOL-SF, BASIS-32, and ASI for participants in MHTC and TAU conditions

	Intake		6 month		12 month	
Condition	*M*	SD	*M*	SD	*M*	SD
Lehman						
MHTC	3.22	1.54	4.14	1.46	4.17	1.45
TAU	3.48	1.46	4.13	1.74	4.08	1.47
BASIS-32						
MHTC	1.94	0.83	1.27	0.80	1.27	0.79
TAU	1.62	0.80	1.33	0.72	1.27	0.75
ASI: drug						
MHTC	0.12	0.12	0.08	0.09	0.08	0.08
TAU	0.09	0.10	0.10	0.11	0.08	0.11
ASI: alcohol						
MHTC	0.23	0.28	0.14	0.18	0.15	0.19
TAU	0.21	0.22	0.18	0.20	0.14	0.18

Higher scores on the Lehman reflect perceptions of a better quality of life; lower scores on the BASIS-32 reflect less distress; lower composite scores on the ASI reflect a lesser problem in that domain.

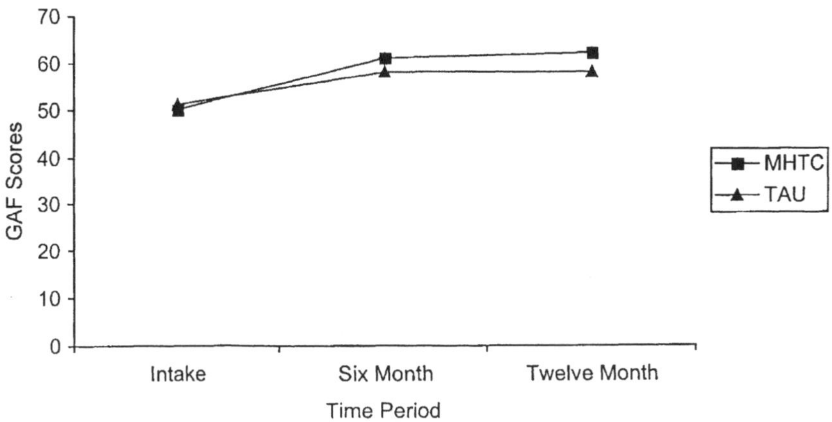

Figure 1. Changes in GAF scores as a function of treatment condition over time.

$\eta^2 = 0.27$, reflecting a relatively large effect size. Overall, participants in both groups who were assessed at the end of 12 months were less distressed than they had been prior to entering either program.

Hypothesis 3 was that clients in the MHTC would show greater improvement in their overall independent functioning than would clients in TAU. A repeated measures analysis found a significant time × condition interaction, Wilks's $\Lambda = 0.97$, $F(2, 147) = 3.39$, $p < 0.05$, $\eta^2 = 0.02$, as well as a significant main effect of time, Wilks's $\Lambda = 0.62$, $F(2, 147) = 44.07$, $p < 0.001$, $\eta^2 = 0.37$. As depicted in Figure 1, clients in both groups had higher GAF scores at their 6 month follow-up than they had at intake, but the MHTC group improved more than the TAU group. Both groups maintained this higher level of functioning at their 12 month follow-up.

Hypothesis 4 examined changes in drug and alcohol problems over time. The composite scores on the ASI were used to measure problem severity. Composite scores range from 0 to 1, with '0' reflecting no problem and '1' the highest need for treatment. A significant time × condition interaction was found for drug problems, Wilks's $\Lambda = 0.95$, $F(2, 147) = 0.35$, $p < 0.05$, $\eta^2 = 0.05$. As noted in Table 3, the MHTC group started by chance with higher composite scores than the TAU group and demonstrated significant change over time, while the TAU scores changed little over the 12 months.

Alcohol composite scores also changed over time for clients, Wilks's $\Lambda = 0.90$, $F(2, 146) = 7.83$, $p = 0.001$, $\eta^2 = 0.09$. Composite scores are provided in Table 3. Clients in the MHTC displayed greater change at 6 months, but both groups had similar composite scores at the end of 12 months.

Finally, criminal outcome data were examined. In order to control for possible variation in prior criminal activities, three ANOVA tests were conducted to assess differences in bookings, convictions, and jail days between MHTC and TAU clients for the 12 month period prior to their entering these programs. There were no significant differences on any of these variables: $F(1, 233) = 0.78$ for bookings; $F(1, 233) = 0.02$ for convictions; and $F(1, 233) = 2.97$ for jail days. Thus, comparisons of criminal activities since entry to the program were not biased by differences in clients' histories.

Data on 12 month outcomes, in terms of number of new bookings, convictions, and jail days, were available for 191 clients (all except those who were deceased and those who were in treatment for less time). The data were highly skewed, with the majority of clients in each condition receiving no new bookings, convictions, or jail days. Thus, the data were recoded into dichotomous variables indicating the presence or absence of any criminal activity during that time period, and analyzed using chi-square analysis. At 12 months, a similar proportion of clients in each condition had been booked at least once and spent some time in jail (76% in MHTC; 72% in TAU). However, there were differences in the proportion of clients convicted of a new crime (47% for MHTC; 60% for TAU, $\chi^2(N=191)=2.98$, $p=0.05$. Further inquiry also found that 51% of convictions for clients in the MHTC were for a probation violation, while only 35% of clients in TAU were convicted for a probation violation, and the rest for more serious charges.

The overall pattern of criminal activity suggests that while clients in both conditions spent time in jail, that time occurred for different reasons. Clients in the MHTC were more likely to be booked but not convicted, and to have convictions related to a probation violation. Clients in TAU were more likely to commit, and be convicted of, a new crime.

DISCUSSION

There were a number of significant outcomes from this study. Clients in both MHTC and TAU demonstrated improvements in life satisfaction, psychological distress, independent functioning, and drug problems. Participants in the MHTC demonstrated greater gain in terms of developing independent living skills and reducing their problems with drugs. While participants in both groups were equally likely to spend some time in jail, the reasons for their arrests differed. Interpretation of these findings requires understanding of the complexities involved in providing intensive services to clients with serious mental illnesses.

As found in other studies (e.g. Clarke et al., 2000; Hamernik & Pakenham, 1999), both groups of participants (i.e. those receiving intensive case management and those receiving regular case management) demonstrated gains in a number of areas. This suggests that either form of treatment can have a beneficial impact on participants. While all participants had serious mental illnesses and are likely to have qualified for mental health services (treatment as usual) prior to the study, their gains can best be explained by the impact of the project on client engagement in treatment. That is, prior to their participation in the project, at the time they were booked, these adults were not actively involved in the mental health system. Program engagement was encouraged in several ways. After group assignment, clients either met with their MHTC case manager, or were given an appointment with the mental health long-term care team. Further, clients in both conditions signed a consent form to participate in the study. Thus, even clients assigned to "treatment as usual" were contacted, assessed, and paid for their assessments every 6 months. Anecdotal reports from the interviewer suggest that many of these clients felt that they were getting special treatment by virtue of being part of the project. That perception, in itself, may have had a positive impact on client behavior.

It is also possible that the changes in outcomes for clients receiving "treatment as usual" were due, in part, to changes in the community during this period. That is, several aspects of "usual" service delivery changed as a function of this project, so that the "treatment as usual" experienced by clients in this investigation was not the same treatment that these same clients would have experienced prior to the project. Given the joint, collaborative nature of this project, there were many community discussions, and trainings, on the needs of offenders with mental illnesses. Anecdotal reports from the judges, public defenders, prosecutors, and members of the sheriff's department, who became better trained and more informed about this population as a function of this project, indicated that offenders with mental illness outside of the MHTC were also being treated differently, with greater thought to their clinical needs and the resources available to them. Olfson (1990) noted that the integration of ACT principles into standard care was one of the reasons that ACT outcomes were no longer as significant as they were in early studies of this intervention.

Although clients in both groups showed gains over time, greater improvement in GAF scores and the need for substance abuse treatment were found for clients in the MHTC. It is possible that the enhanced treatment was more effective than TAU in terms of helping clients to gain stability in the community. In particular, the MHTC offered a more structured approach (through the substance abuse maintenance management groups) for providing clients with substance abuse treatment. Given the high percentage of clients in this study, and in the general mental health population, with concomitant substance abuse problems, this is clearly a critical component of treatment.

Outcomes related to criminal activity require careful interpretation. While clients in both conditions were equally likely to spend time in jail, clients in the MHTC were less likely to be convicted, and more likely to be cited for a probation violation. This pattern can be explained by the fact that clients participating in the MHTC were under greater scrutiny than clients in TAU, and were more likely to be caught on a probation violation. In addition, participants in the MHTC were often given time in jail as a "sanction" when they did not comply with program requirements. This "therapeutic" use of jail time, in order to protect, stabilize, or punish clients, has become common in drug courts as well as some mental health courts. Thus, clients in TAU were more likely to be booked and convicted on a new crime, while clients in the MHTC were more likely to serve jail time because of a probation violation or sanction.

Despite the use of an experimental design, there were several methodological limitations to the study. The relatively small number of clients in each group resulted in chance variation on some of the intake measures, which affected the analyses. Further, the lack of differential findings between MHTC and TAU groups may be a result of regression to the mean for both groups of clients, as all started at very low performance levels. The interviewer was not blind to the condition of the client, which could have biased her perception of clients on the GAF, although the more structured Kennedy-Axis method for obtaining a GAF was used to reduce this problem. In addition, 25% of the initial population could not be relocated at the end of 12 months. This still represents a high response rate from the initial participants, but does limit the generalizability of the findings to clients who could be maintained in the community. Finally, there are concerns about the validity of self-report measures with this particular population. However, it must be noted that in order to participate in the study clients had to be cogent enough to give informed consent, which should reflect their ability to give accurate responses on their questionnaires.

Future research needs to consider the longitudinal impact of the program as well as its strengths and weakness for different sub-populations. This study only allowed clients to be part of the MHTC with its intensive case management for 18 months. After this time, if they still needed treatment, they were transferred to the long-term care team (i.e. "treatment as usual"). The impact of this transfer process on clients, and whether or not continued intensive treatment was needed for some individuals, will be further examined over the course of this study. Further, while clients in both groups demonstrate improvements, clients "peak" in their functioning at "satisfactory" levels on the assessments. While programs such as this may not help clients go beyond obtaining basic stability, clients may need to feel greater satisfaction with their lives in order to maintain this stability over time. The use of formal programs, such as these, to engage "informal" supports, such as family and friends, may be key to helping clients remain in treatment and in the community (Lam & Rosenheck, 1999), and requires further study.

The MHTC/ACT model of treatment effectively helped clients improve their quality of life, reduce distress, and engage in fewer new criminal activities. While usual treatment also had positive findings, this is likely due to changes in the quality of care, and efforts for client engagement, that ensued subsequent to implementing the project. Further understanding of how to help clients with serious mental illness remain in the community with different levels of treatment is needed.

REFERENCES

Belenko, S. R. (2001). Research on drug courts: A critical review, 2001 update. *National Drug Court Institute Review, 3*, 1–59.

Bond, G. R., McGrew, J. H., & Fekete, D. M. (1995). Assertive outreach for frequent users of psychiatric hospitals: A meta-analysis. *Journal of Mental Health Administration, 22*(1), 4–16.

Cacciola, J. S., Koppenhaver, J. M., McKay, J. R., & Alterman, A. I. (1999). Test–retest reliability of the lifetime items on the Addiction Severity Index. *Psychological Assessment, 11*, 86–93.

Chow, J. C., Snowden, L. R., & McConnell, W. (2001). A confirmatory factor analysis of the BASIS-32 in racial and ethnic samples. *Journal of Behavioral Health Services and Research, 28*, 400–411.

Clarke, G. N., Herinckx, H. A., Kinney, R. F., Paulson, R. I., Cutler, D. L., Lewis, K., & Oxman, E. (2000). Psychiatric hospitalizations, arrests, emergency room visits and homelessness of clients with serious and persistent mental illness: Findings from a randomized trial of two ACT programs vs. usual care. *Mental Health Services Research, 2*(3), 155–164.

Eisen, S. V. (1996). Behavior and Symptom Identification Scale (BASIS-32). In L. I. Sederer, & B. Dickey (Eds.), *Outcomes assessment in clinical practice* (pp. 65–69). Baltimore, MD: Williams and Wilkins.

Eisen, S. V., Dill, D. L., & Grob, M. C. (1994). Reliability and validity of a brief patient report instrument for psychiatric outcome evaluation. *Hospital and Community Psychiatry, 45*, 242–247.

Eisen, S. V., Wilcox, M., Leff, H. S., Schaefer, E., & Cuhlane, M. A. (1999). Assessing behavioral health outcomes in outpatient programs: Reliability and validity of the BASIS-32. *Journal of Behavioral Healthcare Management, 26*, 5–17.

Green, S. B., Salkind, N. J., & Akey, T. M. (2000). *Using SPSS for windows: Analyzing and understanding data*. Englewood Cliffs, NJ: Prentice-Hall.

Hall, R. C. W. (1995). Global assessment of functioning: A modified scale. *Psychosomatics, 36*, 267–275.

Hamernik, E., & Pakenham, K. I. (1999). Assertive community treatment for persons with severe mental disorders: A controlled treatment outcome study. *Behaviour Change, 16*(4), 259–268.

Heilbrun, K., & Griffin, P. A. (1998). Community-based forensic treatment. In R. M. Wettstein (Ed.), *Treatment of offenders with mental disorders* (pp. 168–210). New York: Guilford.

Hoffmann, F. L., Capelli, K., & Mastrianni, X. (1997). Measuring treatment outcome for adults and adolescents: Reliability and validity of BASIS-32. *The Journal of Mental Health Administration, 24*, 316–331.

Joyner, L. M., Wright, J. D., & Devine, J. A. (1996). Reliability and validity of the Addiction Severity Index among homeless substance misusers. *Substance Use and Misuse, 31*, 729–751.

Lam, J. A., & Rosenheck, R. (1999). Social support and service use among homeless persons with serious mental illness. *International Journal of Social Psychiatry, 45*(1), 13–28.

Lehman, A. F. (1988). A quality of life interview for the chronically mentally ill. *Evaluation and Program Planning, 11*, 51–62.

Leonhard, C., Mulvey, K., Gastfriend, D. R., & Schwartz, M. (2000). The Addiction Severity Index: A field study of internal consistency and validity. *Journal of Substance Abuse Treatment, 18*, 129–135.

Marshall, M., & Lockwood, A. (2001). The effectiveness of case management and assertive community treatment for people with severe mental disorders. In H. D. Brenner, W. Böker and R. Genner (Eds.), *The Treatment of Schizophrenia—Status and Emerging Trends* (pp. 181–194). Kirkland, WA: Hogrefe and Huber.

McGaha, A., Boothroyd, R. A., Poythress, N. G., Petrila, J., & Ort, R. G. (2002). Lessons from the Broward County Mental Health Court Evaluation. *Evaluation and Program Planning, 25*, 125–135.

McGrew, J. H., & Bond, G. R. (1995). Critical ingredients of assertive community treatment: Judgments of the experts. *Journal of Mental Health Administration, 22*(2), 113–125.

McLellan, A. T., Kushner, H., Metzger, D., Peters, R., Smith, I., Grissom, G., Pettinati, J., & Argeriou, M. (1992). The fifth edition of the Addiction Severity Index. *Journal of Substance Abuse Treatment, 9*, 199–213.

McLellan, A. T., Luborsky, L., Cacciola, J., Griffith, J., Evans, F., Barr, H. L., & O'Brien, C. P. (1985). New data from the Addiction Severity Index. *The Journal of Nervous and Mental Disease, 173*, 412–423.

Olfson, M. (1990). Assertive community treatment: An evaluation of the experimental evidence. *Hospital and Community Psychiatry, 41*(6), 634–641.

Poythress, N. G., Petrila, J., McGaha, A., & Boothroyd, R. (2002). Perceived coercion and procedural justice in the Broward mental health court. *International Journal of Law and Psychiatry, 25*, 517–533.

Roy-Byrne, P., Dagadakis, C., Unutzer, J., & Ries, R. (1996). Evidence for limited validity of the revised Global Assessment of Functioning Scale. *Psychiatric Services, 47*, 864–866.

Russo, J., Reeder, D., Alexander, M., Dwyer-O'Connor, E., Dagadakis, C., Ries, R., & Patrick, D. (1997). Longitudinal assessment of quality of life in acute psychiatric inpatients: Reliability and validity. *The Journal of Nervous and Mental Disease, 185*, 166–175.

Steadman, H. J., Davidson, S., & Brown, C. (2001). Law and psychiatry: Mental health courts: Their promise and unanswered questions. *Psychiatric Services, 52*(4), 457–458.

Stein, L. I., & Test, M. A. (1980). An alternative to mental hospital treatment: I: Conceptual model, treatment program, and clinical evaluation. *Archives of General Psychiatry, 37*, 392–397.

Turnbo, C., & Murray, D. W., Jr. (1997). The state of mental health services to criminal offenders. In T. R. Watkins, & J. W. Callicut (Eds.), *Mental health policy and practice today* (pp. 298–311). Thousand Oaks, CA: Sage.

Wexler, D. B. (2001). The development of therapeutic jurisprudence: From theory to practice. In L. E. Frost, & R. J. Bonnie (Eds.), *The evolution of mental health law* (pp. 279–289). Washington, DC: American Psychological Association Press.

Zanis, D. A., McLellan, A. T., Cnaan, R. A., & Randall, M. (1994). Reliability and validity of the Addiction Severity Index with a homeless sample. *Journal of Substance Abuse Treatment, 11*, 541–548.

Part IV
Youth Assessment And Intervention

[17]

Young children who commit crime: Epidemiology, developmental origins, risk factors, early interventions, and policy implications

ROLF LOEBER[a,b] AND DAVID P. FARRINGTON[c]

[a]*University of Pittsburgh;* [b]*Free University, Amsterdam; and* [c]*University of Cambridge*

Abstract

An early onset of delinquency prior to age 13 years increases the risk of later serious, violent, and chronic offending by a factor of 2–3. Also child delinquents, compared to juveniles who start offending at a later age, tend to have longer delinquent careers. This article summarizes the report of the Office of Juvenile Justice and Delinquency Prevention's Study Group on Very Young Offenders, chaired by Rolf Loeber and David P. Farrington. The Study Group, consisting of 16 scholars and 23 coauthors, worked for 2 years on preparing a report, undertaking extensive secondary data analyses, and writing chapters in different speciality areas. The report consists of a state of the art review of the developmental background of child delinquents. The report also summarizes risk and protective factors in the individual, family, peer group, school, and neighborhood that affect that development. Lastly, the report renews relevant preventive and remedial interventions in the juvenile justice system, families, peer groups, schools, and neighborhoods, and makes a case for improvement in the integration of services for child delinquents. Policy recommendations are presented to improve methods of dealing with child delinquents by juvenile justice, child welfare, and mental health agencies.

The Study Group on Very Young Offenders was chaired by Rolf Loeber and David P. Farrington. We are much indebted to the study group members and their coauthors for their extraordinary efforts to make the study group report highly informative and practical. The initial members of the study group were Barbara J. Burns, John D. Coie, J. David Hawkins, James C. Howell, David Huizinga, Kate Keenan, Darnell F. Hawkins, David R. Offord, Howard N. Snyder, Terence P. Thornberry, and Gail A. Wasserman. They were later joined by Leena K. Augimeri, Brandon C. Welsh, and Janet K. Wiig. The study group members enlisted many coauthors to help them with their chapters, including Meda Chesney-Lind, Ick-Joong Chung, Anne Crawford, Erik K. Duku, Rachele C. Espiritu, Leyla Faw, Kenneth Goldberg, Andrea Hazen, Todd I. Herrenkohl, Karl G. Hill, Larry M. Kalb, Kelly Kelleher, Gordon Keeler, Kimberly Kempf-Leonard, Christopher J. Koegl, Marvin D. Krohn, John Landsverk, David LeMarquand, Marc Le Blanc, Ellen L. Lipman, Shari Miller-Johnson, Craig Rivera, and Angela Seracini. We also owe much to our informal group of advisors, including Alfred Blumstein, Dante Cicchetti, Nancy Crowell, Bernadine Dohrn, Joan McCord, and Christy Visher. We are also grateful to many colleagues and practitioners who gave us advice, including Menke Bol, Theo Dorelijers, Hans Heiner, Eric Joy, Willem Koops, Jim Reiland, Evelyn Wei, and Cathy Spatz Widom, and to over 100 attendees at the National Conference on Juvenile Justice conference in Minneapolis, Minnesota, who in March 1999 responded to our survey on very young offenders, and the attendees of the meeting on "Delinquents Under 10: Targeting the Young Offender," in Minneapolis, Minnesota, September–October 1999. Special thanks are due to Magda Stouthamer-Loeber for her continuing support and encouragement throughout the project. The Study Group on Very Young Offenders has been sponsored by the Office of Juvenile Justice and Delinquency Prevention (OJJDP; grant 95-JD-FX-0018). Points of view or opinions in this paper are ours and do not necessarily represent the official position of OJJDP. Throughout this project we received consistent encouragement and superior counsel from OJJDP's staff, particularly Barbara Allen-Hagen, Shay Bilchik, Betty Chemers, Charlotte Kerr, and John Wilson.

Address correspondence and reprint requests to: Rolf Loeber, Ph.D., WPIC, 3811 O'Hara St., Pittsburgh, PA 15213; E-mail: loeberr@msx.upmc.edu.

Child delinquents have a 2- to 3-fold increased risk of becoming tomorrow's serious, violent, and chronic offenders. Child delinquents also tend to have a longer delinquency career than those with a later onset of offending. For these reasons alone, child delinquents constitute a disproportionate threat to the safety and property of citizens across the nation. The main aim of this paper is to summarize the results of the Study Group on Very Young Offenders, sponsored by the Office of Juvenile Justice and Delinquency Prevention (OJJDP). The principal aims of the Study Group were to advance knowledge about child delinquents, address factors that contribute to offending starting at an early age, and show what types of interventions are effective. We define child delinquents as children who have committed a delinquent act between ages 7 and 12 years inclusive.

The Study Group on Very Young Offenders consisted of 16 scholars on juvenile delinquency and child problem behaviors. They and 23 coauthors have worked for 2 years on the preparation of a volume, entitled *Child Delinquents: Development, Interventions, and Service Needs* (Loeber & Farrington, in press), through regular meetings, special data analyses, and the writing and joint revision of the chapters. The present paper presents highlights from that volume and discusses policy implications.

Juvenile offending is an enduring phenomenon in our society, and it persists from generation to generation of juveniles. Increasingly scholars (e.g., Cicchetti, 1993) have realized that juvenile delinquency, like many other forms of child problem behaviors that wax and wane with age, can best be studied from a developmental point of view. However, scholars differ in their developmental focus and their choice of specific high-risk categories of youth. Initially, pioneering work during the 1980s and 1990s focused on chronic offenders—that is, those with at least four or five arrests or convictions (e.g., Blumstein, Cohen, Roth, & Visher, 1986; Farrington, Ohlin, & Wilson, 1986). The main rationale for this was that chronic offenders are responsible for a disproportionately large amount of crime (and especially serious crime) in communities. Although valuable, the problem with this approach is that, without screening methods, chronic offenders become recognizable only when they have accrued multiple offenses, which usually is late in their criminal careers when they have already inflicted much harm and property loss on others and possibly are beginning to deescalate and desist. It is a waste of criminal justice resources to focus on offenders who are about to stop offending.

Focusing on an earlier stage of criminal careers, Loeber and Farrington (1998) published the results of the Study Group on Serious and Violent Juvenile Offenders, which summarized knowledge about development, risk factors, and interventions for serious and violent juvenile offenders. The Study Group concluded that many of these offenders began their careers of antisocial behavior before the teenage years, but that little was known about child delinquency and few resources were devoted to the prevention either of child delinquency or of escalation in the severity of offending after the onset of child delinquency. These conclusions from the first Study Group on Serious and Violent Juvenile Offenders led logically to the second Study Group on Very Young Offenders. Thus, scientific and policy concerns about serious crime have gradually moved the main focus earlier and earlier in life.

The second Study Group focused on child delinquents. As mentioned, child delinquents, compared to juveniles with a later onset of delinquents, are at risk of becoming serious, violent, and chronic offenders, and have longer delinquency careers (Espiritu, Huizinga, Crawford, & Loeber, in press; Farrington, Loeber, Elliott, Hawkins, Kondel, Klein, McCord, Rower, & Tremblay, 1990; Krohn, Thornberry, Rivera, & Le Blanc, in press; Loeber, 1982, 1988; Loeber & Farrington, 1998; Moffitt, 1993). The main advantage of concentrating on child delinquents is the identification of and possible intervention with children at a much earlier age, *prior to* the accumulation of multiple offenses. In addition, the second Study Group focused on persistently disruptive children, who are not yet engaged in delinquent acts but whose behavior puts them at risk of becoming child delinquents. Disruptive child behaviors are defined first as a recurrent pattern of negativistic, defiant, disobedient, and hostile behavior toward authority figures, and second as a disturbance of children's conduct lasting at least 6 months (American Psychiatric Association, 1994).

Figure 1 summarizes the developmental links between the three groups of youth that concern us most. Children showing persistent disruptive behavior are likely to become child delinquents, while child delinquents are likely to become serious, violent, or chronic offenders. In summary, although many delinquency studies have focused on adolescence when the prevalence of delinquency usually peaks, the search for the early origins of serious, violent, and chronic offending necessarily focuses on the elementary school years and even the preschool years.

Many issues surrounding early onset and child delinquency are unclear. Not all early onset delinquents become chronic offenders. Therefore, the key question is who will and under what conditions. Also, we need to know whether early onset bodes equally ill for offenders from different ethnic or racial backgrounds, and for female as opposed to male offenders. Further, what are the causes of child delinquency, and are they different from the causes of a later onset of delinquency? Given the young age of child delinquents, what types of agencies, other than the juvenile justice system, are dealing with them, and how successful are their efforts in reducing early onset offending? What are the best intervention methods for child delinquents, and what are the best opportunities to prevent delinquency in this high-risk group?

Early Problem Behavior and Delinquency

How are child delinquents legally defined?

Child delinquents are not necessarily legally defined in the same way across states in the United States (Snyder & Sickmund, 1999; Wiig, in press). If child delinquents were defined according to the age of criminal responsibility, information for 1997 shows that this was age 6 years in North Carolina, age 7 years in Maryland, Massachusetts, and New York, age 8 years in Arizona, and age 10 years in the states of Arkansas, Colorado, Kansas, Minnesota, Mississippi, Pennsylvania, South Dakota, Texas, Vermont, and Wisconsin. The remaining states do not have a minimum age of criminal responsibility for children, but according to common law the minimum age is 7 years (Griffin, Torbert, & Szymanski, 1998). Canada has a minimum age of 12 years, with a minimum age of 14 years for juveniles' referral to adult court. England has a minimum age of 10 years. In this article, we define child delinquency as offending between the ages of 7 and 12 years inclusive.

What are important distinctions between problematic children?

We are particularly interested in three categories of problematic children up to age 12 years: (a) *serious child delinquents,* who have committed one or more of the following acts: homicide, aggravated assault, robbery, rape, or serious arson; (b) *other child delinquents* (excluding serious delinquents); and (c) *children showing persistent disruptive behavior,* who are at risk of offending.

We will briefly discuss the importance of these three groups.

Serious child delinquents. It has become increasingly clear that child delinquents can commit very serious crimes, that offenders up to age 12 years constitute a surprisingly high (10%) proportion of all juvenile cases (Butts & Snyder, 1997; Puzzanchera, 1998; Snyder, in press), and that the number of arrested child delinquents increased considerably between 1980 and 1997 (Snyder, 1997, in press).

Homicide. Rightly or wrongly, serious child delinquents are increasingly featured in the news media, especially after unusual and serious crimes committed in parental homes, schools, or the community (e.g., Gegax, Adler, & Pederson, 1998; Cowley, 1998; James & Jenks, 1996; Welch, Fenwick, & Roberts, 1997), including the recent murder by a 6-

year-old boy who fired a gun and killed a classmate in school (Barboza, 2000).

Between 1980 and 1997, 27,000 murders were committed by juveniles; in about 2% of these cases (or about 600 murders), at least one of the identified offenders was age 12 years or less. Thus, murders by child delinquents are uncommon but are still large in absolute numbers. Weapons are frequently used by child offenders: guns were used in over half of the murders committed by child offenders (Snyder, in press). In the Pittsburgh Youth Study (Loeber, Farrington, Stouthamer–Loeber, & Van Kammen, 1998), juvenile gun owners had a lower age of onset of moderately serious delinquency (shoplifting, vandalism, minor fraud) than juveniles not owning guns (average onset age 9.2 vs. 10.3 years, respectively; Drinkwater, 1998). School killings are often featured in the media, but homicide at school committed by juveniles appears very rare (Kachur, Stennies, Powell, Modzeleski, Stephens, Murphy, Kresnow, Sleet, & Lowry, 1996), and appears particularly rare for children younger than age 13 years.

There are few studies of the background of children below age 13 years who committed homicide. In the majority of these cases (59%), the homicide is the first recorded offense, and in about a third of the cases (36%) the child's guardian or teachers described the offender as a discipline problem (Goetting, 1989; see also Cornell, Benedek, & Benedek, 1987, Heide, 1999).[1] It is clear that adolescent murderers are a heterogeneous group of offenders (Benedek & Cornell, 1989; Ewing, 1990; Hardwick & Rowton–Lee, 1996; Heide, 1999). Some commit murder as part of a criminal enterprise and others because of personal conflict, often with relatives or peers (Myers, Scott, Burgess, & Burgess, 1995; Rowley, Ewing, & Singer, 1987). Homicidal victims of child delinquents are mostly younger siblings and infants (Adelson, 1972; Ewing, 1990). Child delinquents rarely commit sexual homicides (Myers, & Blashfield, 1997), and it is very uncommon for them to kill more than one person. Children under age 9 years who kill, in contrast to older youth, "do not fully understand the concept of death" and "have great difficulties comprehending that their actions are irreversible" (Heide, 1999, p. 30).

Nonserious child delinquents. Most child delinquents commit less serious forms of delinquency, such as shoplifting of items of low monetary value, or other acts for which they rarely are prosecuted (e.g., cruelty to animals, setting fires). However, for some young children less serious delinquency is a stepping stone to more serious offending (e.g., Loeber & Dishion, 1983; Lipsey & Derzon, 1998; Loeber, Wung, Keenan, Giroux, Stouthamer–Loeber, Van Kammen, & Maughan, 1993). Better screening devices are needed to enable juvenile justice officials and others dealing with child delinquents to discriminate between those who will escalate to more serious offending and those who will not (Howell, in press-a).

Disruptive children. Many youth who become serious and violent offenders have a long history of nondelinquent, disruptive problem behaviors during childhood (Loeber & Farrington, 1998; Robins, 1966). Typical disruptive behaviors are serious and persistent disobedience, frequent lying, aggressive behaviors, minor forms of theft, truancy during elementary school, and early substance use. Longitudinal studies show that a quarter to a third of these disruptive children are at risk of becoming child delinquents (Loeber & Dishion, 1983; Offord, Lipman, & Duku, in press; Tremblay, Pihl, Vitaro, & Dobkin, 1994).

In addition, already early in life, disruptive children tend to show multiple problems in a diversity of areas, including, attention-deficit hyperactivity disorder (ADHD), ungovernability in the home, poor school performance, internalizing problems (e.g., depressed mood), and, at a later point, substance use, spousal abuse, and young parenthood (Espiritu et al., in press; Farrington, 1994; Loeber, Farring-

1. In contrast, adolescent murderers tend to have a history of one or more prior arrests (Bailey, 1996; Lewis, Moy, Jackson, Aaronson, Restifo, Serra, & Simos, 1985; Myers, Scott, Burgess, & Burgess, 1995).

ton, et al., 1998; Offord et al., in press). Moreover, child delinquents are disproportionally victims of child abuse (Howell, in press-b; Wasserman & Seracini, in press; Wiig, in press).

Epidemiology

How prevalent are child delinquents?

Child delinquency is quite common. Two inner-city studies (Denver and Pittsburgh) show that at 11–12 years of age, about 10% of boys and girls have a police contact because of delinquency (Espiritu et al., in press). The total volume of child delinquents handled in the juvenile courts is large: in 1997 an estimated 181,300 delinquents were below age 13 years at the time of the court intake (Butts & Snyder, 1997; Puzzanchera, 1998; Snyder, in press). Disturbingly, the National Longitudinal Survey of Youth in 1997 found that 7% of all American 12-year-olds reported that they had carried a handgun in the past year (Puzzanchera, 2000). In summary, child delinquents constitute a surprisingly high danger and burden for society and for the juvenile courts.

Race differences. The rate of referral of African American child delinquents to the juvenile court in 1997 was 3 times higher than the referral rate for Caucasian child delinquents (Snyder, in press; Kempf–Leonard, Chesney–Lind, & Hawkins, in press). These differences in referral rates and disruptive behavior need to be examined in the context of children's exposure to risk factors, particularly in the worst inner-city neighborhoods and with regard to the greater police patrolling and likelihood of detection in these areas.

Sex differences. The male referral rate of child delinquents to the juvenile court in 1997 was over 3 times the female rate. Over the years, however, the sex gap has been narrowing. Between 1988 and 1997, court referrals of female child delinquents increased by 69%, compared with the male increase of 26% (Snyder, in press). Sex differences in disruptive child behavior already tend to emerge after age 2 years (Loeber & Hay, 1997). Studies confirm the generally held belief that already at an early age more boys than girls show disruptive behavior, such as aggression. However, the prevalence of indirect aggression (e.g., ostracizing others and spreading malicious rumors) is about the same for each gender, and if anything slightly higher for females (Offord et al., in press). Official records and self-reports of delinquent acts show that early onset offending is more common among males than females (Snyder, in press; Kempf–Leonard et al., in press). For example, self-reports of two inner-city samples of children below age 13 years show that 7–9% of boys and 3% of girls had committed serious aggravated assaults or robberies (Espiritu et al., in press).

What are the most common delinquent acts committed by child delinquents?

In general, child delinquents commit a similar pattern of delinquent acts to older delinquents (Espiritu et al., in press; Snyder, in press). However, the proportion of juvenile arrests involving child delinquents is highest for arson (35%), followed by sex offenses and vandalism (18–19%), larceny or theft, minor assault, burglary, and forcible rape (12–14%). The proportion of child delinquents arrested for status offenses (running away from home, curfew violation, liquor law violations) is lower (about 10%), but this may reflect current practices to avoid processing children under age 13 years for status offenses. National surveys report that 6–9% of children below age 13 years commit status offenses (Espiritu et al., in press). In summary, child delinquency is common and includes serious offenses, as well as status offenses.

Are there geographic concentrations of child delinquents?

It is likely that child delinquents are not randomly distributed across the nation, but the evidence for their concentration in certain states and cities is incomplete. Child delinquents in secure juvenile facilities are unequally distributed across the nation, with the highest concentrations found in Florida, Georgia, Wyoming, South Dakota, and Alaska (Snyder, in press).

It is impossible to say whether the geographic concentration of child delinquents in those states reflects the prevalence of child delinquents, availability of residential and nonresidential services, or routine judicial practices unique to those states. However, we know that juvenile homicides (and probably other serious offenses) committed by juveniles of *any* age are concentrated in large cities (e.g., Los Angeles, Houston, Chicago, Detroit, New York; see Snyder & Sickmund, 1999). Since a high proportion of serious violent offenders start their delinquency careers at an early age, it follows that child delinquents probably are also concentrated in the same locations. This would agree with findings showing that the prevalence of aggression is particularly elevated in children from the lowest income groups and concentrated in inner-city children growing up in poverty (Offord et al., in press). We know that many of the child delinquents had been highly aggressive when younger (Lipsey & Derzon, 1998; Loeber & Dishion, 1983).

Has the prevalence of child delinquents increased in recent years?

Between 1988 and 1997, the number of arrested child delinquents only increased by 6%, although the number dealt with by the juvenile court increased by 33%, showing that law enforcement agencies were increasingly likely to refer child delinquents to the juvenile court. Over two-thirds (69%) of the practitioners we surveyed said that it is now more common than in the recent past for children to become delinquent at a very young age.[2] However, a comparison of self-reported delinquency over the past 20 years does not indicate any increase by young offenders in the United States (Espiritu et al., in press). Moreover, between 1980 and 1997 the number of murders by an offender up to age 12 years remained about the same, averaging about 30 per year (Snyder, in press).

Have child delinquents become more violent?

The recorded offense pattern of child delinquents changed between 1988 and 1997. During that period arrests for violent crimes increased by 45%, arrests for simple assaults increased by 79%, and arrests for weapons law violations increased by 76%. These increases in arrests parallel the increases in these behaviors seen for older juvenile offenders. However, the increases in violence and drug abuse violations by child delinquents has received scant attention so far. The number of violence cases involving child delinquents in the courts more than doubled (up 113%), and the number of drug offenses over the period increased even more (163%; Snyder, in press). It is debatable whether these changes reflect true secular changes in society or changes in prosecution practices in the juvenile justice system. Arrests of child delinquents for property crimes decreased by 17% between 1988 and 1997 (Snyder, in press).

Development

What is the developmental context of child delinquency?

Some children engage in minor delinquent acts for excitement, adventure, or other emotions common among children. For these children, offending may be considered as part of the context of child development in which youngsters learn prosocial behaviors by trial and error. This may be the case for a propor-

2. On March 22, 1999, Rolf Loeber, David P. Farrington, Darnell F. Hawkins, Melissa H. Sickmund, and Gail A. Wasserman made presentations describing the work of the OJJDP Study Group on Very Young Offenders at the 26th National Conference on Juvenile Justice in Minneapolis. During this session, a questionnaire was given out to the audience soliciting their opinions on eight policy issues relevant to child delinquents (see Loeber, Farrington, & Kalb, 1999). Out of about 150 persons in the audience, 111 completed the questionnaire. About three-quarters were juvenile justice workers (juvenile court officers, juvenile probation officers, prosecutors, public defenders, court administrators, child advocates, etc.), while one-quarter were mental health workers (psychologists, psychiatrists, social workers, court clinicians, etc.).

tion of the early onset offenders. However, several important points should be kept in mind: (a) many of the children who come to the attention of the police and the court because of minor delinquent acts also, unknown to the juvenile justice system, engage in more serious acts (Snyder, 1998); (b) for some child offenders, early status offenses and delinquency are stepping stones in pathways to serious, violent, and chronic offending, particularly when the status offenses first appear at a young age (e.g., Loeber & Dishion, 1983; Lipsey & Derzon, 1998; Loeber et al., 1993); (c) about a quarter to a half of children who engage in disruptive behavior are at risk of escalating to delinquent acts (Farrington, 1991; Loeber & Dishion, 1983; Offord et al., in press; Tremblay et al., 1994); (d) about a third to a half of child delinquents are at risk of escalating to serious delinquency (Hawkins, Laub, & Lauritsen, 1998; Lipsey & Derzon, 1998; Loeber & Dishion, 1983), and 40–60% run the risk of becoming chronic offenders (Blumstein, Farrington, & Moitra, 1965; Kempf–Leonard et al., in press); and (e) screening procedures are needed to distinguish prospectively (rather than after the fact) between those youth whose early offending is temporary and those who will either persist in offending over time or escalate to serious offenses (Howell, in press-a).

In summary, research findings support the notion that the development of offending is part of a broader pattern of deviant development that usually starts with disruptive nondelinquent behavior (see Figure 1). Although some of the predictions may refer to similar behaviors (e.g., aggression predicting violence), some types of disruptive behaviors may also predict different types of delinquent acts. For example, research shows that boys who are aggressive by 8–9 years of age, compared to nonaggressive boys, have 5 times as high a risk of engaging in property offenses by ages 12 and 13 years (Offord et al., in press).

What are developmental pathways to disruptive and delinquent behavior?

We hypothesize that disruptive behavior, status offenses, and delinquent acts of different severity levels are different manifestations of the same "underlying" deviancy, and children differ in the extent that they progress over time on developmental pathways to serious delinquent behaviors. The term *pathway* is defined as "a common pattern of development shared by a group of individuals which is distinct from the behavioral development experienced by other groups of individuals" (Loeber, 1991, p. 98). A key thesis is that a proportion of child delinquents develop into serious and violent offenders but that individuals' pathways leading to a similar outcome (i.e., serious and violent offending) can be diverse (called equifinality; Cicchetti & Rogosch, 1996).

Empirical work by Loeber and his colleagues, initially on the three samples of the Pittsburgh Youth Study and since then replicated in several other studies, has demonstrated three pathways in male disruptive and delinquent child behavior, as shown in Figure 2 (Kelley, Huizinga, Thornberry & Loeber, 1997; Loeber, Keenan, & Zhang, 1997; Loeber, DeLamatre, Keenan, & Zhang, 1998a; Loeber, Wei, Stouthamer–Loeber, Huizinga, & Thornberry, 1999; Loeber, Wung, et al., 1993; Tolan, 1998; Tolan & Gorman–Smith, 1998; Tolan, Gorman–Smith, & Loeber, in press): (a) an *overt* pathway, starting with minor aggression, followed by physical fighting, and followed in turn by violence; (b) a *covert* pathway prior to age 15 years, consisting of a sequence of minor covert behaviors (e.g., shoplifting), followed by property damage (fire setting or vandalism) and moderate to serious forms of delinquency; and (c) an *authority conflict* pathway prior to age 12 years, consisting of a sequence of stubborn behavior, defiance, and authority avoidance (truancy, running away, staying out late at night), and which, at the highest level, concerns behaviors that can be construed as status offenses.

Only a minority of boys, especially those with persistent problem behaviors, advance to the most serious level within a pathway. Boys can advance on one or more pathways at the same time. Those with an early onset of disruptive or delinquent behavior are more likely to progress to the highest level of a pathway (Tolan, 1998; Tolan & Gorman–Smith, 1998).

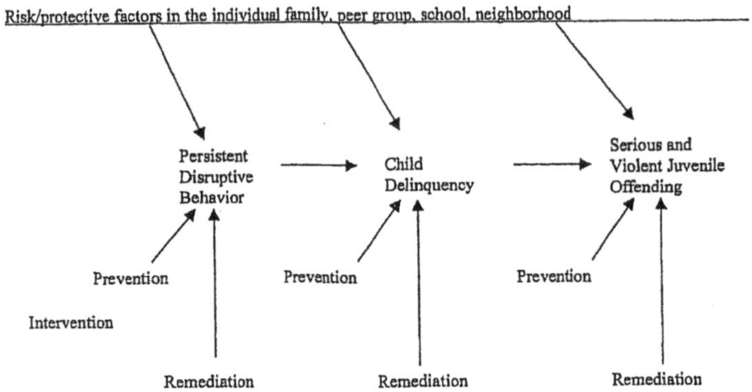

Figure 1. Relationship between risk and protective factors, development of child problem behavior, and interventions.

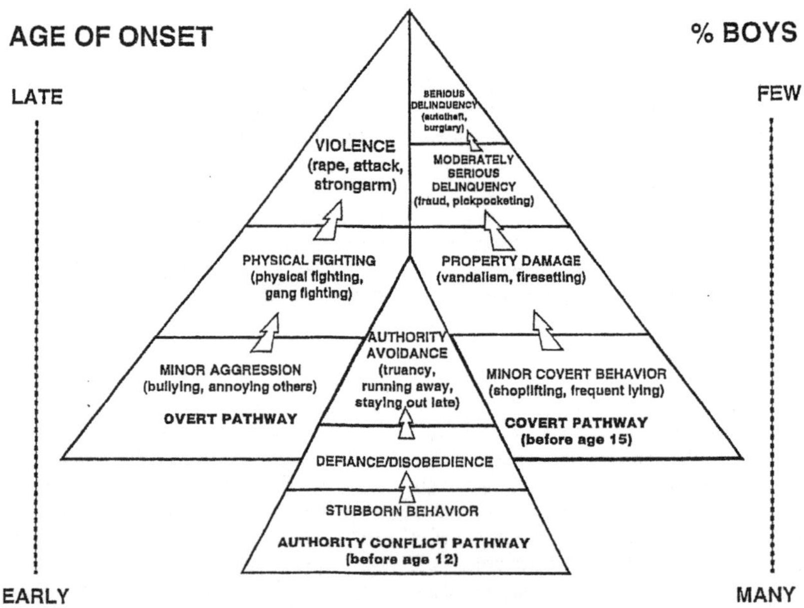

Figure 2. Three developmental pathways in disruptive behavior, status offenses, and delinquent acts (Loeber, Wei, et al., 1999).

Truancy, curfew violation, and running away from home all constitute the last step in the authority conflict pathway (Loeber et al., 1993) and denote avoidance of authority figures such as parents and teachers (Figure 2). Research findings show that boys' advancement in this pathway increases their risk of escalating in the overt or covert pathways leading to violence or serious property offenses, respectively (Loeber et al., 1993).

There are two qualitative changes that take place when children advance from the lower to the higher levels within pathways. First, there is *development of disruptive or delin-*

	Minor Problem Behavior	Moderately Serious Problem Behavior	Serious Delinquency	First Court Contact for Index Offenses
Age	7.0	9.5	11.9	14.5

Figure 3. Age of onset of earlier problem behaviors for boys brought before the juvenile court for and index offense (Office of Juvenile Justice and Delinquency Prevention, 1998).

quent behavior starting in the home and spreading to the school and the community. Often, a developmental pathway towards serious offending starts with persistent disruptive behavior in the home, which then spreads to delinquent acts outside of the home—that is, at school and in the community. The reverse—that is, serious delinquent acts starting in the community (without prior disruptive behavior in the family home) and then spilling over into disruptive or delinquent behavior at home—appears rare. Second, there is *development from infliction of harm on relatives and peers to infliction of harm on strangers.* Typically, early disruptive behavior in the preschool period is directed at adults, especially parents and other caretakers, but often same-age and younger siblings and peers are victimized as well. For example, the majority of murders committed by child delinquents are of acquaintances and relatives. Usually during adolescence, youth start to inflict harm on strangers in the neighborhood close to the youth's home and then, as transportation becomes available, in neighborhoods further away from home.

The study of developmental pathways has shown that there is a relatively wide time window of opportunities for early intervention. For example, research (Office of Juvenile Justice and Delinquency Prevention, 1998) shows that the average age of boys first brought before the juvenile court for an index offense was 14.5 years (Figure 3). Most of these boys had a longstanding history of earlier problem behavior. The average age of onset of minor problem behavior (Step 1 in any of the pathways) for this category of offenders was 7.0 years. The average age of onset of moderately serious problem behavior (Step 2 in the pathways) was 9.5 years, while the average age of onset of serious delinquency was 11.9 years (Step 3 in the pathways). Thus, about 7 years elapsed between the onset of minor problem behavior and boys' first court appearance for an index offense. This means that there is a wide window of opportunity for intervention during the interim period. However, early intervention is preferable to prevent all the antisocial acts committed during this time period.

What are the consequences of an early onset of a delinquent career for the offenders?

There are many negative consequences for children who start their delinquency career early in life (Farrington et al., 1990). We list the most important ones:

1. It is likely that the repeated practice of disruptive behaviors and delinquent acts during a formative period of life contributes to the subsequent stability and continuation of such acts over time.
2. Desistance from offending is less likely for early onset offenders, especially for those who advance to the more serious forms of offending (Loeber, 1988).
3. Years of engaging in delinquency tend to rob youth of many opportunities to learn and practice prosocial behaviors.
4. Engaging in persistent disruptive behavior and delinquency often is associated with poor social skills, leading to major and continued disturbances in social relationships with relatives, peers, partners, and later, employers and coworkers in places of work.
5. Low interest and motivation in educational matters associated with early onset offending leads to major disruption in classrooms, exposure to remedial and often alternative special education services, and,

eventually, to chronic truancy and early school dropout. The resulting poor educational achievement has negative effects on later employment opportunities and lifetime income.

6. Young male repeat offenders are more likely to become fathers at a young age and often are unable or unwilling to fulfill the father role or assume financial responsibilities for their partner and child. In addition, they often provide undesirable role models for their children (Wei & Stouthamer–Loeber, 1999).
7. Young aggressive delinquents have a high risk of depression and suicide (e.g., Lewis, Shanok, Grant, & Ritvo, 1983).
8. Young offenders often are at high risk of criminal victimization in the community and, as a consequence, have a relatively high likelihood of being killed or maimed for life (Loeber, Farrington, & Kalb, 1999).
9. Early onset offenders often start using illicit substances at a young age (Le Blanc & Loeber, 1998), and children who use substances at an early age are at risk of becoming persistent substance abusers (Grant & Dawson, 1998).

In summary, early and persistent involvement in disruptive and delinquent behavior generates cumulative and cascading negative consequences for a person's life (Thornberry & Krohn, in press).

How early can we identify children at risk for child delinquency?

Some researchers have argued that we need to identify during the preschool years or in early childhood those who will later become child delinquents. Although in some ways it is laudable to conduct research on criteria that would facilitate such identification, there are several important complications attached to this strategy. The development of disruptive behavior and early forms of delinquency often takes years and is a function of juveniles' exposure to risk and protective factors during that period (see below). Thus, although some have proposed that "life-course persistent" offenders can be identified very early in life (Moffitt, 1993), this discrimination is far from perfect because many children show some problem behavior early in life. Childhood is a period in which most youth learn about what is good and bad, what is permissible and not permissible in the acquisition of goods, and how to solve interpersonal conflicts without resorting to violence. Childhood is also characterized by age-normative problem behaviors which most children give up as they grow up. Usually, in this period of trial and error learning, many children engage in problem behaviors of a relatively minor nature for a short time and, therefore, are not of major concern. The fact is, however, that currently we have few tools to distinguish between those young children who will continue with their problem behavior and those who will not (see, e.g., Walker, Severson, Stiller, Williams, Haring, Shinn, & Todis, 1988; Walker, Severson, Todis, Block–Pedego, Williams, Haring, & Barckley, 1990; Feil, Severson, & Walker, 1995, 1998). Third, it is unlikely that a single screening method would be of the greatest utility in identifying those at highest risk; instead, it is much more likely that screening methods applied in sequence over time would have a greater utility. Yet researchers are not in agreement about at what age(s) such screening should be accomplished (Le Blanc, 1998; Howell, in press-a).

What are early warning signs?

Generally, the foundations for both prosocial and disruptive behaviors are laid in the first 5 years of life (Keenan, in press). Deviations from normal developmental processes can be identified during this period. In subsequent years child behavior can undergo major changes, with some youth developing more serious disruptive and delinquent behavior and others who had an early onset of disruptive behavior eventually ceasing.

Some level of disruptive behavior is common during the preschool years, especially during the "terrible twos and threes" when many children of both sexes show high levels of aggression and noncompliance. However, the following are important warning signs of later problems: (a) disruptive behavior that is either more frequent or more severe than that of children of the same age; (b) disruptive behavior, such as temper tantrums and aggression, that persists beyond the first 2 to 3 years of life; (c) the majority of early onset antisocial youth had a history of aggressive, inattentive, or sensation-seeking behavior in the preschool years; (d) the reverse, however, was not true—the majority of preschoolers with behavior problems do not go on to become child delinquents .

In summary, in the case of many offenders disruptive behavior becomes apparent during the preschool years and certainly during the elementary school years (Keenan, in press). The question of "how early can we tell" is critical from a scientific as well as a policy standpoint. Specific early warning signs for the development of delinquency at a young age include overt acts, such as physical fighting, cruelty to people or animals, and not getting along with others; covert acts, such as frequent lying, theft, and fire setting; school problem behaviors including low school motivation; and substance use without parental permission (Lipsey & Derzon, 1998; Loeber, Green, Lahey, Frick, & McBurnett, 2000; Loeber, Stouthamer–Loeber, Van Kammen, & Farrington, 1991). In addition, repeated victimization plays a role in an unknown proportion of cases of child delinquents. This victimization may take the form of child abuse by adults or extended exposure to bullying by peers.

How different are early onset offenders?

Advances have been made in the theoretical underpinnings of the distinction between early and later onset offenders, particularly Moffitt's (1993) distinction between life course persistent and adolescent-limited delinquency, Patterson's coercion theory as it applies to early onset offending (Patterson, 1996; Patterson, Capaldi, & Bank, 1991), Thornberry and Krohn's interactional theory (Thornberry & Krohn, in press), and Gottfredson and Hirschi's (1990) self-control theory (for a review of these theories, see Krohn et al., in press). In addition, several other developmental theories contain aspects relevant to early onset offending: Sampson and Laub's age-graded theory of informal social control (1993), Elliott's integration of strain, social learning, and social control perspectives (Elliott, Ageton, & Canter, 1979; Elliott, Huizinga, & Ageton, 1985), and Catalano and Hawkins' Social Development Model (Catalano & Hawkins, 1996). Summaries of these theories can be found in Krohn et al. (in press) and Herrenkohl, Hawkins, Chung, Hill, and Battin–Pearson (in press).

Theoreticians such as Moffitt (1993) have argued cogently for the importance of the distinction between early and later onset of child problem behavior. However, what may be a somewhat clear concept for an individual child may not be so clear for populations of children. Are there differences evident in onset data for populations of children? And at what ages can such distinctions best be made?

First, studies do not always agree whether age 10 years or higher should be used as a cutoff to distinguish between early and later onset groups of youth (e.g., American Psychiatric Association, 1994; Farrington et al., 1990; Loeber & Farrington, 1998). Second, the onset of disruptive behaviors in populations of children is not stepwise but, instead, takes place gradually. This is revealed by the onset curves of serious delinquency for male persistent juvenile offenders in three inner-city, longitudinal studies (Loeber & Farrington, 1998). As shown in Figure 4, in Pittsburgh half of the persistent juvenile offenders experienced the *onset* of serious delinquency by ages 12–13 years. Two years later (ages 14–15 years) over 80% had begun to commit serious delinquency.

Figure 4 does not show the onset curves for disruptive child behavior (such as physical fighting) and nonserious forms of delinquency. For example, the onset curve for moderate to serious conduct disorder symptoms (e.g., theft, fire setting, cruelty to animals or people, physical fighting) in a clinic-referred sample of boys before the age of 13 years shows that by age 6 years over 40% already showed one or more of such symptoms, and this increased

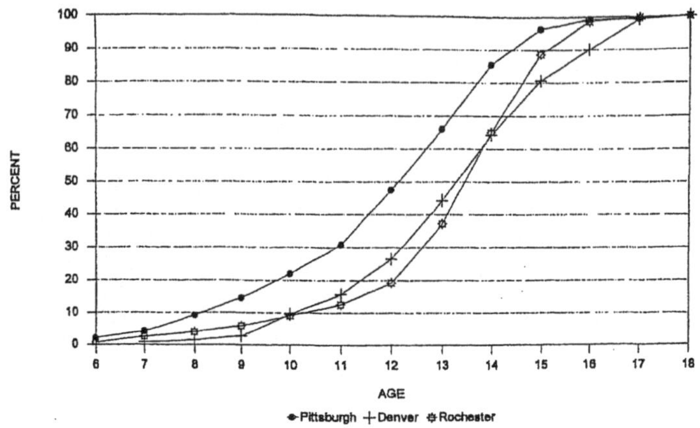

Figure 4. Cumulative onset of persistent serious and violent delinquency in three inner-city studies (Loeber & Farrington, 1998).

to almost 90% by age 10 years (Loeber, Mutchko, & Burke, 2000). In summary, research findings show that the onset of many conduct problems usually predates the onset of serious delinquency by several years (Loeber et al., 1993; Loeber & Stouthamer–Loeber, 1998; Loeber, Wei, Stouthamer–Loeber, Huizinga, & Thornberry, 1999b). Also, the findings do not support a simple dichotomy of early versus later onset in populations of children.

Population onset curves do not show individual children's trajectories in disruptive and delinquent behavior over time. Differences in the within-individual development of various problem behaviors are much better captured by the conceptualization of developmental pathways (Figure 2). The study of the onset of disruptive and delinquent child behavior is important, however. Even though the prevalence of delinquency peaks at ages 17–18 years, many of the most seriously delinquent offenders start their deviant career prior to adolescence.

Causes and Risk Factors

What are the causes of child offending?

Experts, as reported in the media, are not in agreement about the causes of serious crimes committed by child delinquents (Sleek, 1998). Many of the risk factors and predictors (and, possibly, the causes) of child delinquency tend to be partly different from the causes of juveniles' offending starting at a later age. For example, Loeber (1988), who focused on early precursor behaviors, postulated that juveniles who eventually commit both property and violent crime, compared to less serious offenders with an onset during adolescence, often begin showing the onset of conduct problems in the preschool years, and show aggressive and covert problem behaviors and hyperactive or impulsive behavior at a young age. These children often have educational problems, display poor social skills, and demonstrate poor relationships with peers and adults. Importantly, this group of juveniles has a lower remission rate than the later onset offenders. The male to female ratio is higher for early compared to later onset offenders. Further support for many of these propositions has come from several studies and one meta-analysis (see, e.g., Lipsey & Derzon, 1998; Loeber, Farrington, et al., 1998; Moffitt, 1993).

Many risk factors (listed in Table 1) are associated with child delinquency. An extensive summary of knowledge about these risk factors can be found in Loeber and Farrington (in press). That summary is inspired by Bron-

Table 1. *Childhood risk factors for child delinquency and later serious and violent juvenile offending*

- Child factors
  - Difficult temperament
  - Impulsive behavior
  - Hyperactivity (but only when co-occurring with disruptive behavior)
  - Impulsivity
  - Substance use
  - Aggression
  - Early onset disruptive behavior
  - Withdrawn behavior
  - Low intelligence
  - Lead toxicity
- Family factors
  - Parental antisocial or delinquent behavior
  - Parental substance abuse
  - Parents' poor child rearing practices
    - Poor supervision
    - Physical punishment
    - Poor communication
  - Poor parent–child relations
  - Parental physical and sexual abuse
  - Parental neglect
  - Maternal depression
  - Mother's smoking during pregnancy
  - Teenage motherhood
  - Parents disagree on child discipline
  - Single parenthood
  - Large family
  - High turn-over of caretakers
  - Low socioeconomic status of the family
  - Unemployed parent
  - Poorly educated mother
  - Family members' carelessness in allowing children access to weapons, especially guns
- School factors
  - Poor academic performance
  - Old for grade
  - Weak bonding to school
  - Low educational aspirations
  - Low school motivation
  - Poorly organized and functioning schools.
- Peer factors
  - Association with deviant or delinquent siblings and peers
  - Rejection by peers
- Neighborhood factors
  - Neighborhood disadvantage and poverty
  - Disorganized neighborhoods
  - Availability of weapons
  - Media portrayal of violence

Note: Adapted from Loeber and Farrington (in press) and based on Hawkins et al. (1998), Lipsey and Derzon (1998), Loeber, Stouthamer-Loeber, Van Kammen, and Farrington (1991), and Loeber, Farrington, et al. (1998).

fenbrenner's (1979) conceptualization of the different spheres of influence that affect child behavior, such as the family, the peer group, and community. However, a more distinctive developmental model is preferable in which certain domains of risk factors (and possible causes) initially promote early forms of child deviancy, and in which subsequent deviant development is affected by additional domains of risk factors. Specifically, we hypothesize that the *initial* risk factors for child delinquency lie, first, within the individual child (such as impulsive behavior; see Tremblay & LeMarquand, in press) and, second, within the family (such as parents' child-rearing practices; see Keenan, in press, and Wasserman & Seracini, in press). Starting in the preschool years, and certainly from the elementary school period onward, the array of risk factors expands, because some children will be exposed to negative peer influences outside of the home (see Coie & Miller–Johnson, in press). Also during this period, some children will be exposed to additional risk factors situated within schools or in the community at large (see Herrenkohl et al., in press).

Research findings agree that no single risk factor explains serious and violent offending. Instead, studies indicate that the higher the number of risk factors, the greater the likelihood of these outcomes later (summarized in Loeber & Farrington, 1998). Second, research also suggests that the risk of later offending is dependent on the number of risk factors *and* the number of protective or promotive factors (i.e., factors associated with a positive outcome). Recent research on the Pittsburgh Youth Study confirms that this is the case for risk domains (such as the individual child and the family; Stouthamer–Loeber, Loeber, Wei, Farrington, & Wikströlm, in press). As shown in Figure 5, there is an almost linear relationship between the number of promotive or risk domains and the likelihood of persistent serious offending 5 years later. In the youngest sample, first studied at age 7 years, *none* of the

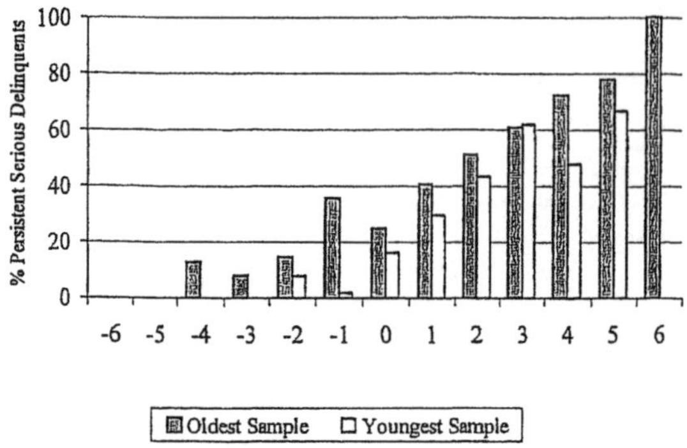

Figure 5. Prediction of male persistent serious offending as a function of the number of domains of risk and promotive factors (Stouthamer–Loeber et al., in press).

boys with a score of −2 or lower (meaning a preponderance of promotive domains) became a persistent serious offender later, compared to two thirds of those with a score of 5 (meaning a greater preponderance of risk domains). The results show that promotive domains may counteract the impact of risk domains.

Interventions

What are the opinions of practitioners about interventions with child delinquents?

Loeber et al. (1999) conducted a survey of practitioners' opinions about child delinquents. Nearly three quarters (71%) thought that there were effective ways of dealing with child delinquents to reduce their risk of offending in the future. However, only 3–6% thought that current juvenile court procedures were effective in achieving this aim, that current mental health programs were effective, or that current child welfare, dependency, and neglect programs were effective. Almost all practitioners (88%) agreed that there was an acute problem for juvenile courts concerning how best to deal with child delinquents.

Why do child delinquents pose a special challenge to agencies?

In the juvenile justice system, procedures for dealing with child delinquents are not always as straightforward as with older delinquents, and rules for interrogation and prosecution have been challenged (Geraghty, 1997; "Police Charge Methods," 1998; Wiig, in press). Child delinquents are often difficult to deal with in the juvenile courts, because of their less than average intelligence, poor understanding of court procedures, and general immaturity (Geraghty, 1997). Crucial issues are the degree to which child delinquents are competent enough to undergo the legal procedures of the juvenile court, whether they understand their own culpability, and whether they understand the reasons for sanctions.

In addition, judges' options for the disposition of child delinquents are often restricted because of characteristics of parents. More of the child delinquents, compared to later onset delinquents, come from dysfunctional families with one or more of the following: family disruption, especially a succession of different caretakers; parental antisocial behavior; parental substance use; mother's depression; and child abuse and neglect (Hennepin County Attorney's Office, 1995; Wasserman & Seracini, in press). These characteristics pose special challenges to agencies, such as the juvenile court, mental health clinics, schools, and child welfare agencies, dealing with these problematic children. Therefore, a lack of resources in the home environment increases the risk of child delinquents being institutionalized or permanently removed from the home.

Developmentally informed interventions

Figure 1 schematically presents our model of developmentally informed interventions, consisting of three components: (a) problem behavior develops from persistent disruptive behavior to, first, child delinquency and, second, serious and violent juvenile offending; (b) this development is thought to be a function of risk and protective factors in the individual, family, peer group, school, and neighborhood; and (c) preventive and remedial interventions based on knowledge of (a) and (b) can reduce children's deviant behavior.

As shown in Figure 1, preventive interventions can be aimed, first, at the prevention of persistent disruptive behavior in children in general; second, at the prevention of child delinquency, particularly among persistent disruptive children; and, third, at the prevention of serious and violent juvenile offending, particularly among child delinquents. At the same time, remedial interventions to address current problem behaviors can be implemented at the level of either persistent disruptive behavior, child delinquency, or serious and violent juvenile offending. Both preventive and remedial interventions can be aimed at the reduction of child problem behavior *and* the reduction of risk factors in each domain of the individual child, family, peer group, school, and neighborhood. Interventions can also be aimed at promoting protective factors in each of the domains associated with prosocial behavior.

Are interventions for child delinquents taking place sufficiently early?

We saw that three key aspects that justify an early and preventive approach to child delinquency are clear from the preceding (Keenan, in press). First, the foundations for developing prosocial and antisocial behavior are established in the first 5 years of life. Second, some preschool children engage in very serious antisocial behavior. Third, in some cases disruptive behavior problems occurring as early as age 2–3 years predicted child delinquency between ages 7 and 12 years.

Is this knowledge generally translated into early preventive interventions? Overall, society appears more prepared to carry the huge costs of dealing with serious and violent juvenile offenders in adolescence and adulthood rather than to take cost-effective preventive measures in childhood (Early years study: Reversing the real brain drain , 1999). Currently, most juvenile justice resources are spent on adolescent juvenile offenders rather than on child delinquents, and are not spent in proportion to the risk of long-term serious outcomes. The same typically applies to schools, where most of the resources of special education and behavior management are funneled into middle and high schools, rather than elementary schools or preschools. Similarly, programs for child delinquents undertaken by welfare agencies often are directed at children whose disruptive behavior is already persistent. We strongly argue that professionals in schools and those working with families should shift their perception of an "early intervention" time frame from elementary school to infancy and toddlerhood.

Of all known interventions to reduce juvenile delinquency, preventive interventions that focus on child delinquents probably will take the largest "bite" out of crime. Yet, as we will show later, the responses of institutions dealing with child delinquents (the juvenile justice system, mental health, child welfare and child protection agencies, schools, parents) often are inadequate on their own and fail to intercept the life course of high-rate offending that commonly follows child offending. In summary, a reorientation of agencies toward "early" prevention is urgently needed to redirect resources to deal with youth at a younger age. This needs to be accomplished along with interventions for serious forms of delinquency by juveniles of any age.

Effectiveness of interventions

One of the important issues is whether preventive and remedial interventions (Figure 1) are effective in reducing the likelihood of long-term serious problem behaviors (e.g., serious and violent offending) and are effective in reducing current disruptive behavior. We will briefly discuss interventions by each of the principal agencies that deal with child delinquents and with children with persistent disruptive behavior.

Juvenile justice. In practice, children are referred to the juvenile court if (a) their offense is thought to be sufficiently serious (which depends on the judgment of a police officer or a court intake officer); and (b) they are old enough to be held criminally responsible (this applies only to those states which have statutes to that effect). If these conditions are not met, children may either be sent back home (with or without a message to their parent; see Espiritu et al., in press) or be classified as dependent, resulting in a referral to Children and Youth Services. National figures about the prevalence of these referrals are not available.

Snyder (in press), in reviewing the response of the juvenile court to child delinquents, found that the number of child delinquency cases that resulted in formal court-ordered probation increased by 73% between 1980 and 1997, while placements of child delinquents to residential facilities increased by 49%. Juvenile courts in 1997 placed nearly 23,000 child delinquents on formal, court-ordered probation and placed another 7,000 child delinquents in a residential facility for committing a delinquent act. In addition, 18,000 child delinquents were held in secure detention facilities in 1997, an increase of 47% compared to 1988. Residential placement for status offenses is relatively more common among child delinquents compared to older delinquents. According to the Census of Juveniles in Residential Placement in 1997, 19% of child delinquents were held for a status offense (all of the above and truancy), compared with 6% of older juveniles (Snyder, in press). There are no evaluations of the effects of juvenile court actions upon the recidivism of child delinquents, nor is it clear whether some actions by the juvenile court are more effective than other actions.

Child delinquents, compared to older offenders, often have special needs and pose many challenges to the juvenile justice system. Very young children, compared to older children, are often less well equipped to comprehend their own culpability and the consequences of their actions. Also, there are large individual differences in the cognitive functioning of older children, with some, because of immaturity or low intelligence, lagging behind their age-mates. We mentioned that states differ very much in the minimum age of criminal responsibility. It is not clear how rigorously these age cutoffs are enforced or followed, and what mechanisms are in place to deal with those children who, although at or above the cutoff, are not competent in one or several ways.

Thus, child delinquents in the juvenile court have a need to be assessed for their competence before being processed through the juvenile justice system (Wiig, in press). In the court and also in their contact with the police and probation departments, child delinquents need to have an advocate, especially in case of the absence or impairment of their parents. Once program decisions are made, child delinquents need to be protected from the negative and criminogenic influences of older delinquent youth in institutions or in delinquency programs outside of institutions. The juvenile justice system also has a responsibility to protect child delinquents from physical and sexual abuse in institutions. Importantly, child delinquents have a need to benefit from the least intrusive program to reduce the risk of disruptive behavior escalating to delinquency and to reduce the risk of early onset, first-time offenders becoming recidivists.

Legislation. Several countries have new juvenile justice acts (e.g., Canada and England) or have such acts in the making (United States). Currently, the effectiveness of legislation to reduce recidivism of child delinquents is far from clear. Some politicians have suggested stiffer legal sanctions for child delinquents within the juvenile court. Others have proposed transfer of juvenile offenders to the adult court. However, in both cases it is unclear to what extent these measures are appropriate for what types of offenses, appropriate to what minimum age, and whether legal sanctions are effective for child delinquents. Also, proposals have been put forward to make parents more legally responsible for the lawbreaking of their children, and especially to provide sanctions for parents who do not prevent children' access to guns (Seelye, 1999). Theoretically, parents who are deficient in their supervision of their child (or practice poor child-rearing methods, such as harsh punishment) could be forced by court order or legislation to participate in parent training (Wiig, in press). The effectiveness of such compulsory methods, however, remains uncertain.

Child welfare agencies. Children with persisting disruptive or delinquent behavior, such as curfew violations, truancy, and underage drinking, can be referred to child welfare agencies. However, often these agencies appear understaffed and overloaded with child abuse investigations. When children are not physically at risk (which applies to the majority of child delinquents), they are given a low priority, resulting in a lack of programs to prevent further offending. For example, Augimeri, Koegl, & Goldberg, (in press) conducted a survey of directors of child welfare in 13 provinces and territories in Canada. The results indicated that "the emphasis in child welfare is on child protection, not offending behavior *per se*. For example, child welfare assesses only the child's need of protection from parental abuse or neglect. Furthermore, we found no consistent tracking of the number of referrals child welfare receives from the police for children under 12 who commit offenses" (p. xx). Although such a survey appears not available in the United States, it is our impression that the same applies in this country.

Parents. Keenan (in press), in reviewing early child disruptive behaviors, concluded that such behaviors are the most common source of referral of preschool children for mental health services. Parenting practices are among the most powerful predictors of later outcomes in children and constitute opportunities for interventions (Wasserman & Seracini, in press). Effective interventions for disruptive and delinquent juveniles include parent management training (PMT), functional family therapy, and multisystemic therapy (MST), although the latter two programs still need to be evaluated with child delinquents (Alexander, Barton, Schiavo, & Parsons, 1976; Borduin, Cone, Mann, Henggeler, Fucci, Blaske, & Williams, 1995; Kazdin, 1995).

In addition, interventions targeted on known and malleable risk factors within the family have been developed and evaluated, such as marital conflict and violence and child abuse, but the effectiveness of these interventions in preventing or reducing disruptive or delinquent behavior in young children remains to be established. Stimulant medication for ADHD often can reduce both on-task behavior of children and disruptive behavior. Often such medication is used in conjunction with family intervention aimed at increasing skills both of the parents and the child. However, there is no empirical evidence that medication alone prevents delinquency in childhood or prevents serious and violent offending later (Wasserman & Seracini, in press).

Peers. Demonstrated peer interventions in schools have largely focused on the reduction of bullying and associated aggression (e.g., Conduct Problems Prevention Research Group, 1999a, 1999b). Interventions to reduce rejection by peers remain to be undertaken (Coie & Miller–Johnson, in press). Not all peer-focused interventions are beneficial. An example is programs that bring delinquent or highly disruptive children together for group therapy (Dishion, McCord, & Poulin, 2000). Knowledge about the effectiveness of routine interventions is an absolute necessity to eliminate interventions that can have deleterious effects. The more widely used interventions are, the more urgent is this knowledge. Peer interventions can be best undertaken in conjunction with other types of programs, such a training program for parents, as has been undertaken in the Fast Track Project (Coie & Miller–Johnson, in press).

Schools. Herrenkohl et al. (in press) reviewed school programs and found several interventions with demonstrated effectiveness in reducing child disruptive behavior. Examples are the Good Behavior Game (Kellam & Rebok, 1992; Kellam, Rebok, Ialongo, & Mayer, 1994), the Seattle Social Development Project (Hawkins, Catalano, Morrison, O'Donnell, Abbott, & Day, 1992; Hawkins, Von Cleve, & Catalano, 1991; Hawkins, Catalano, Kosterman, Abbott, & Hill, 1999; O'Donnell, Hawkins, Catalano, Abbott, & Day, 1995), the Child Development Program, and Fast Track (Conduct Problems Prevention Research Group, 1999a, 1999b; Greenberg, 1998). Most of the programs aim at increasing social skills and improving conflict resolution, especially by promoting skills that are incompatible with aggression. Some programs also improve teachers' teaching skills (e.g., the Seattle Social Development Project). Several programs have been evaluated for elementary and middle school students, such as the Second Step curriculum (Grossman, Neckerman, Koepsell, Asher, Liu, Beland, Frey, & Rivara, 1997) and the Responding in Peaceful and Positive Ways curriculum (Farrell & Meyer, 1997, 1998).

Community. Increasingly, interventions are aimed at reducing risk factors in communities. An example is the Communities That Care program (Hawkins & Catalano, 1992). However, the effectiveness of community programs in reducing persistent disruptive child behavior and preventing child delinquency and later serious and violent offending remains to be evaluated.

Cost–benefit analysis of programs

Welsh (in press) reviewed cost–benefit analyses of programs to prevent or intervene with children showing persistent disruptive behavior. Most intervention programs have not been evaluated using cost–benefit analysis. However, this type of analysis is needed if the benefits of the programs are to be properly evaluated. For several programs, the monetary benefits exceed the monetary costs. This is true, for example, for home visits to disadvantaged women in pregnancy and with infant children (e.g., Olds, Henderson, Cole, Eckenrode, Kitzman, Luckey, Pettitt, Sidora, Morris, Powers, 1998), for preschool intellectual enrichment programs (e.g., Schweinhart, Barnes, & Weikart, 1993), and for child skills training (Hawkins et al., 1999). More cost–benefit analyses of prevention and intervention programs for child delinquents should be carried out.

The need for integrated services

Child delinquents, because of their misbehavior, often are seen by a greater variety of agencies than later onset offenders, including the juvenile justice system, schools, child welfare and child welfare agencies, and mental health clinics (Augimeri, et. al., in press; Herrenkohl et al., in press; Wasserman & Seracini, in press; Wiig, in press). In addition, child delinquents frequently have other problems such as learning difficulties, ADHD, mood problems, and exposure to child abuse and neglect. Different agencies also provide remedial services to child delinquents in these areas. Together, this means that child delinquents consume during their youth a disproportionately large amount of funds and resources of several agencies.

Our survey of practitioners (Loeber et al., 1999) indicated that they were almost unanimous (99%) in agreeing that more integration between agencies (juvenile justice, child welfare, mental health, schools, etc.) was needed to deal with very young offenders. However, such integrated programs are extremely rare. Of the few programs for child delinquents that came to our attention, those in the cities of Toronto and Minneapolis achieved a successful integration of services for child delinquents (Augimeri et al., in press; Howell, in press-b), but their effectiveness in reducing recidivism and preventing serious and violent juvenile offending remains to be evaluated.

There are three possible models for improving coordination between different agencies. First, an interagency coordinating council could be set up, including representatives from all the different agencies. Second, a single agency (i.e., a Community Assessment Center) could be set up to coordinate service provision from different agencies, to provide a single point of entry for all children, and to track the progress of all children in an integrated case management system. Third, wraparound services could be established, in which one person is designated to be responsible for coordinating all service provision for each family. The Toronto and Minneapolis projects were more like the second model, including integrated service delivery teams in the projects.

The need for a comprehensive strategy to reduce child delinquency

The need for the integration of services is all the more important because of changing manifestations of disruptive or delinquent behavior as children grow up (Figure 1). Therefore, a comprehensive strategy within and across agencies is needed. The Study Group on Very Young Offenders was inspired by OJJDP's Comprehensive Strategy for Serious, Violent, and Chronic Juvenile Offenders (Howell, 1995; Howell, in press-b; Howell, Krisberg, Hawkins, & Wilson, 1995; Wilson & Howell, 1993). The conceptual and practical thrust of this strategy lies in an integration of forces in the family and core social institutions (schools, religious institutions, and community organizations) in their roles of developing capable, mature, and responsible youth.

One of the strengths of the Comprehensive Strategy is its orientation to promote prevention as the most cost-effective approach to dealing with juvenile delinquency, and its emphasis on intervening immediately and effectively when delinquent behavior occurs, to prevent delinquents from becoming chronic offenders or progressively committing more serious and violent crimes. A second strength is that it views the juvenile justice system as a second screen, after family and core institutions, to deal with those child delinquents who cannot be handled by other systems. The Comprehensive Strategy aims to improve the juvenile justice system response to delinquent offenders through a system of graduated sanctions, based on risk and needs assessments (Howell, in press-b). Attached to these assessments is a continuum of treatment alternatives that includes immediate intervention, intermediate sanctions, community-based corrections including restitution and community service, and secure corrections including community confinement and incarceration in training schools. In summary, the Comprehensive Strategy offers a promising approach to integrate the efforts of different institutions in society in their efforts to prevent and deal with child delinquents effectively.

Are there effective screening methods to identify high risk child delinquents?

Our practitioner survey indicated that the vast majority (85%) agreed that better screening instruments were needed to discriminate between child delinquents who are at high risk of becoming serious and violent juvenile offenders and those who are not. Currently, a few screening methods for child delinquents are available, but, although they are based on known risk factors, their predictive utility remains to be evaluated (Howell, in press-a). One of the most promising is the EARL-20B, developed in Toronto, which is an empirically based screening instrument constructed to "red flag" certain areas of the child and family's life for services, help match services with the child's level of risk, and promote multidisciplinary team assessment of the risk of aggression and violence (Augimeri, Goldberg, & Koegl, 1999). More research is needed on the development of screening instruments to identify child delinquents who are likely to escalate in the future. It is important to establish how early and how accurately future serious and violent juvenile offenders can be predicted.

Policy Implications

Child delinquents constitute a population not usually recognized as needing services to prevent them becoming tomorrow's serious, violent, and chronic offenders. The Study Group's work has clear implications for policymakers on town, city, county, state, and federal levels. The policymakers referred to here are those who can influence the day to day and long-term operation of agencies or their funding to maintain, improve, or create new programs.

The Study Group indirectly also addresses the "frontline" workers who everyday deal with child delinquents and children with persistent disruptive behavior, and whose voices and concerns should be heard by policymakers.

The Study Group focused on three interlinked categories of children, who should receive *more attention* from policymakers: (a) very serious offenders at ages 7–12 years (committing homicide, robbery, rape, aggravated assault, or serious arson); (b) identified offenders at ages 7–12 years (excluding very serious offenders); (c) children with persistent disruptive behavior up to age 12 years who are at risk of offending but who have not been identified as offenders.

There are several key reasons why policymakers should be concerned about child delinquents and children with persistent disruptive behavior: (a) child delinquents are a significant public health risk, (b) better information is needed about child delinquents, (c) child delinquents are highly costly to taxpayers and society, and (d) early intervention with child delinquents is essential. We will briefly discuss each of these points.

Child delinquents are a significant public health risk

Child delinquents and children with persistent disruptive behavior constitute a serious public health risk of a magnitude that is directly comparable to other, more widely recognized public health risks. As mentioned, child delinquents, compared to later onset offenders, have 2–3 times the risk of becoming tomorrow's serious offenders. To put this in perspective, this risk is about the same as that of adults developing coronary heart disease when they have high blood pressure (Gordon & Shurtleff, 1973, cited in Kahn & Sempos, 1989). To return to child problem behavior and risk factors, Stouthamer–Loeber et al. (in press) found that children with three risk domains more than protective domains, compared to children with a balance of fewer risk domains, have an 8-fold increase in the likelihood of becoming a persistent serious delinquent in adolescence.

In summary, the risk of some children becoming serious offenders is as high as other more widely known public health threats. What is different is that such risks for children are not general public knowledge and, consequently, are rarely acted on to prevent the development of serious, violent, and chronic offending.

Better information is needed about child delinquents

The question is whether we as a society have the information about child delinquents that is needed to reduce this pervasive social problem. Such knowledge is crucial for the planning of services for child offenders at an early stage in children's delinquency careers. Specifically, information addressing the following questions is important: Are child delinquents included in national, regional, or citywide surveys of offenders or victims? How common are very serious child delinquents? Are they qualitatively or quantitatively different from other child delinquents?

Currently, we know less about children in the United States than about farm animals. Information about the numbers of animals (such as cattle, pigs, sheep, and goats) and their offspring is collected monthly and is readily available on the World Wide Web for each state and for the whole country (http://jan.mannlib.cornell.edu/reports/nassr/livestock/pct-bbc/). In contrast, the Study Group noted the absence of annual surveys of the prevalence of persistent disruptive children in elementary schools. In addition, there appears to be no consistent tracking of the number of referrals child welfare offices receive from the police for children under 12 years of age who commit delinquent acts. On the other hand, annual police reports of juvenile delinquency are available. However, it is not clear how accurate and comprehensive this information is collected on child delinquents is because of differences among jurisdictions in the minimal age of criminal responsibility of children and, possibly, differences in police recording practices of delinquent acts committed by children.

There is an urgent need for policymakers to step forward and insist on informing our society in a timely fashion about (a) the prevalence of child delinquency and persistent disruptive behaviors, (b) the proportion of such children who receive services for their problem behaviors, (c) the proportion of risk factors for these children that are routinely targeted for intervention, and (d) the dissemination of effective and replicated interventions.

Child delinquents are highly costly to taxpayers and society

Child delinquents tend to be highly costly to society because of the number of interventions they receive from different agencies, such as special school services, services by child welfare and agencies, mental health agencies, and family counseling services. Child delinquents are likely to receive service from the *majority* of agencies dealing with children. Although not all of these children are engaged by all of these services at the same time, many of the young problematic children require the attention and intervention of a succession of several of the agencies.

Given the barriers that often exist between different agencies and given poor data sharing among agencies, it is highly likely that assessments are duplicated. Also, many practitioners complain about the lack of an integrated and coordinated approach by multiple agencies trying to deal with the multiple problems of child delinquents. Although precise figures are needed, the cost of unintegrated and uncoordinated services must be higher than that of integrated services. Also, the effectiveness of unintegrated services can be expected to be lower than that of integrated services, especially when well-planned and evaluated services are used.

The other major aspect of cost is the fact that 6 in 10 child delinquents become later chronic offenders (Blumstein, et al. 1985). We know that the cost to society of a single high-risk youth engaging in 4 years of offending as a juvenile and 10 years as an adult ranged from $1.7 to $2.3 million (in 1997 dollars; Cohen, 1998). Given that many of these high-rate offenders start their delinquent and disruptive career early in life, we can safely assume that the cost to society of child delinquents is considerable.

Early intervention with child delinquents is essential

Currently, there is a whole array of effective interventions to reduce persistent disruptive child behavior and early onset delinquency. Also, there are well-tested interventions to prevent delinquent juveniles from escalating to serious, violent, and chronic offending. Much needed, however, are evaluations of well-tried integrated programs for child delinquents, such as the ones developed in Minneapolis and in Toronto (Howell, in press-a).

Policymakers tend to fund more plentiful programs for adolescent than for child delinquents, and for programs that confine serious adolescent offenders in costly institutions rather than prevent high-risk children from becoming tomorrow's incarcerated offenders. We do not imply that adolescent delinquents should be ignored and that all the attention and funds should be given to child delinquents. Instead, we make a case for a more effective balance of resources so that the roots of adolescent serious delinquency can be addressed better in childhood than is the case now.

Unfortunately, policymakers appear rarely cognizant of the efficacy and cost effectiveness of alternative interventions. We find that very often policymakers do not choose to fund prevention methods that can benefit juveniles in general, and taxpayers and citizens in particular. As a parallel, nowadays no policymaker in his or her right mind would argue that an optimal public health strategy to deal with nicotine addiction is the removal of a cancerous lungs in large numbers of affected smokers. Fortunately, prevention strategies have been developed and are now widely endorsed and enforced. The same type of strategies that are applied to smoking and other public health risks should be undertaken now to prevent serious and violent juvenile delinquency by focusing on early risk factors associated with child delinquency and persistent disruptive child behavior. In more and more communities, the increase in the number of child delinquents (and disruptive youth) is reaching the level of critical mass—the point at which system professionals and policymakers realize that the problem has become too large to be ignored and that special programs are needed. The time for action is now.

References

Adelson, L. (1972). The battering child. *Journal of the American Medical Association, 222,* 159–161.

Alexander, J. F., Barton, C., Schiavo, R. S., & Parsons, B. V. (1976). Systems-behavioral intervention with families of delinquents: Therapist characteristics, family behavior and outcome. *Journal of Consulting and Clinical Psychology, 44,* 656–664.

American Psychiatric Association. (1994). *Diagnostic and statistical manual for mental disorders* (4th ed.). Washington, DC: American Psychiatric Association Press.

Augimeri, L. K., Koegl, C. J., & Goldberg, K. (in press). Children under 12 committing offenses: Canadian legal and treatment approaches. In R. Loeber & D. P. Farrington (Eds.), *Child delinquents: Development, interventions, and service needs.* Thousand Oaks, CA: Sage.

Augimeri, L. K., Goldberg, K., & Koegl, C. (1999). *Canadian children under 12 committing offenses: Police protocols.* Toronto: Earlscourt Child and Family Centre.

Bailey, S. (1996). Adolescents who murder. *Journal of Adolescence, 19,* 19–39.

Barboza, D. (2000, March 2). A life of guns, drugs and now, killing, all at 6. *The New York Times,* pp. A1, A8.

Benedek, E. P., & Cornell, D. G. (1989). *Juvenile homicide.* Washington, DC: American Psychiatric Press.

Blumstein, A., Cohen, J., Roth, J. A., & Visher, C. A. (1986). *Criminal careers and "career criminals"* (Vol. II). Washington, DC: National Academy Press.

Blumstein, A., Farrington, D. P., & Moitra, S. (1985). Delinquency careers: Innocents, desisters, and persisters. In M. Tonry & N. Morris (Eds.), *Crime and Justice* (Vol. 6, pp. 137–168). Chicago: University of Chicago Press.

Bronfenbrenner, U. (1979). *The ecology of human development. Experiments by nature and design.* Cambridge, MA: Harvard University Press.

Borduin, C. M., Cone, L. T., Mann, B. J., Henggeler, S. W., Fucci, B. R., Blaske, D. M., & Williams, R. A. (1995). Multisystemic treatment of serious juvenile offenders: Long-term prevention of criminality and violence. *Journal of Consulting and Clinical Psychology, 63,* 569–578.

Butts, J. A., & Snyder, H. N. (1997). The youngest delinquents: Offenders under age 15. *OJJDP Bulletin.* Washington, DC: U.S. Department of Justice, Office of Juvenile Justice and Delinquency Prevention.

Catalano, R. F., & Hawkins, J. D. (1996). The social development model: A theory of antisocial behavior. In J. D. Hawkins (Ed.), *Delinquency and crime: Current theories* (pp. 149–197). New York: Cambridge University Press.

Cicchetti, D. (1993). Developmental psychopathology: Reactions, reflections, projections. *Developmental Review, 13,* 471–502.

Cicchetti, D., & Rogosch, F. A. (1996). Equifinality and multifinality in developmental psychopathology. *Development and Psychopathology, 8,* 597–600.

Cohen, M. A. (1998). The monetary value of saving a high-risk youth. *Journal of Quantitative Criminology, 14,* 5–33.

Coie, J. D., & Miller–Johnson, S. (in press). Peer factors and interventions. In R. Loeber & D. P. Farrington (Eds.), *Child delinquents: Development, interventions, and service needs.* Thousand Oaks, CA: Sage.

Conduct Problems Prevention Research Group. (1999a). Initial impact of the Fast Track Prevention Trial for Conduct Problems: I. The high-risk sample. *Journal of Consulting and Clinical Psychology, 65,* 631–647.

Conduct Problems Prevention Research Group. (1999b). Initial impact of the Fast Track Prevention Trial for Conduct Problems: II. Classroom effects. *Journal of Consulting and Clinical Psychology, 67,* 648–657.

Cornell, D. G., Benedek, E. P., & Benedek, D. M. (1987). Juvenile homicide: Prior adjustment and a proposed typology. *American Journal of Orthopsychiatry, 57,* 383–393.

Cowley, G. (1998, April 6). Why children turn violent. *Newsweek,* 24–26.

Dishion, T. J., McCord, J., & Poulin, F. (1999). When interventions harms: Peer groups and problem behavior. *American Psychologist, 54,* 755–764.

Drinkwater, M. (1998). The relationship between onset of delinquency and gun ownership. Unpublished analyses on data from the Pittsburgh Youth Study. Pittsburgh, PA: University of Pittsburgh, School of Medicine.

Elliott, D. S., Ageton, S. S., & Canter, R. J. (1979). An integrated theoretical perspective on delinquent behavior. *Journal of Research in Crime and Delinquency, 16,* 3–27.

Elliott, D. S., Huizinga, D., & Ageton, S. S. (1985). *Explaining delinquency and drug use.* Beverly Hills, CA: Sage.

Espiritu, R. C., Huizinga, D., Crawford, A., & Loeber, R. (in press). Epidemiology of self-reported delinquency. In R. Loeber & D. P. Farrington (Eds.), *Child delinquents: Development, interventions, and service needs.* Thousand Oaks, CA: Sage.

Ewing, C. P. (1990). *When children kill. The dynamics of juvenile homicide.* Lexington, MA: D. C. Heath.

Farrell, A. D., & Meyer, A. L. (1997). The effectiveness of a school-based curriculum for reducing violence among urban sixth-grade students. *American Journal of Public Health, 87,* 979–984.

Farrell, A. D., & Meyer, A. L. (1998). *Social skills training to promote resilience in urban sixth-grade students: One product of an action strategy to prevent youth violence in high-risk environments.* Richmond, VA: Unpublished manuscript, Virginia Commonwealth University.

Farrington, D. P. (1991). Childhood aggression and adult violence: Early precursors and later-life outcomes. In D. J. Pepler & K. H. Rubin (Eds.), *The development and treatment of childhood aggression* (pp. 5–29). Hillsdale, NJ: Erlbaum.

Farrington, D. P. (1994). Childhood, adolescent, and adult features of violent males. In L. R. Huesmann (Ed.), *Aggressive behavior: Current perspectives* (pp. 215–240). New York: Plenum Press.

Farrington, D. P., Loeber, R., Elliott, D. S., Hawkins, J. D., Kandel, D. B., Klein, M. W., McCord, J., Rowe, D. C., & Tremblay, R. E. (1990). Advancing knowledge about the onset of delinquency and crime. In B. B. Lahey & A. E. Kazdin (Eds.), *Advances in clinical child psychology* (Vol. 13, pp. 283–342). New York, NY: Plenum Press.

Farrington, D. P., Loeber, R., & Kalb, L. M. (in press). Key research and policy issues. In R. Loeber & D. P. Farrington (Eds.), *Child delinquents: Development, interventions, and service needs*. Thousand Oaks, CA: Sage .

Farrington, D. P., Ohlin, L. E., & Wilson, J. Q. (1986). *Understanding and controlling crime: Towards a new research strategy*. New York: Springer–Verlag.

Feil, E. G., Severson, H. H., & Walker, H. M. (1995). The Early Screening Project for young children with behavior problems. *Journal of Emotional and Behavior Disorders, 3,* 194–202.

Feil, E. G., Severson, H. H., & Walker, H. M. (1998). Screening for emotional and behavioral delays: The Early Screening Project. *Journal of Early Intervention, 21,* 252–266.

Gegax, T. T., Adler, J., & Pederson, D. (1998). The boys behind the ambush. *Newsweek,* pp. 20–26.

Geraghty, T. F. (1997). Justice for children: How do we get there? *The Journal of Criminal Law and Criminology, 88,* 190–241.

Goetting, A. (1989). Patterns of homicide among children. *Criminal Justice and Behavior, 16,* 63–80.

Gordon, T., & Schurtleff, D. (1973). *The Framingham Study* (NIH Publication No. 74–478). Washington, DC: Department of Health, Education and Welfare.

Gottfredson, M. R., & Hirschi, T. (1990). *A general theory of crime*. Stanford, CA: Stanford University Press.

Grant, B. F., & Dawson, D. A. (1998). Age of onset of drug use and its association with DSM-IV drug use and dependence: Results from the National Longitudinal Alcohol Epidemiology Survey. *Journal of Substance Abuse, 10,* 163–178.

Greenberg, M. T. (1998, August). *Testing developmental theory of antisocial behavior with outcomes from the Fast Track Prevention Project*. Paper presented at the Annual Meeting of the American Psychological Association, Chicago.

Griffin, P., Torbet, P., & Szymanski, L. (1998). Trying juveniles as adults in criminal court: An analysis of state transfer provisions. Washington, DC: Office of Juvenile Justice and Delinquency Prevention.

Grossman, D. C., Neckerman, H. J., Koepsell, T., Asher, K., Liu, P. Y., Beland, K., Frey, K., & Rivara, F. P. (1997). Effectiveness of a violence prevention curriculum among children in elementary school. *Journal of the American Medical Association, 277,* 1605–1611.

Hardwick, P. J., & Rowton–Lee, M. A. (1996). Adolescent homicide: towards assessment of risk. *Journal of Adolescence, 19,* 263–276.

Hawkins, J. D., & Catalano, R. F. (1992). *Communities that care*. San Francisco: Jossey–Bass,

Hawkins, J. D., Catalano, R. F., Kosterman, R., Abbott, R., & Hill, K. G. (1999). Preventing adolescent health-risk behaviors by strengthening protection during childhood. *Archives of Pediatrics and Adolescent Medicine, 153,* 226–234.

Hawkins, J. D., Catalano, R. F., Morrison, D. M., O'Donnell, J., Abbott, R. D., & Day, L. E. (1992). The Seattle Social Development Project: Effects of the first four years on protective factors and problem behaviors. In J. McCord & R. E. Tremblay (Eds.), *Preventing antisocial behavior: Interventions from birth through adolescence* (pp. 139–161). New York: Guilford Press.

Hawkins, D. F., Laub, J. H., & Lauritsen, J. L. (1998). Race, ethnicity, and serious juvenile offending. In R. Loeber & D. P. Farrington (Eds.), *Serious & violent juvenile offenders* (pp. 30–46). Thousand Oaks, CA: Sage.

Hawkins, J. D., Von Cleve, E., & Catalano, R. F. (1991). Reducing early childhood aggression: results of a primary prevention program. *Journal of the American Academy of Child and Adolescent Psychiatry, 30,* 208–217.

Heide, K. M. (1999). *Young killers: The challenge of juvenile homicide*. Thousand Oaks, CA: Sage.

Hennepin County Attorney's Office. (1995). *Delinquents under 10 in Hennepin County: A statistical analysis and practices and experiences of police jurisdiction*. Minneapolis, MN: Hennepin County Attorney's Office.

Herrenkohl, T. I., Hawkins, J. D., Chung, I. J., Hill, K. G., & Sara Battin–Pearson, S. (in press). School and community risk factors and interventions. In R. Loeber & D. P. Farrington (Eds.), *Child delinquents: Development, interventions, and service needs*. Thousand Oaks, CA: Sage.

Howell, J. C. (in press-a). Juvenile justice programs and strategies. In R. Loeber & D. P. Farrington (Eds.), *Child delinquents: Development, interventions, and service needs*. Thousand Oaks, CA: Sage.

Howell, J. C. (in press-b). Risk-needs assessment and screening devices. In R. Loeber & D. P. Farrington (Eds.), *Child delinquents: Development, interventions, and service needs*. Thousand Oaks, CA: Sage.

Howell, J. C. (1995). *Guide for implementing the comprehensive strategy for serious, violent, and chronic juvenile offenders*. Washington, DC: U.S. Department of Justice, Office of Juvenile Justice and Delinquency Prevention.

Howell, J. C., Krisberg, B., Hawkins, J. D., & Wilson, J. J. (1995). *A source book: Serious, violent, and chronic juvenile offenders*. Thousand Oaks, CA: Sage.

James, A., & Jenks, C. (1996). Public perceptions of childhood criminality. *British Journal of Criminology, 47,* 315–331.

Kachur, S. P., Stennies, G. M., Powell, K. E., Modzeleski, W., Stephens, R., Murphy, R., Kresnow, M., Sleet, D., & Lowry, R. (1996). School-associated violent deaths in the United States, 1992 to 1994. *Journal of the American Medical Association, 275,* 1729–1733.

Kahn, H. A., & Sempos, C. T. (1989). *Statistical methods in epidemiology*. Oxford: Oxford University Press.

Kazdin, A. E. (1985). *Treatment of antisocial behavior in children and adolescents*. Homewood, IL: Dorsey Press.

Keenan, K. (in press). Uncovering preschool precursor problem behaviors. In R. Loeber & D. P. Farrington

(Eds.), *Child delinquents: Development, interventions, and service needs*. Thousand Oaks, CA: Sage.

Kellam, S. G., & Rebok, G. W. (1992). Building developmental and etiological theory through epidemiologically based preventive intervention trials. In J. McCord & R. E. Tremblay (Eds.), *Preventing antisocial behavior: Interventions from birth through adolescence* (pp. 162–195). New York: Guilford Press.

Kellam, S. G., Rebok, G. W., Ialongo, N., & Mayer, L. S. (1994). The course and malleability of aggressive behavior from early first grade into middle school: Results of a developmental epidemiologically-based preventive trial. *Journal of Child Psychology and Psychiatry, 35*, 259–281.

Kelley, B. T., Huizinga, D., Thornberry, T. P., & Loeber, R. (1997). Developmental pathways in disruptive and delinquent behavior. *Juvenile Justice Bulletin, Office of Juvenile Justice and Delinquency Prevention*.

Kempf-Leonard, K., Chesney-Lind, M., & Hawkins, D. F. (in press). Race and gender issues. In R. Loeber & D. P. Farrington (Eds.), *Child delinquents: Development, interventions, and service needs*. Thousand Oaks, CA: Sage.

Krohn, M. D., Thornberry, T. P., Rivera, C., & Le Blanc, M. (in press). Later delinquency careers. In R. Loeber & D. P. Farrington (Eds.), *Child delinquents: Development, interventions, and service needs*. Thousand Oaks, CA: Sage.

Le Blanc, M. (1998). Screening of serious and violent juvenile offenders: Identification, classification, and prediction. In R. Loeber & D. P. Farrington (Eds.), *Serious and violent juvenile offenders: Risk factors and successful interventions* (pp. 167–196). Thousand Oaks, CA: Sage.

Le Blanc, M., & Loeber, R. (1998). Developmental criminology updated. In M. Tonry (Ed.), *Crime and justice: A review of research* (Vol. 23, pp. 115–198). Chicago: University of Chicago Press.

Lewis, D. O., Moy, E., Jackson, L. D., Aaronson, R., Restifo, N., Serra, S., & Simos, A. (1985). Biopsychological characteristics of children who later murder: A prospective study. *American Journal of Psychiatry, 142*, 1161–1167.

Lewis, D. O., Shanok, S. S., Grant, M., & Ritvo, E. (1983). Homicidally aggressive young children: Neuropsychiatric and experiential correlates. *The American Journal of Psychiatry, 140*, 148–153.

Lipsey, M. W., & Derzon, J. H. (1998). Predictors of violent or serious delinquency in adolescence and early adulthood: A synthesis of longitudinal research. In R. Loeber & D. P. Farrington (Eds.), *Serious and violent juvenile offenders: Risk factors and successful interventions* (pp. 313–345). Thousand Oaks, CA: Sage.

Loeber, R. (1982). The stability of antisocial and delinquent and child behavior: A review. *Child Development, 53*, 1431–1446.

Loeber, R. (1988). The natural histories of juvenile conduct problems, substance use and delinquency: Evidence for developmental progressions. In B. Lahey & A. E. Kazdin (Eds.), *Advances in clinical child psychology* (Vol. 11, pp. 73–124). New York: Plenum Press.

Loeber, R. (1991). Questions and advances in the study of developmental pathways. In D. Cicchetti & S. Toth (Eds.), *Rochester Symposium on Developmental Psychopathology* (Vol. 3, pp. 97–115). Rochester, NY: Rochester University Press.

Loeber, R., DeLamatre, M., Keenan, K., & Zhang, Q. (1998). A prospective replication of developmental pathways in disruptive and delinquent behavior. In R. Cairns, L. Bergman, & J. Kagan (Eds.), *Methods and models for studying the individual* (pp. 185–215). Thousand Oaks, CA: Sage.

Loeber, R., DeLamatre, M., Tita, G., Cohen, J., Van Kammen, W. B., & Stouthamer-Loeber, M. (1999). Gun injury and mortality: The delinquent background of its juvenile victims. *Violence and Victims, 14*, 339–352.

Loeber, R., & Dishion, T. J. (1983). Early predictors of male delinquency: A review. *Psychological Bulletin, 94*, 68–99.

Loeber, R., & Farrington, D. (1998). *Serious and violent juvenile offenders: Risk factors and successful interventions*. Thousand Oaks, CA: Sage.

Loeber, R., & Farrington, D. P. (in press). *Child delinquents: Development, interventions, and service needs*. Thousand Oaks, CA: Sage.

Loeber, R., Farrington, D. P., & Kalb, L. (1999). *Findings from a questionnaire administered at the 26th National Conference on Juvenile Justice, Minneapolis, MN*. Unpublished manuscript, Western Psychiatric Institute and Clinic, University of Pittsburgh, Pittsburgh, PA.

Loeber, R., Farrington, D. P., Stouthamer-Loeber, M., & Van Kammen, W. B. (1998). *Antisocial behavior and mental health problems: Explanatory factors in childhood and adolescence*. Mawhaw, NJ: Erlbaum.

Loeber, R., Green, S. M., Lahey, B. B., Frick, P. J., & McBurnett, K. (2000). Findings on disruptive behavior disorders from the first decade of the Developmental Trends Studies. *Clinical Child and Family Psychology Review, 3*, 37–60.

Loeber, R., & Hay, D. (1997). Key issues in the development of aggression and violence from childhood to early adulthood. *Annual Review of Psychology, 48*, 371–410.

Loeber, R., Keenan, K., & Zhang, Q. (1987). Boys' experimentation and persistence in developmental pathways toward serious delinquency. *Journal of Child and Family Studies, 6*, 321–357.

Loeber, R., Mutchko, J., & Burke, J. (2000). [Analyses from the Developmental Trends Study] Unpublished data, Western Psychiatric Institute and Clinic, University of Pittsburgh, Pittsburgh, PA.

Loeber, R., & Southamer-Loeber, M. (1998). Development of juvenile aggression and violence: Some common misconceptions and controversies. *American Psychologist, 53*, 242–259.

Loeber, R., Stouthamer-Loeber, M., Van Kammen, W. B., & Farrington, D. P. (1991). Initiation, escalation and desistance in juvenile offending and their correlates. *Journal of Criminal Law and Criminology, 82*, 36–82.

Loeber, R., Wei, E., Stouthamer-Loeber, M., Huizinga, D., & Thornberry, T. (1999). Behavioral antecedents to serious and violent juvenile offending: Joint analyses from the Denver Youth Survey, Pittsburgh Youth Study, and the Rochester Development Study. *Studies in Crime and Crime Prevention, 8*, 245–263.

Loeber, R., Wung, P., Keenan, K., Giroux, A., Stouthamer-Loeber, M., Van Kammen, W. B., & Maughan, B. (1993). Developmental pathways in disruptive child behavior. *Development and Psychopathology, 5*, 101–132.

Moffitt, T. E. (1993). Adolescence-limited and life-course-persistent antisocial behavior: A developmental taxonomy. *Psychological Review, 100,* 674–701.

Myers, W. C., & Blashfield, R. (1997). Psychopathology and personality in juvenile sexual homicide offenders. *Journal of the American Academy of Psychiatry and Law, 25,* 497–508.

Myers, W. C., Scott, K., Burgess, A. W., & Burgess, A. G. (1995). Psychopathy, biopsychological factors, crime characteristics, and classification of 25 homicidal youths. *Journal of the American Academy of Child and Adolescent Psychiatry, 34,* 1483–1489.

O'Donnell, J., Hawkins, J. D., Catalano, R. F., Abbott, R. D., & Day, L. E. (1995). Preventing school failure, drug use, and delinquency among low-income children: Long-term intervention in elementary schools. *American Journal of Orthopsychiatry, 65,* 87–100.

Office of Juvenile Justice and Delinquency Prevention (OJJDP). (1998). *Serious and violence juvenile offenders* (Juvenile Justice Bulletin No. 00). Washington, DC: U.S. Department of Justice, OJJDP.

Offord, D. R., Lipman, E. L., & Duku, E. K. (in press). Epidemiology of problem behavior up to age 12. In R. Loeber & D. P. Farrington (Eds.), *Child delinquents: Development, interventions, and service needs.* Thousand Oaks, CA: Sage.

Olds, D., Henderson, C. R., Cole, R., Eckenrode, J., Kitzman, H., Luckey, D., Pettitt, L., Sidora, K., Morris, P., & Powers, J. (1998). Long-term effects of nurse home visitation on children's criminal and antisocial behavior: Fifteen-year follow-up of a randomized controlled trial. *Journal of the American Medical Association, 280,* 1238–1244.

Patterson, G. R. (1996). Some characteristics of a developmental theory for early-onset delinquency. In M. F. Lenzenweger & J. J. Haugaard (Eds.), *Frontiers of developmental psychopathology* (pp. 81–124). New York: Oxford University Press.

Patterson, G. R., Capaldi, D. M., & Bank, L. (1991). An early starter model for predicting delinquency. In D. J. Pepler & K. H. Rubin (Eds.), *The development and treatment of childhood aggression* (pp. 139–168). Hillsdale, NJ: Erlbaum.

Police charge methods for very young suspects. (1998, October 2). *The New York Times,* p. .

Puzzanchera, C. M. (1998, November). The youngest offenders. *OJJDP fact sheet* (Nos. 1–2).

Puzzanchera, C. M. (2000, February). Self-reported delinquency by 12-year olds, 1997. *OJJDP fact sheet* (No. 3). *Early years study: Reversing the real brain drain* (1999). Toronto: Children's Secretariat.

Robins, L. N. (1966). *Deviant children grown up.* Baltimore, MD: Williams & Wilkins.

Rowley, J. C., Ewing, C. P., & Singer, S. I. (1987). Juvenile homicide: The need for an interdisciplinary approach. *Behavioral Sciences & the Law, 5,* 1–10.

Sampson, R. J., & Laub, J. H. (1993). *Crime in the making: Pathways and turning points through life.* Cambridge, MA: Harvard University Press.

Schweinhart, L. J., Barnes, H. V., & Weikart, D. P. (1993). *Significant benefits: The High/Scope Perry preschool study through age 27.* Ypsilanti, MI: High/Scope Press.

Seelye, K. Q. (1999, April). Clinton's new gun proposal include charging parents of children who commit gun crimes. *The New York Times,* p. .

Sleek, S. (1998, August). Experts scrambling on school shootings. *APA Monitor, 1,* 35–36.

Snyder, H. N. (1997). *Juvenile Arrests 1996.* Washington, DC: U.S. Department of Justice, Office Justice Programs, Office of Juvenile Justice and Delinquency Prevention.

Snyder, H. N. (1998). Serious, violent, and chronic juvenile offenders: An assessment of the extent of and trends in officially-recognized serious criminal behavior in a delinquent population. In R. Loeber & D. P. Farrington (Eds.), *Serious and violent juvenile offenders: Risk factors and successful interventions* (pp. 428–444). Thousand Oaks, CA: Sage.

Snyder, H. N. (in press). Epidemiology of official offending. In R. Loeber & D. P. Farrington (Eds.), *Child delinquents: Development, interventions, and service needs.* Thousand Oaks, CA: Sage.

Snyder, H. N., & Sickmund, M. (1999). *Juvenile offenders and victims: 1999 national report.* Washington, DC: U.S. Department of Justice, Office of Juvenile Justice and Delinquency Prevention.

Stouthamer-Loeber, M., Loeber, R., Wei, E., Farrington, D. P., & Wikström, P.-O. H. (in press). Risk and promotive effects in the explanation of persistent serious delinquency in boys. *Journal of Clinical and Consulting Psychology.*

Thornberry, T. P. & Krohn, M. D. (in press). The development of delinquency: An interactional perspective. In S. O. White (Ed.), *Handbook of law and social science: Youth and justice.* New York: Plenum Press.

Tolan, P. H. (1998). Voorspellen van gewelddadig gedrag bij jongeren. In W. Koops & W. Slot (Eds.), *Van lastig to misdadig* (pp. 52–64). Houten/Diegem, Netherlands: Bohn Stafleu Van Loghem.

Tolan, P. H., & Gorman-Smith, D. (1998). Development of serious and violent offending careers. In R. Loeber & D. P. Farrington (Eds.), *Serious and violent juvenile offenders: Risk factors and successful interventions* (pp. 68–85). Thousand Oaks, CA: Sage.

Tolan, P. H., Gorman-Smith, D., & Loeber, R. (in press). Developmental timing of onsets of disruptive behaviors and later delinquency of inner-city youth. *Journal of Child and Family Studies.*

Tremblay, R. E., & LeMarquand, D. (in press). Individual risk and protective factors. In R. Loeber & D. P. Farrington (Eds.), *Child delinquents: Development, interventions, and service needs.* Thousand Oaks, CA: Sage.

Tremblay, R. E., Pihl, R. O., Vitaro, F., & Dobkin, P. L. (1994). Predicting early onset of male antisocial behavior from preschool behavior. *Archives of General Psychiatry, 51,* 732–739.

Walker, H. M., Severson, H., Stiller, B., Williams, G., Haring, N., Shinn, M., & Todis, B. (1988). Systematic screening of pupils in the elementary age range at risk for behavior disorders: Development and trial testing of a multiple gating model. *Remedial and Special Education, 9,* 8–20.

Walker, H. M., Severson, H. H., Todis, B. J., Block-Pedego, A. E., Williams, G. J., Haring, N. G., & Barckley, M. (1990). Systematic Screening for Behavior Disorders (SSBD): Further validation, replication, and normative data. *Remedial and Special Education, 11,* 32–46.

Wasserman, G. A. & Seracini, A. M. (in press). Family risk factors and interventions. In R. Loeber & D. P. Farrington (Eds.), *Child delinquents: Development, interventions, and service needs.* Thousand Oaks, CA: Sage.

Wei, E., & Stouthamer-Loeber, M. (1999). *Sexual activity and fatherhood among persistent & violent offend-*

ers. Paper presented at the meeting of the American Society of Criminology, Toronto.

Welch, M., Fenwick, M., & Roberts, M. (1997). Primary definitions of crime and moral panic: A content analysis of experts' quotes in feature newspaper articles on crime. *Journal of Research in Crime and Delinquency, 34*, 474–494.

Welsh, B. C. (in press). Economic costs and benefits of early developmental prevention. In R. Loeber & D. P. Farrington (Eds.), *Child delinquents: Development, interventions, and service needs*. Thousand Oaks, CA: Sage.

Wiig, J. K. (in press). Legal issues. In R. Loeber & D. P. Farrington (Eds.), *Child delinquents: Development, interventions, and service needs*. Thousand Oaks, CA: Sage.

Wilson, J. J., & Howell, J. C. (1993). *A comprehensive strategy for serious, violent, and chronic juvenile offenders*. Washington, DC: U.S. Department of Justice, Office of Juvenile Justice and Delinquency Prevention.

[18]

Psychiatric Disorders in Youth in Juvenile Detention

Linda A. Teplin, PhD; Karen M. Abram, PhD; Gary M. McClelland, PhD; Mina K. Dulcan, MD; Amy A. Mericle, PhD

Background: Given the growth of juvenile detainee populations, epidemiologic data on their psychiatric disorders are increasingly important. Yet, there are few empirical studies. Until we have better epidemiologic data, we cannot know how best to use the system's scarce mental health resources.

Methods: Using the Diagnostic Interview Schedule for Children version 2.3, interviewers assessed a randomly selected, stratified sample of 1829 African American, non-Hispanic white, and Hispanic youth (1172 males, 657 females, ages 10-18 years) who were arrested and detained in Cook County, Illinois (which includes Chicago and surrounding suburbs). We present 6-month prevalence estimates by demographic subgroups (sex, race/ethnicity, and age) for the following disorders: affective disorders (major depressive episode, dysthymia, manic episode), anxiety (panic, separation anxiety, overanxious, generalized anxiety, and obsessive-compulsive disorders), psychosis, attention-deficit/hyperactivity disorder, disruptive behavior disorders (oppositional defiant disorder, conduct disorder), and substance use disorders (alcohol and other drugs).

Results: Nearly two thirds of males and nearly three quarters of females met diagnostic criteria for one or more psychiatric disorders. Excluding conduct disorder (common among detained youth), nearly 60% of males and more than two thirds of females met diagnostic criteria and had diagnosis-specific impairment for one or more psychiatric disorders. Half of males and almost half of females had a substance use disorder, and more than 40% of males and females met criteria for disruptive behavior disorders. Affective disorders were also prevalent, especially among females; more than 20% of females met criteria for a major depressive episode. Rates of many disorders were higher among females, non-Hispanic whites, and older adolescents.

Conclusions: These results suggest substantial psychiatric morbidity among juvenile detainees. Youth with psychiatric disorders pose a challenge for the juvenile justice system and, after their release, for the larger mental health system.

Arch Gen Psychiatry. 2002;59:1133-1143

A GREAT PROPORTION of this country's young people are now involved in the juvenile justice system. In 1999, the Federal Bureau of Investigation estimated that there were 2.5 million arrests of juveniles.[1] In 1997, juvenile courts handled almost 1800000 delinquency cases.[2] On an average day, more than 106000 youth are in custody in juvenile facilities.[3] Almost 60% of detained youth are African American or Hispanic.[3] Moreover, recent changes in the laws, such as mandatory penalties for drug crimes and lowering the age that juveniles can be tried as adults, have resulted in more juveniles serving time than ever before. There are currently 163200 cases per year of juveniles convicted and serving sentences.[2] Many are incarcerated in adult prisons, which do not have psychiatric services designed for juveniles. The number of females in the juvenile justice system is increasing at an even faster rate than the number of males[3] and is at an all time high.[2]

Given the growth of juvenile detainee populations,[4] epidemiologic data on their psychiatric disorders are increasingly important. Like adult detainees, juvenile detainees with serious mental disorders have a constitutional right (under the Eighth and Fourteenth Amendments) to receive needed treatment.[5] Mental health professionals believe that providing psychiatric services to juvenile detainees could improve their quality of life and help reduce recidivism.[6-8] Until we have better data, we cannot know how best to use the system's scarce mental health resources.[9,10]

Despite the importance of psychiatric epidemiologic data on juvenile detain-

From The Feinberg School of Medicine, Northwestern University Department of Psychiatry and Behavioral Sciences (Drs Teplin, Abram, McClelland, and Dulcan); Psycho-Legal Studies Program (Drs Teplin, Abram, and McClelland); Children's Memorial Hospital (Dr Dulcan); and the School of Social Service Administration, University of Chicago (Dr Mericle), Chicago, Ill.

ees, there are few empirical studies[10] and little consistency in results. Among studies[7,11-28] published since 1980 (summary table available from authors), rates for affective disorder varied from 2%[15] to 88%.[7] Rates of substance use disorders ranged from 13%[14] to 88%.[7] This disparity in findings may be because youth were sampled at various points in the juvenile justice system (eg, at admission, after conviction). In addition, there are 3 methodologic problems.

1. *Biased Samples.* Previous studies[11] used disparate exclusion criteria (eg, excluding juveniles with psychotic symptoms, mental retardation, or physical handicaps). Many studies excluded females entirely[16,21] or sampled too few to analyze them.[25]
2. *Small Samples.* Some severe disorders have low base rates, between 1% and 4%.[29,30] Low base rates require large sample sizes to generate reliable estimates.[31] Some studies sampled too few subjects to generate reliable rates even for the more common disorders.[18,21]
3. *Problems in Measurement.* Some studies did not specify the diagnostic criteria,[18] used nonstandard or untested instruments,[16] or extracted diagnoses from case records.[17]

This study overcomes these methodologic limitations. We have a large, random sample of juvenile detainees and used a reliable measure, version 2.3 of the Diagnostic Interview Schedule for Children (DISC),[32] to determine psychiatric diagnoses.

METHODS

PARTICIPANTS AND SAMPLING PROCEDURES

Participants in the Northwestern Juvenile Project included 1829 male and female youth (aged 10-18 years) who were randomly sampled from intake into the Cook County Juvenile Temporary Detention Center (CCJTDC) from November 1995 through June 1998. The sample was stratified by sex, race/ethnicity (African American, non-Hispanic white, Hispanic), age (10-13 years or ≥14 years), and legal status (processed as a juvenile or as an adult) to obtain enough participants to compare key subgroups (eg, females, Hispanics, and younger children).

The CCJTDC receives approximately 8500 admissions each year (John Howard Association, unpublished data, 1992) and is used solely for pretrial detention and for offenders sentenced for fewer than 30 days. All detainees younger than 17 years are held at CCJTDC, including youth processed as adults (automatic transfers to adult court). Juveniles up to age 21 years may be detained in the CCJTDC if they are still being prosecuted for an arrest that occurred when they were younger than 17 years.

Like juvenile detainees nationwide, approximately 90% of the CCJTDC detainees are males, and most are racial/ethnic minorities.[3] The CCJTDC population is 77.9% African American, 5.6% non-Hispanic white, 16.0% Hispanic, and 0.5% other racial or ethnic groups. The age and offense distributions of CCJTDC detainees are also similar to detained juveniles nationwide.[3]

We chose the detention center in Cook County (which includes Chicago and surrounding suburbs) for 3 reasons. First, nationwide, most juvenile detainees live in and are detained in urban areas.[33] Second, Cook County is ethnically diverse and has the third largest Hispanic population in the United States.[34] Studying Hispanics is important because they are the largest minority group in the United States[35] and they are overrepresented in the justice systems.[3] Finally, the detention center's size (daily census of approximately 650 youth and intake of 20 youth per day) ensured that enough participants would be available.

No single site can represent the entire country because jurisdictions may have different options for diversion.[36,37] Nevertheless, Illinois' criteria for detaining juveniles are similar to the criteria of other states.[36] All states allow pretrial detention if the juvenile needs protection, is likely to flee, or is considered a danger to the community.[36,37]

Detainees were eligible to participate, regardless of their psychiatric morbidity, state of alcohol or other drug intoxication, or fitness to stand trial. Within each stratum, we used a random-numbers table to select names from the CCJTDC's intake log. Throughout the study, we tracked how many participants were still needed to fill each stratum. Project staff sampled the rarest cells first. When more than one participant was available for a stratum, a random-numbers table was used. The final sampling fractions ranged from 0.018 to 0.689. (Additional information on the sample is available from the authors.)

Studying detained youth requires special procedures because they are minors, they are detained, and many do not have a parent or guardian who can provide appropriate consent.[38] Project staff approached participants on their units, explained the project, and assured them that anything they told us (except comments implying imminent danger to self or others) would be confidential. Detainees who chose to participate signed an assent form (if they were younger than 18 years) or consent form (if they were 18 years or older). Federal regulations allow parental consent to be waived if the research involves minimal risk (45 CFR [Code of Federal Regulations] 46.116[c], 45 CFR 46.116[d], and 45 CFR 46.408[c]).[38,39] The Northwestern University Institutional Review Board, the Centers for Disease Control and Prevention Institutional Review Board, and the US Office of Protection From Research Risks waived parental consent. However, as ethicists recommend, we nevertheless tried to contact parents to provide them an opportunity to decline participation and to offer them additional information (45 CFR 46.116[d][4]).[40,41] Despite repeated attempts to contact the parent or guardian, for 43.8% of participants, none could be found. In lieu of parental consent, assent from the juvenile subject was overseen by a participant advocate who represented the interests of the participants. Federal regulations allow for a participant advocate if parental consent is not feasible (45 CFR 46.116[d]).[40] Of the 2275 names selected, 4.2% (34 youth and 62 parents or guardians) refused to participate. There were no significant differences in refusal rates by sex, race/ethnicity, or age. Some youth processed as adults (automatic transfers) were counseled by their lawyers to refuse participation; in this stratum, the refusal rate was 7.1% (26 of 368 youth). Twenty-seven youth left the detention center before we could schedule an interview; 312 were not interviewed because they left while we were locating their caretakers for consent. Eleven others were excluded: 9 participants who became physically ill during the interview and could not finish it, 1 participant who was too cognitively impaired to be interviewed, and 1 participant who seemed to be lying. The final sample size was 1829. This sample size allows us to reliably detect disorders (ie, distinguish them from zero) that have a base rate in the general population of 1.0% or greater with a power of 0.80.[31]

Participants were interviewed in a private area, almost always within 2 days of intake. Most interviews lasted 2 to 3 hours, depending on how many symptoms were reported. We used both male and female interviewers. Female participants were always interviewed by female interviewers. Interviewers were trained for at least a month; most had a master's degree in psychology or an associated field and experience interviewing high-risk youth. One third of our interviewers were fluent in Spanish. We maintained consistency throughout the study by monitoring scripted interviews with mock subjects.

PSYCHIATRIC DIAGNOSES

We used version 2.3 of the DISC,[32,42] the most recent English and Spanish versions then available. The DISC assesses the presence of disorders in the past 6 months. The DISC is highly structured, contains detailed symptom probes, has acceptable reliability and validity,[32,43-46] and requires relatively brief training.

Two diagnoses required special management. The psychosis module, a broad symptom screen, does not generate a specific diagnosis. Instead, this module flags participants if they endorse any "possible" or "probable" pathognomonic symptoms or at least 3 nonpathognomonic symptoms. More than one quarter of our participants scored positive on the screen. To be conservative, we counted these participants as psychotic only if (1) their symptoms persisted for at least 1 week; (2) they had not used alcohol, illicit drugs, or medication during this time; and (3) a project clinician (a psychiatrist or clinical psychologist) reviewed the case and judged that the symptoms were "probably indicative of psychosis." Twelve participants met these criteria. Project clinicians also included another 8 participants as psychotic who, although they denied symptoms, appeared to have auditory hallucinations, thought disorders, or delusions during the interview.

Attention-deficit/hyperactivity disorder (ADHD) is difficult to assess via self-report[47] and is even more challenging to diagnose among delinquent youth.[48] In addition, *DSM-III-R* requires that symptoms of ADHD be present before the age of 7 years. Age of onset is usually reported by the caretaker. Most of our participants, even if they reported symptoms of ADHD, could not remember when their symptoms began. To avoid underreporting ADHD, we calculated rates in 2 ways: in the conventional manner (requiring that the subject report that symptoms were present before the age of 7 years) and counting the disorder as present regardless of the reported age of onset, as long as the duration criterion was met. (We present only the latter; the former rates are available from the authors.)

We determined rates of disorders in 2 ways. First, as most investigators have done, we used the DISC standard computer algorithms to calculate rates using *DSM-III-R* criteria. We then calculated more conservative (less inclusive) rates for diagnoses that met both *DSM-III-R* criteria and diagnosis-specific impairment criteria, reported by participants.[32] Although young people are poor reporters of their own impairment,[32,49] we calculated these latter rates because recent reviews[32,50,51] suggest that psychiatric diagnoses are more accurately determined by the presence of both symptoms and functional impairment. (We also examined rates using *DSM-III-R* criteria and a global measure of functional impairment, the Children's Global Assessment Scale.[52,53] These rates, substantially similar to those reported herein, are available from the authors.)

STATISTICAL ANALYSIS

Because we stratified our sample by sex, race/ethnicity, age, and legal status, we weighted all prevalence estimates to reflect the distributions of these variables in the detention center's population. All reported SEs and tests of significance have been corrected for design characteristics with Taylor series linearization.[54,55] We used 2-tailed tests; our level of significance for all tests was .05. We report all disorders for males and females separately because combining them masks important differences.

Table 1. Unweighted Sample Characteristics*

Characteristic	No. (%) of Participants (N = 1829)
Race/ethnicity	
African American	1005 (54.9)
Non-Hispanic white	296 (16.2)
Hispanic	524 (28.7)
Other	4 (0.2)
Sex	
Male	1172 (64.1)
Female	657 (35.9)
Age, y	
Mean	14.9
Median	15
Mode	16
Specific ages, y	
10	7 (0.4)
11	20 (1.1)
12	87 (4.8)
13	258 (14.1)
14	217 (11.9)
15	498 (27.2)
16	644 (35.2)
17	89 (4.9)
18	9 (0.5)
Education, grade	
≤6th	89 (4.9)
7th	171 (9.3)
8th	306 (16.7)
9th	568 (31.1)
10th	455 (24.9)
11th	172 (9.4)
12th	27 (1.5)
Currently in general equivalency diploma classes	31 (1.7)
Alternative or home schooling	5 (0.3)
Unknown	5 (0.3)
Legal status	
Processed in adult court (automatic transfer)	275 (15.0)
Processed in juvenile court	1554 (85.0)

*Percentages may not sum to 100% because of rounding error.

RESULTS

Table 1 presents unweighted demographic characteristics of our sample. **Table 2** provides data showing that nearly two thirds of the males and nearly three quarters of females met diagnostic criteria for 1 or more of the disorders listed. The more conservative estimates using the diagnosis-specific impairment criteria are only slightly lower. We also calculated overall rates excluding conduct disorder because many symptoms are related to delinquent behaviors; Table 2 also shows overall rates, excluding conduct disorder (with and without diagnosis-specific impairment criteria); rates decreased only slightly.

The most common disorders among both males and females were substance use disorders and disruptive behavior disorders (oppositional defiant disorder and conduct disorder). Half of males and almost half of females met criteria for a substance use disorder, and more than 40% of males and females met criteria for disruptive behavior

Table 2. Six-Month Prevalence and Odds Ratios (ORs) of *DSM-III-R* Diagnoses by Sex With and Without Diagnosis-Specific Impairment Criteria*

Disorder	Male, % (95% CI) (n = 1170)		Female, % (95% CI) (n = 656)		Female-Male ORs (95% CI)	
	Diagnosis	Diagnosis With Impairment	Diagnosis	Diagnosis With Impairment	Diagnosis	Diagnosis With Impairment
Any of the listed disorders	66.3 (61.6-70.7)	63.3 (58.6-67.8)	73.8 (70.1-77.1)	71.2 (67.5-74.7)	1.43 (1.09-1.88)	1.43 (1.10-1.87)
Any except conduct disorder	60.9 (56.2-65.5)	59.7 (54.9-64.3)	70.0 (66.2-73.5)	68.2 (64.4-71.8)	1.49 (1.15-1.94)	1.45 (1.12-1.88)
Any affective disorder	18.7 (15.2-22.8)	16.1 (12.8-20.0)	27.6 (23.6-32.0)	22.9 (19.0-27.2)	1.66 (1.20-2.29)	1.55 (1.09-2.20)
Major depressive episode	13.0 (10.0-16.6)	11.0 (8.3-14.5)	21.6 (17.8-25.9)	18.9 (15.2-23.2)	1.85 (1.27-2.70)	1.88 (1.25-2.82)
Dysthymia	12.2 (9.3-15.8)	9.9 (7.3-13.2)	15.8 (13.1-18.8)	12.5 (10.2-15.3)	1.34 (0.93-1.95)	1.31 (0.87-1.96)
Manic episode	2.2 (1.1-4.3)	2.0 (1.0-4.1)	1.8 (1.0-3.2)	1.2 (0.6-2.4)	0.81 (0.33-1.99)	0.58 (0.21-1.63)
Psychotic disorders	1.0 (0.4-2.6)	...	1.0 (0.5-2.1)	...	0.98 (0.30-3.25)	...
Any anxiety disorder	21.3 (17.6-25.6)	20.7 (17.0-24.9)	30.8 (27.2-34.6)	28.9 (25.5-32.7)	1.64 (1.22-2.20)	1.56 (1.16-2.10)
Panic disorder	0.3 (0.1-0.6)	0.1 (0.0-0.4)	1.5 (0.8-2.7)	1.0 (0.5-2.0)	5.65 (2.04-15.65)	8.13 (2.01-32.85)
Separation anxiety disorder	12.9 (9.9-16.5)	10.8 (8.1-14.2)	18.6 (15.7-21.9)	16.3 (13.6-19.4)	1.55 (1.08-2.21)	1.61 (1.10-2.34)
Overanxious disorder	6.7 (4.6-9.7)	5.9 (4.0-8.7)	12.3 (9.9-15.1)	11.5 (9.2-14.2)	1.95 (1.23-3.10)	2.06 (1.27-3.35)
Generalized anxiety disorder	7.1 (4.9-10.2)	6.4 (4.3-9.4)	7.3 (5.6-9.6)	6.8 (5.1-9.0)	1.03 (0.63-1.69)	1.07 (0.64-1.79)
Obsessive-compulsive disorder	8.3 (6.1-11.3)	...	10.6 (8.4-13.2)	...	1.31 (0.86-2.00)	...
Attention-deficit/hyperactivity disorder†	16.6 (13.3-20.5)	11.2 (8.5-14.6)	21.4 (18.4-24.8)	16.4 (13.7-19.5)	1.37 (0.99-1.89)	1.55 (1.07-2.25)
Any disruptive behavior disorder	41.4 (36.8-46.2)	31.4 (27.2-36.0)	45.6 (41.4-49.8)	38.0 (33.9-42.2)	1.19 (0.92-1.53)	1.33 (1.02-1.75)
Oppositional-defiant disorder	14.5 (11.4-18.2)	12.6 (9.8-16.2)	17.5 (14.7-20.6)	15.1 (12.5-18.1)	1.25 (0.89-1.76)	1.23 (0.86-1.76)
Conduct disorder	37.8 (33.3-42.6)	24.3 (20.5-28.5)	40.6 (36.5-44.8)	28.5 (24.6-32.8)	1.12 (0.86-1.46)	1.24 (0.92-1.67)
Any substance use disorder	50.7 (45.9-55.5)	...	46.8 (42.6-51.1)	...	0.86 (0.66-1.11)	...
Alcohol use disorder	25.9 (21.9-30.4)	...	26.5 (22.6-30.9)	...	1.03 (0.76-1.40)	...
Marijuana use disorder	44.8 (40.1-49.6)	...	40.5 (36.8-44.4)	...	0.84 (0.65-1.08)	...
Other substance use disorder	2.4 (1.7-3.4)	...	6.9 (4.1-11.4)	...	3.00 (1.57-5.74)	...
Both alcohol and other drug use disorders	20.7 (17.0-24.9)	...	20.9 (18.0-24.2)	...	1.01 (0.75-1.38)	...

*CI indicates confidence interval. Ellipses indicate that diagnosis and diagnosis with impairment are identical because the diagnostic criteria for psychotic disorders, obsessive-compulsive disorder, and substance use disorders include impairment.

†Attention-deficit/hyperactivity disorder is reported without the criterion of onset before age 7 years because caretaker information is not available and self-report of symptoms before age 7 years is unreliable.

disorders. Rates of disorder using diagnosis-specific impairment criteria for conduct disorder are more than 10% lower than conduct disorder without impairment. More than one fourth of females and almost one fifth of males met criteria for 1 or more affective disorders.

Table 2 also reports the female-male odds ratios. Odds ratios greater than 1.0 indicate that females had higher odds of having the disorder than males; those less than 1.0 show that females had lower odds of having the disorder. Females had significantly higher odds than males of having any disorder, any disorder except conduct disorder, any affective disorder, major depressive episode, any anxiety disorder, panic disorder, separation anxiety disorder, overanxious disorder, and substance use disorder other than alcohol or marijuana.

Table 3 and **Table 4** show the prevalence rates of disorders for males and females by race/ethnicity. Cases in these and subsequent tables met *DSM-III-R* criteria. (Tables of disorders that meet diagnosis-specific impairment criteria also are available from the authors.) We report protected tests of significance for specific racial/ethnic contrasts only when the overall test was significant. Table 3 shows that among males, non-Hispanic whites had the highest rates of many disorders and African Americans the lowest. Specifically, compared with African Americans, non-Hispanic whites had significantly higher rates of any disorder, any disorder except conduct disorder, any disruptive behavior disorder, conduct disorder, any substance use disorder, and substance use disorder other than alcohol or marijuana. The only disorder for which African Americans had significantly higher rates than non-Hispanic whites was separation anxiety disorder. Hispanics had significantly higher rates than non-Hispanic whites of any anxiety disorder and separation anxiety disorder. Hispanics had higher rates than African Americans of panic disorder, obsessive-compulsive disorder, and substance use other than alcohol or marijuana disorders. Non-Hispanic whites had higher rates than Hispanics of any disorder, any disruptive behavior disorder, conduct disorder, and substance use disorder other than alcohol or marijuana.

Table 4 compares rates by race/ethnicity for females. Non-Hispanic white females had significantly higher rates than African Americans of any disorder, any disorder except conduct disorder, any disruptive behavior disorder, conduct disorder, and all substance use disorders and higher rates than Hispanics of any disorder except conduct disorder. Hispanic females had higher rates of generalized anxiety disorder than either African American or white females. Compared with African Americans, Hispanic females had higher rates of all disruptive behavior disorders, conduct disorder, alcohol use disorder, substance use disorder other than alcohol or marijuana, and both alcohol and drug use disorder.

Table 5 and **Table 6** show the prevalence rates of disorders for males and females by age. Among males, Table 5 indicates that the youngest age group had the lowest rates of many disorders. They had significantly lower rates than both older age groups of any disorder, any dis-

Table 3. Six-Month Prevalence of *DSM-III-R* Diagnoses for Males by Race/Ethnicity*

Disorder	Prevalence, % (95% CI)			Overall Significance	Protected Tests†
	African American (n = 574)	Non-Hispanic White (n = 207)	Hispanic (n = 386)		
Any of the listed disorders	64.6 (58.8-69.9)	82.0 (76.2-86.7)	70.4 (63.3-76.7)	<.001	White > African American; white > Hispanic
Any except conduct disorder	59.4 (53.5-65.0)	72.9 (66.5-78.6)	65.3 (58.1-71.9)	.009	White > African American
Any affective disorder	18.6 (14.4-23.6)	13.8 (9.6-19.5)	21.5 (15.3-29.3)	.19	
Major depressive episode	12.5 (9.1-17.0)	9.5 (6.0-14.6)	16.6 (10.8-24.7)	.20	
Dysthymia	12.2 (8.8-16.7)	9.5 (6.1-14.5)	13.3 (8.4-20.6)	.53	
Manic episode	2.5 (1.2-5.2)	0.5 (0.1-3.7)	1.4 (0.6-3.2)	.27	
Psychotic disorders	1.0 (0.3-3.2)	2.6 (1.1-6.2)	0.7 (0.2-2.6)	.19	
Any anxiety disorder	20.9 (16.5-26.1)	14.4 (10.1-20.2)	25.5 (18.7-33.7)	.046	Hispanic > white
Panic disorder	0.1 (0.0-0.4)	0.5 (0.1-3.7)	1.0 (0.3-3.1)	.04	Hispanic > African American
Separation anxiety disorder	12.7 (9.3-17.2)	5.9 (3.3-10.3)	15.5 (9.8-23.6)	.02	African American > white; Hispanic > white
Overanxious disorder	6.9 (4.4-10.7)	2.9 (1.3-6.6)	7.0 (3.6-13.0)	.16	
Generalized anxiety disorder	7.5 (4.8-11.4)	2.5 (1.0-5.9)	7.2 (3.7-13.3)	.08	
Obsessive-compulsive disorder	6.5 (4.2-10.0)	9.3 (5.8-14.4)	17.0 (10.7-25.9)	.01	Hispanic > African American
Attention-deficit/hyperactivity disorder‡	17.0 (13.0-21.9)	20.9 (15.8-27.3)	13.7 (9.4-19.5)	.18	
Any disruptive behavior disorder	39.8 (34.2-45.7)	60.3 (53.3-66.9)	43.3 (36.1-50.8)	<.001	White > African American; white > Hispanic
Oppositional-defiant disorder	14.4 (10.7-19.1)	19.4 (14.4-25.6)	13.6 (9.3-19.5)	.23	
Conduct disorder	35.6 (30.1-41.5)	59.9 (53.0-66.5)	41.7 (34.5-49.2)	<.001	White > African American; white > Hispanic
Any substance use disorder	49.1 (43.2-55.0)	62.6 (55.7-69.0)	55.4 (47.8-62.7)	.01	White > African American
Alcohol use disorder	24.6 (19.8-30.2)	30.1 (24.0-36.9)	30.8 (24.1-38.5)	.28	
Marijuana use disorder	44.4 (38.6-50.4)	53.8 (46.8-60.6)	45.4 (38.0-52.9)	.11	
Other substance use disorder	0.5 (0.1-2.8)	21.1 (15.9-27.4)	6.0 (3.9-9.1)	<.001	White > African American; white > Hispanic; Hispanic > African American
Both alcohol and other drug use disorders	20.4 (16.0-25.7)	24.0 (18.5-30.6)	21.7 (16.5-28.0)	.65	

*CI indicates confidence interval. Two cases of "other" race/ethnicity are excluded from this table.
†Protected tests are performed only if the α for the overall test is less than .05.
‡Attention-deficit/hyperactivity disorder is reported without the criterion of onset before the age of 7 years because caretaker information is not available and self-report of symptoms before the age of 7 years is unreliable.

order except conduct disorder, generalized anxiety disorder, and all the substance use disorders. The 14- to 15-year-old group had higher rates of psychotic disorders than the 16 years or older age group.

Table 6 shows somewhat different patterns of disorder for females. The oldest age group had significantly lower rates of oppositional defiant disorder than the younger age groups. The youngest age group had significantly lower rates of any substance use disorder and marijuana use disorder than either of the older age groups.

COMMENT

Our study shows that youth with psychiatric disorders pose a challenge for the juvenile justice system and, after their release, for the larger mental health system. Even after excluding conduct disorder, nearly 60% of male juvenile detainees and more than two thirds of females met diagnostic criteria and had diagnosis-specific impairment for one or more psychiatric disorders.

These rates may underestimate the true prevalence among youth entering the juvenile justice system for 2 reasons. First, our sample included only detainees; it excluded youth who were not detained because their charges were less serious, they were immediately released, or they were referred directly into the mental health system. Second, underreporting of symptoms and impairments by youth is common, especially for disruptive behavior disorders.[47]

It is difficult to compare our findings with studies of general population youth because rates vary widely, depending on the sample, the method, the source of data (participant or collaterals), and whether functional impairment was required for diagnosis.[50] Despite these differences, our overall rates are substantially higher than the median rate reported in a major review article (15%)[50] and other more recent investigations: the Great Smoky Mountains Study (20.3%),[56] the Virginia Twin Study of Adolescent Behavioral Development (142 cases per 1000 persons),[57] the Methods for the Epidemiology of Child and Adolescent Mental Disorders (6.1%),[32] and the Miami–Dade County Public School Study (38%).[58] We are especially concerned about the high rates of depression and dysthymia among detained youth (17.2% of males, 26.3% of females), which are also higher than general population rates.[51,56-61] Depressive disorders are difficult to detect (and treat) in the chaos of the corrections milieu. Overall, our prevalence rates are comparable to rates in other high-risk populations (eg, maltreated or runaway youth).[62,63]

Table 4. Six-Month Prevalence of *DSM-III-R* Diagnoses for Females by Race/Ethnicity*

Disorder	Prevalence, % (95% CI) African American (n = 430)	Non-Hispanic White (n = 89)	Hispanic (n = 136)	Overall Significance	Protected Tests†
Any of the listed disorders	70.9 (66.4-75.0)	86.1 (77.1-92.0)	75.9 (67.9-82.5)	.01	White > African American
Any except conduct disorders	67.4 (62.8-71.6)	83.9 (74.6-90.3)	69.5 (61.2-76.7)	.01	White > African American; white > Hispanic
Any affective disorder	26.2 (22.2-30.5)	23.4 (15.8-33.4)	28.7 (21.8-36.9)	.68	
Major depressive episode	19.7 (16.2-23.7)	19.0 (12.1-28.5)	22.8 (16.5-30.5)	.70	
Dysthymia	15.5 (12.4-19.2)	17.9 (11.2-27.3)	17.2 (11.8-24.5)	.80	
Manic episode	1.9 (0.9-3.7)	1.1 (0.2-7.5)	2.1 (0.7-6.4)	.85	
Psychotic disorders	0.9 (0.4-2.5)	0.0	2.1 (0.7-6.3)	.29‡	
Any anxiety disorder	31.2 (27.0-35.8)	30.0 (21.4-40.3)	32.6 (25.2-40.9)	.92	
Panic disorder	0.9 (0.4-2.5)	3.4 (1.1-10.0)	2.8 (1.0-7.1)	.17	
Separation anxiety disorder	18.9 (15.5-22.9)	14.5 (8.6-23.4)	21.7 (15.5-29.4)	.41	
Overanxious disorder	12.5 (9.7-16.0)	11.1 (6.1-19.5)	13.2 (8.4-20.1)	.90	
Generalized anxiety disorder	6.6 (4.6-9.4)	4.4 (1.7-11.3)	13.1 (8.4-19.9)	.03	Hispanic > African American; Hispanic > white
Obsessive-compulsive disorder	10.3 (7.8-13.6)	12.4 (7.0-21.1)	10.6 (6.5-16.9)	.84	
Attention-deficit/hyperactivity disorder§	20.0 (16.5-24.1)	22.2 (14.7-32.0)	29.3 (22.2-37.5)	.08	
Any disruptive behavior disorder	39.4 (34.9-44.1)	61.6 (51.0-71.1)	56.5 (47.9-64.6)	<.001	White > African American; Hispanic > African American
Oppositional-defiant disorder	15.8 (12.7-19.6)	17.8 (11.1-27.1)	26.2 (19.5-34.3)	.03	Hispanic > African American
Conduct disorder	34.3 (29.9-38.9)	58.9 (48.3-68.7)	50.2 (41.8-58.6)	<.001	White > African American; Hispanic > African American
Any substance use disorder	42.3 (37.6-47.1)	61.9 (51.2-71.6)	51.7 (43.1-60.1)	.002	White > African American
Alcohol use disorder	21.2 (17.5-25.3)	39.2 (29.5-49.9)	34.0 (26.4-42.5)	<.001	White > African American; Hispanic > African American
Marijuana use disorder	37.8 (33.3-42.5)	53.4 (42.9-63.6)	44.7 (36.3-53.3)	.02	White > African American
Other substance use disorder	0.9 (0.4-2.5)	20.0 (12.9-29.6)	14.7 (9.7-21.5)	<.001	White > African American; Hispanic > African American
Both alcohol and other drug use disorders	17.2 (13.9-21.1)	35.1 (25.7-45.8)	28.3 (21.2-36.7)	<.001	White > African American; Hispanic > African American

*CI indicates confidence interval. Two cases of "other" race/ethnicity are excluded from this table.
†Protected tests are performed only if the α for the overall test is less than .05.
‡Test computed with 1 *df* because of empty cells.
§Attention-deficit/hyperactivity disorder is reported without the criterion of onset before the age of 7 years because caretaker information is not available and self-report of symptoms before the age of 7 years is unreliable.

Our data highlight an important paradox regarding race/ethnicity. More than half of the youth in our juvenile justice system are African American or Hispanic. Therefore, most detained youth with psychiatric disorders are minorities. The prevalence, however, of many disorders is highest among non-Hispanic whites. Thus, white youth in the juvenile justice system may, on average, be more dysfunctional (have greater psychiatric morbidity) than minority youth.

Females had higher rates than males of many psychiatric disorders, including major depressive episode, some anxiety disorders, and "other substance use disorders" (eg, cocaine and hallucinogens). Our findings confirm those of prior studies of adult female detainees and females with conduct disorders, which found that females have higher rates of psychiatric disorders than males.[64,65]

Overall, the youngest age group (≤13 years) had the lowest prevalence rates of most disorders, confirming studies[57,66-68] of general population youth. Many youth in the juvenile justice system may develop new or additional disorders as they age.

LIMITATIONS

Our study provides only a "snapshot" of our participants' psychiatric disorders immediately after arrest and detention. We cannot know whether mental disorder causes delinquency, increases the likelihood of arrest and detention, or is merely a frequent trait among delinquent youth. Some symptoms could be a reaction to incarceration. Moreover, our rates might differ somewhat if we had been able to use *DSM-IV* instead of *DSM-III-R* criteria. Our findings, drawn from only one site, may pertain only to youth in urban detention centers with similar demographic composition. Finally, because it was not feasible to interview caretakers, our data are subject to the limitations of self-report. Despite these limitations, our study has important implications for research on delinquent youth and mental health policy.

FUTURE RESEARCH

We suggest 3 directions for future research.

1. *Studies of Patterns and Sequences of Comorbidity*. Examining comorbidity is critical because it is so prevalent among juveniles in the general population,[69,70] adult jail detainees,[71] and adults who have high arrest rates, such as substance abusers,[72] young, long-term psychiatric patients,[73] and homeless, mentally ill persons.[74] Moreover, studies[71] of adults suggest that juveniles with comorbid disorders may be especially vulnerable to arrest, particularly if they are poor and

Table 5. Six-Month Prevalence of *DSM-III-R* Diagnosis for Males by Age*

Disorder	Prevalence, % (95% CI) Age ≤13 Years (n = 315)	Age 14 and 15 Years (n = 361)	Age ≥16 Years (n = 494)	Overall Significance	Protected Tests†
Any of the listed disorders	52.7 (46.5-58.8)	68.0 (60.3-74.8)	67.3 (60.3-73.7)	.001	14 and 15 years > 13 years and younger; 16 years and older > 13 years and younger
Any except conduct disorder	44.9 (38.9-51.0)	63.4 (55.6-70.6)	61.8 (54.7-68.5)	<.001	14 and 15 years > 13 years and younger; 16 years and older > 13 years and younger
Any affective disorder	13.0 (9.4-17.6)	21.2 (15.4-28.4)	17.7 (12.9-23.7)	.09	
Major depressive episode	7.5 (4.9-11.4)	14.8 (10.0-21.5)	12.4 (8.5-17.8)	.06	
Dysthymia	7.3 (4.7-11.3)	14.5 (9.7-21.1)	11.2 (7.4-16.4)	.08	
Manic episode	1.6 (0.7-4.0)	2.6 (0.9-7.2)	2.0 (0.7-5.1)	.80	
Psychotic disorders	0.0	2.1 (0.7-6.0)	0.3 (0.2-0.8)	.01‡	14 and 15 years > 16 years and older
Any anxiety disorder	17.7 (13.6-22.9)	23.0 (16.9-30.4)	20.6 (15.5-26.7)	.42	
Panic disorder	0.8 (0.2-3.3)	0.1 (0.0-0.9)	0.3 (0.1-0.9)	.25	
Separation anxiety disorder	10.0 (6.9-14.3)	14.5 (9.7-21.1)	12.0 (8.1-17.5)	.40	
Overanxious disorder	4.8 (2.8-8.0)	5.1 (2.6-9.9)	8.4 (5.1-13.5)	.25	
Generalized anxiety disorder	1.3 (0.5-3.4)	5.9 (3.1-11.0)	9.2 (5.8-14.4)	.001	14 and 15 years > 13 years and younger; 16 years and older > 13 years and younger
Obsessive-compulsive disorder	6.0 (3.7-9.7)	9.4 (5.7-15.0)	7.8 (4.9-12.2)	.43	
Attention-deficit/hyperactivity disorder§	12.5 (9.1-16.9)	20.9 (15.1-28.0)	13.8 (9.7-19.2)	.06	
Any disruptive behavior disorder	32.9 (27.5-38.8)	43.5 (35.9-51.3)	41.2 (34.5-48.2)	.06	
Oppositional-defiant disorder	10.7 (7.5-14.9)	18.2 (12.8-25.1)	12.1 (8.3-17.3)	.08	
Conduct disorder	30.8 (25.6-36.6)	41.1 (33.6-49.1)	36.4 (30.0-43.3)	.10	
Any substance use disorder	28.3 (23.1-34.0)	51.3 (43.5-59.1)	54.4 (47.3-61.3)	<.001	14 and 15 years > 13 years and younger; 16 years and older > 13 years and younger
Alcohol use disorder	12.9 (9.5-17.4)	25.6 (19.3-33.0)	28.7 (22.8-35.4)	<.001	14 and 15 years > 13 years and younger; 16 years and older > 13 years and younger
Marijuana use disorder	25.1 (20.3-30.5)	46.9 (39.1-54.8)	46.8 (39.8-53.9)	<.001	14 and 15 years > 13 years and younger; 16 years and older > 13 years and younger
Other substance use disorder	0.8 (0.4-1.7)	2.5 (1.2-5.0)	2.6 (1.9-3.6)	.01	14 and 15 years > 13 years and younger; 16 years and older > 13 years and younger
Both alcohol and other drug use disorders	10.2 (7.2-14.3)	21.5 (15.7-28.7)	22.0 (16.7-28.3)	<.001	14 and 15 years > 13 years and younger; 16 years and older > 13 years and younger

*CI indicates confidence interval.
†Protected tests are performed only if the α for the overall test is less than .05.
‡Test computed with 1 *df* because of empty cells.
§Attention-deficit/hyperactivity disorder is reported without the criterion of onset before the age of 7 years because caretaker information is not available and self-report of symptoms before the age of 7 years is unreliable.

cannot afford treatment. Data on the sequences of comorbidity would help provide the foundation for innovative treatments and tailor services for special populations such as females and minorities.

2. *Studies of Females in the Juvenile Justice System*. Females are increasingly arrested for crimes against persons and violent crimes[75] and make up an increasingly large proportion of delinquent youth.[1,2] Prior studies[76,77] of youth with conduct disorders (many of whom will become delinquent) suggest that females have greater persistence of emotional disorder and worse outcomes than males. Moreover, their problem behaviors often persist beyond adolescence. As they age, they may become suicidal, addicted to alcohol or other drugs, enmeshed in violent relationships, and unable to care for their children.[64,76] Delinquent females also engage in sexual activity at an earlier age than nonoffenders, placing them at greater risk for unwanted pregnancy and human immunodeficiency virus.[78] Understanding psychiatric morbidity and associated risk factors among delinquent females could help us to improve treatment and reduce the cycle of disorder and dysfunction.
3. *Longitudinal Studies*. Many youth in the juvenile justice population may develop new disorders as they age. Risk factors for the development of disorders[79] are common among delinquent youth, including physical and sexual abuse, a troubled family environment, parental substance abuse, poverty, poor education, neighborhood disintegration, and neglect.[80-84] Delinquent youth have few protective factors to offset these risks.[85] Thus, most youth in the juvenile justice system are at

Table 6. Six-Month Prevalence of *DSM-III-R* Diagnosis for Females by Age*

Disorder	Prevalence, % (95% CI) Age ≤13 Years (n = 56)	Age 14 and 15 Years (n = 353)	Age ≥16 Years (n = 247)	Overall Significance	Protected Tests†
Any of the listed disorders	66.7 (53.2-77.9)	72.2 (67.2-76.7)	77.6 (71.6-82.7)	.18	
Any except conduct disorder	64.7 (51.2-76.2)	67.4 (62.2-72.1)	74.8 (68.6-80.2)	.13	
Any affective disorder	20.7 (12.0-33.3)	27.9 (23.5-32.9)	28.8 (21.2-37.8)	.50	
Major depressive episode	13.0 (6.5-24.2)	21.6 (17.6-26.3)	23.4 (16.0-32.9)	.27	
Dysthymia	10.4 (4.7-21.4)	15.6 (12.2-19.8)	17.2 (12.8-22.6)	.46	
Manic episode	3.9 (1.0-14.4)	1.4 (0.6-3.3)	1.9 (0.8-4.7)	.45	
Psychotic disorders	0.0	0.6 (0.2-2.5)	1.8 (0.7-4.3)	.21‡	
Any anxiety disorder	26.6 (16.7-39.7)	32.6 (27.8-37.7)	29.2 (23.4-35.7)	.55	
Panic disorder	1.9 (0.3-12.4)	1.7 (0.8-3.6)	1.0 (0.3-3.2)	.75	
Separation anxiety disorder	18.1 (10.0-30.6)	19.7 (15.8-24.2)	17.2 (12.9-22.7)	.77	
Overanxious disorder	7.1 (2.7-17.7)	13.8 (10.5-17.8)	11.4 (7.9-16.1)	.34	
Generalized anxiety disorder	3.8 (1.0-14.1)	7.1 (4.9-10.3)	8.4 (5.5-12.7)	.51	
Obsessive-compulsive disorder	10.4 (4.7-21.5)	11.8 (8.8-15.7)	8.8 (5.8-13.1)	.51	
Attention-deficit/hyperactivity disorder§	26.6 (16.6-39.7)	22.7 (18.6-27.4)	18.5 (14.0-24.0)	.30	
Any disruptive behavior disorder	44.7 (32.2-57.9)	50.0 (44.8-55.2)	39.6 (32.0-47.8)	.11	
Oppositional-defiant disorder	30.5 (19.9-43.6)	20.2 (16.4-24.7)	10.7 (7.3-15.2)	<.001	13 years and younger > 16 years and older; 14 and 15 years > 16 years and older
Conduct disorder	33.0 (22.0-46.3)	45.3 (40.2-50.5)	35.7 (28.1-44.2)	.06	
Any substance use disorder	30.5 (19.9-43.7)	45.8 (40.6-51.2)	52.0 (44.5-59.4)	.02	14 and 15 years > 13 years and younger; 16 years and older > 13 years and younger
Alcohol use disorder	16.7 (9.1-28.6)	25.4 (21.1-30.3)	30.3 (22.7-39.2)	.16	
Marijuana use disorder	24.8 (15.3-37.5)	41.3 (36.2-46.6)	43.3 (37.1-49.7)	.04	14 and 15 years > 13 years and younger; 16 years and older > 13 years and younger
Other substance use disorder	5.9 (2.2-14.9)	5.3 (3.5-7.8)	9.5 (3.7-22.2)	.52	
Both alcohol and other drug use disorders	11.5 (5.5-22.5)	21.8 (17.7-26.4)	22.0 (17.2-27.6)	.20	

*CI indicates confidence interval.
†Protected tests are performed only if the α for the overall test is less than .05.
‡Test computed with 1 *df* because of empty cells.
§Attention-deficit/hyperactivity disorder is reported without the criterion of onset before the age of 7 years because caretaker information is not available and self-report of symptoms before the age of 7 years is unreliable.

great risk for psychiatric disorders, problem behaviors, and even early death.[86,87] Longitudinal studies are needed to examine why some delinquent youth develop new psychiatric disorders and others do not, to investigate protective factors, and to determine how vulnerability and risk differ by key variables such as sex and race/ethnicity. We are now collecting longitudinal data on our participants. Future articles will address persistence and change in psychiatric disorders (including onset, remission, and recurrence), comorbidity, associated functional impairments, and the risk and protective factors related to these disorders and impairments.

IMPLICATIONS FOR MENTAL HEALTH POLICY

Advocacy groups, researchers, and public policy experts believe that the juvenile justice system has become the only alternative for many poor and minority youth with psychiatric disorders.[88-92] Many states have imposed more severe sanctions for delinquent youth and transfer increasing numbers of juveniles to adult court,[93-95] policies that disproportionately affect minority youth.[94,96] In addition, 2 recent changes in public health policy may have inadvertently contributed to the criminalization of youth with mental disorders.

1. *Welfare Reform.* Welfare reform has disrupted Medicaid benefits for millions of children who need treatment.[97,98] Medicaid enables many youth to receive psychiatric treatment.[99] Many parents who left welfare to go to work found their new jobs did not provide insurance or, when available, they could not afford copayments.[100,101] The State Children's Health Insurance Program, designed to offset the loss of Medicaid, did not fulfill its intended purpose.[98,102] Moreover, welfare reform has not substantially decreased poverty[103]; many poor children have become even poorer.[104] Poor children are vulnerable to poor outcomes,[105] including involvement with the juvenile justice system.
2. *Managed Care.* Managed care now dominates the private insurance industry[92] and increasingly controls public insurance benefits, such as Medicaid.[106,107] Many disorders prevalent among delinquent youth, such as conduct disorder, ADHD, and substance use disorders, are often not covered or have restrictive treatment guidelines.[108] As the public health system re-

duces services, youth with psychiatric disorders may increasingly fall through the cracks into the juvenile justice system.[109]

These changes (welfare reform and managed care) have the most serious consequences for poor and minority children, groups overrepresented in the juvenile justice system. Our findings are even more sobering because the prevalence of psychosocial problems among youth seems to be increasing.[110,111] The US Surgeon General reports that the unmet need for services is as high now as it was 20 years ago.[112] Even youth who are insured often cannot obtain treatment because few child and adolescent psychiatrists practice in poor and minority neighborhoods.[113,114]

The juvenile justice system is not equipped to provide adequate mental health services for the large numbers of detainees with psychiatric disorders.[115,116] Although the mental health needs of youth in the juvenile justice system have been given much attention recently,[10,117,118] there are still few empirical studies of the effectiveness of treatment and outcomes.[10] This omission is critical. We need research to guide mental health policy and to understand the complex interplay among the many systems—primary care, mental health, education, child welfare, and justice—that treat delinquent youth.

Submitted for publication October 11, 2001; final revision received March 7, 2002; accepted March 12, 2002.

This work was supported by National Institute of Mental Health (NIMH) grants R01MH54197 and R01MH59463, and grant 1999-JE-FX-1001 from the Office of Juvenile Justice and Delinquency Prevention. Major funding was also provided by the National Institute on Drug Abuse (Bethesda, Md), the Center for Mental Health Services (Rockville, Md), the Centers for Disease Control and Prevention (CDC) National Center for HIV, STD, and TB Prevention (Atlanta, Ga), the National Institute on Alcohol Abuse and Alcoholism (Bethesda), the National Institutes of Health (NIH) Office of Research on Women's Health (Bethesda), the Center for Substance Abuse Prevention (Rockville, Md), the NIH Center on Minority Health and Health Disparities (Bethesda), NIH Office of Rare Diseases (Bethesda), CDC National Center on Injury Prevention and Control (Atlanta), the Center for Substance Abuse Treatment, The William T. Grant Foundation (New York, NY), and The Robert Wood Johnson Foundation (Princeton, NJ). Additional funds were provided by The John D. and Catherine T. MacArthur Foundation (Chicago), the Open Society Institute (New York), and The Chicago Community Trust. We thank all our agencies for their collaborative spirit and steadfast support.

Many more people than the authors contributed to this project. From the NIMH, Ann Hohmann, PhD, and Kimberly Hoagwood, PhD, provided technical assistance and moral support that went beyond the call of duty; Eve Moscicki, ScD, and Heather Ringeisen, PhD, critiqued earlier versions of the article; Grayson Norquist, MD, and Delores Parron, PhD (now at NIH), provided steadfast support throughout. Celia Fisher, PhD, guided our human subjects procedures. We thank all project staff, especially Amy E. Lansing, PhD, for supervising the data collection. We also thank Laura Coats, our expert editor and research assistant, and Kate Elkington for her meticulous library work. We also greatly appreciate the cooperation of everyone working in the Cook County systems, especially David H. Lux, our project liaison. Without the county's cooperation, this study would not have been possible. Finally, we thank our participants for their time and willingness to participate.

Corresponding author and reprints: Linda A. Teplin, PhD, Psycho-Legal Studies Program, Department of Psychiatry and Behavioral Sciences, The Feinberg School of Medicine, Northwestern Univerity, 710 N Lake Shore Dr, Suite 900, Chicago, IL 60611 (e-mail: psycho-legal@northwestern.edu).

REFERENCES

1. Snyder HN. *Juvenile Arrests 1999.* Washington, DC: Office of Juvenile Justice and Delinquency Prevention; 2000.
2. Puzzanchera C, Stahl AL, Finnegan TA, Snyder HN, Poole RS, Tierney N. *Juvenile Court Statistics 1997.* Washington DC: Office of Juvenile Justice and Delinquency Prevention; 2000.
3. Snyder HN, Sickmund M. *Juvenile Offenders and Victims: 1999 National Report.* Washington, DC: Office of Juvenile Justice and Delinquency Prevention; 1999.
4. Porter G. *Detention in Delinquency Cases, 1988-1997.* Washington, DC: Office of Juvenile Justice and Delinquency Prevention; 2000.
5. Costello JC, Jameson EJ. Legal and ethical duties of health care professionals to incarcerated children. *J Leg Med.* 1987;8:191-263.
6. Dembo R, Schmeidler J, Pacheco K, Cooper S, Williams LW. The relationships between youth's identified substance use, mental health or other problems at a juvenile assessment center and their referrals to needed services. *J Child Adolesc Subst Abuse.* 1997;6:23-54.
7. Timmons-Mitchell J, Brown C, Schulz SC, Webster SE, Underwood LA, Semple WE. Comparing the mental health needs of female and male incarcerated juvenile delinquents. *Behav Sci Law.* 1997;15:195-202.
8. McCord J, Widom CS, Crowell NA, eds. *Juvenile Crime, Juvenile Justice.* Washington, DC: National Academy Press; 2001
9. General Accounting Office. *Mentally Ill Inmates: Better Data Would Help Determine Protection and Advocacy Needs.* Washington, DC: General Accounting Office; 1991.
10. Cocozza JJ, Skowyra KR. Youth with mental health disorders: issues and emerging responses. *Juvenile Justice.* 2000;7:3-13.
11. Chiles JA, Miller ML, Cox GB. Depression in an adolescent delinquent population. *Arch Gen Psychiatry.* 1980;37:1179-1184.
12. Miller ML, Chiles JA, Barnes VE. Suicide attempters within a delinquent population. *J Consult Clin Psychol.* 1982;50:491-498.
13. McManus M, Alessi NE, Grapentine WL, Brickman A. Psychiatric disturbance in serious delinquents. *J Am Acad Child Adolesc Psychiatry.* 1984;23:602-615.
14. McManus M, Brickman A, Alessi NE, Grapentine WL. Borderline personality in serious delinquents. *Comp Psychiatry.* 1984;25:446-454.
15. Cocozza JJ, Ingalls RP. *Out of Home Care.* Albany: New York State Council on Children and Families; 1984.
16. Hollander HE, Turner FD. Characteristics of incarcerated delinquents: relationship between development disorders, environmental and family factors, and patterns of offense and recidivism. *J Am Acad Child Adol Psychiatry.* 1985;24:221-226.
17. Friedman RM, Kutash K. *Mad, Bad, Sad, Can't Add: Florida Adolescent and Child Treatment Study (FACTS).* Tampa: University of South Florida, Florida Mental Health Institute; 1986.
18. Lewis DO, Pincus JH, Lovely R, Spitzer E, Moy E. Biopsychosocial characteristics of matched samples of delinquents and nondelinquents. *J Am Acad Child Adolesc Psychiatry.* 1987;26:744-752.
19. Davis DL, Bean GJ, Schumacher JE, Stringer TL. Prevalence of emotional disorders in a juvenile justice institutional population. *Am J Forensic Psychol.* 1991;9:5-17.
20. Eppright TD, Kashani JH, Robison BD, Reid JC. Comorbidity of conduct disorder and personality disorders in an incarcerated juvenile population. *Am J Psychiatry.* 1993;150:1233-1236.
21. Steiner H, Garcia IG, Mathews Z. Posttraumatic stress disorder in incarcerated juvenile delinquents. *J Am Acad Child Adolesc Psychiatry.* 1997;36:357-365.
22. Duclos CW, Beals J, Novins DK, Martin C, Jewett CS, Manson SM. Prevalence

of common psychiatric disorders among American Indian adolescent detainees. *J Am Acad Child Adolesc Psychiatry.* 1998;37:866-873.

23. Gray TA, Wish ED. *Substance Abuse Need for Treatment Among Arrestees (SANTA) in Maryland: Youth in the Juvenile Justice System.* College Park, Md: Center for Substance Abuse Research; 1998.
24. Cauffman E, Feldman S, Waterman J, Steiner H. Posttraumatic stress disorder among female juvenile offenders. *J Am Acad Child Adolesc Psychiatry.* 1998; 37:1209-1216.
25. Atkins DL, Pumariega AJ, Rogers K, Montgomery L, Nybro C, Jeffers G, Sease F. Mental health and incarcerated youth, I: prevalence and nature of psychopathology. *J Child Fam Stud.* 1999;8:193-204.
26. Pliszka SR, Sherman JO, Barrow MV, Irick S. Affective disorder in juvenile offenders: a preliminary study. *Am J Psychiatry.* 2000;157:130-132.
27. Aarons GA, Brown SA, Hough RL, Garland AF, Wood PA. Prevalence of adolescent substance use disorders across five sectors of care. *J Am Acad Child Adolesc Psychiatry.* 2001;40:419-426.
28. Garland AF, Hough RL, McCabe KM, Yeh M, Wood PA, Aarons GA. Prevalence of psychiatric disorders in youth across five sectors of care. *J Am Acad Child Adolesc Psychiatry.* 2001;40:409-418.
29. Whitaker A, Johnson J, Shaffer D, Rapoport JL, Kalikow K, Walsh BT, Davies M, Braiman S, Dolinsky A. Uncommon troubles in young people: prevalence estimates of selected psychiatric disorders in a nonreferred adolescent population. *Arch Gen Psychiatry.* 1990;47:487-496.
30. Christie KA, Burke JD, Regier DA, Rae DS, Boyd JH, Locke BZ. Epidemiologic evidence for early onset of mental disorders and higher risk of drug abuse in young adults. *Am J Psychiatry.* 1988;145:971-975.
31. Cohen J. *Statistical Power Analysis for the Behavioral Sciences.* 2nd ed. Hillsdale, NJ: Lawrence Earlbaum Associates; 1988.
32. Shaffer D, Fisher P, Dulcan MK, Davies M, Piacentini J, Schwab-Stone ME, Lahey BB, Bourdon K, Jensen PS, Bird HR, Canino G, Regier DA. The NIMH Diagnostic Interview Schedule for Children Version 2.3 (DISC-2.3): description, acceptability, prevalence rates, and performance in the MECA Study. *J Am Acad Child Adolesc Psychiatry.* 1996;35:865-877.
33. Pastore AL, Maguire K. *Sourcebook of Criminal Justice Statistics—1999.* Washington, DC: US Dept of Justice; 2000.
34. US Bureau of the Census. *The Hispanic Population.* Washington, DC: US Dept of Commerce; 2001.
35. US Bureau of the Census. *Population by Race and Hispanic or Latino Origin for the United States: 1990 and 2000.* Washington, DC: US Dept of Commerce; 2001: table 1. Available at: http://www.census.gov/population/www/cen2000 /phc-t1.html. Accessed June 6, 2002.
36. Grisso T, Tomkins A, Casey P. Psychosocial concepts in juvenile law. *Law Hum Behav.* 1988;12:403-437.
37. Illinois Criminal Justice Information Authority. *Trends and Issues 1997.* Chicago: Illinois Criminal Justice Information Authority; 1997.
38. Federal Policy for the Protection of Human Subjects: Notices and Rules, part 2, Vol 56, No. 117 (18 June 1991), 56 *Federal Register* 28002-32.
39. Shaffer D. Use of passive consent in child/adolescent mental health research—effect of letter from Dr Charles R. McCarthy, Director of the Office for Protection from Research Risks, NIH [editorial]. *Res Notes Child Adolesc Psychiatry.* Summer 1992:10.
40. Fisher CB. Integrating science and ethics in research with high-risk children and youth. *Soc Res Child Dev.* 1993;7:1-27.
41. Nolan K. Ethical issues: assent, consent, and behavioral research with adolescents. *Res Notes Child Psychiatry.* Summer 1992:7-10.
42. Bravo M, Woodbury-Farina M, Canino GJ, Rubio-Stipec M. The Spanish translation and cultural adaptation of the Diagnostic Interview Schedule for Children (DISC) in Puerto Rico. *Cult Med Psychiatry.* 1993;17:329-344.
43. Fisher PW, Shaffer D, Piacentini JC, Lapkin J, Kafantaris V, Leonard H, Herzog DB. Sensitivity of the Diagnostic Interview Schedule for Children, 2nd edition (DISC-2.1), for specific diagnoses of children and adolescents. *J Am Acad Child Adolesc Psychiatry.* 1993;32:666-673.
44. Piacentini J, Shaffer D, Fisher PW, Schwab-Stone ME, Davies M, Gioia P. The Diagnostic Interview Schedule for Children–Revised Version (DISC-R), III: concurrent criterion validity. *J Am Acad Child Adolesc Psychiatry.* 1993;32:658-665.
45. Schwab-Stone M, Fisher PW, Piacentini J, Shaffer D, Davies M, Briggs M. The Diagnostic Interview Schedule for Children–Revised Version (DISC-R), II: test-retest reliability. *J Am Acad Child Adolesc Psychiatry.* 1993;32:651-657.
46. Shaffer D, Schwab-Stone ME, Fisher PW, Cohen P, Piacentini J, Davies M, Conners CK, Regier D. The Diagnostic Interview Schedule for Children–Revised Version (DISC-R), I: preparation, field testing, interrater reliability, and acceptability. *J Am Acad Child Adolesc Psychiatry.* 1993;32:643-650.
47. Schwab-Stone ME, Shaffer D, Dulcan MK, Jensen PS, Fisher P, Bird HR, Goodman SH, Lahey BB, Lichtman JH, Canino G, Rubio-Stipec M, Rae DS. Criterion validity of the NIMH Diagnostic Interview Schedule for Children Version 2.3 (DISC-2.3). *J Am Acad Child Adolesc Psychiatry.* 1996;35:878-888.
48. Thompson LL, Riggs PD, Mikulich SK, Crowley TJ. Contribution of ADHD symptoms to substance problems and delinquency in conduct-disordered adolescents. *J Abnorm Child Psychol.* 1996;24:325-347.
49. Bird HR, Davies M, Fisher P, Narrow WE, Jensen PS, Hoven C, Cohen P, Dulcan MK. How specific is specific impairment? *J Am Acad Child Adolesc Psychiatry.* 2000;39:1182-1189.
50. Roberts RE, Attkisson C, Rosenblatt A. Prevalence of psychopathology among children and adolescents. *Am J Psychiatry.* 1998;155:715-725.
51. Costello EJ, Angold A, Burns BJ, Erkanli A, Stangle DK, Tweed DL. The Great Smoky Mountains Study of Youth: functional impairment and serious emotional disturbance. *Arch Gen Psychiatry.* 1996;53:1137-1143.
52. Bird HR, Canino G, Rubio-Stipec M, Ribera JC. Further measures of the psychometric properties of the Children's Global Assessment Scale. *Arch Gen Psychiatry.* 1987;44:821-824.
53. Shaffer D, Gould MS, Brasic J, Ambrosini P, Fisher P, Bird HR, Aluwahlia S. A Children's Global Assessment Scale (CGAS). *Arch Gen Psychiatry.* 1983;40: 1228-1231.
54. Cochran WG. *Sampling Techniques.* New York, NY: John Wiley & Sons; 1997.
55. Levy PS, Lemeshow S. *Sampling of Populations: Methods and Applications.* New York, NY: John Wiley & Sons; 1999.
56. Costello EJ, Angold A, Burns BJ, Stangle DK, Tweed DL, Erkanli A, Worthman CM. The Great Smoky Mountains Study of Youth: goals, design, methods, and the prevalence of *DSM-III-R* disorders. *Arch Gen Psychiatry.* 1996;53:1129-1136.
57. Simonoff E, Pickles A, Meyer JM, Silberg JL, Maes HH, Loeber R, Rutter M, Hewitt JK, Eaves LJ. The Virginia Twin Study of Adolescent Behavioral Development: influences of age, sex, and impairment on rates of disorder. *Arch Gen Psychiatry.* 1997;54:801-808.
58. Turner RJ, Gil AG. Psychiatric and substance use disorders in South Florida: racial/ethnic and gender contrasts in a young adult cohort. *Arch Gen Psychiatry.* 2002;59:43-50.
59. Kessler RC, Walters EE. Epidemiology of *DSM-III-R* major depression and minor depression among adolescents and young adults in the National Comorbidity Survey. *Depress Anxiety.* 1998;7:3-14.
60. McGee R, Feehan M, Williams S, Anderson J. *DSM-III* disorders from age 11 to age 15 years. *J Am Acad Child Adolesc Psychiatry.* 1992;31:50-59.
61. Garrison CZ, Waller JL, Cuffe SP, McKeown RE, Addy CL, Jackson KL. Incidence of major depressive disorder and dysthymia in young adolescents. *J Am Acad Child Adolesc Psychiatry.* 1997;36:458-465.
62. Feitel B, Margetson N, Chamas J, Lipman C. Psychosocial background and behavioral and emotional disorders of homeless and runaway youth. *Hosp Comm Psychiatry.* 1992;43:155-159.
63. Famularo R, Kinscherff R, Fenton T. Psychiatric diagnoses of maltreated children: preliminary findings. *J Am Acad Child Adolesc Psychiatry.* 1992;31:863-867.
64. Lewis DO, Yeager CA, Cobham-Portorreal CS, Klein N, Showalter C, Anthony A. A follow-up of female delinquents: maternal contributions to the perpetuation of deviance. *J Am Acad Child Adolesc Psychiatry.* 1991;30:197-201.
65. Teplin LA, Abram KM, McClelland GM. Prevalence of psychiatric disorders among incarcerated women, I: pretrial jail detainees. *Arch Gen Psychiatry.* 1996;53: 505-512.
66. Cohen P, Cohen J, Brook JS. An epidemiological study of disorders in late childhood and adolescence, II: persistence of disorders. *J Child Psychol Psychiatry.* 1993;34:869-877.
67. Kandel DB, Johnson JG, Bird HR, Canino G, Goodman SH, Lahey BB, Regier DA, Schwab-Stone M. Psychiatric disorders associated with substance use among children and adolescents: findings from the Methods for the Epidemiology of Child and Adolescent Mental Disorders (MECA) Study. *J Abnorm Child Psychol.* 1997;25:121-132.
68. Newman DL, Moffitt TE, Caspi A, Magdol L, Silva PA, Stanton WR. Psychiatric disorder in a birth cohort of young adults: prevalence, comorbidity, clinical significance, and new case incidence from ages 11 to 21. *J Consult Clin Psychol.* 1996;64:552-562.
69. Angold A, Costello EJ. Depressive comorbidity in children and adolescents: empirical, theoretical, and methodological issues. *Am J Psychiatry.* 1993;150: 1779-1791.
70. Bukstein OG, Brent DA, Kaminer Y. Comorbidity of substance abuse and other psychiatric disorders in adolescents. *Am J Psychiatry.* 1989;146:1131-1141.
71. Abram KM, Teplin LA. Co-occurring disorders among mentally ill jail detainees: implications for public policy. *Am Psychol.* 1991;46:1036-1045.
72. Hesselbrock MN, Meyer RE, Keener JJ. Psychopathology in hospitalized alcoholics. *Arch Gen Psychiatry.* 1985;42:1050-1055.
73. Caton CLM, Gralnick A, Bender S, Simon R. Young chronic patients and substance abuse. *Hosp Comm Psychiatry.* 1989;40:1037-1040.

74. Breakey WR, Fischer PJ, Kramer M, Nestadt G, Romanoski AJ, Ross A, Royal RM, Stine OC. Health and mental health problems of homeless men and women. *JAMA*. 1989;262:1352-1357.
75. Poe-Yamagata E, Butts JA. *Female Offenders in the Juvenile Justice System*. Washington, DC: Office of Juvenile Justice and Delinquency Prevention; 1996.
76. Zoccolillo M. Co-occurrence of conduct disorder and its adult outcomes with depressive and anxiety disorders: a review. *J Am Acad Child Adolesc Psychiatry*. 1992;31:547-556.
77. Loeber R, Stouthamer-Loeber M. Development of juvenile aggression and violence. *Am Psychol*. 1998;53:242-259.
78. Gender-Specific Programming for Girls Advisory Committee. *Guiding Principles for Promising Female Programming*. Washington, DC: Office of Juvenile Justice and Delinquency Prevention; 1998. Available at: http://www.ojjdp.ncjrs.org /pubs/principles/contents.html. Accessed July 30, 2001.
79. Werner EE. High-risk children in young adulthood: a longitudinal study from birth to 32 years. *Am J Orthopsychiatry*. 1989;59:72-81.
80. National Research Council. *Losing Generations: Adolescents in High-Risk Settings*. Washington, DC: National Academy Press; 1993.
81. Lewis DO, Yeager CA, Lovely R, Stein A, Cobham-Portorreal CS. A clinical follow-up of delinquent males: ignored vulnerabilities, unmet needs, and the perpetuation of violence. *J Am Acad Child Adolesc Psychiatry*. 1994;33:518-528.
82. Leventhal T, Brooks-Gunn J. The neighborhoods they live in: the effects of neighborhood residence on child and adolescent outcomes. *Psychol Bull*. 2000;126: 309-337.
83. Buckner JC, Bassuk EL. Mental disorders and service utilization among youths from homeless and low-income housed families. *J Am Acad Child Adolesc Psychiatry*. 1997;36:890-900.
84. Dembo R, Williams L, Schmeidler J. Gender differences in mental health service needs among youths entering a juvenile detention center. *J Prison Jail Health*. 1993;12:73-101.
85. Cocozza JJ. *Responding to the Mental Health Needs of Youth in the Juvenile Justice System*. Seattle, Wash: National Coalition for the Mentally Ill in the Criminal Justice System; 1992.
86. Lattimore PK, Linster RL, MacDonald JM. Risk of death among serious young offenders. *J Res Crime Delinq*. 1997;34:187-209.
87. Loeber R, DeLamatre M, Tita G, Cohen J, Stouthamer-Loeber M, Farrington DP. Gun injury and mortality: the delinquent backgrounds of juvenile victims. *Violence Vict*. 1999;14:339-352.
88. National Alliance for the Mentally Ill. *Families on the Brink: The Impact of Ignoring Children With Serious Mental Illness: Results of a National Survey of Parents and Other Caregivers*. Arlington, Va: National Alliance for the Mentally Ill; 1999.
89. Knitzer J. Children's mental health: changing paradigms and policies. In: Zigler EF, Kagan SL, Hall NW, eds. *Children, Families, and Government: Preparing for the Twenty-first Century*. New York, NY: Cambridge University Press; 1996: 207-232.
90. Srebnik D, Cauce AM, Baydar N. Help-seeking pathways for children and adolescents. *J Emotional Behav Dis*. 1996;4:210-220.
91. Redding RE. Juvenile offenders in criminal court and adult prison: legal, psychological, and behavioral outcomes. *Juvenile Fam Court J*. Winter 1999:1-20.
92. US Department of Health and Human Services. *Mental Health: A Report of the Surgeon General*. Rockville, Md: US Dept of Health and Human Services; 1999.
93. Grisso T. What we know about youths' capacities as trial defendants. In: Grisso T, Schwartz RG, eds. *Youth on Trial: A Developmental Perspective on Juvenile Justice*. Chicago, Ill: University of Chicago Press; 2000:139-171.
94. Bishop DM. Juvenile offenders in the adult criminal justice system. *Crime Justice*. 2000;27:81-167.
95. Mears DP. Getting tough with juvenile offenders: explaining support for sanctioning youths as adults. *Criminal Justice Behav*. 2001;28:206-226.
96. Hamparian DM, Estep LK, Muntean SM, Priestino RR, Swisher RG, Wallace PL, White TL. *Major Issues in Juvenile Justice Information and Training*. Washington, DC: US Dept of Justice; 1982.
97. Heymann SJ, Earle A. The impact of welfare reform on parents' ability to care for their children's health. *Am J Public Health*. 1999;89:502-505.
98. Center for Mental Health Services. *Mental Health and Substance Abuse Services Under the State Children's Health Insurance Program*. Rockville, Md: US Dept of Health and Human Services, Substance Abuse and Mental Health Services Administration; 2000.
99. Burns BJ, Costello EJ, Erkanli A, Tweed DL, Farmer EMZ, Angold A. Insurance coverage and mental health service use by adolescents with serious emotional disturbance. *J Child Fam Studies*. 1997;6:89-111.
100. Children's Defense Fund. *Families Struggling to Make It in the Workforce: A Post Welfare Report*. Washington, DC: Children's Defense Fund; 2000. Available at: http://www.childrensdefense.org/pdf/CMPreport.pdf. Accessed June 5, 2002.
101. Sherman A, Amey C, Duffield B, Ebb N, Weinstein D. *Welfare to What: Early Findings on Family Hardship and Well-Being*. Washington, DC: Children's Defense Fund and National Coalition for the Homeless; 1998. Available at: http:// www.childrensdefense.org/pdf/wlfwhat.pdf. Accessed June 5, 2002.
102. General Accounting Office. *Medicaid and SCHIP: Comparisons of Outreach, Enrollment Practices, and Benefits*. Washington, DC: General Accounting Office; 2000.
103. Zuckerman DM. The evolution of welfare reform: policy changes and current knowledge. *J Soc Issues*. 2000;56:811-820.
104. Porter K, Primus W. *Recent Changes in the Impact of the Safety Net on Child Poverty*. Washington, DC: Center on Budget and Policy Priorities; 1999. Available at: http://www.cbpp.org/12-23-99wel-es.htm. Accessed June 5, 2002.
105. Knitzer J, Yoshikawa H, Cauthen NK, Aber JL. Welfare reform, family support, and child development: perspectives from policy analysis and developmental psychopathology. *Dev Psychopathol*. 2000;12:619-632.
106. Iglehart JK. Managed care and mental health. *N Engl J Med*. 1996;334:131-135.
107. Frank RG. The creation of Medicare and Medicaid: the emergence of insurance and markets for mental health services. *Psychiatr Serv*. 2000;51:465-468.
108. Shirk S, Talmi A, Olds D. A developmental psychopathology perspective on child and adolescent treatment policy. *Dev Psychopathol*. 2000;12:835-855.
109. Mechanic D. Topics for our times: managed care and public health opportunities. *Am J Public Health*. 1998;88:874-875.
110. Kelleher KJ, McInerny TK, Gardner WP, Childs GE, Wasserman RC. Increasing identification of psychosocial problems: 1979-1996. *Pediatrics*. 2000;105:1313-1321.
111. Burns BJ. Mental health service use by adolescents in the 1970s and 1980s. *J Am Acad Child Adolesc Psychiatry*. 1991;30:144-150.
112. US Department of Health and Human Services. *Report of the Surgeon General's Conference on Children's Mental Health: A National Action Agenda*. Washington, DC: US Dept of Health and Human Services; 2000.
113. Thomas CR, Holzer CE III. National distribution of child and adolescent psychiatrists. *J Am Acad Child Adolesc Psychiatry*. 1999;38:9-16.
114. Coalition for Juvenile Justice. *Handle With Care: Serving the Mental Health Needs of Young Offenders*. Washington, DC: Coalition for Juvenile Justice; 2000.
115. Redding RE. Barriers to meeting the mental health needs of juvenile offenders. *Dev Mental Health Law*. 1999;19:1-23.
116. Faenza M, Siegfried C, Wood J. *Community Perspectives on the Mental Health and Substance Abuse Treatment Needs of Youth Involved in the Juvenile Justice System*. Alexandria, Va: National Mental Health Association and the Office of Juvenile Justice and Delinquency Prevention; 2000.
117. Grisso T. Juvenile offenders and mental illness. *Psychiatry Psychol Law*. 1999; 6:143-151.
118. Ulzen TPM, Hamilton H. The nature and characteristics of psychiatric comorbidity in incarcerated adolescents. *Can J Psychiatry*. 1998;43:57-63.

[19]

Examining the Science and Practice of Violence Risk Assessment with Female Adolescents

Candice L. Odgers,[1,3] Marlene M. Moretti,[2] and N. Dickon Reppucci[1]

While the field of violence risk assessment among adult males has progressed rapidly, several questions remain with respect to the application of forensic risk assessment tools within other populations. In this article, we consider the empirical evidence for the assessment, prediction, and management of violence in adolescent girls. We discuss limitations of generalizing violence risk assessment findings from other populations to adolescent girls and point out areas where there is little or no empirical foundation. Critical issues that must be addressed in research prior to the adoption or rejection of such instruments are delineated. Finally, we provide practice guidelines for clinicians currently involved with adolescent females within risk assessment contexts.

KEY WORDS: adolescent females; psychopathy; risk assessment; violence.

Over the two past decades, significant advances have been made in the field of violence risk assessment (see Borum, 1996; Douglas & Ogloff, 2003; Monahan & Steadman, 1994). A plethora of risk assessment instruments have been developed and tested widely among adult male forensic populations (see, e.g., Hare, 1991; Harris, Rice, & Quinsey, 1993; Webster, Douglas, Eaves, & Hart, 1997). Research to date indicates that, when consistently applied, structured violence risk assessment systems increase case management efficiency and allow for predictions of future violence that surpass those made based on unstructured clinical judgment (Kropp, Hart, Webster, & Eaves, 1999; Monahan, Steadman, Silver, Appelbaum, Robbins, Mulvey, et. al., 2001; Otto, 2000). As such, structured assessment tools are now accepted as an important part of violence risk assessments, and are considered by some to be a *necessary* component (Gacono, 2000; Nicholls, Hemphill, Boer, Kropp, & Zapf, 2001).

While the field of violence risk assessment among adult males has progressed rapidly, several questions remain with respect to the application of forensic risk

[1]Department of Psychology, University of Virginia, Charlottesville, Virginia.
[2]Department of Psychology, Simon Fraser University, Burnaby, British Columbia, Canada.
[3]To whom correspondence should be addressed at Department of Psychology, University of Virginia, 102 Gilmer Hall, P.O. Box 400400, Charlottesville, Virginia 22904-4400; e-mail: clo8d@virginia.edu.

assessment tools within other populations. Although researchers have begun to test the utility of violence risk assessment tools with male adolescents (Edens, Skeem, Cruise, & Cauffman, 2001; Forth, 1995; Forth & Mailloux, 2000; Vincent, 2002) and adult women (Forth, 1996; Rutherford, Cacciola, Alterman, & McKay, 1996; Salekin, Rogers, Ustad, & Sewell, 1998), virtually no studies have focused specifically on female adolescents.

Recently, female adolescents have emerged at the forefront of violence-related research and policy agendas due to increases in official violent offending (FBI, 2002; Puzzanchera, Stahl, Finnegan, Tierney, & Snyder, 2003; Statistics Canada, 2003), self-reported violent behaviors (U.S. Department of Health and Human Services, 2001), and entries into juvenile detention facilities (Porter, 2000). Consequently, demands to apply existing risk assessment tools to, and develop gender-specific instruments for, populations of female youth have increased. Unfortunately, empirically validated assessment tools for this population have not met the growing demands.

In this article, we consider the empirical evidence for the assessment, prediction, and case management of violence in adolescent girls. We discuss limitations of generalizing risk assessment findings from other populations to adolescent girls, and point out areas where there is little or no empirical foundation. Finally, we delineate critical issues that must be addressed in research prior to the adoption or rejection of such instruments, and we provide practice guidelines for the clinicians currently involved with this population.

EMPIRICAL SUPPORT FOR THE PREDICTION AND MANAGEMENT OF VIOLENCE IN ADOLESCENT GIRLS

The identification of factors that reliably predict future violence is essential to risk assessment and case management. Indeed, the goals of prediction and case management go hand in hand—one relies on the other. In the case of risk assessment involving adolescent girls, there is a growing body of literature, which suggests that the risk factors, causal mechanisms, and manifestation of violence may not fit the general models that have been designed for boys and men. The implication, therefore, is that the interrelated goals of risk prediction and risk management may, at best, be difficult to reach given the current state of knowledge and practice.

We next consider three questions: (1) what are the unique challenges of predicting violence in girls?, (2) can research on other populations be generalized to prediction of violence in adolescent girls?, and (3) what, if anything, can risk assessment models offer in managing violence among adolescent girls?

What Are the Unique Challenges of Predicting Violence in Girls?

A review of the research related to violence in adolescent females quickly reveals that traditional violence prediction tools may be of limited value when applied to adolescent female offenders. Several factors contribute to this conclusion.

Low Base Rate of Traditional Forms of Violence Among Females

Although female adolescents are the only population that is continuing to experience consistent increases in violent offending, violent crime statistics are still dominated by males. In fact, across both time and context, males are consistently found to be far more likely than females to engage in serious physical forms of violence (Archer & McDaniel, 1995; Boritch, 1997; Dell & Boe, 1998; Savioe, 2000). For example, in 2000, the violent crime index offense arrest rate (murder, robbery, aggravated assault) among female youth was approximately 11.7 charges per 10,000, and for simple assault, the rate was 46.4 charges per 10,000 (FBI, 2002). By comparison, the rate of violence among adolescent boys was 49.2 charges for violent crime index offenses and 96.7 charges for simple assault.

Even if we consider self-report research that suggests female and male rates of violence are more equivalent, girls still linger behind boys with respect to the absolute prevalence, frequency, and severity of their violent behavior. Although the male-to-female ratio for self-reported violence is decreasing, boys still outnumber girls by 3.5 to 1 (US Department of Health and Human Services, 2001). Girls are also less likely to report involvement in serious forms of violence, such as major assault, robbery, and weapon carrying, and tend to engage in violent acts at a lower frequency than their male counterparts (Moffitt, Caspi, Rutter & Silva, 2001; Snyder, & Sickmund, 1999; Webster, Gainer, & Champion, 1993). While the low base rate of violence in general creates challenges for accurate prediction, the extremely low numbers of girls who go on to commit the forms of violence that risk instruments are designed to predict is especially problematic. In fact, being female is typically considered a protective factor and is given a negative weighting within actuarial violence assessment models.

It is important to note that the difficulties in predicting future violence among females cannot be attributed solely to the problem of a lower base rate. There are other problems in clinical judgment that seem to limit accurate prediction of violence in women. For example, within civil psychiatric and inpatient settings, where the likelihood of future violence is typically more equivalent across males and females (Lidz, Mulvey & Gardner, 1993; Newhill, Mulvey & Lidz, 1995; Robbins, Monahan & Silver, 2003; Stueve & Link, 1998) and clinicians generally possess a modest ability to predict future violence among men (Borum, 1996), clinicians have performed poorly when attempting to predict future violence among women. Specifically, they have tended to underestimate the risk of women's future violence (Lidz et al., 1993; McNiel & Binder, 1995; Nicholls, Ogloff & Ledwidge, 2003).

Gender Differences in the Form and Target of Violent Behavior

A growing body of research suggests that the expression of violence among females may differ both quantitatively and qualitatively from that of their male counterparts. For example, females are less likely than males to engage in physical forms of aggression, and more likely to engage in relationally as opposed to physically aggressive acts (Cote, Valliancourt, Farhat, & Tremblay, 2002; Crick & Grotpeter, 1995; Everett & Price, 1995). Nonetheless, in the context of intimate relationships, adult female aggression can escalate to include physical acts of violence, especially assaults against a partner or family member and are less likely to cause injuries that result in medical attention (Newhill et al., 1995; Shaw & Dubois, 1995). It is quite possible that these types of violent acts by females are less likely to be reported than are violent acts perpetrated in public contexts and against strangers (Straus & Gelles, 1986). Thus, the heavy reliance on official measures of violent offending does not allow for the construction of adequate prediction models for alternative, yet equally harmful, forms of violence in which females are more likely to be involved (e.g., violence against partners, children, and other family members).

Gender Differences in Developmental Course

One of the most robust predictors of future violent offending is the presence of a prior history of involvement in aggressive and violent behavior. Specifically, an early age of onset for aggressive and antisocial acts ($r = .21$–$.45$) and a prior history of violence (1.9–6.3 odds ratio) demonstrate a strong relationship to future violence among males as measured by both official records and self-report data (see Lipsey & Derzon, 1998). The strength of these risk factors within female populations, however, is unclear. For instance, a number of longitudinal studies show no relationship between previous offending and future violence, or in some cases a decreased risk of future violence, for females who begin offending prior to age 15 (Stattin & Magnusson, 1989; White, 1992).

The picture of violence among adolescent females is further complicated by the possibility that the developmental course of aggression may differ for females compared to males (Silverthorn & Frick, 1999). It is well documented that the majority of females who engage in antisocial and aggressive behavior during adolescence disappear from the radar when traditional violence measures are used (Lanctot, 2002), with women being more likely to engage in violence within the home and against family members (Estroff & Zimmer, 1994; Robbins et al., 2003). While many of these women are at a high risk for a myriad of other psychological, physical, and social problems (Moffitt et al., 2001), it is unlikely that they will commit a violent act that will be detected by official arrest statistics. Thus, prediction models used to construct the majority of actuarial tools may not include the best linear combination of risk factors for the small number of adolescent females who go on to engage in violence.

Lack of Gender-Specific and Empirically Based Prediction Models

Applying risk prediction tools to female adolescents is also problematic because the risk factors that are selected for inclusion in the majority of existing tools have been chosen based on their robustness as predictors in: (a) retrospective studies of adult male offenders (Hare, 1991; Harris, Rice & Cormier, 1991), (b) large longitudinal studies from juvenile justice that have focused primarily on male offending, or (c) studies involving male and female youth where estimates of the relationships were neither calculated nor reported separately from the results presented for males.

In sum, several interrelated issues create significant challenges in the prediction of violence in adolescent girls. Together, these factors are likely to reduce the predictive accuracy of current assessment tools. Unfortunately, it is not even possible to determine the extent of the problem because there is simply insufficient research. We next turn our attention to research on related populations and examine whether it is reasonable to generalize findings from these groups to support the practice of risk assessment in female adolescents.

What Does Research with Adult Women Tell Us About the Prediction of Violence Risk Among Adolescent Females?

Experts in the risk assessment field have stated that male-based instruments are likely to function similarly within female populations (Hare, 1991; Webster, 1999). The empirical data to support these claims, however, are equivocal at best. While researchers have evaluated a number of different risk instruments with women, (e.g., the *Violence Risk Appraisal Guide* [VRAG] Harris et al, 1993, and the HCR-20, Webster et al., 1997) the *Psychopathy Checklist-Revised* (PCL-R; Hare, 1991) is currently viewed as the gold standard in violence risk assessment. As such, we focus our review primary on psychopathy related research.

A number of researchers have cited the postdictive power the PCL-R as evidence that the instrument applies equally well within populations of adult women (see Rutherford et al., 1996; Weiler & Widom, 1996). However, the degree to which these studies can be seen as providing support for the PCL-R as a risk assessment instrument is highly compromised by the fact that criminal history is specifically used to form a number of PCL item ratings (e.g., early behavioral problems, serious criminal offending, criminal versatility, revocation of conditional release) and carries significant weight in others (e.g., lack of remorse, impulsivity, irresponsibility, poor anger control). Predictive rather than postdictive studies are required and results are much less favorable when researchers attempt to predict *future* offending among women (Salekin et al., 1998).

Among the only *prospective* examinations of structured risk assessment with women, Salekin and colleagues (Salekin, Rogers, & Sewell, 1997; Salekin et al., 1998) found that the classification accuracy of the PCL-R was "moderate to poor." In addition, in one of the most comprehensive reviews of the empirical research on psychopathy and women, Vitale and Newman (2001) concluded that "if clinicians are using the PCL-R for the sole purpose of predicting specific outcomes for any particular women in these areas [predicting criminal recidivism, predicting institutional violence, planning and implementing treatments and interventions], they would be doing so without empirical evidence or the predictive power of the PCL-R in such domains" (p. 128). It should be noted, however, that this review relied heavily on the research by Salekin and colleagues that was comprised of a primarily African American sample, yet ethnic differences were not addressed. Even if one were to factor in these methodological considerations, however, it would be difficult at this point to justify the use of the PCL-R with women for predictive purposes.

Other researchers have argued that a greater understanding of the differences that exist between male and female populations is needed to increase the accuracy of future predictions of violent behavior (Uggen & Kruttschnitt, 1998). Brennan and Austin (1997) charge that gender neutral classification tools tend to overclassify females, while others assert that the bias functions in the opposite direction, producing an underprediction in females (Coontz, Lidz, & Mulvey, 1994). Coulson, Flacqua, Nutbrown, Giulekas, and Cudjoe (1996) concluded that current risk cut-off thresholds that have been normed on samples of men (e.g., *Level of Service Inventory*) are not appropriate for female offenders. In addition, a number of leading authorities in the risk assessment field have stated that factors other than those included in current risk assessment schemes may be necessary to consider in the prediction of violence among women (Monahan, 1996).

The problems associated with predicting violence risk in women are not limited to situations where violence risk assessment instruments and guides are used. Rather, there is a convincing body of research on unstructured clinical judgment which demonstrates that this is part of a more general problem. In one of the most definitive studies, Lidz et al. (1993) found that although clinicians were able to predict with a moderate degree of accuracy whether male civil psychiatric patients would be involved in a violent incident, they were no better than chance when predicting future violence among females. Even though the base rate of future violence was higher among the females versus males in this sample (49% vs. 42%, respectively) clinicians were only able to predict violence in 22% of the females versus 45% of the males. Based on these findings, the authors suggest that the cues considered by clinicians in cases involving women may be inaccurate. A further examination of the judgment processes employed by clinicians suggested that clinical judgments of future violence risk are, in part, dependent on cultural beliefs regarding appropriate gender role behavior, with clinicians being less likely to address the topic of violence with female versus male patients (Coontz et al., 1994). Very little is known, however, regarding why clinicians perform more poorly when evaluating women within an unstructured context. It has been hypothesized that gender-based stereotypes such as the general tendency to perceive females as less threatening and aggressive (Bettencourt & Miller, 1996) and more "mad" than "bad" may have an indirect impact on the assessment process.

In sum, the majority of the research on violence prediction in adult women is extremely limited and the findings are unclear at best. Although many scholars have taken the position that it would be unlikely that current male-based instruments have no application to women (see Hare, 1991; Webster, 1999), the empirical body of research necessary to support the use of these tools for purposes other than research does not exist. In fact, the problems in the field are of such magnitude that researchers have clearly stated that instruments, such as the PCL-R, should not be used for predictive purposes with adult female samples although they recommend continued use of the PCL-R as a research instrument in its current form (Vitale & Newman, 2001). If any generalization can be made downward to adolescent females at all, it would be to view current assessment instruments and the prediction of violence in adolescent girls with extreme caution.

What Does Research with Boys Tell Us About the Prediction of Risk Among Adolescent Females?

Even if research on adult women offers little basis for downward generalization to adolescent girls, it is possible that findings based on adolescent male samples could be generalized laterally to girls. A number of studies using the *Psychopathy Checklist: Youth Version* (PCL:YV; Forth, Kosson, & Hare, 2003) have reported similar psychometric properties to the PCL-R (Hare, 1991) and found that male juveniles scoring high on the PCL:YV are similar to adult male psychopaths with respect both to psychological correlates and behavioral characteristics (see Vincent & Hart, 2002, for a review). The PCL–YV has also demonstrated predictive utility within short-term prospective studies of male adolescents (Forth, Hart, & Hare, 1990; Ridenour, Marchant, & Dean, 2001). However, a review of published PCL–YV studies indicates that only 6 of the 34 studies completed to date have included females, with sample sizes ranging from 11 to 80 females (Forth et al., 2003). Given the lack of empirical data, it is difficult to assess the psychometric properties of the PCL–YV when applied to females.

Although significantly more research has been done with boys, and psychopathy is considered the gold standard in the prediction of both violent and general criminal recidivism in adult males (Hare, 1991; Hare, McPherson, & Forth, 1988; Harris et al., 1991), there is not enough evidence to establish whether this disorder exists or can be assessed prior to early adulthood (Vincent & Hart, 2002). For example, Vincent (2002) reported differential item functioning between male adolescents and adults on interpersonal and behavioral items of the PCL-R and PCL–YV. In this case, adolescents who were rated as psychopathic needed higher levels of the latent trait of psychopathy in order to receive ratings as high as adults on items such as irresponsibility and impulsivity. These findings raise the fundamental question of whether these instruments are measuring the same thing, in this case psychopathy, across adult and adolescent male populations.

Even if we interpret existing research as providing some degree of evidence to support the use of violence risk prediction in adolescent males, it is important to keep in mind that there are significant concerns regarding the assessment of risk in general, and psychopathy in particular, during adolescence (for reviews, see Edens et al., 2001; Vincent & Hart, 2002). Specifically, behaviors that are normative during adolescence, such as impulsivity, may appear pathological from a risk assessment perspective (Seagrave & Grisso, 2002). For example, although the majority of youth engage in antisocial behavior during adolescence, this behavior is largely transient and desists as youths enter young adulthood (Cauffman & Steinberg, 2000; Farrington, 1989; Moffitt, 1993). The normative fluctuations that occur in adolescence raise the question of whether the presentation of disorders and traits may vary significantly with the adolescents' stage of emotional and psychosocial development.

The instability that characterizes adolescence is particularly important in light of the *fundamental assumption* that many of the traits that comprise risk assessment instruments are stable within the individual and can be assessed reliably over time. At the heart of the issue is the question of whether adolescent personality development has stabilized sufficiently to extract the information required to conduct such evaluations, and at present we lack a definitive answer to this question. As such, adolescents have been described as moving targets that are difficult to assess based on single observations (Grisso, 1998).

Should We Overlook Developmental Concerns and Place More Confidence in Research on the Assessment of Psychopathy and Violence Prediction in Adolescent Males?

If we were to place more emphasis on the assessment of psychopathy among adolescent males, this would not necessarily mean that research on this population could be wholly generalized to the prediction of violence in adolescent girls. As previously noted, very little is known regarding the normative developmental course of antisocial and aggressive behavior among girls. Although Moffitt et al. (2001) argue that the Life Course Persistent (LCP) versus Adolescent Limited (AL) taxonomy applies equally well to males and females, research examining gender differences is quite limited and what exists suggests that few females follow the LCP trajectory. For example, only 6 of the approximately 450 females (1%) from the Dunedin Longitudinal Study (Moffitt et al., 2001) were identified as LCP offenders, whereas 78 (18%) were identified as AL. Among males in the sample, 10% of (47) were identified as LCP offenders, and an additional 122 (26%) met the criteria for the AL Pathway. Consistent with this finding, the gender gap in rates of Conduct Disorder (CD) is greater in childhood than in adolescence (for reviews, see Cohen et al., 1993; Lahey et al., 2000; Moffitt et al., 2001; Zoccolillo, 1993).

The fact that adolescent-onset aggression is more common in girls than is childhood-onset aggression has led some researchers to suggest that the classic distinction between LCP versus AL does not apply to girls (Loeber & Stouthamer-Loeber, 1998; Silverthorn & Frick, 1999). Silverthorn and Frick (1999) propose that the delayed-onset pattern in girls is equivalent to the early-onset pattern in boys in terms of risk markers, stability, and persistence into adulthood. The controversy surrounding the developmental course of aggression among girls is especially relevant within risk assessment research due to the heavy reliance on childhood behaviors as markers of future risk for violence. It is possible that the commonly cited early markers of violence may not exist for girls, or that early risk markers may manifest themselves differently across development among females.

In sum, the current use of risk assessment instruments to predict future violence in adult females and adolescent males is not widely supported. Even if there were greater support within each of these populations, questions still remain as to whether the findings could be generalized downward in terms of age, or laterally in terms of gender. Given the current state of the research, it is clear that the traditional practice of risk assessment for the purpose of violence prediction in adolescent girls is not advisable.

What Can Risk Prediction Models Offer to the Field of Adolescent Female Violence?

Although there is no evidence to support the practice of violence prediction with current instruments per se, the literature does confirm that adolescent girls with serious behavioral problems, as reflected in a diagnosis of CD and/or incarceration, are at risk for a variety of poor mental health and social functioning outcomes as they move toward adulthood. For example, in the Dunedin longitudinal study, Moffitt et al. (2001) found that 21-year-old women diagnosed with CD in childhood or adolescence were significantly more likely to show mental health symptoms (anxiety, depression, psychosis, mania, and suicidality), suffer from more medical problems, require social assistance, be victimized by their partners, and perpetrate physical abuse against them in return than were girls not diagnosed with CD. Similar negative outcomes have been found for female juvenile offenders with respect to mental health symptoms of depression, substance abuse, suicidality, as well as social and economic marginalization in young adulthood (Lanctot, 2002; Lewis, Yeager, Cobham-Portorreal, & Klein, 1991).

Given these findings, the social costs of failing to intervene and reduce the risk of violence in forensic populations of adolescent females is likely significant. For example, studies by Robins (1986) verify that girls diagnosed with CD in adolescence went on to be in involved in multiple mental health services as young women. Not only does the financial burden of providing social and mental health support increase over time in the absence of intervention, but there is evidence to suggest that the risk for involvement in criminality is even higher in the offspring of mothers than fathers with a criminal history (Tremblay, 1991). As a result, it makes sense to develop instruments to detect risk for deleterious social-emotional and health outcomes even if there is only a small likelihood that these girls will engage in the typical form of violent behavior that is commonly seen in males. Although current research findings do not support assessment and prediction of violence in girls, it seems important that further research and refinement of assessment measures will be undertaken to enhance accuracy to the point that they become valid and useful.

RESEARCH GUIDELINES: GENDER REFINEMENT OF RISK ASSESSMENT INSTRUMENTS

There are a number of tools that have been developed specifically to assess and manage risk among adolescents (for a review, see Office of Juvenile Justice and Delinquency Prevention, 1995). Although some of these have been developed specifically for adolescents (e.g., the Structured Assessment of Violence Risk in Youth [SAVRY]; Borum, Bartel, & Forth, 2002), most were designed for use with adult offenders and are either directly applied or slightly modified for use with adolescents. Developmental considerations have not been factored into the majority of current risk assessment schemes and prospective studies that would support the use of such instruments during this period are lacking. There have been virtually no attempts to construct tools designed for female populations within forensic settings. In fact, most instruments do not consider gender, and the majority of assessment schemes assume that items apply equally to male and female populations.

The construction of developmentally and gender-sensitive risk management instruments must not only be anchored in research on adolescent development, but it must also take into consideration gender-related factors that are of relevance in understanding the emergence and course of aggressive, violent, and antisocial behavior in girls. These include greater attention to: (a) gender-specific risk and protective factors; (b) psychiatric co-morbidity; (c) social context and relational issues; and (d) gender differences in item sensitivity.

Inclusion of Gender-Specific Risk and Protective Factors

Only recently have researchers begun to empirically assess the form and predictive utility of gender-specific risk factors (Chesney-Lind & Sheldon, 1998; Levene, Augimeri, Pepler, Walsh, Webster, & Koegl, 2001; Reitsma-Street, 1999; Totten, 2000). Cunningham, Baker, Mazaheri, Ashbourne, VanBrunschot, and Currie (2000) have argued that although adolescent women share several risk markers with their male counterparts, there are a number of important risk factors, such as a history of attempted suicide and depression, that are not generally considered in most instruments. For example, Borst and Noam (1993) documented distinct developmental pathways and correlates (e.g., aggression, psychopathology) of suicidal behaviors among a sample of young female psychiatric patients ($n = 139$). Suicidal behaviors may be considered as a marker for distinct types of psychological maladjustment and as a risk factor for future violence towards self and others.

Our recent review of the literature (Odgers & Moretti, 2002) provides little empirical evidence to support the need for gender-specific risk factors among normative samples of children and youth (see also Leschied, Cummings, Van Brunschot, Cunningham, & Saunders, 2000). Instead, the primary message throughout these studies is the remarkable level of similarity with respect to the risk factors that are related to violence among boys and girls (e.g., antisocial peers, academic problems, and antisocial parental behavior). Differences that did exist included higher rates of sexual abuse and depression for females. Clinical experience with forensic populations, however, presents a very different picture with respect to the potential importance of gender-specific risk domains and unique nonlinear combinations of risk factors in explaining and managing violence among high-risk girls.

Data from juvenile justice centers indicate that incarcerated girls are more likely than boys to have a broad array of co-occurring mental health problems (e.g., high rates of suicidal ideation, substance abuse, depression, posttraumatic stress disorder [PTSD], and suicide attempts); be exposed to more severe levels of victimization and maltreatment; experience high levels of distress and preoccupation related to their involvement in abusive and highly conflictual relationships, and come from homes that are characterized by high levels of dysfunction (Bergsmann, 1989; Lewis et al., 1991; Moretti, Holland, & McKay, 2001; Odgers & Moretti, 2002; Rosenbaum, 1989; Viale-Val & Sylvester, 1993). Females within juvenile justice settings are also more likely to be from a minority population and experience other forms of economic and social marginalization (Chesney-Lind & Sheldon, 1998; Corrado, Odgers, & Cohen, 2001).

Clinically, the most salient risk factors for girls relate to their abuse history and the high levels of relationship dysfunction. Although the majority of studies relying on normative populations have *not* shown that aggressive girls and boys differ in exposure to such risk factors as physical maltreatment (Moffitt et al., 2001; Pepler & Sedighdeilami, 1998), and only a weak relationship exists between exposure to abuse and later violence (Lipsey & Derzon, 1998), research conducted within forensic and clinical samples consistently shows that, compared to boys, girls in these populations are significantly more likely to have experienced severe victimization, particularly sexual abuse (Bergsmann, 1989; Corrado et al., 2001; Rivera & Widom, 1990; U.S. Bureau of Justice Statistics, 1997; Viale-Val & Sylvester, 1993). The impact of abuse likely depends on the availability of other supports to children as well as the duration and severity of abusive experiences. Thus, it is important for instruments to go beyond the mere recording of exposure to maltreatment and to more thoroughly assess the type, severity, and duration of abuse, as well as variables such as the relationship to the perpetrator and availability of support. Greater attention to abuse experiences may be helpful in terms of developing management strategies including specific forms of intervention.

It is also the case that current risk assessment instruments could better predict adult outcomes for adolescent girls if they took into account factors that are associated with a *decreased* probability of violence as well. Careful examination of the ways girls are socialized could offer important clues as to why the majority of girls do *not* engage in physical forms of violence. For example, in studies of normative populations, researchers have found that mothers are more likely to discuss others' feelings with their young daughters than their sons, and by age two girls are more likely to talk about feelings than are boys (Dunn, Bretherton, & Munn, 1987). Parents also use more induction techniques with their daughters than their sons to encourage them to consider the feelings of others, and girls are more likely than boys to feel bad if they act aggressively toward others (Boldizar, Perry & Perry, 1989; Cross & Madson, 1997). Although female gendered socialization may increase risk in girls for internalizing disorders (see Moretti & Higgins, 1999; Moretti, Rein & Weibe, 1998), it may provide protection against the development of overt forms of aggressive and violent behavior. To the extent that girls are socialized during early childhood in this way they may be less likely to become involved in overt aggressive and violent behavior during childhood, and more likely to desist in such behavior if it arises during adolescence. It is also likely that socialization practices that are more typically observed in the parenting of girls could potentially provide protection against the development of aggression and violence in boys. On the other hand, traditional forms of female socialization may lead to a reliance on social and relational forms of aggressive behavior. Thus, it is necessary to understand the tradeoffs of gendered socialization in determining which aspects are most likely to contribute to healthy development.

Co-morbidity Issues

Within adult research, the co-morbidity of mental disorders has been cited as a threat to the validity of current risk assessment schemes (Douglas & Webster, 1999) as well as an important consideration in the prediction of future violence (Monahan et al., 2001). Co-morbidity is often viewed as an impediment to research due to questions surrounding the distinctiveness of disorders and diagnostic taxonomy. It is often difficult, for example, to identify the source of multiple symptom patterns and to predict the interactive effect of co-occurring disorders on future behavior. Despite these challenges, the most definitive research in this area has highlighted the importance of considering co-morbid disorders when evaluating risk for future violence. In the MacArthur Risk Assessment Study, Monahan et al. (2001) found that violence committed by people discharged from a mental hospital was very similar to violence committed by other people living in their communities; however, the primary difference was that violence tended to be higher among those with a co-occurring substance abuse.

With respect to adolescents, our current lack of understanding regarding the developmental course and manifestation of co-morbid disorders presents unique challenges for assessments. The precise estimate of mental disorders among youth within the juvenile justice system varies depending on the assessment tool used. For example, Otto, Greenstein, Johnson & Friedman (1992) reported a prevalence rate of 20% among juvenile offenders when only serious mental disorders were included, while others have reported much higher rates when disorders such as substance abuse and conduct disorder are considered (Kazdin, 2000). Regardless of the measure used, a consistent finding is that girls within forensic populations are more likely than their male counterparts to exhibit co-occurring mental health problems (for a review, see Moretti & Odgers, 2002). For example, Teplin (2003) examined the rates of mental disorder in a juvenile detention sample (657 girls and 1,172 boys) and found that approximately 53% of girls versus 41% of boys had two or more disorders, and of the 20 categories of disorders that they examined girls were more likely than boys to be diagnosed in 16 of them.

Girls within high-risk populations also differ with respect to the types of disorders that they exhibit. Specifically, rates of PTSD, depression, attention-deficit hyperactivity disorder, and substance dependency are higher among girls in juvenile justice and mental health settings than among both normative girls and boys in forensic populations (see Cauffman, Feldman, Waterman & Steiner, 1998; Loeber & Keenan, 1994; Zoccolillo, 1993). For example, Cauffman et al. (1998) found that approximately 60% of incarcerated female juvenile offenders met partial (12%) or full (49%) criteria for PTSD. These rates were significantly higher than those noted for male juvenile delinquents.

In sum, the majority of the research points to higher levels of co-morbidity among adolescent girls within forensic settings, as well as a higher prevalence of certain disorders. Arguably, the mental health status of high-risk girls makes prediction more complex. Even if our understanding of the relationship between co-occurring mental problems and later violence among girls was more advanced, the interaction between multiple disorders and complex symptom patterns makes it difficult to predict where their individual developmental course will lead. For example, Sroufe (1990) reported a diversity of developmental trajectories even in the presence of the same risk factors. One possibility is that among high-risk adolescent females, who are characterized by higher levels of psychiatric co-morbidity than their male counterparts, development is skewed toward a pathological course. In other words, once these young women cross a certain threshold of risk their probability of a wide range of negative outcomes, including violence, may increase exponentially. Future research is needed, however, in order to support this assertion.

Increased Focus on Relationship Dynamics

As previously noted, the vast majority of adolescent girls who engage in aggressive and violent behavior are involved in various types of abusive relationships in which they are victimized by their caregivers, romantic partners, and peers, and in which they perpetrate violence upon others. For example, female youths are most likely to aggress against family members, romantic partners, and members of their peer group. Aggression can take the form of physical acts perpetrated toward others, or "relational" acts of aggression that function to coerce and control others in interpersonal relationships (Moretti & Odgers, 2002). Researchers in the field of gender and identity development have argued that, compared to boys, girls' identity development is more contextualized within their close interpersonal relationship (Artz, 1998; Moretti & Higgins, 1999). Consequently, girls may suffer more than boys when their relationships are threatened, and they are more distressed by relational forms of aggression than are boys (Geiger, Zimmer-Gembeck & Crick, 2004; Moretti & Odgers, 2002).

There is also evidence that specific attachment patterns are associated with coercive and aggressive behavior toward others. Allen, Moore, Kuperminc, and Bell (1998) found that preoccupied teens were more likely to engage in delinquent activities, including getting into physical fights and assaulting people, than were secure teens, and their delinquent behavior is more likely to increase between the ages of 16 and 18 years (Allen, Marsh, McFarland, Boykin, Land, Jodl, et al., 2002). Moretti, DaSilva and Holland (2004) have found that preoccupied attachment is more common in adolescent girls than boys diagnosed with CD, and degree of attachment preoccupation is uniquely related to aggressive behavior toward others. This research suggests that aggression among adolescent girls may function as a coercive, albeit dysfunctional, strategy to maintain relationships.

Gender Differences in Item Sensitivity in Assessing Aggression and Violence

There is a growing body of evidence regarding gender differences in the manifestation of violence among females. Qualitative research has provided us with rich descriptions of the ways in which the forms and motivations for aggression among females may differ (Artz, 1998; Chesney-Lind & Sheldon, 1998). Recent quantitative analyses also point to important gender differences when measuring violence among girls. For example, Odgers, Moretti and Pepler (2003) found a different underlying structure of aggression among high-risk girls as compared to the structure for girls in normative settings and boys from both normative and high-risk settings ($n = 1448$). Here, even when the same instrument was used, the *Youth Self Report* (Achenbach, 1991), a different latent trait of aggression was being measured within high-risk females.

Theoretically, it makes sense that violence may differ in both form and function across gender. Now, empirically, there is evidence which questions the ability of commonly used aggression scales to adequately measure aggression among forensic populations of females. The danger is that if equivalent measurement is *not* obtained across gender, the potential for misinterpreting the limited body of research that does exist is high. At best, results could be misconstrued through the reporting of inaccurate estimates in the size of the relationships between various risk factors and violent outcomes and, at worst, researchers may be reporting the wrong size and direction of the effects. With respect to risk assessment, if the weight of various predictors of aggression are calibrated using the results of studies where the dependent variable (aggression/violence) is not comparable across gender, then it does not make sense to compare the relative weight and importance of risk factors between males and females. Thus, until we are confident that the measurement of aggression is invariant across male and female samples, conclusions regarding the relative importance of various risk factors must remain tentative.

Researchers have also pointed to the greater tendency for females to rely on alternative forms of violence—such as relational and social aggression. Studies have shown that relational forms of aggression may be equally as harmful as overt forms (Crick & Bigbee, 1998; Paquette & Underwood, 1999) and are more common in young women than previously believed (Bjorkgvist & Niemela, 1992; Crick & Grotpeter, 1995; Moretti et al., 2001). The recognition of the level and consequences of relational aggression has the potential to inform risk assessment. First, relational aggression may be considered a marker or precursor to more direct and physical forms of violence, as well as providing the context in which acts of physical violence occur. Second, it is advisable to expand the traditional outcome measure of violence within both basic and applied research settings beyond official acts of recidivism. As previously noted, female youths are unlikely to engage in violence that is detected by the criminal justice system. As such, the expansion of the outcome measure of violence and the use of collateral informants to assess the nature and the extent of the damage that is caused by the violence that these women go on to commit against their children, spouses, and themselves will be crucial in completing the complex picture of the developmental course of aggression among females. Finally, there is a need for qualitative research that examines the phenotypic pattern of violence, specifically the relationship between overt and relational forms of aggression among females.

Learn from Tools Developed for Very Young Aggressive Boys and Girls

The challenge of creating a developmentally appropriate and gender-sensitive risk management tools for girls is sizeable. Although we have access to only a limited body of research and practice that is related directly to assessment with female adolescents, there are many important points to be gleaned from the research related to very young boys and girls. For example, the *Early Assessment Risk List for Boys (EARL-20B) Version 2* (Augimeri, Koegl, Webster, & Levene, 2001) and the *Early Assessment Risk List for Girls (EARL-21G) Version 1: Consultation Edition* (Levene et al., 2001) are risk assessment devices designed to promote gender-specific assessment of risk of antisocial, aggressive, or violent conduct in young children under 12 years of age. The EARL-21G includes items on maternal caregiver–daughter interaction and sexual development to capture issues that may be of unique relevance to girls. Although a preliminary study of the predictive validity of the EARL-21G in a sample of 67 girls revealed that 6 (34%) of the 18 girls who went on to offend in adolescence were classified in childhood in the high-risk range versus 4 (20%) classified in the low-risk group, this difference was not significant (Levene, Augimeri & Pepler, 2004). These findings suggest that the EARL-G in its current form should not be used for predictive purposes, even though the scale has proven to be of considerable value in tailoring programing for young girls (Pepler, Walsh, & Levene, 2004).

In sum, while there is a need to search for gender-specific factors and tailor assessment practices to girls, we must keep in mind that many risk factors for aggression and violence influence girls and boys similarly. Therefore, building assessment tools from lessons we have learned from boys, while keeping in mind unique gender issues, is likely to be more productive than ignoring past research. At the same time, recent research suggests that even when we try to operationalize violence the same way across males and females, we may be measuring a different construct. Advancements in both qualitative and quantitative research designs are required in order to modify existing violence measures and coding schemes to account for the diverse nature and patterns of violence among females. Greater attention should also be paid to the contextual and relational factors in which violent acts committed by girls are embedded. Again, the primary goal for those who are invested in this process should be managing and reducing violence and other negative outcomes among young women as opposed to prediction in the absence of appropriate programing and treatment options.

PRACTICE GUIDELINES: SHOULD CLINICIANS EVALUATE RISK IN ADOLESCENT GIRLS?

While the previous section provided direction for researchers and the future development of a field that is in its infancy, the key question for mental health and other professionals is whether clinicians should evaluate risk in adolescent girls, and if so, for what purpose. First, our review concludes that the assessment of risk for violence for predictive purposes with adolescent girls is not supported by empirical research. Given this conclusion, such assessments cannot be ethically justified and should be vigorously discouraged. On the other hand, there appears to be value in the use of current risk instruments for research purposes and as an adjunct to other assessment procedures to inform clinical management strategies.

There are several ways in which risk assessment can be used constructively with adolescent girls. First and foremost, the use of these measures helps to bring the issue of female aggression and violence into focus for clinicians who might otherwise tend to ignore such issues. Second, by applying a method of systematic and structured assessment of risk factors, clinicians are more likely to examine comprehensively those factors that are likely to be of relevance to case management. Although we have argued that risk assessment for predictive purposes is not advisable, many of the factors that are embedded in risk assessment instruments are of relevance to guiding case management. Identifying those domains, which are particularly problematic or appear to have contributed to the instigation of violence in the past, can be extremely helpful in developing more precise management strategies. For example, if delinquent peer affiliation is identified as a precursor to acts of aggression and violence, steps should be taken to reduce the opportunities for and interest in delinquent peers. These may include working with the youth, family, and community to identify ways in which at-risk girls can be integrated into prosocial peer contexts, and can develop social, recreational, and vocational skills that provide a foundation for their success in nondelinquent peer groups. Similarly, the systematic identification of substance-use problems in at-risk girls is of particular importance in ensuring that appropriate programing is put into place to address their needs.

In this article, we have pointed the need to consider gender-related factors that may be of unique importance in risk assessment for girls, but which are often not represented in risk assessment instruments, such as the PCL:YV. Among these are exposure to sexual abuse, psychiatric co-morbidity, threat to interpersonal relationships, and insecure attachment. It is advisable that clinicians who pursue risk assessment for the purpose of clinical case management are mindful of these factors in their work with adolescent girls. Not only may this enhance the "fit" of programing to the needs of girls, but it is also of importance in contributing to research on the question of whether a gendered approach to risk assessment is necessary.

Although we believe that risk assessment is valuable for case management of adolescent girls, we caution clinicians to be aware that assessments are sometimes used for unintended purposes. Even though a clinician may engage in risk assessment with a clear appreciation of the limitations of these risk assessment measures in terms of prediction of future incidents and include a clear statement of such limitations in their reports, it is often difficult to control the use of information that appears in psychological reports and records. In our opinion, given the limitations of the field and the potential deleterious consequences of misuse of risk assessment findings, the burden of responsibility must rest on the shoulders of clinicians who undertake such procedures. Every precaution should be taken to ensure that findings are not used inappropriately, and clinicians must be active in voicing their concerns and informing public bodies about the reality of research findings when assessments are inappropriately conducted or used.

We anticipate that the next decade will bring many new insights into risk management and assessment with diverse populations. It is our hope that the models and tools that are developed for assessing and managing violence among young women will evolve alongside the growing body of empirical research. Although current tools must be used with great caution (if at all), there remains a need for empirically sound and gender-sensitive risk management tools. Thus, the challenge for mental health researchers and clinicians is to proceed with an appreciation of the severe limitations that exist in *both* research and practice and, perhaps more importantly, to allow for alternative ways of approaching violence risk assessment and management with adolescent females.

ACKNOWLEDGMENTS

This research is funded by the CIHR Institute of Gender and Health (IGH) in partnership with the CIHR Institute of Human Development, Child and Youth Health (IHDCYH) though a Newly Emerging Team grant awarded to Dr. M. Moretti (# 31-711036 6319).

REFERENCES

Achenbach, T. M. (1991). *Manual for the youth self-report and 1991 profile.* Burlington: University of Vermont, Department of Psychiatry.

Allen, J. P., Marsh, P., McFarland, C., Boykin, K., Land, D. J., Jodl, K. M., et al. (2002). Attachment and autonomy as predictors of the development of social skills and delinquency during mid-adolescence. *Journal of Consulting and Clinical Psychology, 70,* 55–66.

Allen, J. P., Moore, C., Kuperminc, G., & Bell, K. (1998). Attachment and adolescent functioning. *Child Development, 69,* 1406–1419.

Archer, D., & McDaniel, P. (1995). Violence and gender. In R. B. Ruback & N. A. Weiner (Eds.), *Interpersonal violent behaviors: Social and cultural aspects* (pp. 63–87). New York, NY: Springer.

Artz, S. (1998). *Sex, power, and the violent school girl.* Toronto: Trifolium Press.

Augimeri, L. K., Koegl, C. J., Webster, C. D., & Levene, K. S. (2001). *Early assessment risk list for boys: EARL-20B (Version 2).* Toronto, ON: Earlscourt Child and Family Centre.

Bergsmann, I. R. (1989). The forgotten few: Juvenile female offenders. *Federal Probation, 12,* 73–78.

Bettencourt, B. A., & Miller, N. (1996). Gender differences in aggression as a function of provocation: A meta-analysis. *Psychological Bulletin, 119,* 422–447.

Bjorkqvist, K., & Niemela, P. (1992). *Of mice and women: Aspects of female aggression.* San Diego, CA: Academic Press.

Boldizar, J. P., Perry, D. G., & Perry, L. C. (1989). Outcome values and aggression. *Child Development, 60,* 571–579.

Boritch, H. (1997). *Fallen women: Women and crime and criminal justice.* Toronto, ON: ITP Nelson.

Borst, S. R., & Noam, G. G. (1993). Developmental psychopathology in suicidal and nonsuicidal adolescent girls. *Journal of the American Academy of Child and Adolescent Psychiatry, 32,* 501–521.

Borum, R. (1996). Improving the clinical practice of violence risk assessment: Technology, guidelines, and training. *American Psychologist, 51,* 945–956.

Borum, R., Bartel, P., & Forth, A. (2002). *Manual for the Structured Assessment of Violence Risk in Youth (SAVRY).* University of South Florida.

Brennan, T., & Austin, J. (1997). *Women in jail: Classification issues.* Washington, DC: U.S. Department of Justice, National Institute of Corrections.

Cauffman, E., Feldman, S. S., Waterman, J., & Steiner, H. (1998). Posttraumatic stress disorder among female juvenile offenders. *Journal of the American Academy of Child and Adolescent Psychiatry, 37,* 1209–1216.

Cauffman, E., & Steinberg, L. (2000). The cognitive and affective influences of adolescent decision making. *Temple Law Review, 68,* 1763–1789.

Chesney-Lind, M., & Sheldon, R. (1998). *Girls, delinquency, and juvenile justice* (2nd ed.). Pacific Grove, CA: Brooks/Cole.

Cohen, P., Cohen, J., Kasen, S., Velez, C., Hartmark, C., Johnson, J., et al. (1993). An epidemiological study of disorders in late childhood and adolescence: Age and gender specific prevalence. *Journal of Child Psychology and Psychiatry, 34,* 851–867.

Coontz, P., Lidz, C., & Mulvey, E. (1994). Gender and the assessment of dangerousness in the psychiatric emergency room. *International Journal of Law and Psychiatry, 17,* 369–376.

Corrado, R., Odgers, C., & Cohen, I. (2001). The use of incarceration for female youth: Protection for whom? *Canadian Journal of Criminology, 42,* 189–206.

Cote, S., Valliancourt, T., Farhat, A., & Tremblay, R. (2002, July). *Childhood physical and indirect aggression: Sex difference in developmental trends.* Paper presented at the International Society for Research on Aggression Bi-Annual Meeting, Montreal, Canada.

Coulson, G., Flacqua, G., Nutbrown, V., Giulekas, D., & Cudjoe, F. (1996). Predictive utility of the LSI for incarcerated female offenders. *Criminal Justice and Behavior, 23,* 427–439.

Crick, N. R., & Bigbee, M. A. (1998). Relational and overt forms of peer victimization: A multiinformant approach. *Journal of Consulting and Clinical Psychology, 66,* 337–347.

Crick, N. R., & Grotpeter, J. K. (1995). Relational aggression, gender, and social-psychological adjustment. *Child Development, 66,* 710–722.

Cross, S. E., & Madson, L. (1997). Models of the self: Self-construals and gender. *Psychological Bulletin, 122,* 5–37.

Cunningham, A., Baker, L., Mazaheri, N., Ashbourne, L., VanBrunschot, M., & Currie, M. (2000). *Best practice programming for phase II young offenders: A literature review.* London: Centre for Children and Families in the Justice System.

Dell, A., & Boe, R. (1998). *Female young offenders in Canada* (rev. ed.). Ottawa: Research Branch, Correctional Service of Canada.

Douglas, K. S., & Ogloff, R. P. (2003). Multiple facets of risk for violence: The impact of judgmental specificity on structured decisions about risk. *International Journal of Forensic Mental Health, 2,* 19–34.

Douglas, K. S., & Webster, C. D. (1999). Predicting violence in mentally and personality disordered individuals. In R. Roesch, S. D. Hart, & J. R. P. Ogloff (Eds.), *Psychology and law: The state of the discipline* (pp. 176–239). New York, NY: Kluwer Academic.

Dunn, J., Bretherton, I., & Munn, I. P. (1987). Conversations about feeling states between mothers and their young children. *Developmental Psychology, 23,* 132–139.

Edens, J. F., Skeem, J. L., Cruise, K. R., & Cauffman, E. (2001). Assessment of "juvenile psychopathy" and its association with violence: A critical review. *Behavioral Sciences and the Law, 19,* 53–80.

Estroff, S. E., & Zimmer, C. (1994). Social networks, social support, and violence among persons with severe, persistent mental illness. In J. Monahan & H. J. Steadman (Eds.), *Violence and mental disorder: Developments in risk assessment* (pp. 259–295). Chicago, IL: University of Chicago Press.

Everett, S. A., & Price, J. H. (1995). Students' perceptions of violence in the public schools: The Metlife survey. *Journal of Adolescent Health, 17,* 345–352.

Farrington, D. P. (1989). Predictors, causes, and correlates of male youth violence. In M. Tonry & M. H. Moore (Eds.), *Crime and justice: A review of research: Vol. 24. Youth violence* (pp. 421–476). Chicago: University of Chicago Press.

FBI Uniform Crime Report. (2002, September). Online. Available from http://www.fbi.gov/ucr/ucr.htm.

Forth, A. E. (1995). *Psychopathy and young offenders: Prevalence, family background, and violence.* Unpublished report, Carleton University, Ottawa, Ontario.

Forth, A. E. (1996). Psychopathy in adolescent offenders: Assessment, family background, and violence. In D. J. Cooke, A. E. Forth, J. P. Newman, & R. D. Hare (Eds.), *Issues in criminological and legal psychology: No. 24, International perspectives on psychopathy* (pp. 42–44). Leicester, UK: British Psychological Society.

Forth, A. E., Hart, S. D., & Hare, R. D. (1990). Assessment of psychopathy in male young offenders. *Psychological Assessment, 2,* 342–344.

Forth, A. E., Kosson, D. S., & Hare, R. D. (2003). *Hare Psychopathy Checklist: Youth Version.* Multi-Health Systems Inc.

Forth, A. E., & Mailloux, D. L. (2000). Psychopathy in youth: What do we know? In C. B. Gacono (Ed.), *The clinical and forensic assessment of psychopathy: A practitioner's guide* (pp. 25–54). Mahwah, NJ: Lawrence Erlbaum Associates.

Gacono, C. B. (2000). Suggestions for implementation and use of the psychopathy checklists in forensic and clinical practice. In C. B. Gacono (Ed.), *The clinical and forensic assessment of psychopathy: A practitioner's guide* (pp. 175–201). Mahwah, NJ: Lawrence Erlbaum Associates.

Geiger, T. C., Zimmer-Gembeck, M., & Crick, N. R. (2004). The science of relational aggression: Can we guide intervention? In M. M. Moretti, C. L. Odgers, & M. A. Jackson (Eds.), *Girls and violence: Contributing factors and intervention principles* (pp. 7–25). New York, NY: Plenum Press/Kluwer Academic.

Grisso, T. (1998). *Forensic evaluation of juveniles.* Sarasota, FL: Professional Resource Press/Professional Resource Exchange, Inc.

Hare, R. D. (1991). *The Hare Psychopathy Checklist-Revised.* Toronto: Multi-Health Systems.

Hare, R. D., McPherson, L. E., & Forth, A. E. (1988). Male psychopaths and their criminal careers. *Journal of Consulting and Clinical Psychology, 56,* 710–714.

Harris, G. T., Rice, M. E., & Cormier, C. (1991). Psychopathy and violent recidivism. *Law and Human Behavior, 26,* 377–394.

Harris, G. T., Rice, M. E., & Quinsey, V. L. (1993). Violent recidivism of mentally disordered offenders: The development of a statistical prediction instrument. *Criminal Justice and Behavior, 20,* 315–335.

Kazdin, A. (2000). Adolescent development, mental disorders, and decision making of delinquent youths. In T. Grisso & R. G. Schwartz (Eds.), *Youth on trial: A developmental perspective on juvenile justice* (pp. 33–65). Chicago, IL: University of Chicago Press.

Kropp, R., Hart, S., Webster, C., & Eaves, D. (1999). *Manual for the spousal risk assessment guide* (3rd ed.). Toronto: Multi-Health Systems.

Lahey, B., Schwab-Stone, M., Goodman, S. H., Waldman, I. D., Canino, G., Rathouz, P. J., et al. (2000). Age and gender difference in oppositional behavior and conduct problems: A cross sectional household study of middle childhood and adolescence. *Journal of Abnormal Psychology, 109,* 488–503.

Lanctot, N. (2002, May). *Violence among females from adolescence to adulthood: Results from a longitudinal study.* Paper presented at the Vancouver Conference on Aggressive and Violent Girls, Vancouver, Canada.

Leschied, A., Cummings, A., Van Brunschot, M., Cunningham, A., & Saunders, A. (2000). *Female adolescent aggression: A review of the literature and the correlates of aggression* (User Report No. 2000–04). Ottawa: Solicitor General of Canada.

Levene, K. S., Augimeri, L. K., & Pepler, D. J. (2004). Linking identification and treatment of early risk factors for female delinquency. In M. M. Moretti, C. L. Odgers, & M. A. Jackson (Eds.), *Girls and violence: Contributing factors and intervention principles* (pp. 147–163). Plenum Press/Kluwer Academic.

Levene, K. S., Augimeri, L. K., Pepler, D. J., Walsh, M. M., Webster, C. D., & Koegl, C. J. (2001). *Early assessment risk list for girls (EARL-21G).* Toronto: Earlscourt Child and Family Centre.

Lewis, D. O., Yeager, C. A., Cobham-Portorreal, C. S., & Klein, N. (1991). A follow-up of female delinquents: Maternal contributions to the perpetuation of deviance. *Journal of the American Academy of Child and Adolescent Psychiatry, 30,* 197–201.

Lidz, C., Mulvey, E., & Gardner, W. (1993). The accuracy of predictions of violence to others. *Journal of American Medical Association, 269,* 1007–1011.

Lipsey, M. W., & Derzon, J. H. (1998). Predictors of violence and serious delinquency in adolescence and early adulthood: A synthesis of longitudinal research. In R. Loeber & D. P. Farrington (Eds.), *Serious and violent juvenile offenders: Risk factors and successful interventions* (pp. 86–105). Thousand Oaks, CA: Sage.

Loeber, R., & Keenan, K. (1994). Interaction between conduct disorder and its comorbid conditions: Effects of age and gender. *Clinical Psychology Review, 14,* 497–523.

Loeber, R., & Stouthamer-Loeber, M. (1998). Development of juvenile aggression and violence: Some common misconceptions and controversies. *American Psychologist, 53,* 242–259.

McNiel, D., & Binder, R. (1995). Correlates of accuracy in the assessment of psychiatric inpatients' risk of violence. *American Journal of Psychiatry, 152,* 901–906.

Moffitt, T. E. (1993). Adolescence-limited and life course-persistent antisocial behavior developmental taxonomy. *Psychological Review, 100,* 674–701.

Moffitt, T. E., Caspi, A., Rutter, M., & Silva, P. A. (2001). *Sex differences in antisocial behavior: Conduct disorder, delinquency, and violence in the Dunedin Longitudinal Study.* Cambridge: Cambridge University Press.

Monahan, J. (1996). Violence prediction: The past twenty years and the next twenty years. *Criminal Justice and Behavior, 23,* 107–120.

Monahan, J., & Steadman, H. (1994). *Violence and mental disorder: Developments in risk assessment.* Chicago: University of Chicago Press.

Monahan, J., Steadman, H., Silver, E., Appelbaum, P., Robbins, P., Mulvey, E., et al. (2001). *Rethinking risk assessment: The MacArthur study of mental disorder and violence.* New York, NY: Oxford University Press.

Moretti, M. M., DaSilva, K., & Holland, R. (2004). Aggression and violence from an attachment perspective: Gender issues and therapeutic implications. In M. Moretti, C. Odgers, & M. Jackson (Eds.), *Girls and aggression: Contributing factors and intervention principles* (pp. 41–56). New York, NY: Kluwer Academic Press.

Moretti, M. M., & Higgins, E. T. (1999). Own versus other standpoints in self-regulation: Developmental antecedents and functional consequences. *Review of General Psychology, 3,* 188–223.

Moretti, M. M., Holland, R., & McKay, S. (2001). Self-other representations and relational and overt aggression in adolescent girls and boys. *Behavioral Sciences and the Law, 19,* 109–126.

Moretti, M. M., & Odgers, C. L. (2002). Aggressive and violent girls: Prevalence, profiles and contributing factors. In R. R. Corrado, R. Roesch, S. D. Hart, & J. Gierowski (Eds.), *Multi-problem violent youth: A foundation for comparative research on needs, interventions and outcomes* (pp. 302–329). Amsterdam: IOS Press.

Moretti, M. M., Rein, A.S., & Wiebe, V. (1998). Relational self-regulation: Gender differences in risk for dysphoria. *Canadian Journal of Behavioral Science, 30,* 243–252.

Newhill, C. E., Mulvey, E. P., & Lidz, C. W. (1995). Characteristics of violence in the community by female patients seen in a psychiatric emergency service. *Psychiatric Services, 46,* 785–789.

Nicholls, T. L., Hemphill, J. F., Boer, D. A., Kropp, P. R., & Zapf, P. (2001). Offenders: Assessment and treatment in special populations. In R. Schuller & J. R. P. Ogloff (Eds.), *Introduction to psychology and law: Canadian perspectives* (pp. 248–282). Toronto, ON: University of Toronto Press.

Nicholls, T. L., Ogloff, J. R., & Ledwidge, B. (2003). *Inpatient aggression and clinicians' assessments of violence risk.* Paper present at the meeting of the American Psychology and Law Society and European Association of Psychology and Law, Edinburgh, Scotland.

Odgers, C. L., & Moretti, M. M. (2002). Aggressive and antisocial girls: Research update and future challenges. *International Journal of Forensic and Mental Health, 2,* 17–33.

Odgers, C. L., Moretti, M. M., & Pepler, D. J. (2003, April). *Antisocial and aggressive behavior in girls: Are we measuring the same construct?* Paper present at the International Association of Forensic Mental Health Services. Miami, FL.

Office of Juvenile Justice and Delinquency Prevention. (1995). *Guide for implementing the comprehensive strategy for serious, violent, and chronic juvenile offenders.* Washington, DC: Office of Juvenile Justice and Delinquency Prevention, Department of Justice.

Otto, R. (2000). Assessing and managing violence risk in outpatient settings. *Journal of Clinical Psychology, 56,* 1239–1262.

Otto, R. K., Greenstein, J. J., Johnson, M. K., & Friedman, R. M. (1992). Prevalence of mental disorders among youth in the juvenile justice system. In J. J. Cocozza (Ed.), *Responding to the mental health needs of youth in the juvenile justice system* (pp. 7–48). Seattle, WA: The National Coalition for the Mentally Ill in the Criminal Justice System.

Paquette, J. A., & Underwood, M. K. (1999). Gender differences in young adolescents' experiences of peer victimization: Social and physical aggression. *Merrill-Palmer Quarterly, 45,* 242–266.

Pepler, D. J., & Sedighdeilami, F. (1998). *Aggressive girls in Canada.* Ottawa: Applied Research Branch, Strategic Policy Human Resources Development Canada.

Pepler, D. J., Walsh, M. M., & Levene, K. S. (2004). Interventions for aggressive girls: Tailoring and measuring the fit. In M. Moretti, C. Odgers, & M. Jackson (Eds.), *Girls and aggression: Contributing factors and intervention principles* (pp. 131–145). New York, NY: Kluwer Academic Press.

Porter, G. (2000). *Detention and delinquency cases, 1988–1997.* Washington, DC: Office of Juvenile Justice and Delinquency Prevention.

Puzzanchera, C., Stahl, A. L., Finnegan, T. A., Tierney, N., & Snyder, H. N. (2003). *Juvenile Court Statistics 1998.* Washington, DC: Office of Juvenile Justice and Delinquency Prevention.

Reitsma-Street, M. (1999). Justice for Canadian girls: A 1990s update. *Canadian Journal of Criminology, 41,* 335–364.

Ridenour, T. A., Marchant, G. J., & Dean, R. S. (2001). Is the revised Psychopathy Checklist clinically useful for adolescents? *Journal of Psychoeducational Assessment, 19,* 227–238.

Rivera, B., & Widom, C. S. (1990). Childhood victimization and violent offending. *Violence and Victims, 5,* 19–35.

Robbins, P. C., Monahan, J., & Silver, E. (2003). Mental disorder, violence, and gender. *Law and Human Behavior, 27,* 561–571.

Robins, L. N. (1986). The consequence of conduct disorder in girls. In D. Olweus, J. Block, & M. Radke-Yarrow (Eds.), *Development of antisocial and prosocial behavior* (pp. 385–414). New York: Harcourt Brace Jovanovich.

Rosenbaum, J. L. (1989). Family dysfunction and female delinquency. *Crime and Delinquency, 35,* 31–44.

Rutherford, M. J., Cacciola, J. S., Alterman, A. I., & McKay, J. R. (1996). Reliability and validity of the revised Psychopathy Checklist in women methadone patients. *Assessment, 3,* 145–156.

Salekin, R. T., Rogers, R., & Sewell, K. W. (1997). Construct validity of psychopathy in a female offender sample: A multitrait-multimethod evaluation. *Journal of Abnormal Psychology, 106,* 576–585.

Salekin, R. T., Rogers, R., Ustad, K. L., & Sewell, K. W. (1998). Psychopathy and recidivism among female inmates. *Law and Human Behavior, 22,* 109–127.

Savioe, J. (2000). *Youth violent crime* (Statistics Canada, Catalogue no. 85-002-XPE, Vol. 19, no. 3). Ottawa: Canadian Centre for Justice Statistics.

Seagrave, D., & Grisso, T. (2002). Adolescent development and the measurement of juvenile psychopathy. *Law and Human Behavior, 26,* 219–239.

Shaw, M., & Dubois, S. (1995). *Understanding violence by women: A review of the literature.* Ottawa: Correctional Service of Canada.

Silverthorn, P., & Frick, P. (1999). Developmental pathways to antisocial behavior: The delayed-onset pathway in girls. *Development and Psychopathology, 11,* 101–126.

Snyder, H., & Sickmund, M. (1999). *Juvenile offenders and victims: 1999 National Report.* Washington, DC: Office of Juvenile Justice and Delinquency Prevention.

Sroufe, L. A. (1990). Considering normal and abnormal together: The essence of developmental psychopathology. *Development and Psychopathology, 2,* 335–347.

Statistics Canada. (2003, November 1). Canadian dimensions: Youth and adult crime rates. Retrieved November 1, 2003, from http://www.statcan.ca/english/Pgdb/justic.htm#vic.

Stattin, H., & Magnusson, D. (1989). The role of early aggressive behavior in the frequency, seriousness, and types of later crime. *Journal of Consulting and Clinical Psychology, 57,* 710–718.

Straus, M., & Gelles, R. J. (1986). Societal change and change in family violence from 1975 to 1985 as revealed by two national surveys *Journal of Marriage and the Family, 48,* 465–479.

Stueve, A., & Link, B. G. (1998). Gender differences in the relationship between mental illness and violence: Evidence from a community-based epidemiological study in Israel. *Social Psychiatry and Psychiatric Epidemiology, 33,* 61–67.

Teplin, L. A. (2003, April). *Psychiatric disorders in detained youth: Implication for treatment and public health policy.* Plenary address at the 3rd Annual International Association of Forensic Mental Health Services conference, Miami, FL.

Totten, M. (2000). *The special needs of females in Canada's youth justice system: An account of some young women's experiences and views.* Ottawa: Department of Justice Canada.

Tremblay, R. (1991). Aggression, prosocial behavior, and gender: Three magic words but no magic wands. In D. Pepler & K. Rubin (Eds.), *The Development & Treatment of Childhood Aggression* (pp. 71–79). Hillsdale: Lawrence Erlbaum.

Uggen, C., & Kruttschnitt, C. (1998). Crime in the breaking: Gender differences in desistance. *Law and Society Review, 32,* 339–366.

U.S. Bureau of Justice Statistics. (1997). *Privacy and juvenile justice records: A mid-decade status report.* Annapolis Junction, MD: Bureau of Justice.

U.S. Department of Health and Human Services. (2001). *Youth violence: A report of the Surgeon General.* Rockville, MD: U.S. Department of Health and Human Services, Centers for Disease Control and Prevention, National Center for Injury Prevention and Control; Substance Abuse and Mental Health Services Administration, Center for Mental Health Services; and National Institutes of Health, National Institute of Mental Health.

Viale-Val, G., & Sylvester, C. (1993). Female delinquency. In M. Sugar (Ed.), *Female adolescent development* (pp. 169–191). New York: Brunner-Mazel.

Vincent, G. M. (2002). *Investigating the legitimacy of adolescent psychopathy assessment: Contributions of item response theory.* Unpublished dissertation, Simon Fraser University.

Vincent, G. M., & Hart, S. (2002). Psychopathy and youth. In R. R. Corrado, R. Roesch, S. D. Hart, & J. Gierowski (Eds.), *Multi-problem violent youth: A foundation for comparative research on needs, interventions and outcomes* (pp. 302–329). Amsterdam: IOS Press.

Vitale, J. E., & Newman, J. P. (2001). Using the Psychopathy Checklist-Revised with female samples: Reliability, validity, and implications for clinical utility. *Clinical Psychology: Science and Practice, 8,* 117–132.

Webster, C. D. (1999, December). *Risk assessment and risk management with women offenders.* Report to the National Parole Board, Ottawa, Canada.

Webster, C. D., Douglas, K. S., Eaves, D., & Hart, S. D. (1997). *HCR-20 assessing risk for violence: Version 2.* Burnaby, British Columbia: Mental Health, Law, and Policy Institute, Simon Fraser University.

Webster, D. W., Gainer, P. S., & Champion, H. R. (1993). Weapon carrying among inner-city junior high school students: Defensive behavior versus aggressive delinquency. *American Journal of Public Health, 83,* 1604–1608.

Weiler, B. L., & Widom, C. S. (1996). Psychopathy and violent behaviour in abused and neglected young adults. *Criminal Behavior and Mental Health, 6,* 253–271.

White, H. R. (1992). Early problem behavior and later drug problems. *Journal of Research in Crime and Delinquency, 29,* 41–429.

Zoccolillo, M. (1993). Gender and the development of conduct disorder. *Development and Psychopathology, 5,* 65–78.

[20]

The Inherent Limits of Predicting School Violence

Edward P. Mulvey and Elizabeth Cauffman
University of Pittsburgh

The recent media hype over school shootings has led to demands for methods of identifying school shooters before they act. Despite the fact that schools remain one of the safest places for youths to be, schools are beginning to adopt identification systems to determine which students could be future killers. The methods used to accomplish this not only are unproven but are inherently limited in usefulness and often do more harm than good for both the children and the school setting. The authors' goals in the present article are to place school shootings in perspective relative to other risks of violence that children face and to provide a reasonable and scientifically defensible approach to improving the safety of schools.

School violence, having been dubbed a crisis, permeates the national consciousness and media outlets. This concern, moreover, has gone beyond simple statements and speculations. A heightened awareness of the potential tragedy of a school-related violent incident has prompted school administrators, law enforcement professionals, and mental health professionals to put into place methods for identifying and intervening proactively with potentially violent students and situations. Many communities have seen curriculum changes, the adoption of "safe school" policies, new weapons-reporting requirements, and increased efforts to refer problem students to mental health professionals. For example, several years ago, New York City spent over $28 million dollars on metal detectors (Kemper, 1993), and numerous school districts have implemented mandatory school uniform policies to cut down on gang identification (Stephens, 1998). After the shooting at Columbine High School, the principal distributed a memorandum requesting students to report on other students whom they deemed to be demonstrating maladaptive behavior (e.g., dressing oddly, being loners; Aronson, 2000). Currently, professionals seem open to trying just about anything to combat the perceived dangers of school violence.

In the midst of these activities, it is important to note that such policy changes are fueled primarily by graphic images of children killing and being killed at school rather than by actual numbers indicating an epidemic of violence. Data from the National Crime Victimization Survey and the School Crime Supplement, for example, suggest that there is virtually no difference between the rates of criminal victimization in schools in 1989 and the rates of victimization in 1995 (Snyder & Sickmund, 1999). Other examinations of the figures regarding adolescent deaths indicate that violent deaths are a rare event, with less than 1% of the homicides and suicides among school-age children occurring in or around school grounds (Kachur et al., 1996). Moreover, the rate of violent crimes committed by juveniles remains low during the school day, but it spikes at the close of the school day and declines throughout the evening hours (Snyder & Sickmund, 1999), indicating that school hours are probably the safest time of the day for adolescents.

Yet, somehow, the images of the violence at Columbine, Padukah, and Santee are more persistent than the realities of the situations connected with the 99% of school-age victims who meet their fate when school is not in session. That students are very unlikely to be assaulted in the school setting and that urban adolescents are safer in their schools than on their way to or from school do not emerge as key points in most discussions of school violence. As Joseph Stalin, of all people, noted in another time, "A single death is a tragedy, a million deaths is a statistic" (as quoted in Bartlett, 1980, p. 766). Unfortunately, there now may have been enough tragedies to precipitate action.

An attractive strategy for addressing school violence is to increase efforts at early detection of and intervention with adolescents who are likely to commit these horrible acts. One of the most common reactions to the adolescents who opened fire in Padukah, Columbine, or Santee is to ask, "How could someone not have known that this adolescent was in trouble?" The problem, of course, is that it is not often clear exactly what to look for, who should have looked for it, or what should have been done if someone had seen something. Indeed, in postmortems of these situations, one often picks up signs of distress or despair in these adolescents, but one is rarely sure if the level or types of indicators found would have been enough to make even a vigilant and caring adult do something markedly different than what was done. After all, for every killer youth, there

---

Edward P. Mulvey and Elizabeth Cauffman, Law and Psychiatry Program, Western Psychiatric Institute and Clinic, University of Pittsburgh.

Preparation of this article was supported by the John D. and Catherine T. MacArthur Foundation Research Network on Adolescent Development and Juvenile Justice. This article was presented as part of a symposium at the 1999 Annual Meeting of the American Society of Criminology held on November 18, 1999, in Toronto, Ontario, Canada.

Correspondence concerning this article should be addressed to Edward P. Mulvey, Law and Psychiatry Program, Western Psychiatric Institute and Clinic, University of Pittsburgh, 3811 O'Hara Street, Pittsburgh, PA 15213. Electronic mail may be sent to mulveyep@msx.upmc.edu.

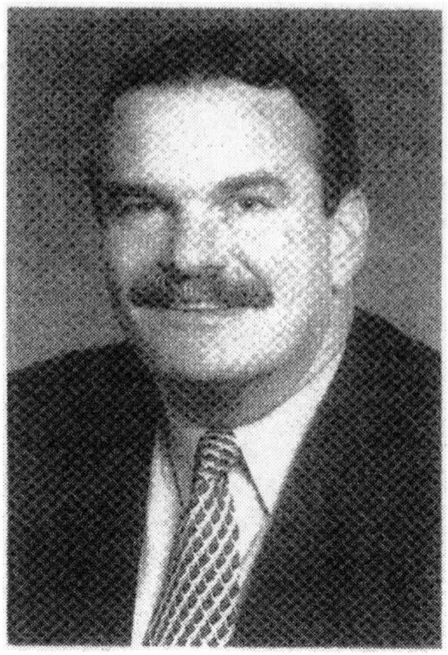

Edward P. Mulvey

are many others with the same behaviors or attitudes who never come close to killing their classmates.

The inability to see clear markers of trouble in these cases should reveal something. It should make clear the daunting nature of the identification task taken on by many school administrators and mental health professionals. Identification of adolescents who are at high risk for committing serious, public acts of violence poses many inherent challenges; considering these can lead psychologists to think more realistically about where to direct their energies for interventions for school violence.

The Characteristics of Adolescent Violence and the Identification Process

The first challenge facing any system for identifying adolescents who could commit serious acts of violence in school is that the behavior being predicted is a rare event. There are severe restrictions on the ability of any predictive strategy (even if reasonably accurate) to identify true positives for a low base-rate behavior without also identifying a large number of false positives (Hart, Webster, & Menzies, 1993; Meehl, 1954). Identification of large numbers of false positives is not a problem if such identification causes no harm (Morris & Miller, 1985), but the ratio of true positives to false positives matters greatly if all identified individuals are stigmatized or if their opportunities are limited. One way to avoid the low base-rate problem is to expand the definition of the violent outcome being predicted, effectively converting many false positives into true positives. If one includes bullying, threats, and fistfights in the definition of school violence, the base rate increases dramatically, and the ability to predict who might be involved in these activities may increase. According to the Centers for Disease Controls and Prevention's 1997 Youth Risk Behavior Surveillance System, 37% of high school students said they had been in a physical fight during the past school year (Centers for Disease Control and Prevention, 1997); approximately 80% of youths have indicated that they engage in some form of bullying behavior such as pushing, teasing, or threatening others (Bosworth, Espelage, & Simon, 1999). With this expanded definition, however, comes a blurring of the behavior being examined and a good chance that the processes behind these behaviors will become more heterogeneous. Taken to extremes, this approach amounts to dealing with a problem that is hard to solve by choosing to solve a different problem. If the identified problems are too broadly defined, the intervention strategy is reduced to meeting the needs of the general pool of troubled adolescents found in any school, and the hard-to-solve problem of identifying potentially violent adolescents is dealt with by choosing to solve the problem of disruptive students.

The second major obstacle to identifying students who are likely to be involved in serious school violence is that the event being predicted is usually embedded in a social and transactional sequence of events. One thing that is clear about youth violence in general and seemingly about many of the recent tragedies is that this behavior has a heavy social component (Staub & Rosenthal, 1994). Youths who engage in criminal behavior, both violent and nonviolent, are not usually loners. For example, 60% of juvenile offenders who committed assault were with peers at the time, and 90% of juvenile offenders who committed robbery were with adolescent peers (Zimring, 1981, 1998). Moreover, youths who are aggressive not only seek each other out but also form coercive cliques (Cairns, Cairns, Neckerman, Gest, & Gariepy, 1988; Coie & Dodge, 1998), which in turn provide a training ground for subsequent delinquent behaviors (Parker & Asher, 1987; Patterson, Reid, & Dishion, 1992). Predictably, then, it appears that for both lethal and nonlethal incidents, school violence is more likely to occur in larger rather than smaller schools and in "unowned" areas such as hallways, dining areas, and parking lots (Astor, Meyer, & Behre, 1999). Furthermore, violent events in the schools are part of a chain of actions and reactions, often among numerous other individuals (e.g., taunting peers, disinterested girlfriends or boyfriends, uninterested parents; see Fagan & Wilkinson, 1998), and bystanders appear to be a critical component of the escalation of disputes into violence (Decker, 1996; Tedeschi & Felson, 1994). Previous research has shown that these events do not occur in a vacuum and that there are numerous rationales for and pathways to the violent act. Identification based only on the characteristics of an individual neglects these highly salient social and transactional aspects of school violence.

The third major obstacle to the task of identification is that the individuals being assessed are adolescents whose characters are often not yet fully formed. Research in the areas of physical development (Buchanan, Eccles, & Becker, 1992), psychosocial development (Cauffman & Steinberg, 2000; Steinberg & Cauffman, 1996), and even

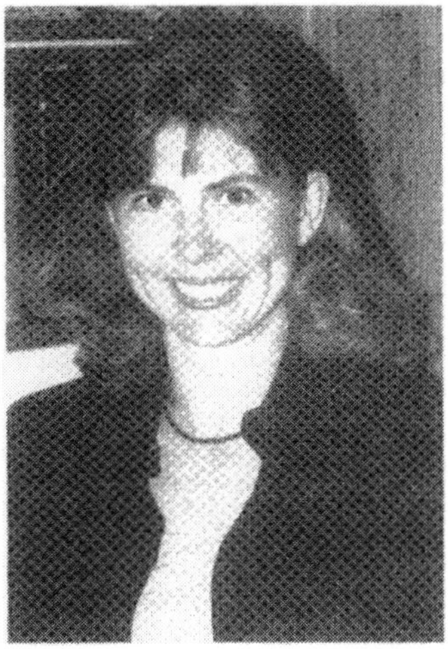

Elizabeth Cauffman

brain development (Baird et al., 1999; Giedd et al., 1999; Sowell, Thompson, Holmes, Jernigan, & Toga, 1999) suggests that adolescents are still changing and that their characters are not yet fully formed. Assessing adolescents, therefore, presents the formidable challenge of trying to capture a rapidly changing process with few trustworthy markers. Diagnostic systems for adolescents are not as well developed as those for adult disorders, many disorders do not emerge clearly until young adulthood, and the diagnostic tools used to assess adults are often of questionable value when applied to adolescents. Despite these limitations, adult diagnoses or concepts periodically have been applied to children, adolescents, or both without taking into account important developmental factors that may affect the applicability or validity of these constructs (for a review, see Achenbach, 1995). For example, some characteristics that are viewed as risk factors for psychopathy among adults (e.g., impulsivity, little concern for future consequences) are common and transitory aspects of normal adolescent development and may be easily misinterpreted when using standard approaches (Edens, Skeem, Cruise, & Cauffman, 2001). These realities make assessments of adolescents by mental health professionals using tools designed for adults difficult to interpret meaningfully.

Finally, it is not clear what interventions are likely to work with violence-prone adolescents. Part of the reason for identifying an adolescent who is at high risk for serious violence is to prevent the occurrence of an incident. This can be done either by imposing restrictions on the adolescent (e.g., enforcing some schedule or activity restrictions) or by altering the processes within the adolescent or in his or her life that might be contributing to the violence (e.g., enrolling the adolescent in an anger-management group). Unfortunately, most of the single-focus interventions for violent adolescents have demonstrated limited effectiveness (McCord, Widom, & Crowell, 2001; U.S. Department of Health and Human Services, 2001), and the most successful interventions with antisocial adolescents work in multiple community settings and focus on building specific skills (Lipsey & Wilson, 1998). Schools can certainly provide valuable prevention programs, such as social skills training, but these settings are not generally well equipped to deliver individualized, broadly based services to small numbers of identified students.

Recasting the Problem as Risk Management

This dismal picture does not justify inaction. The limits of identification and intervention are real and substantial, but they should be used to inform people about reasonable strategies rather than discourage them from facing the problem. They highlight the need for professionals to take a realistic view of what might be accomplished through the development of early identification systems and to focus planning and programming in a way that increases the likelihood of success.

Perhaps the first step is to approach the problem as one of ongoing risk assessment rather than prediction. A great deal can be learned in this regard from the progress that has been made over the past 20 years regarding management of violence in mentally ill adults (see Borum, 1996; Otto, 1992). In this area, as in the area of school violence, the goal is to predict and prevent rare, socially embedded violence for which little effective intervention technology exists. Trends in preventing violence in mentally ill adults, however, have been moving away from framing the problem as one of predicting an event and toward the approach of managing risk (Heilbrun, 1997). Ongoing risk assessment and management have replaced prediction of dangerousness, a shift with subtle but important implications for policy, practice, and research (Skeem & Mulvey, in press).

This new approach recognizes that violence risk is a dynamic, rather than static, process. Although it is possible to sort individuals into high- and low-risk groups generally, the task of managing risk effectively requires an ongoing evaluation of the factors that increase or decrease the likelihood of a violent incident in individuals at relatively high risk already (Monahan & Steadman, 1996; Mulvey & Lidz, 1998). A risk management approach thus starts out much like a more traditional predictive strategy by using available indicators of generalized risk for adolescents and some structured data-collection scheme to sort individuals into a high- or low-risk status. This identification process, however, is only the first step toward avoiding violent incidents. The next step is to monitor the ongoing changes in the lives of these individuals for transitions or turning points that may further increase the likelihood of violence.

Framing the problem in this way might well change the focus of school violence programs. Rather than developing more elaborate and potentially discriminatory or arbitrary approaches to choosing those who might be at highest risk, researchers could direct more resources into ongoing involvement with the group of individuals who are clearly high risk. The natural reaction in the face of disastrous violence in schools is to look for a system that can pick out the people who may react similarly in the future. The reality of prediction, however, is that this is a largely futile task. The fuzziness of the categories, the base rate of the behavior being predicted, and the time frame to which the prediction applies must always compromise any identification scheme for schoolyard killers. Therefore, rather than being used to make a marginal improvement in a sorting algorithm to identify troubled students, resources may well be better spent monitoring the activities of those students who would be identified under just about any risk-assessment method.

Need for a Focus on School Environment

Although easier to do than accurately modeling individual behavior using a violence-prediction machine, keeping abreast of the ongoing activities of troubled and troubling adolescents is no easy feat. Now, as always, the best source of information about the activities of students in a school is other students. A long line of research has demonstrated that students are well aware of the problem children in their own classrooms (for a review, see Hartup, 1992). For example, since the advent of sociometric research in 1934, researchers have been able to identify which youths are liked or disliked by their peers, as well as future delinquent behaviors among youths (Rubin, Bukowski, & Parker, 1998). Ignoring this potentially rich source of information in favor of structured psychological assessment places unwarranted faith in the powers of individual assessment. Peers and teachers who talk with problem students can often provide the most useful information about when such students are in trouble.

For such information to flow from students to administrators requires an atmosphere where sharing in good faith is respected and honored. Giving information about the problems that another student is having or about threats or scary activities going on in a school environment can occur only if students feel that they are (and will remain) safe and that a reasoned response will result from their reporting. Getting accurate information about the activities of high-risk students on an ongoing basis, therefore, rests heavily on establishing and maintaining a supportive school environment.

Ironically, many schools appear to be taking the opposite approach. Instead of working to foster a sense of belonging, schools are implementing zero-tolerance policies that virtually guarantee an unreasoned response to any reported problem. For example, when a student is expelled or suspended for carrying aspirin (in violation of a zero-tolerance drug policy), that student is likely to hold the school administration in contempt. It is also likely that other students will withhold information from the administration to avoid such disproportionate punishments. This change in school atmosphere is all too real. For example, in a *New York Times* op-ed piece written by a high school student from Littleton, Colorado, the student remarked as follows:

> High school students in Littleton now have a new excuse to get out of class for a few extra minutes: the lockdown drill. . . . Apart from the lockdown drills, there have been few changes in security procedures. The greatest change has been the increase of paranoia. For example, a few weeks after the shooting I was working on a graph assignment with a friend. We arranged the points on the graph to spell out a humorous but inappropriate message. A month earlier, my friend would have said, "The teacher's going to be mad." This time he said, "If we turn this in, we'll be expelled." There's the difference. (Black, 2001, p. A23)

Empirical evidence, meanwhile, seems to support the contention that promoting healthy relationships and environments is more effective for reducing school misconduct and crime than instituting punitive penalties (Nettles, Mucherah, & Jones, 2000). For example, a study of 7th-, 8th-, and 9th-grade students found that commitment to school and belief in the fairness and consistent enforcement of school rules are the most important elements in reducing school crime (Jenkins, 1997). Similarly, the National Longitudinal Study of Adolescent Health found that among a nationally representative sample of 7th–12th graders, attachment to family and school served as protective factors against violence (Franke, 2000), a result consistent with earlier research indicating that adolescents with a low commitment to school are at increased risk of engaging in violent behavior (Cernkovich & Giordano, 1992; Farrington, 1991). Also, a study of school-based violence-prevention interventions found that between 1993 and 1997, elementary schools that focused on the broader school environment appeared successful in changing violence-related behavior (Howard, Flora, & Griffin, 1999). Finally, the most powerful predictor of adolescent well-being is a feeling of connection to school (Resnick et al., 1997), and students who feel close to others, fairly treated, and vested in school are less likely to engage in risky behaviors than those who do not (Resnick et al., 1997). Each of these studies suggests that a key factor in preventing school violence is students' positive relations to their school environments. Students who are committed to school, feel that they belong, and trust the administration are less likely to commit violent acts than those who are uninvolved, alienated, or distrustful.

Conclusion

In sum, preventing violent incidents in school does not require either more sophisticated methods for assessing students individually or a magical, uniform method for intervening with them for a short while after they have been identified. It seems instead to rest largely on developing a positive and supportive organizational climate in a school. A crucial component of any school violence program is thus a school environment where ongoing activities and problems of students are discussed, rather than tallied with structured assessment instruments. Such an environment promotes ongoing risk management, which can be achieved only with the support and involvement of those closest to the indicators of trouble.

It is also worth noting that school violence is rarely just about what happens in school. Gun-related violence outside the school is a better predictor of weapon-related victimization at or during travel to and from school than is the dangerousness of the school environment itself (Sheley, McGee, & Wright, 1995), and neighborhood conditions such as poverty, population turnover, and crime rates are the strongest predictors of school violence (Laub & Lauritsen, 1998). Community incidents are carried into the school environment, just as the effects of the school day's events linger on after dismissal.

Although connecting schools with families and communities is often given as a mantra for school reform, it is worth chanting once more when discussing interventions to prevent school violence. The indicators of trouble for violence-prone adolescents can come from a variety of sources, and often, the only way one can obtain a clear picture of what is moving an adolescent toward violence is by looking at the adolescent's world from the broadest perspective. Strategies designed to address school violence must recognize the interdependence of school violence with neighborhood and family conditions.

This call for an emphasis on organizational issues for the prevention of school violence reflects a recognition that there will never be a technology that matches the desire to find and control the uncontrollable events of life. Violence of the sort seen recently in schools is horrific and compels society to reestablish order in the face of chaos. Unfortunately, the technology of predicting rare events will always be a poor substitute for solid human relations and sound organizational management. Establishing school environments where students feel connected and trusted will build the critical link between those who often know when trouble is brewing and those who can act to prevent it.

REFERENCES

Achenbach, T. M. (1995). Developmental issues in assessment, taxonomy, and diagnosis of child and adolescent psychopathology. In D. Cicchetti & D. J. Cohen (Eds.), *Developmental psychopathology, Vol. 1: Theory and methods* (pp. 57–80). New York: Wiley.

Aronson, E. (2000). *Nobody left to hate: Teach compassion after Columbine.* New York: Worth.

Astor, R., Meyer, H., & Behre, W. (1999). Unowned places and times: Maps and interviews about violence in high schools. *American Educational Research Journal, 36,* 3–42.

Baird, A., Gruber, S., Fein, D., Maas, L., Steingard, R., Renshaw, P., Cohen, B., & Yurgelun-Todd, D. (1999). Functional magnetic resonance imaging of facial affect recognition in children and adolescents. *Journal of the American Academy of Child and Adolescent Psychiatry, 38,* 195–199.

Bartlett, J. (1980). *Bartlett's familiar quotations* (15th ed.). Boston: Little, Brown.

Black, N. (2001, March 8). After a shooting. *The New York Times,* p. A23.

Borum, R. (1996). Improving the clinical practice of violence risk assessment: Technology, guidelines, and training. *American Psychologist, 51,* 945–948.

Bosworth, K., Espelage, D., & Simon, T. (1999). Factors associated with bullying behavior in middle school students. *Journal of Early Adolescence, 19,* 341–362.

Buchanan, C. M., Eccles, J. S., & Becker, J. B. (1992). Are adolescents victims of raging hormones? Evidence for activational effects of hormones on moods and behavior at adolescence. *Psychological Bulletin, 111,* 62–107.

Cairns, R., Cairns, B., Neckerman, H., Gest, S., & Gariepy, J. (1988). Social networks and aggressive behavior: Peer support or peer rejection? *Developmental Psychology, 24,* 815–823.

Cauffman, E., & Steinberg, L. (2000). (Im)maturity of judgment in adolescence: Why adolescents may be less culpable than adults. *Behavioral Sciences and the Law, 18,* 741–760.

Centers for Disease Control and Prevention. (1997). Rates of homicide, suicide, and firearm-related death among children—26 industrialized countries. *Morbidity and Mortality Weekly Report, 46,* 101–105.

Cernkovich, S. A., & Giordano, P. C. (1992). School bonding, race, and delinquency. *Criminology, 31,* 261–291.

Coie, J., & Dodge, K. (1998). Aggression and antisocial behavior. In W. Damon & N. Eisenberg (Eds.), *Handbook of child psychology* (pp. 779–862). New York: Wiley.

Decker, S. (1996). Reconstructing homicide events: The role of witnesses in fatal encounters. *Journal of Criminal Justice, 23,* 439–450.

Edens, J., Skeem, J., Cruise, K., & Cauffman, E. (2001). The assessment of juvenile psychopathy and its association with violence: A critical review. *Behavioral Sciences and the Law, 19,* 53–80.

Fagan, J., & Wilkinson, D. (1998). Social contexts and functions of adolescent violence. In D. Elliott, B. Hamburg, & K. Williams (Eds.), *Violence in American schools* (pp. 55–93). New York: Cambridge University Press.

Farrington, D. (1991). Childhood aggression and adult violence: Early precursors and later life outcomes. In D. Pepper & K. Rubin (Eds.), *The development and treatment of childhood aggression* (pp. 5–29). Hillsdale, NJ: Erlbaum.

Franke, T. (2000). The role of attachment as a protective factor in adolescent violent behavior. *Adolescent and Family Health, 1,* 40–51.

Giedd, J., Blumenthal, J., Jeffries, N., Castellanos, F., Liu, H., Zijdenbos, A., Paus, T., Evans, A., & Rapoport, J. (1999). Brain development during childhood and adolescence: A longitudinal MRI study. *Nature Neuroscience, 2,* 861–863.

Hart, S. D., Webster, C. D., & Menzies, R. J. (1993). A note on portraying the accuracy of violence predictions. *Law and Human Behavior, 17,* 695–700.

Hartup, W. (1992). Peer relations in early and middle childhood. In V. B. Van Hasselt & M. Hersen (Eds.), *Handbook of social development: A lifespan perspective* (pp. 257–281). New York: Plenum.

Heilbrun, K. (1997). Prediction versus management models relevant to risk assessment: The importance of legal decision-making context. *Law and Human Behavior, 21,* 347–359.

Howard, K., Flora, J., & Griffin, M. (1999). Violence-prevention programs in schools: State of the science and implications for future research. *Applied and Preventive Psychology, 8,* 197–215.

Jenkins, P. (1997). School delinquency and the school social bond. *Journal of Research in Crime and Delinquency, 34,* 337–367.

Kachur, S. P., Stennies, G., Powell, K., Modzeleski, W., Stephens, R., Murphy, R., Kresnow, M., Sleet, D., & Lowry, R. (1996). School-associated deaths in the United States, 1992–1994. *JAMA, 275,* 1729–1733.

Kemper, P. (1993, Fall). Disarming youth. *California School Boards Journal,* 25–33.

Laub, J., & Lauritsen, J. (1998). The interdependence of school violence with neighborhood and family conditions. In D. Elliott, B. Hamburg, & K. Williams (Eds.), *Violence in American schools* (pp. 55–93). New York: Cambridge University Press.

Lipsey, M., & Wilson, D. (1998). Effective intervention for serious juvenile offenders: A synthesis of research. In R. Loeber & D. Farrington (Eds.), *Serious and violent juvenile offenders: Risk factors and successful interventions* (pp. 313–345). Thousand Oaks, CA: Sage.

McCord, J., Widom, C. S., & Crowell, N. A. (Eds.). (2001). *Juvenile crime, juvenile justice.* Washington, DC: National Academy Press.

Meehl, P. E. (1954). *Clinical versus statistical prediction: A theoretical analysis and a review of the evidence.* Minneapolis: University of Minnesota Press.

Monahan, J., & Steadman, H. (1996). Violent storms and violent people: How meteorology can inform risk communication in mental health law. *American Psychologist, 51,* 931–938.

Morris, N., & Miller, M. (1985). Predictions of dangerousness. In M. Tonry & N. Morris (Eds.), *Crime and justice: An annual review of research* (Vol. 6, pp. 1–50). Chicago: University of Chicago Press.

Mulvey, E. P., & Lidz, C. W. (1998). The clinical prediction of violence as a conditional judgment. *Social Psychiatry and Psychiatric Epidemiology, 33,* 107–113.

Nettles, S., Mucherah, W., & Jones, D. (2000). Understanding resilience: The role of social resources. *Journal of Education for Students Placed at Risk, 5,* 47–60.

Otto, R. K. (1992). Prediction of dangerous behavior: A review and analysis of "second-generation" research. *Forensic Reports, 5,* 103–133.

Parker, J., & Asher, S. (1987). Peer relations and later personal adjustment: Are low-accepted children at risk? *Psychological Bulletin, 102,* 357–389.

Patterson, G., Reid, J., & Dishion, T. (1992). *Antisocial boys.* Eugene, OR: Castalia.

Resnick, M., Bearman, P., Blum, R., Bauman, K., Harris, K., Jones, J., Tabor, J., Beuhring, T., Sieving, R., Shew, M., Ireland, M., Bearinger, L., & Udry, R. (1997). Protecting adolescents from harm: Findings from the National Longitudinal Study on Adolescent Health. *JAMA, 278,* 823–832.

Rubin, K., Bukowski, W., & Parker, J. (1998). Peer interactions, relationships, and groups. In W. Damon & N. Eisenberg (Eds.), *Handbook of child psychology* (pp. 619–700). New York: Wiley.

Sheley, J., McGee, Z., & Wright, J. (1995). Gun-related violence in and around inner-city schools. *American Journal of Diseases of Children, 146,* 677–682.

Skeem, J., & Mulvey, E. (in press). Assessing the violence potential of mentally disordered offenders being treated in the community. In A. Buchanan (Ed.), *Care of the mentally disordered offender in the community.* Oxford, England: Oxford University Press.

Snyder, H., & Sickmund, M. (1999). *Juvenile offenders and victims: 1999 national report.* Washington, DC: Office of Juvenile Justice and Delinquency Prevention.

Sowell, E., Thompson, P., Holmes, C., Jernigan, T., & Toga, A. (1999). In vivo evidence for post-adolescent brain maturation in frontal and striatal regions. *Nature Neuroscience, 2,* 859–861.

Staub, E., & Rosenthal, L. (1994). Mob violence: Cultural–societal sources, instigators, group processes, and participants. In L. Eron & J. Gentry (Eds.), *Reason to hope: A psychosocial perspective on violence and youth* (pp. 281–313). Washington, DC: American Psychological Association.

Steinberg, L., & Cauffman, E. (1996). Maturity of judgment in adolescence: Psychosocial factors in adolescent decision making. *Law and Human Behavior, 20,* 249–272.

Stephens, R. (1998). Safe school planning. In D. Elliott, B. Hamburg, & K. Williams (Eds.), *Violence in American schools* (pp. 253–289). New York: Cambridge University Press.

Tedeschi, J., & Felson, R. (1994). *Violence, aggression, and coercive actions.* Washington, DC: American Psychological Association.

U.S. Department of Health and Human Services. (2001). *Youth violence: A report of the Surgeon General.* Washington, DC: Author.

Zimring, F. (1981). Kids, groups, and crime: Some implications of a well-known secret. *Journal of Criminal Law and Criminology, 72,* 867.

Zimring, F. (1998). *American youth violence.* New York: Oxford University Press.

[21]

Juveniles' Competence to Stand Trial: A Comparison of Adolescents' and Adults' Capacities as Trial Defendants

Thomas Grisso,[1,9] Laurence Steinberg,[2] Jennifer Woolard,[3] Elizabeth Cauffman,[4] Elizabeth Scott,[5] Sandra Graham,[6] Fran Lexcen,[1] N. Dickon Reppucci,[7] and Robert Schwartz[8]

Abilities associated with adjudicative competence were assessed among 927 adolescents in juvenile detention facilities and community settings. Adolescents' abilities were compared to those of 466 young adults in jails and in the community. Participants at 4 locations across the United States completed a standardized measure of abilities relevant for competence to stand trial (the MacArthur Competence Assessment Tool—Criminal Adjudication*) as well as a new procedure for assessing psychosocial influences on legal decisions often required of defendants (*MacArthur Judgment Evaluation*). Youths aged 15 and younger performed more poorly than young adults, with a greater proportion manifesting a level of impairment consistent with that of persons found incompetent to stand trial. Adolescents also tended more often than young adults to make choices (e.g., about plea agreements) that reflected compliance with authority, as well as influences of psychosocial immaturity. Implications of these results for policy and practice are discussed, with an emphasis on the development of legal standards that recognize immaturity as a potential predicate of incompetence to stand trial.*

KEY WORDS: adolescence; legal competence; delinquency; juvenile justice.

During the 1990s, nationwide legal reforms lowered the age at which youths could be tried in adult criminal court and expanded the range of young offenders subject to adult adjudication and punishment (Snyder & Sickmund, 1999); at the same time, the severity of penalties available to the juvenile court increased (Torbet et al., 1996).

[1]University of Massachusetts Medical School, Worcester, Massachusetts.
[2]Department of Psychology, Temple University, Philadelphia, Pennsylvania.
[3]Department of Psychology, Georgetown University, Washington, DC.
[4]Western Psychiatric Institute and Clinic, University of Pittsburgh, Pittsburgh, Pennsylvania.
[5]School of Law, University of Virginia, Charlottesville, Virginia.
[6]Graduate School of Education and Information Studies, University of California – Los Angeles, Los Angeles, California.
[7]Department of Psychology, University of Virginia, Charlottesville, Virginia.
[8]Juvenile Law Center, Philadelphia, Pennsylvania.
[9]To whom correspondence should be addressed at Department of Psychiatry, University of Massachusetts Medical School, 55 Lake Avenue North, Worcester, Massachusetts 01655.

These legal developments raise an important issue that has received surprisingly little attention: whether youths charged with crimes have the developmental capacities needed to participate effectively in their trials.

It is well established that a criminal proceeding meets the constitutional requirements of due process only when the defendant is competent to stand trial, which includes capacities to assist counsel and to understand the nature of the proceeding sufficiently to participate in it and make decisions about rights afforded all defendants (*Dusky v. U.S.*, 1960; *Godinez v. Moran*, 1993). Although courts and legislatures in some states have determined that youths adjudicated in juvenile and criminal courts must be competent to stand trial, the conventional standard that has been applied focuses on mental illness and disability. In general, there has been little recognition that youths in criminal court may be incompetent because of developmental immaturity (Bonnie & Grisso, 2000; Redding & Frost, 2002).

Until now, little meaningful data have been available regarding the capacities of adolescents relevant for adjudicative competence. A few studies have examined youths' understanding of the nature of trials and trial procedures (for reviews, see Grisso, 1997, 2000; Mumley, Tillbrook, & Grisso, in press), but typically they have included small sample sizes, measures that are seriously limited in content or known reliability, or no comparison between the capacities of adolescents and adults. Similarly, exploratory studies have found significant age-related increases in youths' performance on tasks that parallel decisions that defendants are expected to make (Abramovitch, Peterson-Badali, & Rohan, 1995; Peterson-Badali & Abramovitch, 1993; Peterson-Badali, Abramovitch, & Duda, 1997), but without comparison to adults.

Information about youths' competence to stand trial (CST) is needed for several reasons. First, states need guidance for the development of meaningful laws in this area. The doctrine regulating CST has focused on adult criminal defendants impaired by mental illness and mental retardation. Yet basic research on cognitive and psychosocial development suggests that some youths will manifest deficits in legally relevant abilities similar to deficits seen in adults with mental disabilities, but for reasons of immaturity rather than mental disorder (see generally Grisso & Schwartz, 2000). If there were empirical evidence for this, it would suggest that the criminal law should take immaturity into consideration when evaluating the adjudicative competence of youths in criminal court.

Second, practitioners need information about youths' capacities as trial defendants, including their CST. Prosecutors and defense attorneys must make case-by-case decisions about whether to raise this issue. Mental health professionals who are asked to perform evaluations of youths' CST need guidance regarding the potential implications of youths' developmental status for assessing deficits in the legally relevant abilities. This may require attention to different constructs (immaturity, not only disorder) and a different logic (e.g., the "achievement" rather than "restoration" of competence among those found incompetent) than in adult CST evaluations prompted by putative mental illnesses. Finally, judges need guidance in interpreting the law to protect young defendants who may be incompetent, especially in their abilities to make decisions to waive important rights in the context of their potentially immature perspectives regarding the implications of their choices.

Past analyses of the legal concept of adjudicative competence have outlined the specific functional abilities about which the law is concerned in competence cases (Grisso, 2002), as well as their classification into broader psycholegal constructs (e.g., Understanding, Reasoning, Appreciation; see Grisso & Appelbaum, 1998; Hoge et al., 1997; Otto et al., 1998; Poythress et al., 1999). These abilities focus on the fundamental aspects of adjudicative competence, or what Bonnie (1992, 1993) called "competence to proceed": a basic comprehension of the purpose and nature of the trial process (Understanding), the capacity to provide relevant information to counsel and to process information (Reasoning), and the ability to apply information to one's own situation in a manner that is neither distorted nor irrational (Appreciation).

Some studies have suggested that preadolescents have less knowledge of trials and legal concepts than do older adolescents (e.g., Peterson-Badali et al., 1997) or adults (Grisso, 1981). General developmental research on adolescents' cognitive abilities (see Keating, 1990), however, would not lead us to expect substantial differences between "average" adolescents and adults in their ability to grasp everyday factual or conceptual information that is provided to them, or their ability to cognitively process it to make decisions. In addition, results of basic developmental research on youths' cognitive abilities do not necessarily generalize to abilities to deal specifically with trial-related tasks of comprehension and information processing, and to the abilities of the population of juveniles facing adjudication for alleged offenses, many of whom are of below-average intelligence. A few studies have employed brief, specialized "competency screening" measures (e.g., Cooper, 1997) to assess the abilities of youths in this relevant population, but these measures typically focus on "understanding," failing to assess the wider range of abilities associated with trial competence.

Bonnie (1992, 1993) suggested that, in addition to defendants' basic understanding and reasoning abilities, their "decisional competence" may be significant in cases in which defendants must make important decisions about the waiver of constitutional rights. A potentially important difference between adolescents and adults in this regard involves maturity of judgment. Differences between adolescents and adults not only are cognitive, but also involve aspects of psychosocial maturation that include progress toward greater future orientation, better risk perception, and less susceptibility to peer influence. Several authors have hypothesized that these developmental factors could result in differences between adolescents' and adults' decision making about important rights in the adjudicative process (Cauffman & Steinberg, 2000; Scott, 1992; Scott, Reppucci, & Woolard, 1995; Steinberg & Cauffman, 1996).

Current law does not include these developmental factors as relevant when considering a defendant's adjudicative competence. For example, when making a decision about waiver of important rights, defendants are free to place a primary value on their immediate gratification at the expense of their future welfare, or to opt to please their friends rather than act in their best interests, as long as they adequately understand and grasp the consequences of their choices. But if adolescents place a relatively higher value on immediate gratification than do adults as a consequence of their developmental immaturity, they may make different legal decisions than they themselves would make in their adult years. Although psychosocial immaturity is not addressed in the formal legal construct of competence to stand trial, it needs to be investigated in this context to provide a comprehensive account of adolescents' capacities to participate in the trial process.

In this study, we used two tools to examine the two types of capacities outlined previously. The *MacArthur Competence Assessment Tool–Criminal Adjudication* (MacCAT-CA) focuses primarily on the formal functional abilities typically associated with the legal construct of CST (Bonnie's "competence to proceed"). In a large-scale study, the instrument manifested meaningful differences among adult defendants with and without findings of incompetence to stand trial (Otto et al., 1998), and a MacCAT-CA manual subsequently was published with adult norms (Poythress et al., 1999). Although the instrument is now widely known among forensic mental health professionals, the extent of its use is not known, and its recent publication has not yet produced additional research findings. There are no reports of its use with youths.

In contrast to the MacCAT-CA, the *MacArthur Judgment Evaluation* (MacJEN) was designed for this study as a research tool to examine the question of immaturity of judgment, especially the potential relation between immaturity and choices that defendants make in the course of adjudication. As described later, the MacJEN uses three vignettes and structured interview questions with objective categories of responses. It allows for examination of differences in choices across ages, as well as the relation between choices and three psychosocial factors (risk appraisal, future orientation, and resistance to peer influence) with theoretical developmental significance (i.e., are theoretically expected to change from childhood to adulthood). The MacJEN measures these factors as features of respondents' reasons for their choices. We anticipated that adolescents and adults might differ on these developmental dimensions in the reasons for their choices, and thus in the maturity of their judgment.

Research to address the major policy and practical questions about juveniles' adjudicative competence requires data from youths representing the relevant adolescent age range, as well as from adults to whom their performance can be compared. In this study, we selected 11–17 as the adolescent age range, because very few youths are arrested on delinquencies below 11 and because juvenile justice jurisdiction in most states does not exceed 17. Our comparison group included young adults aged 18–24 because this represents the age range most commonly seen by the criminal courts and permits a legally relevant, although conservative, test of the differences between adolescents and adults in abilities related to adjudicative competence.

Two groups of youths and two groups of young adults were studied: those currently detained within the juvenile detention centers or adult jails, and those in the community with no current (and little past) juvenile or criminal court involvement. We reasoned that any age differences in competence-relevant abilities could be more reliably interpreted if they were found in both justice system and community samples.

In summary, this study was designed to address three basic questions:

- Do adolescents differ from young adults in abilities to participate in their trials?
- If so, what types of youths manifest significant differences from young adults?
- What kinds of deficits in abilities are salient for law, policy, and practice in this area?

METHOD

Greater detail regarding the study's sample, instruments, and procedures is available in an archival report of the study's method, available at www.mac-adoldev-juvjustice.org.

Participants and Sites

The study used a four-group design of adolescents and young adults, drawn from the justice system and the general community. Participants included 927 "youths" aged 11–17 and 466 "young adults" ages 18–24. (Youths' ages were further grouped 11–13, 14–15, and 16–17 during data analysis.) "Detained" participants (detained youths = 453; detained adults = 233) resided in juvenile detention facilities or adult jails. "Community" participants (community youths = 474; community adults = 233) were individuals residing in the same or similar communities as the Detained participants, and who reported during recruitment that they had never been held overnight in a justice system facility and were not currently charged with any offenses. (Recruitment of these participants is described under "Procedure.")

These 1,393 participants were among 1,429 individuals originally enrolled in the study; 10 participants were dropped from the analyses because of excessive missing data, 2 because they were 25 years of age, and 24 because they obtained IQ scores below 60 (for which one of the study's dependent measures had not been normed).

Tables 1 and 2 show the demographic composition of the study groups. Males composed 66.3% of the Detained sample and 56.8% of the Community sample. The ethnic composition of the sample was about 40% African American, 23% Hispanic, 35% non-Hispanic White, 1% Asian, and 1% from other ethnic identities; these proportions were similar across age and Detained/Community groups. Most participants in both the Detained samples (75 and 77%) and Community samples (62 and 73%) were classified in the two lowest socioeconomic classes by using the Hollingshead

Table 1. Sample Demographics

	Detained					Community				
	Youth age groups			Youth adults		Youth age groups			Youth adults	
	11–13	14–15	16–17	11–17	18–24	11–13	14–15	16–17	11–17	18–24
Participants (n)	74	186	193	453	233	116	159	199	474	233
Male (% of age group)	74	62	62	64	71	52	60	57	57	57
Ethnicity (% of age group)										
African American	56	32	38	39	43	41	52	33	41	37
Hispanic	21	28	25	26	25	20	20	21	20	24
Non-Hispanic White	21	35	35	32	32	36	28	44	37	37
Asian and Other	2	5	2	3	0	3	0	2	2	2
Socioeconomic Status (% of age group)										
I–II	8	7	11	9	7	15	13	15	14	9
III	12	16	18	16	16	23	26	24	24	18
IV–V	80	77	71	75	77	62	61	61	62	73

Table 2. Number of Participants in Gender/Ethnicity by Age Groups (% of Age Group in Parentheses)

	Detained				Community			
	11–13	14–15	16–17	18–24	11–13	14–15	16–17	18–24
Males								
African American	27 (37)	40 (22)	47 (24)	70 (30)	24 (21)	49 (31)	32 (16)	47 (20)
Hispanic	12 (16)	30 (16)	25 (13)	47 (20)	15 (13)	16 (10)	22 (11)	32 (14)
Non-Hispanic White	13 (18)	41 (22)	46 (24)	48 (21)	20 (17)	30 (19)	55 (28)	50 (21)
Asian and other	2 (3)	4 (2)	2 (1)	0	1 (1)	1 (1)	4 (2)	3 (1)
Females								
African American	14 (19)	20 (11)	27 (14)	29 (12)	23 (20)	33 (21)	33 (17)	39 (17)
Hispanic	3 (4)	23 (12)	23 (12)	12 (5)	8 (7)	15 (9)	19 (10)	24 (10)
Non-Hispanic White	2 (3)	24 (13)	21 (11)	27 (12)	22 (19)	15 (9)	33 (17)	37 (16)
Asian and other	0	4 (2)	1 (1)	0	3 (2)	0	0	1 (1)

(1975) system. Current charges for the Detained youths were primarily (about 80%) offenses against persons and offenses against property, in about equal proportions. Charges for the Detained adults were primarily (about 80%) drug-related, against persons, or against property, in about equal proportions. The distribution of charges did not differ between the youth and young adult groups, except that drug-related charges were more frequent in the Detained adult sample (32%) than in the Detained youth sample (10%).

To enhance ethnic diversity and minimize bias due to geographic location, the study employed four data collection sites. (A project coordinating team at a fifth site was responsible for cross-site training, consultation, monitoring data collection procedures, and managing the data base.) Data were collected in Los Angeles ($n = 404$; 29% of total sample), Philadelphia ($n = 390$; 28%), northern Florida ($n = 223$; 16%) and northern, central, and western Virginia ($n = 376$; 27%) at 11 juvenile detention centers, 8 adult jails, and their surrounding communities. Each site contributed an approximately equal number of Detained and Community participants. Each site contributed participants to every age/gender/ethnicity cell, although site contributions to ethnic groups were disproportionate, reflecting the ethnic composition of each site.

It was not possible to compare the demographic characteristics of the Detained participants to the characteristics of the total detained population of each detainment facility, because total admissions data were unavailable. The age proportions in our Detained youth samples, however, appeared to be representative of juvenile detention centers generally, and the proportions of different ethnic groups in the Detained youth sample were nearly identical to those reported in a national survey of juvenile detention centers (Snyder & Sickmund, 1995).

Independent Variables

Demographic and Justice System Experience Variables

We obtained data regarding age, gender, ethnicity, offense charged (for Detained participants), and socioeconomic status by self-report. SES was determined using education and occupation according to the Hollingshead system (1975), which provides five classifications ranging from I (*highest class*) to V (*lowest class*). In analyses in which the interaction between SES and a second variable (e.g., age) was of interest, SES was treated as either a five-level or a three-level (Hollingshead classes I–II, III, and IV–V) categorical variable. In analyses in which SES was covaried, SES was treated as a continuous variable, with scores ranging from 1 to 5. For the Detained samples, experience in the justice system was coded from answers to two questions: whether the participant had (a) ever before been "found guilty" of a delinquency or crime and (b) ever before been "locked up" in a detention center or jail (coding "no" to both questions as "0," "yes" to only one of the questions as "1," and "yes" to both questions as "2").

Intelligence

The *Wechsler Abbreviated Scale of Intelligence*(WASI; Psychological Corporation, 1999) produces an estimate of general intellectual ability on the basis of two subtests (Vocabulary and Matrix Reasoning) that can be administered in approximately 15 min. The WASI is linked to the Wechsler Intelligence Scale for Children (WISC-III) and the Wechsler Adult Intelligence Scale (WAIS-III), and has been normed for individuals aged 6–89 years.

Mental Health Problems

The *Massachusetts Youth Screening Instrument-Second Version* (MAYSI-2; Grisso & Barnum, 2000; Grisso, Barnum, Fletcher, Cauffman, & Peuschold, 2001) is a 52-item, six-scale *yes/no* self-report mental health screening inventory that provides indexes of degree of disturbance on six clinical scales (Alcohol/Drug Use, Angry-Irritable, Depressed-Anxious, Somatic Complaints, Suicide Ideation, Thought Disturbance). Two items were modified for use with young adults in this study; in both, the word "school" was replaced with the word "work." Alpha coefficients for Detained and Community youth and young adult samples were comparable to acceptable coefficients published in earlier MAYSI-2 reports (Grisso et al., 2001; Grisso & Barnum, 2000), with the exception of one scale (Thought Disturbance), which did not achieve acceptable alpha coefficients for any of the subgroups.

Dependent Variables

Functional Abilities Related to Competence to Stand Trial

The primary dependent variable was the MacCAT-CA, designed to assess criminal defendants' abilities to participate in their defense ("competence to stand trial"; Otto et al., 1998; Poythress et al., 1999). The instrument's scoring criteria, as well as norms based on large, national samples of pretrial adult defendants, are provided in the MacCAT-CA manual. At the time of the present study, there were no publications reporting use of the MacCAT-CA with adolescents. The standard administration and content of the MacCAT-CA were unaltered for this study.

The 22 MacCAT-CA items are grouped into three subscales: *Understanding*, *Reasoning*, and *Appreciation*. *Understanding* assesses comprehension of courtroom procedures and personnel and the defendant's rights at trial. *Reasoning* assesses the recognition of information relevant to a legal defense and the ability to process information for legal decision making. The *Appreciation* subscale, referring to a person's ability to recognize the relevance of information for one's own situation, assesses whether a defendant's legal decision making is influenced by symptoms of mental illness, such as delusional thinking.

This study employed mean subscale scores on the three MacCAT-CA scales, as well as a system of classifying MacCAT-CA subscale scores into three hierarchical categories using cutoff scores provided in the MacCAT-CA manual indicating "minimal or no impairment," "mild impairment," or "clinically significant impairment." The cutoff score for "clinically significant impairment" is set at the score equaling 1.5 standard deviations below the mean of the "presumed competent" samples in the original MacCAT-CA norming study (Poythress et al., 1999). Performance above 1.0 standard deviation below the mean for those samples is considered to represent "minimal or no impairment." Scores between those two cutoffs were labeled "mild impairment."

Inter-rater reliability for the MacCAT-CA was assessed twice using all scorers (25 research assistants) at all four of the study sites. For *Understanding* and *Reasoning*, intra-class correlations for youth data were marginally adequate early in the data collection process (.63 and .60, respectively), and better at a later point in the study (.91 and .80; for young adults, .88 and .70). Intra-class correlations for *Appreciation* were much more variable, ranging from .86 for youths early in the study to .17 for young adults later in the study. The latter result apparently was due to highly truncated scores on Appreciation items, with almost no young adult participants producing 0-credit responses.

Decisions and Judgment in the Adjudicative Process

The MacJEN, developed for this study and based on an earlier instrument (Woolard, 1998), was designed to provide data regarding age-related differences in choices and the psychosocial factors that might influence those choices. The MacJEN uses vignettes to pose three legal decisions common in the delinquency/criminal process: (a) responding to police interrogation, (b) disclosing information during consultation with a defense attorney (one half of the participants were administered a vignette about a public defender and one half a vignette about a privately retained attorney); and (c) responding to a plea agreement for reduced consequences in exchange for a guilty plea and testimony against other defendants.

Respondents are given several response choices and asked to recommend a "best choice" and "worst choice" for the vignette character. Choices for the police interrogation vignette include confessing to the offense, denying the offense, and refusing to speak. Choices for the attorney consultation vignette include full disclosure, partial disclosure, denying the offense, and refusing to cooperate. Choices for the plea agreement vignette include accepting or rejecting the offer for reduced charges in exchange for testimony against other defendants. Participants' "best choice" recommendations for the vignette character were used to create a variable indicating readiness to comply with authority figures.

MacJEN responses were also scored according to criteria designed to identify three variables representing aspects of psychosocial maturity: *risk appraisal* (represented by three indexes), *future orientation*, and *resistance to peer influence*.

To assess *risk appraisal,* participants were asked to identify all positive and negative consequences, or risks, of each best and worst choice recommendation, the likelihood of a given set of risks, and the unpleasantness of those risks. These responses contributed to three separate indexes conceptualized as different aspects of *risk appraisal*: (a) "risk recognition," which summed the total number of risks identified across the best and worst choices in each vignette and then averaged across vignettes; (b) "risk likelihood," which summed participants' Likert-type responses to questions that asked about the likelihood that possible negative consequences would occur; and (c) "risk impact," which summed participants' Likert-type responses to questions regarding how unpleasant the negative consequences would be if they did occur.

The second psychosocial maturity variable, *future orientation*, was assessed by coding all of the risks identified by each participant as reflecting the short- or long-range nature of their consequences (employing a standardized classification system). Long-range risks were averaged across vignettes to produce an index of future orientation.

The third psychosocial maturity variable, *resistance to peer influence,* was assessed with questions asked after participants had made their original choices, posing new information to them about peers' recommendations that were contrary to the participants' choices. For each decision-making vignette, peer resistance was measured as a dichotomous variable (retained original choice versus switched to peers' choice).

Procedure

Prior to data collection, all site project directors and research assistants met at one location for several days of training by the project coordinating team. The project coordinators then supervised research teams on site during practice protocol administrations at cooperating facilities.

Research assistants visited the participating juvenile detention centers and adult jails once or twice a week for about 11 months. They were assisted by staff to identify new detainees who had arrived since the previous visit, and to determine whether any detainees had been "screened out" by staff or participant advocates regarding potential research participation. Special protections for human subjects in research were required because Detained participants were identified as belonging to "vulnerable" populations. Independent participant advocates monitored the solicitation of Detained youths, assuring conditions of voluntary youth assent and vetoing specific youths' participation if it might pose unnecessary stress. In addition, parents in some sites were notified by mail prior to approaching Detained youths, and youths whose parents responded indicating that they objected were not included. All human participants procedures were approved by the IRB of the university at which the coordinating site was located as well as the IRB of the university associated with each data collection site.

Any detainees who had not been screened out were approached by research assistants with an explanation of the study, the procedure, and a request for assent to participate. As the study period progressed, Detained youths and adults were approached more selectively to augment contributions to age, gender, and/or ethnicity subsamples that accrued in smaller proportions in detained settings. Females and very young adolescents especially were oversampled in proportion to their actual representation in detention and jail facilities.

Community youths and young adults were solicited in neighborhoods served by the relevant youth detention or adult jail facilities. Community youths were solicited in schools, youth programs, and Girls' and Boys' Clubs, whereas community adults were solicited in community clubs, agencies and shelters, and at community colleges, using posters, leaflets, and/or direct contact by research assistants. Human participants considerations required parental consent for Community youths. As data collection proceeded, the Age × Gender × Ethnic proportions that were accruing in the Detained samples were examined periodically to guide a more selective approach to the recruitment of potential Community participants, aiming at final Community samples that were demographically similar to their respective Detained samples.

It was not possible to determine participation rates for either the detained or community samples because of the way in which participants were recruited in each group. In the case of detained participants, detainees in each facility were periodically informed of the study by facility staff persons and asked if they were interested in speaking with a research staff member about the project; this was done on a regular basis because the population of detainees changed daily. Facility staff did not approach detainees who they believed were especially vulnerable or otherwise unqualified to participate in the study (e.g., due to mental illness, recent trauma, etc.). It was not possible to monitor how many detainees were approached by facility staff and what proportion refused to speak with the research staff. Generally speaking, however, very few detainees with whom we were permitted to speak refused to participate. The recruitment of the community participants was done by posting advertisements about the study in community centers, schools, and recreation centers. Individuals who were interested in the study were asked to call our research office.

All participation was voluntary. Detained youths and adults received $10 for their participation (or snacks in some facilities that did not allow monetary awards); community youths and adults received $25. Informed and signed consent (assent for youths) was required for all participants. Confidentiality was assured with the exception of the researchers' obligation to report to others in cases in which information was obtained that suggested imminent risk of harm to self or others, or danger of harm from others. Participants endorsing two out of three critical "Suicide Ideation" items on the MAYSI-2 were screened further by research assistants using a structured process to obtain data on seriousness and recency of suicidal intent. Responses were evaluated in consultation with the site project director or a site clinician, as well as the project coordinator, to determine the need to breach confidentiality. (For details on frequency with which breaching confidentiality was required, see an archival report of the study's method at www.mac-adoldev-juvjustice.org.)

Table 3. Means (*SD*) for MacCAT-CA Understanding, Reasoning, and Appreciation Subscales

Age groups (*N*)	Understanding	Reasoning	Appreciation
11–13 (190)	10.45 (3.31)[a]	11.30 (2.82)[a]	9.68 (2.34)[a]
14–15 (345)	11.27 (2.97)[b]	12.10 (2.55)[b]	10.33 (1.79)[b]
16–17 (392)	12.00 (2.82)[c]	12.76 (2.34)[c]	10.65 (1.66)[b,c]
18–24 (466)	12.13 (2.92)[c]	12.57 (2.51)[b,c]	10.77 (1.57)[c]

Note. Superscripts refer to age group comparisons for each subscale considered separately. Age groups with different superscripts differed significantly on that subscale, at $p < .05$.

When a participant had consented/assented, the research assistant administered the study protocol, obtaining demographic and justice experience data first, followed by the MacCAT-CA, the WASI, the MAYSI-2, and the MacJEN. The protocol typically required between 90 and 180 min to administer. The project coordination team continuously monitored the data collection process and compliance with ethical procedures at the four data collection sites. Research assistants at each site scored their own protocols, and scored copies were sent to the coordinating site for quality checks, data entry, and database management.

RESULTS

MacCAT-CA: Age Differences in Performance[10]

Preliminary analyses indicated that the four age groups did not differ significantly with respect to gender or ethnicity, but did differ significantly, albeit slightly, with respect to social class and intelligence. As a consequence, all comparisons between age groups controlled for these latter two variables.

To examine age differences in MacCAT-CA performance, a multiple analysis of covariance (MANCOVA) was conducted with the three MacCAT-CA subscale scores (Understanding, Reasoning, and Appreciation) as the dependent variables, age group as the independent variable, and the continuous measure of SES and IQ as covariates. The analysis indicated a significant multivariate effect for age, multivariate $F(9, 3263) = 11.32$, $p < .001$, with significant univariate effects for age on all three subscales, for Understanding, $F(3, 1343) = 16.24$, $p < .001$; for Reasoning, $F(3, 1343) = 19.33$, $p < .001$; for Appreciation, $F(3, 1343) = 18.06$, $p < .001$. As shown in Table 3, post hoc contrasts indicated that, on the Understanding subscale, the 11- to 13-year-olds performed significantly worse than the 14- to 15-year-olds, who performed significantly worse than the two older groups; 16- to 17-year-olds and young adults did not differ. On Reasoning, 11- to 13-year-olds performed significantly worse than 14- to 15-year-olds, who performed significantly worse than the 16- to 17-year-olds; 14- to 15-year-olds and 16- to 17-year-olds did not differ from young adults. On the Appreciation subscale, 11- to 13-year-olds performed significantly worse than 14- to 15-year-olds, who scored lower than young adults, but did not

[10]Various stages of the following analyses examined youths' and young adults' performance on the MacCAT-CA by study site across the demographic variables. Very few site differences were found, no more than would be expected by chance.

differ from 16- to 17-year-olds; as with the other two subscales, 16- to 17-year-olds and young adults did not differ. In general, the magnitude of the difference (i.e., the effect size) between the scores of the 11- to 13-year-olds versus adults was moderate by conventional statistical standards (e.g., *d*s between .5 and .6) whereas the differences between the scores of the 14- to 15-year-olds and adults were small (e.g., *d*s between .2 and .3).

These patterns of age differences were also seen when chi-square analyses were used to compare age groups (both with and without controlling for IQ and SES) with respect to the proportions of individuals showing various levels of impairment—"no impairment," "mild impairment," or "significant impairment" (Poythress et al., 1999)—in Understanding, $\chi^2(6) = 49.60$, $p < .001$, and Reasoning, $\chi^2(6) = 37.56$, $p < .001$; see Fig. 1).[11] For example, whereas 20% of 11- to 13-year-olds, and 13% of 14- to 15-year-olds, showed significantly impaired Understanding, only 7% of the 16- to 17-year-olds and this same proportion of adults scored in this range. Similarly, proportions of individuals showing significantly impaired Reasoning declined from 16% among 11- to 13-year-olds to 9% among 14- to 15-year-olds, to less than 7% among 16- to 17-year-olds and young adults.

It is important to examine the proportions of each age group who show significantly impaired Understanding or Reasoning (or both), because significant impairment in either could raise doubts about competence. These results are presented in Fig. 2, illustrating that 30% of 11- to 13-year-olds, and 19% of 14- to 15-year-olds, were significantly impaired on one or both of these subscales; the figures for 16- to 17-year-olds and for young adults were both 12%.

To examine whether these patterns of age differences varied as a function of gender, ethnicity, or Detained versus Community status, a 4 (age group) × 2 (gender) × 3 (ethnicity) × 2 (Detained/Community status) multiple analysis of covariance (MANCOVA) was conducted with the three MacCAT-CA subscale scores (Understanding, Reasoning, and Appreciation) as the dependent variables and SES and IQ as covariates. MacCAT-CA performance was unrelated to Detained/Community status, gender, and ethnicity. More importantly, the only interaction to reach significance was the two-way interaction between age and Detained/Community status, multivariate $F(9, 3157) = 2.465$, $p < .01$, and the univariate effect was significant only for scores on the Understanding subscale, $F(3, 1299) = 6.09$, $p < .001$. Follow-up analyses indicated that whereas Detained and Community young adults differed significantly in Understanding scores, Detained and Community juveniles (of any age) did not.

In a separate analysis that treated socioeconomic status as a three-level independent variable rather than as a covariate, we did not find significant main effects for SES or a significant interaction between SES and age. The absence of significant interactions between age and gender, age and ethnicity, and age and SES indicates

[11] We do not report proportions of individuals showing impaired appreciation, because it is not clear what such impairment means in a sample of individuals without serious mental illness. This subscale of the MacCAT-CA was developed to identify individuals whose beliefs about their trial were highly irrational or distorted as a result of serious mental disorder. In this study, the majority of individuals who showed "impaired" appreciation did so because they could not articulate reasons for their responses to certain interview questions, not because they demonstrated distorted or irrational thinking.

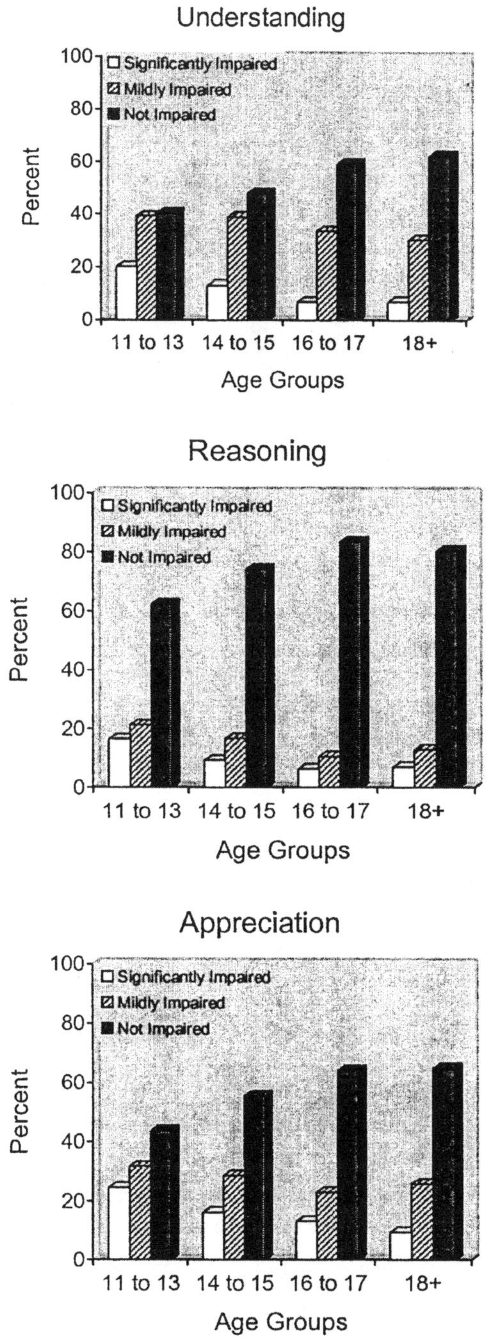

Fig. 1. Degree of impairment on MacCAT-CA Understanding, Reasoning, and Appreciation subscales as a function of age.

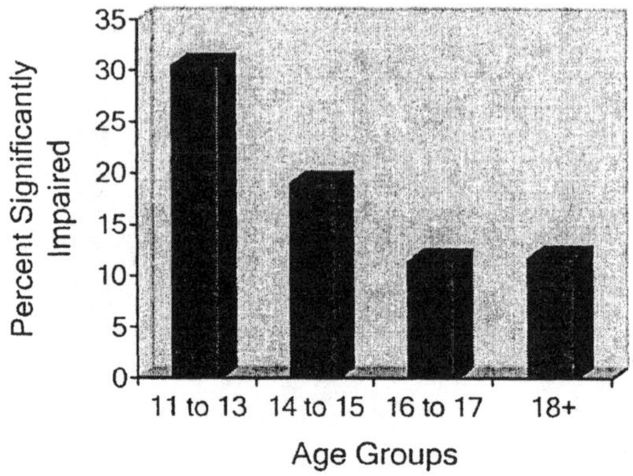

Fig. 2. Proportion of individuals at different ages who are significantly impaired with respect to either or both MacCAT-CA Understanding and Reasoning.

that age differences in MacCAT-CA performance were consistent between males and females, across individuals from different ethnic groups, and across individuals from different socioeconomic backgrounds when controlled for IQ.

Patterns of age differences in the proportions of individuals showing no impairment, mild impairment, or significant impairment on Understanding are shown separately for the Detained and Community samples in Fig. 3. As the figure illustrates, the proportions of individuals showing mild or significant impairment in Understanding differed between Detained and Community adults but were relatively similar among Detained and Community juveniles.

When chi-square analyses were used to compare the Detained and Community groups with respect to the proportions of individuals in each age group who demonstrate significantly impaired Understanding *or* Reasoning (or both), similar patterns of age differences in the two groups emerged (both with and without controlling for IQ and SES). As Fig. 4 illustrates, although impairment was more common among Detained than Community individuals, in both groups, 11- to 13-year-olds, and to a lesser extent 14- to 15-year-olds, were more likely than adults to show deficits in the capacities related to CTS, for Community participants, $\chi^2(3) = 32.37$, $p < .001$; for Detained participants, $\chi^2(3) = 17.10$, $p < .001$. In both groups, the performance of 16- to 17-year-olds was comparable to that of young adults.

MacCAT-CA: Intelligence, Prior Justice System Experience, Mental Health Problems

MacCAT-CA performance may be influenced by factors other than age, including intelligence (which one would be expected to be positively related to MacCAT performance), mental health problems (expected to be negatively related to MacCAT-CA performance), and prior experience in the justice system (expected to be positively related to MacCAT-CA performance). To examine these relations, we conducted a series of multiple regression analyses, regressing scores for each of

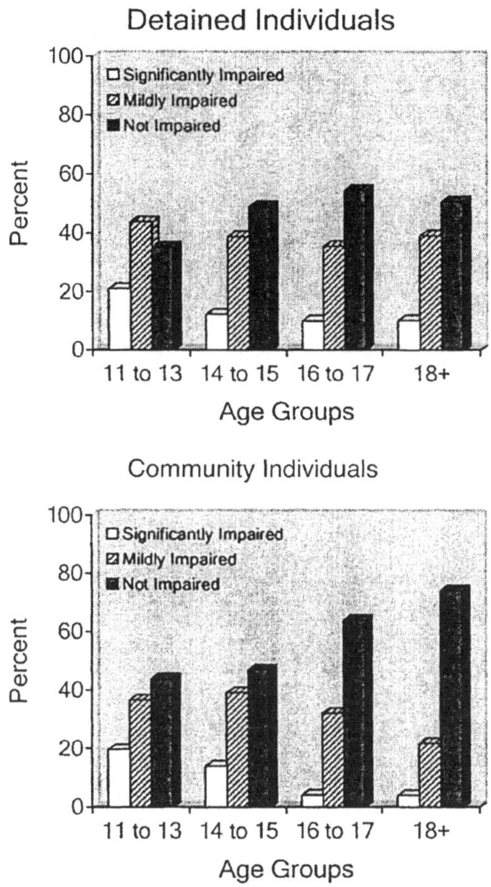

Fig. 3. Impairment on MacCAT-CA Understanding subscale as a function of age and justice system status.

the MacCAT-CA subscales on age (as a continuous variable), IQ, each of the six subscales of the MAYSI-2, and our measure of prior experience in the justice system (for justice system participants only). As expected, IQ was significantly correlated with Understanding, $\beta = .415$, $t(1358) = 15.96$, $p < .001$; Reasoning, $\beta = .421$, $t(1358) = 16.17$, $p < .001$; and Appreciation, $\beta = .328$, $t(1358) = 12.10$, $p < .001$. Contrary to expectancy, MacCAT-CA performance was unrelated to our measure of prior experience in the justice system and largely unrelated to MAYSI-2 mental health problems.

Figure 5 shows the relation between IQ, treated as a three-level categorical variable (IQ = 60–74, 75–89, or 90 and above) and impairment on the three MacCAT-CA subscales. As expected, chi-square analyses showed that individuals of lower intelligence were more likely to have impaired Understanding, $\chi^2(4) = 211.27$, $p <$

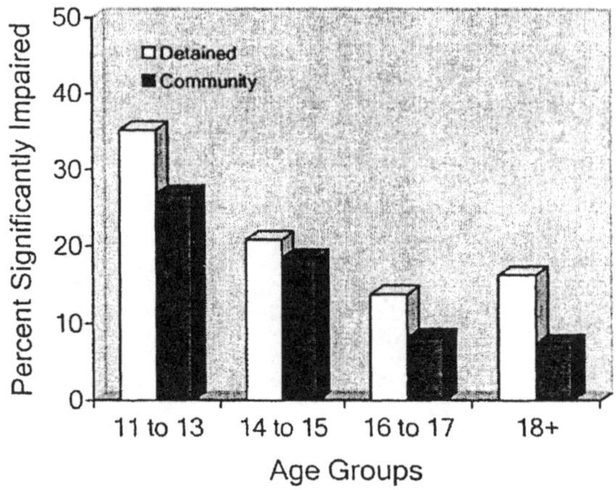

Fig. 4. Proportion of individuals at different ages who are significantly impaired with respect to either or both MacCAT-CA Understanding and Reasoning as a function of age and justice system status.

.001, Reasoning, $\chi^2(4) = 130.50$, $p < .001$, and Appreciation, $\chi^2(4) = 119.55$, $p < .001$. Figure 6 displays the proportions of individuals in each IQ group who were significantly impaired on either the Understanding or the Reasoning scale (or both). Again, individuals of lower intelligence were far more likely to lack these capacities related to participation in trials as defendants.

To examine whether the relations between MacCAT-CA performance and intelligence and justice system experience varied with age, we conducted a second series of regressions, in which the main effects of these variables, along with age (as a continuous variable), were entered into the equation followed by the terms representing the interactions between each variable and age. Age remained a significant predictor of MacCAT-CA performance on all three scales, even when intelligence and prior justice system experience were controlled. There were marginally significant interactions between age and IQ for both Understanding, $\beta = .324$, $t(1361) = 1.696$, $p = .09$, and Appreciation, $\beta = -.382$, $t(1361) = -1.909$, $p = .06$, but no age by experience interaction.

To examine the nature of these interactions, follow-up analyses were conducted in which correlations between MacCAT-CA performance and IQ were computed separately for each age group. The interaction between age and IQ in the prediction of MacCAT-CA performance is difficult to interpret; the correlation between IQ and Understanding generally increased with age, but the correlation between IQ and Appreciation generally decreased with age.

MacCAT-CA Performance as a Function of Intelligence, Age, and Detained/Community Status

It is widely established that, on average, individuals who are detained in the justice system score lower on intelligence tests than demographically comparable

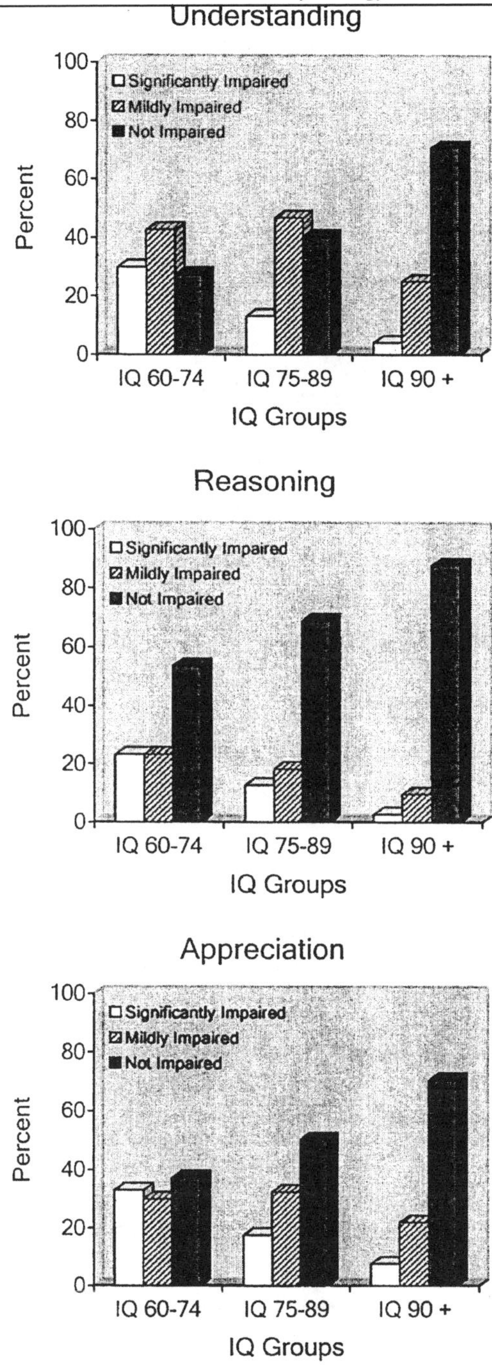

Fig. 5. Impairment on MacCAT-CA Understanding, Reasoning, and Appreciation subscales as a function of IQ.

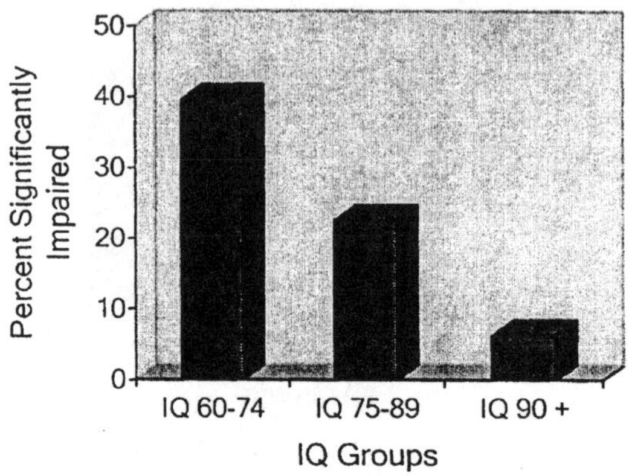

Fig. 6. Proportion of individuals who are significantly impaired with respect to either or both MacCAT-CA Understanding and Reasoning as a function of IQ.

samples of individuals drawn from the community. As expected, an analysis of variance showed that the average IQ score of detained individuals in this study ($M = 86.28$, $SD = 12.95$) was substantially lower than that of individuals from the community, $M = 97.46$, $SD = 15.63$; $F(3, 1385) = 5.64$, $p < .001$, a finding that did not vary as a function of age, $F(3, 1385) = .48$, *ns*). In light of this, and in view of the strong relation between IQ and MacCAT-CA performance, we examined the associations between IQ and MacCAT-CA performance separately within each age group, focusing on proportions with scores in the seriously impaired range.

Figure 7 shows the proportions of individuals of different levels of intelligence, within each age group, who were seriously impaired with respect to Understanding or Reasoning or both. Younger individuals of lower intelligence were especially likely to be deficient in the necessary capacities associated with trial competence. Indeed, among 11- to 13-year-olds, more than one half with an IQ between 60 and 74, and more than one third with an IQ between 75 and 89, were significantly impaired. Among 14- to 15-year-olds, approximately 40% of those with an IQ between 60 and 74, and more than one in four with an IQ between 75 and 89, were comparably impaired. These figures are important because, as Fig. 8 illustrates, between one fifth and one quarter of juveniles aged 15 and younger in the Detained sample had IQ scores between 60 and 74, and approximately 40% of Detained juveniles aged 15 and younger had IQ scores between 75 and 89. In other words, approximately two thirds of the Detained juveniles aged 15 and younger had an IQ that was associated with a significant risk of being incompetent to stand trial because of impaired Understanding or Reasoning or both.

MacJEN: Age Differences in Choices on Decision-Making Vignettes

Turning now to MacJEN results related to questions about participants' legal decision making, we examined age differences in the participants' recommended best choice, using separate chi-square analyses for each of the three decision-making

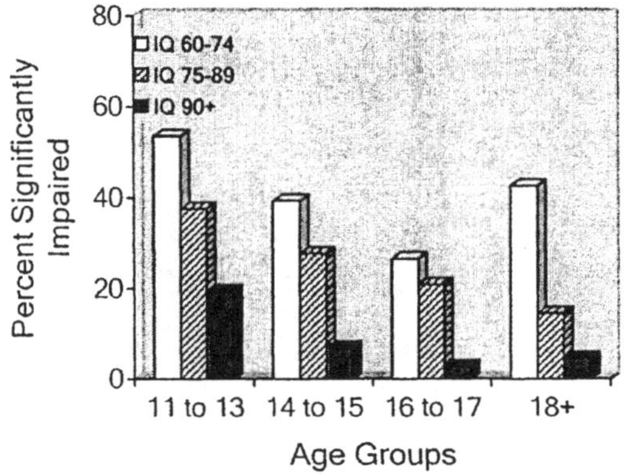

Fig. 7. Proportion of individuals at different ages who are significantly impaired with respect to either or both MacCAT-CA Understanding and Reasoning as a function of age and IQ.

vignettes (police interrogation, attorney consultation, plea agreement; see Fig. 9). Analyses indicated significant age differences for choices regarding police interrogation, $\chi^2(6) = 158.73$, $p < .001$. The proportion of participants who chose confession as the best choice decreased with age, from about one half of the 11- to 13-year-olds to only one fifth of young adults. No age differences were found for the second vignette regarding consultation with a public defender, $\chi^2(9) = 11.59$, *ns*, or a private attorney, $\chi^2(9) = 11.32$, *ns*); over 75% of each age group recommended full disclosure. Significant age differences were found for the plea agreement vignette, $\chi^2(3) = 45.58$, $p < .001$, the proportion accepting the plea agreement decreasing from 74% among 11- to 13-year-olds to 50% of young adults.

Because the four age groups differed significantly with respect to social class and intelligence, separate chi-square analyses examined age differences within three

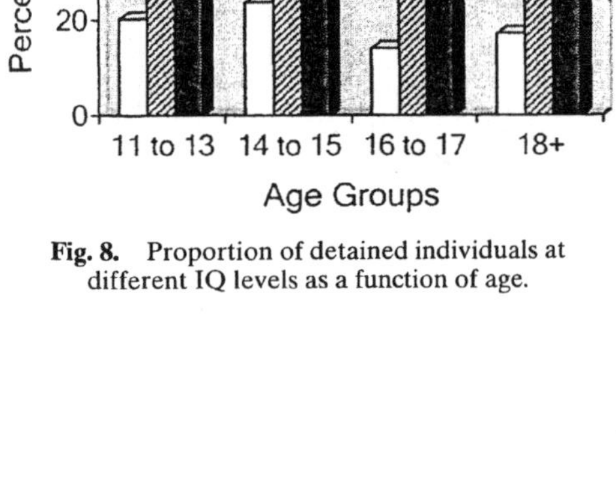

Fig. 8. Proportion of detained individuals at different IQ levels as a function of age.

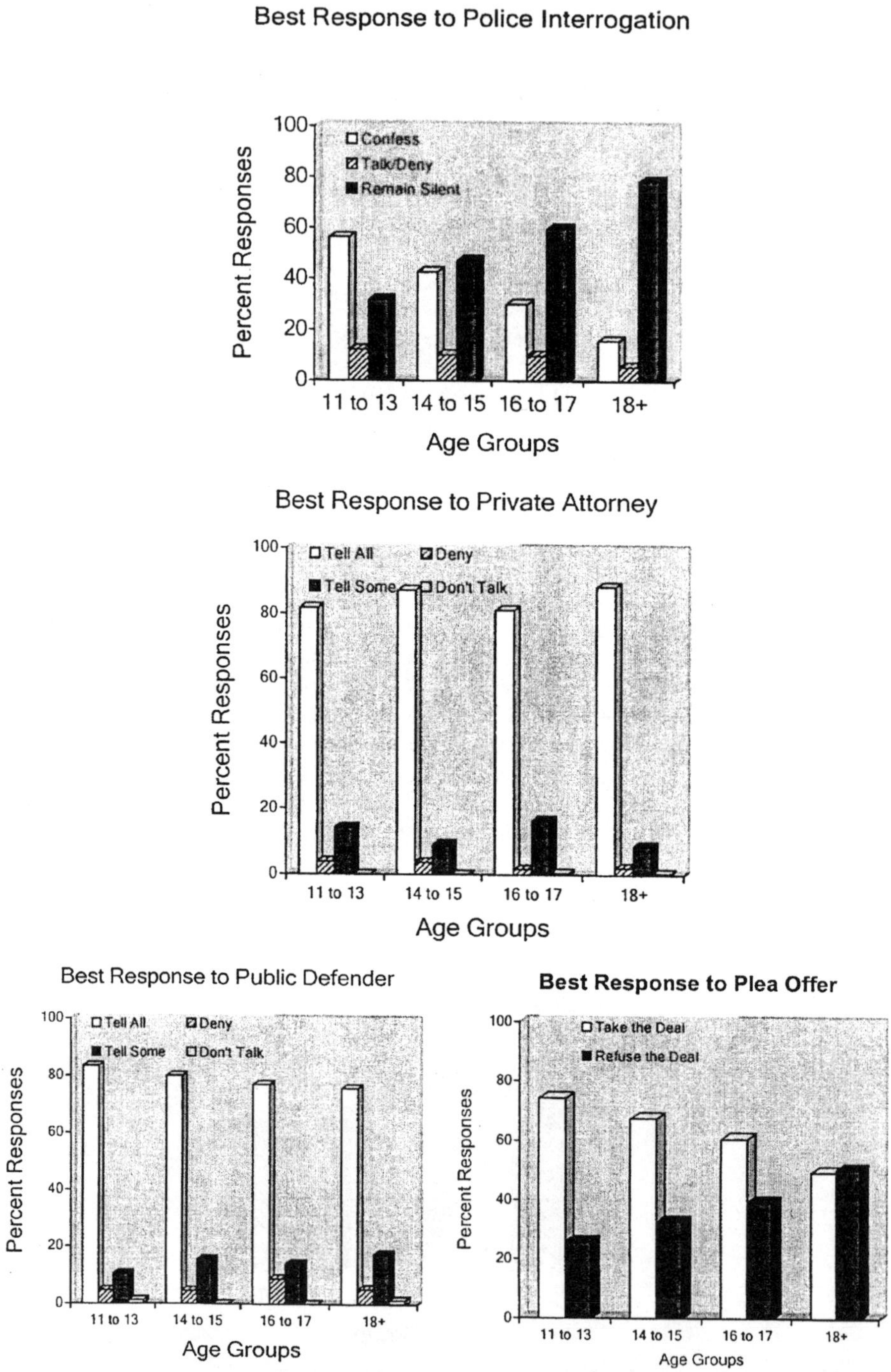

Fig. 9. Decision choices for Police Interrogation, Attorney Consultation, and Plea Agreement vignettes as a function of age.

IQ categories (60–74, 75–89, 90 and above) and five SES categories. The proportion of confession and plea recommendations decreased with age for each IQ category ($p < .005$ or smaller for each analysis), except for the plea recommendation among low IQ participants in which no age-based differences were found. The proportion of confession and plea recommendations decreased with age for each SES category ($p < .05$ or smaller for each analysis) except for those in the highest socioeconomic class, which was not statistically significant.

To examine whether the age effects varied across the other demographic variables, a hierarchical logistical regression was run for each of the three dependent variables (confess/other, full disclosure/less than full, accept plea/refuse plea) with all two-way age interaction terms included in the second step. None of the interactions were significant for the confession, disclosure to public defender, or plea agreement vignettes, indicating that age differences in these choices remain consistent across gender, ethnicity, and Detained/Community status, as well as intelligence and SES. An Ethnicity (White/other) × Age interaction was significant for the regression on full disclosure to a private attorney. Specifically, there were no ethnic differences for 11- to 13-year-olds and 14- to 15-year-olds, but a higher proportion of non-Hispanic White 16- to 17-year-olds (90%) recommended full disclosure than other ethnic groups of the same ages (75% of 16- to 17-year-olds and 85% of young adults).

MacJEN: Age and Compliance With Authorities

In each vignette, one decision choice represents compliance with authority—confessing to police, fully disclosing to the attorney, and accepting the prosecutor's plea agreement. An *authority compliance* score summed the number of compliant choices made across the three vignettes. An Analysis of Variance (ANOVA) was conducted with compliance as the dependent variable, and age, intelligence, and SES as independent variables. The results demonstrated a significant effect for age, $F(3, 1352) = 88.71$, $p < .001$. Post hoc tests indicated that the 11- to 13-year-olds ($M = 2.0$) did not differ from the 14- to 15-year-olds ($M = 1.8$), but both groups were more compliant with authority than the two older groups; the 16- to 17-year-olds ($M = 1.5$) did not differ from the young adults ($M = 1.3$; see Fig. 10).

A 4 (age group) × 2 (gender) × 3 (ethnicity) × 2 (Detained/Community status) ANOVA tested whether age differences in authority compliance varied by gender, ethnicity, and Detained/Community status when SES and intelligence were included as covariates. The main effect of age was significant and post hoc tests were consistent with results reported previously. No significant two-way interactions with age were found, indicating that age differences in authority compliance remained constant across gender, ethnicity, and Detained/Community status.

MacJEN: Psychosocial Factors and Legal Decision Making

Risk Appraisal

Three variables assessed risk appraisal in the decision-making vignettes: (a) risk recognition, (b) risk likelihood (as perceived by the participant), and (c) risk impact (how unpleasant the negative consequences would be if they did occur).

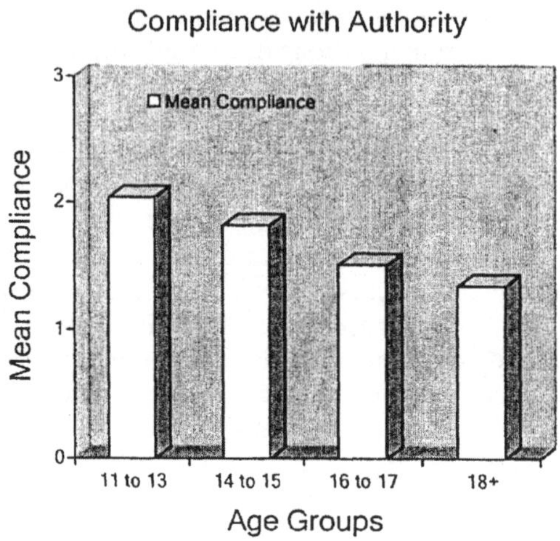

Fig. 10. Authority compliance scores as a function of age.

An ANOVA with age, IQ, and SES as independent variables and *risk recognition* as the dependent variable resulted in main effects for all three independent variables. post hoc tests of the age effect, $F(3, 1368) = 5.18$, $p < .001$, indicated that 11- to 13-year-olds ($M = 3.0$) scored lower than 16- to 17-year-olds ($M = 3.3$) and young adults ($M = 3.3$); the 14- to 15-year-olds ($M = 3.1$) were not significantly different from any other age group.

Main effects for age, $F(3, 1368) = 14.26$, $p < .001$, and SES, $F(4, 1368) = 4.08$, $p < .01$, were found in an ANOVA with average *risk likelihood* as the dependent variable. Young adults reported significantly higher likelihood of risk ($M = 13.7$) than the three adolescent groups, which did not differ from each other.

In the analysis of age, intelligence, and SES with average *risk impact* as the dependent variable, only a main effect of age was significant, $F(3, 1368) = 8.37$, $p < .001$. The youngest participants ($M = 14.5$) and 14- to 15-year-olds ($M = 14.6$) scored lower than young adults ($M = 15.2$). The 16- 17-year-olds (15.0) were significantly higher than 14- to 15-year-olds but did not differ from young adults.

Future Orientation

Recognition of future consequences was indexed by the average number of long-range consequences identified across vignettes. An ANOVA resulted in main effects for age, $F(3, 1368) = 3.56$, $p < .01$, and intelligence, $F(2, 1368) = 28.46$, $p < .001$, but not SES, $F(4, 1368) = 11.54$, *ns*. The 11- to 13-year-olds reported fewer long-range consequences ($M = 7.8$) than the 16- to 17-year-olds ($M = 8.6$). The 14- to 15-year-olds ($M = 8.1$) and young adults ($M = 8.5$) were not significantly different from any other group. All three intelligence categories were significantly different from each other; average long-range consequence scores increased as intelligence increased ($Ms = 7.3, 8.2, 9.2$).

Resistance to Peer Influence

Resistance to peer influence was measured by comparing the participants' original choice in each decision-making vignette to their choice under a condition of peer influence in which peers recommended the opposite course of action (e.g., if a participant stated that they would confess to the police, peers recommended remaining silent). For each decision-making vignette, resistance to peer influence was measured as a dichotomous variable (resisted influence and retained original choice versus influenced by peers and switched to peers' choice). We used age group, gender, ethnicity, detained/community status, intelligence, SES, the original vignette choice, and all two-way age interaction terms in a hierarchical logistic regression to predict whether a participant resisted peer pressure.

In the police interrogation vignette, there was a significant effect for original vignette choice (odds ratio = 4.36), in which those who said they would confess were more resistant than those who would have done something else (denied or remained silent). In addition, there was an Age × Original Choice interaction (odds ratio = 0.44), indicating that resistance to peers depended in part on what participants originally chose to do (see Fig. 11). Among participants who said they would confess, young adults were more likely to change their minds and remain silent than were youths, who were more likely to resist peer influence and confess anyway. Of those who originally said they would remain silent, however, resistance increased with age.

Only the original vignette choice predicted resistance to peer influence in the attorney consultation vignette. Those who reported they would not fully disclose to their attorney were much less likely to resist peer influence than those who said they would fully disclose. Similarly, only the original vignette choice predicted resistance to peer influence in the plea agreement vignette. Those who reported they would

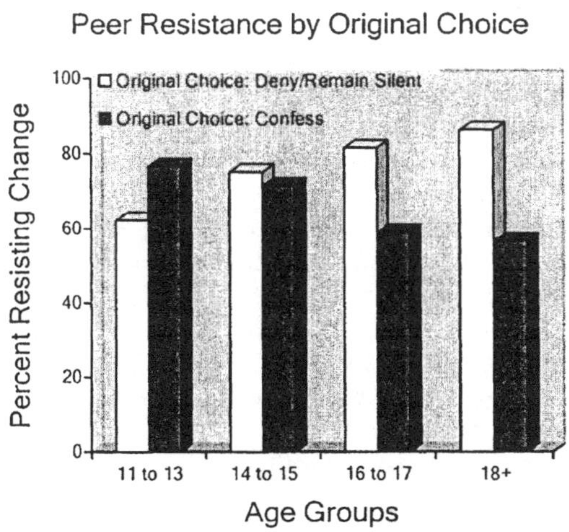

Fig. 11. Peer resistance in the police interrogation vignette as a function of age and original vignette choice.

accept the plea agreement were more resistant to peer influence than those who refused the plea agreement.

Summarizing the age-related findings with the MacJEN, (a) age was significantly related to *choices* in two of the three legal contexts (police questioning, plea agreement), at all IQ levels; (b) youths aged 15 and younger were significantly more likely to choose options that represented *compliance with authorities* in the three legal contexts; (c) compared to young adults, younger adolescents significantly less often recognized *risks*, thought that risks were likely, or thought that risks would be serious if they happened, with the three legal contexts; (d) youths under 14 were significantly less likely than other groups to provide long-range *future consequences* in explaining their choices; and (e) the relation between age and changing one's choices in response to peer suggestions varied in complex ways with the nature of participants' original choices.

DISCUSSION

Review of Findings

Our results indicate that juveniles aged 15 and younger are significantly more likely than older adolescents and young adults to be impaired in ways that compromise their ability to serve as competent defendants in a criminal proceeding. On the basis of criteria established in studies of mentally ill adult offenders (Otto et al, 1998; Poythress et al., 1999), approximately one third of 11- to 13-year-olds, and approximately one fifth of 14- to 15-year-olds are as impaired in capacities relevant to adjudicative competence as are seriously mentally ill adults who would likely be considered incompetent to stand trial by clinicians who perform evaluations for courts. Our results also indicate that the competence-relevant capacities of 16- and 17-year-olds as a group do not differ significantly from those of young adults. These patterns of age differences are robust across groups defined by gender, ethnicity, and SES, and they are evident among individuals in the justice system and in the community. Not surprisingly, juveniles of below-average intelligence are more likely than juveniles of average intelligence to be impaired in abilities relevant for competence to stand trial. Because a greater proportion of youths in the juvenile justice system than in the community are of below-average intelligence, the risk for incompetence to stand trial is therefore even greater among adolescents who are in the justice system than it is among adolescents in the community.

The results are consistent with findings from earlier studies of youths' capacities in legal contexts. For example, in a study of youths' abilities to understand and appreciate *Miranda* warnings, Grisso (1981) found that "understanding... was significantly poorer among juveniles who were 14 years of age or younger than among 15–16-year-old juveniles or adult offenders..." (p. 192), and that those deficits were even more pronounced among youths with low IQ scores, including youths who were 15 and 16 years of age. Similarly, prior research on youths' understanding and reasoning related to trial participation, although fragmentary, has been fairly consistent in suggesting poorer abilities among youths under 14 years of age (for a review, see Grisso, 1997, 2000).

Moving beyond formal competence to stand trial criteria, the results of our examination of adolescents' and young adults' responses to decisionmaking vignettes (the MacJEN procedure) indicate that psychosocial immaturity may affect the performance of youths as defendants in ways that extend beyond the elements of understanding and reasoning that are explicitly relevant to competence to stand trial. Adolescents are more likely than young adults to make choices that reflect a propensity to comply with authority figures, such as confessing to the police rather than remaining silent or accepting a prosecutor's offer of a plea agreement. In addition, when being interrogated by the police, consulting with an attorney, or evaluating a plea agreement, younger adolescents are less likely, or perhaps less able, than others to recognize the risks inherent in the various choices they face or to consider the long-term, and not merely the immediate, consequences of their legal decisions. As is the case with capacities relevant for competence to stand trial, these patterns of age differences in legal decision making generally do not vary with gender, ethnicity, or SES.

It is difficult to compare our results on decision making and psychosocial maturity with past studies, because there has been little research on this relationship and only one study with youths in juvenile or adult justice system custody. In that study, Woolard, Fried, and Reppucci (2001) found that decision options, outcomes, and judgment factors in legally relevant vignettes changed across age. The closest other parallel to our effort was a study of high school students' decisions (in nondefendant contexts), which found relationships between decisions and psychosocial maturity similar to those in the present study (Cauffman & Steinberg, 2000).

Three limits of the study must be kept in mind when interpreting our results. They pertain to *measurement*, *sampling*, and the *application* of the data for juvenile justice policy.

Concerning *measurement*, no set of standardized observations regarding abilities associated with competence to stand trial can identify all of the abilities that courts might consider when making decisions about defendants' competence. The MacCAT-CA, for example, does not assess defendants' abilities to assist counsel in reconstructing events at the time of the offense or to manage their behavior in the courtroom. One must also be careful not to interpret our proportions of youths with "serious impairments" on the MacCAT-CA as the percentage of juveniles who are actually incompetent to stand trial; the instrument assesses capacities that are relevant for the competence question, but not legal competence itself. Neither the law nor the social sciences recognize any psychometric definition of legal incompetence.

Concerning the variables in the MacJEN (risk appraisal, future orientation, and resistance to peer influence), this report provides evidence regarding their psychometric properties but not their construct validity. A subsequent report will describe their relation to other developmental measures that examine similar constructs measured as general developmental concepts, in contrast to the MacJEN's measurement of the concepts manifested in decision making in legal contexts. Further research will be required, however, to examine whether youths' performance on the MacJEN is related to their perceptions and choices in real-life legal circumstances.

Three aspects of the study's *sample* potentially affect the generalizability of the findings. First, although we oversampled younger adolescents in detention centers, detention populations typically do not have large numbers of 11- to 13-year-old youths; as a consequence, we obtained relatively smaller samples of Detained youths who were younger than 14 than those 14 years or older. Second, we were unable to obtain sufficient numbers of Asian youths across sites to analyze data separately for that ethnic group. Third, our method for obtaining the Detained samples may have reduced the number of youths in our samples with serious (e.g., psychotic) mental disorders. Such youths are often diverted from detention to psychiatric services, or they may have been screened out of study participation by participant advocates, in either case making them unavailable to the study interviewers; this might not have been the case for the jailed adults. If this is so, the present results should be seen as conservative age-related estimates of proportions of youths with serious impairments on the MacCAT-CA, since inclusion of youths with serious mental disorders would likely have increased those proportions.

Finally, we caution against the *application* of these results to legal issues other than competence to stand trial. Society is engaged in active debate concerning whether adolescents should be held responsible for their offenses to the same degree, and punished to the same extent, as adults (Fagan & Zimring, 2000). Given the results of the present study, policymakers and practitioners may wish to consider whether the proportion of very young adolescents with deficits in abilities to participate in their trials is sufficiently great to warrant special protections against unfair adjudication as adults. However, our results say nothing about whether youths' developmental capacities render them more or less culpable than adults in terms of their behavior at the time of the alleged offense.

Implications

The issue that the study addresses—the relationship between immaturity and competence to stand trial—has been largely unnoticed (at least in policy circles) during the last decade or so, as legislatures around the country have moved to facilitate the adjudication of younger and younger offenders in adult criminal court (Bonnie & Grisso, 2000). On reflection, however, it is obvious that the same due process constraints that prohibit the adjudication of mentally ill and mentally retarded defendants who do not understand the process they face or cannot assist their attorneys also apply to juveniles who are incompetent because of immaturity alone. The standard announced by the Supreme Court in *Dusky v. United States* (1960) is a functional test, and functionally it should make no difference whether the source of the defendant's incompetency is mental illness or immaturity. This study confronts policymakers and courts with an uncomfortable reality. Under well-accepted constitutional restrictions on the state's authority to adjudicate those charged with crimes, many young offenders—particularly among those under 14—may not be appropriate participants for criminal adjudication.

The findings of this study raise several important issues. Most obvious, perhaps, are the policy and practice implications for the adjudication of youths in adult criminal court. If one in three 11- to 13-year-old defendants potentially may not be competent to stand trial, this should be a concern whenever a youth in this age group is subject to adjudication in adult criminal court. When youths are considered for transfer to criminal court on the basis of judicial discretion, the simplest response would be to make a determination of competence a condition of criminal adjudication for younger defendants. A few states, such as Virginia, already require a finding of competence to stand trial as a predicate condition before a court may consider the transfer of youths from juvenile to adult court (Va. Code Ann. Sect. 16.1-269.1 (A)(3)(2001)).

When youths are charged directly in criminal court, the proper mechanism might be a requirement that an evaluation and determination of competence to stand trial would automatically precede the adjudication. The optimal age boundary for an automatic inquiry into competence is not obvious; clearly jurisdictions and courts will vary. It does seem clear, however, that at some minimal age, the risk of incompetence is so great that a determination should always be a predicate to adjudication in adult court. Even with youths older than this minimum age, defense attorneys, prosecutors, and judges should be concerned about a defendant's competence to stand trial whenever adult adjudication is proposed for a juvenile.

The findings of the study may also be relevant to the legislative determination of the minimum age for adjudication of youths in adult court. Many jurisdictions have set the age bar very low for adult prosecution of youths for serious crimes, usually without consideration of the likelihood that many youths of the specified minimum age may be incompetent (Bonnie & Grisso, 2000). Because the evaluation and judicial determination of competence are likely to be costly in both time and money (and because the risk of incompetence is substantial below age 14), a legislature might well conclude that an efficient and just approach is to set the minimum age of adult adjudication at an age at which competence to stand trial is not potentially an issue in every case.

The findings of the study should also focus attention on the issue of competence to stand trial in juvenile court delinquency proceedings. Many states extend the competence requirement to juvenile court adjudications, but most focus on mental illness and disability as the sources of incapacity (Redding & Frost, 2002). An important consideration in expanding the doctrinal framework to include incompetence as a result of immaturity is whether the competence standard applied in juvenile court should be less demanding than that applied in adult criminal court. This is important because the standard for competence in juvenile court will determine whether youths adjudicated incompetent as adults can be tried as juveniles. If a less demanding standard operates in juvenile court proceedings, many younger defendants who lack the capacity to be adjudicated as adults can be tried in this venue. Otherwise, the question of how to respond to these immature defendants presents a daunting challenge.

We believe that a more relaxed competence standard in juvenile court is compatible with the demands of constitutional due process. The Supreme Court has made it clear that the requirements of due process in delinquency proceedings are not identical to those that regulate criminal trials (*McKeiver v. Pennsylvania*, 1971). The justification for a separate juvenile court rests in part on the fact that it is not an exact replica of criminal court. If juvenile court jurisdiction ends when the minor reaches adulthood (an important "if"), then the stakes of a delinquency proceeding are not as high as those faced by a youth charged with a felony in adult court. Under these conditions, no constitutional bar would restrict the use of a more relaxed standard of adjudicative competence in juvenile court. As Bonnie and Grisso (2000) have argued, in an ordinary juvenile court delinquency proceeding, the minimal criteria for adjudication are satisfied if the youth "has a basic understanding of the purpose of the proceedings and can communicate rationally with counsel" (p. 97).

This approach not only is constitutionally legitimate, but also offers a practical solution to the challenges that may follow when courts recognize incompetence due to developmental immaturity. Most children and adolescents who are found incompetent to proceed in criminal court because of immaturity could likely be adjudicated in a juvenile delinquency proceeding under a more relaxed competence standard. In most cases, this avoids the dispositional problem of dealing with young defendants who cannot be tried as adults and are not likely to become competent in a reasonable time. Several courts that have considered competence to stand trial in juvenile court assume that the competence demands of a delinquency proceeding are lower than in an adult trial, and that youths who cannot be transferred to criminal court because of incompetence can be tried in juvenile court (e.g., *In the Matter of W.A.F*, 1990; *Ohio v. Settles*, 1998).

The two-tier standard also minimizes the extent to which delinquency proceedings will be burdened by the incorporation of developmental immaturity as a basis for incompetence. If youths in juvenile court must meet adult standards of competence, prosecutors legitimately might worry that defense attorneys in delinquency proceedings will routinely petition for competence assessments. This will be unlikely if the competency standard in juvenile court is understood to be a modest one. Those who care about the welfare of youths and those who worry about the efficiency of the justice process share a common interest in promoting practices that implement due process without creating an undue burden on the court system.

Careful attention must be directed toward devising dispositions for youths who are found to be incompetent as a result of developmental immaturity, in part to allay fears that might arise about the possibility that some dangerous youths would be immune from prosecution because of immaturity—a specter that will alarm many people. Whereas the disposition of mentally ill defendants is directed toward restoration to competence, this goal is not appropriate for immature youths who have never achieved competence. A disposition that simply waits for a youth to mature until he or she is competent to stand trial is both politically inconceivable and constitutionally problematic.[12] Unless other dispositions are offered, courts and legislatures are unlikely to deal seriously with developmental incompetence.

This challenge may be less daunting than it at first appears. As suggested earlier, most youths who are not competent to stand trial as adults because of immaturity could likely be adjudicated in juvenile court. Moreover, some defendants whose

[12]In *Jackson v. Indiana*, 406 U.S. 715 (1972), the Supreme Court held that due process requires that the state must either restore the incompetent defendant in a reasonable period of time or release him.

incompetence is based solely on deficient understanding (rather than immature reasoning) could likely be tried as adults after a period of instruction about the matters they do not comprehend. Thus, the great majority of youths would be subject to adjudication on their criminal charges with little delay even when an assessment of their abilities indicates they do not meet adult competence standards.

The more difficult questions involve appropriate dispositions for those defendants who are (a) charged with serious crimes and (b) incompetent to stand trial even in juvenile court on the basis of their immaturity. At least a few options other than the dismissal of charges suggest themselves as possible responses to this very small group of offenders. First, if the youth is a danger to self or others, civil commitment procedures can be initiated. Confinement for an indefinite period to achieve sufficient maturity to stand trial is another option, but one that must have outer time limits. As the Supreme Court made it clear in *Jackson v. Indiana* (1972) (at least for adults), indefinite confinement of incompetent defendants is analogous to punishment without a trial. Finally, a social service or an educational intervention may be warranted as a response to problems manifested by the child's behavior. For example, failure of parental supervision may result in removal of the child to state custody and foster care placement. None of these responses are ideal; they may be more restrictive than dispositions that are appropriate for adults. Nonetheless, they deserve careful consideration as responses to the unique developmental status of children.

This study compared juveniles and adults in their capacities to function in the trial process under established doctrinal requirements that focus on reasoning, understanding, and appreciation. But questions about how minors function as criminal defendants compared to adults go beyond those that are captured by the narrow focus of the ordinary competence inquiry. The study indicates that psychosocial immaturity may affect a young person's decisions, attitudes, and behavior in the role of defendant in ways that do not directly implicate competence to stand trial, but that may be quite important to how they make choices, interact with police, relate to their attorneys, and respond to the trial context.

Policymakers and practitioners should be concerned about these matters, and special procedures and strategies may be warranted when youths face criminal jeopardy. For example, if young persons are more likely to talk to the police than are adults because of different attitudes toward adult authority figures, they may be more vulnerable to police coercion. If so, youths may need special protection of their Fifth Amendment rights in the custodial context, such as a per se rule that requires the presence of an attorney as a predicate to interrogation (Grisso, 1980). In the plea agreement context, judicial inquiry that goes beyond the standard colloquy may be needed when courts are presented with a guilty plea by a young defendant. In general, those who deal with young persons charged with crimes—and particularly their attorneys—should be alert to the impact of psychosocial factors on youths' attitudes and decisions, even when their understanding and reasoning appear to be adequate. Deficiencies in risk perception and future orientation, as well as immature attitudes toward authority figures, may undermine competent decision making in ways that standard assessments of competence to stand trial do not capture.

ACKNOWLEDGMENTS

The authors are pleased to acknowledge the special assistance provided during the project by Richard Bonnie, Tom Hecker, Dan Keating, Edward Mulvey, Dawn Peuschold, and Norman Poythress. This project was an initiative of the John D. and Catherine T. MacArthur Foundation Research Network on Adolescent Development and Juvenile Justice and was supported by grants from the MacArthur Foundation and the Open Society Institute. Network members offered important guidance for the study; those not listed as authors or as special contributors above include Jeffrey Fagan, Amy Hehn, Patricia Lee, Paul McGill, and Franklin Zimring.

REFERENCES

Abramovitch, R., Peterson-Badali, J., & Rohan, M. (1995). Young people's understanding and assertion of their rights to silence and legal counsel. *Canadian Journal of Criminology*, *37*, 1–18.

Bonnie, R. (1992). The competence of criminal defendants: A theoretical reformulation. *Behavioral Sciences and the Law*, *10*, 291–316.

Bonnie, R. (1993). The competence of criminal defendants: Beyond Dusky and Drope. *Miami Law Review*, *47*, 539–601.

Bonnie, R., & Grisso, T. (2000). Adjudicative competence and youthful offenders. In T. Grisso & R. Schwartz (Eds.), *Youth on trial: A developmental perspective on juvenile justice* (pp. 73–103). Chicago: University of Chicago Press.

Cooper, D. (1997). Juveniles' understanding of trial-related information: Are they competent defendants? *Behavioral Sciences and the Law*, *15*, 167–180.

Cauffman, E., & Steinberg, L. (2000). (Im)maturity of judgment in adolescence: Why adolescents may be less culpable than adults. *Behavioral Sciences and the Law*, *18*, 741–760. *Dusky v. United States*, 362 U.S. 402 (1960).

Fagan, J., & Zimring, F. (Eds.). (2000). *The changing borders of juvenile justice: Transfer of adolescents to the criminal court.* Chicago: University of Chicago Press.

Godinez v. Moran, 509 U.S. 389 (1993).

Grisso, T. (1980). Juveniles' capacities to waive *Miranda* rights: An empirical analysis. *California Law Review*, *68*, 1134–1166.

Grisso, T. (1981). *Juveniles' waiver of rights: Legal and psychological competence.* New York: Plenum.

Grisso, T. (1997). The competence of adolescents as trial defendants. *Psychology, Public Policy, and Law*, *3*, 3–32.

Grisso, T. (2000). What we know about youths' capacities as trial defendants. In T. Grisso & R. Schwartz (Eds.), *Youth on trial: A developmental perspective on juvenile justice* (pp. 139–171). Chicago: University of Chicago Press.

Grisso, T. (2002). *Evaluating competencies: Forensic assessments and instruments* (2nd en.). New York: Kluwer/Plenum.

Grisso, T., & Appelbaum, P. (1998). *Assessing competence to consent to treatment: A guide for physicians and other health care professionals.* New York: Oxford University Press.

Grisso, T., & Barnum, R. (2000). *Massachusetts Youth Screening Instrument—Second Version: User's manual and technical report.* Worcester: University of Massachusetts Medical School.

Grisso, T., Barnum, R., Fletcher, K., Cauffman, E., & Peuschold, D. (2001). Massachusetts Youth Screening Instrument for mental health needs of juvenile justice youths. *Journal of the American Academy of Child and Adolescent Psychiatry*, *40*, 541–548.

Grisso, T., & Schwartz, R. (Eds.). (2000). *Youth on trial: A developmental perspective on juvenile justice.* Chicago: University of Chicago Press.

Hollingshead, A. (1975). *Four factor index of social status*. New Haven, CT: Department of Sociology, Yale University.

In the Matter of W.A.F., 573 A2d 1264 (D.C. 1990).

Jackson v. Indiana, 406 U.S. 715 (1972).

Keating, D. (1990). Adolescent thinking. In S. Feldman and G. Elliott (Eds.), *At the threshold: The developing adolescent* (pp. 54–89). Cambridge: Harvard University Press.

McKeiver v. Pennsylvania, 403 U.S. 538 (1971).

Mumley, D., Tillbrook, C., & Grisso, T. (in press). Five year research update (1996–2000): Evaluations for competence to stand trial (adjudicative competence). *Behavioral Sciences and the Law.*

Ohio v. Settles, 13-97-50 (1998) Ohio App. LEXIS 4973 (Ohio App. 3rd Sept. 30, 1998).

Otto, R., Poythress, N., Edens, N., Nicholson, R., Monahan, J., Bonnie, R., Hoge, S., & Eisenberg, M. (1998). Psychometric properties of the MacArthur Competence Assessment Tool-Criminal Adjudication. *Psychological Assessment, 10,* 435–443.

Peterson-Badali, M., & Abramovitch, R. (1993). Grade related changes in young people's reasoning about plea decisions. *Law and Human Behavior, 17,* 537–552.

Peterson-Badali, M., Abramovitch, R., & Duda, J. (1997). Young children's legal knowledge and reasoning ability. *Canadian Journal of Criminology, 39,* 145–170.

Poythress, N., Nicholson, R., Otto, R., Edens, J., Bonnie, R., Monahan, J., & Hoge, S. (1999). *The MacArthur Competence Assessment Tool—Criminal Adjudication: Professional manual.* Odessa, FL: Psychological Assessment Resources.

Psychological Corporation. (1999). *Wechsler Abbreviated Scale of Intelligence.* San Antonio, TX: Psychological Corportation.

Redding, R., & Frost, L. (2002). Adjudicative competence in the modern juvenile court. *Virginia Journal of Social Policy and the Law, 9,* 353–410.

Scott, E. (1992). Judgment and reasoning in adolescent decision making. *Villanova Law Review, 37,* 1607–1669.

Scott, E., Reppucci, N., & Woolard, J. (1995). Evaluating adolescent decision-making in legal contexts. *Law and Human Behavior, 19,* 221–244.

Snyder, H., & Sickmund, M. (1995). *Juvenile offenders and victims: A national report.* Washington, DC: Office of Juvenile Justice and Delinquency Prevention.

Snyder, H., & Sickmund, M. (1999). *Juvenile offenders and victims: 1999 national report.* Washington, DC: Office of Juvenile Justice and Delinquency Prevention.

Steinberg, L., & Cauffman, E. (1996). Maturity of judgment in adolescence: Psychosocial factors in adolescent decision-making. *Law and Human Behavior, 20,* 249–272.

Torbet, P., Gable, R., Hurst, H., Montgomery, I., Szymanski, L., & Thomas, D. (1996). *State responses to serious and violent juvenile crime.* Washington, DC: Office of Juvenile Justice and Delinquency Prevention.

Woolard, J. (1998). *Developmental aspects of judgment and competence in legally relevant contexts.* Unpublished doctoral dissertation, Psychology Department, University of Virginia.

Woolard, J., Fried, C., & Reppucci, N. (2001). Toward an expanded definition of adolescent competence in legal situations. In R. Roesch, R. Corrado, & R. Dempster (Eds.), *Psychology in the courts: International advances in knowledge* (pp. 21–40). London: Routledge.

[22]

Multisystemic Treatment of Criminality and Violence in Adolescents

CHARLES M. BORDUIN, PH.D.

ABSTRACT

Objective: To discuss the emergent success of multisystemic therapy (MST), a family-based therapeutic approach that has been viewed as a promising treatment for violence and other serious antisocial behaviors in adolescents. **Method:** The empirical underpinnings, theoretical foundation, and clinical features of MST are described, followed by a brief review of studies of MST effectiveness with serious juvenile offenders. **Results:** The theoretical foundation and clinical features of MST draw upon empirical findings regarding the multidetermined nature of serious antisocial behavior as well as upon social-ecological models of behavior in which the youth and family's school, work, peers, and neighborhood are viewed as interconnected systems with dynamic and reciprocal influences on the behavior of family members. In controlled studies with serious juvenile offenders, MST has demonstrated long-term reductions in criminal activity, violent offenses, drug-related arrests, and incarceration. **Conclusions:** The success of MST can be attributed primarily to (1) the match between MST intervention foci and empirically identified correlates/causes of criminality and violence in adolescents (e.g., parental discipline, family affective relations, peer associations, school performance) and (2) the flexible use of well-validated intervention strategies in the natural environment. *J. Am. Acad. Child Adolesc. Psychiatry,* 1999, 38(3):242–249. **Key Words:** crime, violence, delinquency, multisystemic therapy, treatment outcome.

Violent criminal acts and other serious crimes (i.e., index offenses) committed by adolescents present significant problems at several levels of analysis, and these problems argue for the development of effective treatment approaches. On a personal level, adolescents who commit serious crimes experience numerous psychosocial problems as well as reduced educational and occupational opportunities (Melton and Pagliocca, 1992). Moreover, serious criminal activity perpetrated by adolescents has extremely detrimental emotional, physical, and economic effects on victims, the families of victims and perpetrators, and the larger community (Gottfredson, 1989; Miller et al., 1993; Oswald and Singh, 1996). Therefore, effective treatment may not only benefit the youth and his or her family, but may also save many persons from victimization.

On an epidemiological level, youths under the age of 18 years account for approximately 30% of all arrests for index offenses, including 19% of violent crimes and 35% of property crimes (Federal Bureau of Investigation, 1996), and such arrests greatly underestimate the prevalence of youth criminal activity (Elliott et al., 1987; Loeber et al., 1998). In addition, although only about a fourth of youths arrested for delinquent acts could be characterized as serious offenders and even fewer (approximately 15%) could be characterized as chronic offenders, serious and chronic juvenile offenders account for more than half of the total volume of youth crime in a community (Farrington et al., 1986; Loeber et al., 1998; Moffitt, 1993). Thus, if one purpose of treating juvenile offenders is to decrease crime, then serious and chronic juvenile offenders are a logical target for intervention efforts.

On a social services level, juvenile offenders, especially those who are violent, consume much of the resources of the child mental health, juvenile justice, and special education systems and are overrepresented in the "deep end" of these systems (Melton et al., 1998), with considerable cost to the public treasury and intrusion on family integrity and youth autonomy. Moreover, serious and violent adolescent offenders often have continued contact with the mental health and criminal justice systems well into

Accepted September 16, 1998.

Dr. Borduin is Professor, Department of Psychology, University of Missouri, Columbia.

Reprint requests to Dr. Borduin, Department of Psychology, 210 McAlester Hall, University of Missouri, Columbia, MO 65211-2500.

0890-8567/99/3803–0242/$03.00/0©1999 by the American Academy of Child and Adolescent Psychiatry.

adulthood (Borduin and Schaeffer, 1998). Therefore, the development of effective treatments for adolescent criminality and violence may help to free resources to address other important problems of children and their families.

Unfortunately, the development of effective treatments for violence and criminality in adolescents has been an extremely difficult task. Indeed, several reviews of the delinquency treatment literature in the 1970s concluded that "nothing works" (Henggeler, 1989). More recently, Kazdin (1995) has described several empirically driven treatments as "promising" (e.g., behavioral parent training, cognitive-behavioral therapy, functional family therapy), and Lipsey (1992) argued that such structured, skill-oriented treatments have demonstrated the largest effects on delinquents in general. However, although such treatments have demonstrated efficacy with relatively mild forms of antisocial behavior, they have been unsuccessful in treating serious antisocial behavior (see, e.g., Bank et al., 1991; Weisz et al., 1990). Findings such as these have led many mental health professionals and policymakers to virtually give up on the possibility of attenuating further criminal activity in those youths who are already serious perpetrators.

Multisystemic therapy (MST) (Borduin and Henggeler, 1990; Henggeler and Borduin, 1990) was developed to address major limitations of existing mental health services for juvenile offenders and has received the most empirical support as an effective treatment for serious and violent criminal behavior in adolescents (see Levesque, 1996; Tate et al., 1995). The primary purpose of this article is to address the empirical rationale for the application of MST as well as the features of MST that make it well-suited for treating serious antisocial behavior in adolescents. More specifically, this article begins with a brief review of empirical findings regarding the correlates and causes of violent and other serious criminal behaviors in adolescents. Next, the theoretical foundation of MST is described, followed by a brief description of the clinical features and guiding principles of MST interventions. Findings from controlled evaluations that demonstrate the efficacy of MST with violent and chronic juvenile offenders are then summarized. Finally, important aspects of MST that contribute to its success and that distinguish MST from commonly available treatments and service programs for serious juvenile offenders are discussed.

CORRELATES AND CAUSES OF ANTISOCIAL BEHAVIOR

A large number of studies have evaluated correlates of antisocial and violent behavior in adolescents. In general, these correlates pertain to the individual adolescent and to the key social systems (family, peers, school, neighborhood) in which the adolescent is embedded. Table 1 lists the correlates that have consistently emerged in the literature (for reviews, see Borduin and Schaeffer, 1998; Henggeler, 1989; Kazdin, 1995; Thornberry et al., 1995).

In light of the numerous correlates of violent and other serious antisocial behavior in adolescents, several research groups have developed empirically based multidimensional causal models of delinquent behavior. These research groups have used path analysis or structural equation modeling to examine the interrelations among variables from several of the psychosocial domains (i.e., individual, family, peer, school, neighborhood) that have been linked with antisocial behavior. Such causal modeling studies allow a determination of which variables have direct versus indirect effects on antisocial behavior, and which variables are no longer linked with

TABLE 1
Correlates of Antisocial Behavior

Individual adolescent characteristics
- Low Verbal IQ
- Immature moral reasoning
- Cognitive bias to attribute hostile intentions to others
- Favorable attitudes toward antisocial behavior

Family characteristics
- Low affection and cohesion
- High conflict and hostility
- Lax and ineffective parental discipline
- Poor parental monitoring
- Parental difficulties, such as substance abuse, psychiatric conditions, and criminality

Peer relations
- High involvement with deviant peers
- Poor social skills
- Low involvement with prosocial peers

School factors
- Poor academic performance
- Dropout
- Low commitment to education
- Poor academic quality and weak structure of school

Neighborhood and community characteristics
- Criminal subculture (e.g., drug dealing, prostitution)
- Low organizational participation among residents
- Low social support available from church, neighbors, and the like
- High mobility

antisocial behavior when the effects of other correlates are controlled.

Elliott et al. (1985) conducted a longitudinal evaluation of a representative national sample of adolescents (N = 1,725) to assess the psychosocial determinants of delinquent behavior, including violent and other serious crimes. Path analyses showed that serious delinquency (i.e., index offenses) at time 1 and involvement with delinquent peers at time 2 (1 year later) had direct effects on serious delinquent behavior at time 2, especially for males; in addition, serious delinquent behavior at time 2 was predicted indirectly by family and school difficulties, which predicted involvement with delinquent peers. Similarly, in a cross-sectional study using 553 male adolescents and their mothers from 12 New York City neighborhoods, Simcha-Fagan and Schwartz (1986) found that association with delinquent peers, school attachment, neighborhood criminal subculture, and age had direct effects on severe delinquent behavior, including violent crime; furthermore, family residential stability, neighborhood organizational participation, and neighborhood residential stability had indirect effects on severe delinquency through their direct association with school attachment. These and other causal modeling studies (for a review, see Henggeler, 1991) provide consistent support for the view that variance in violent and other serious delinquent behavior is contributed to directly or indirectly by variables at the individual, familial, and extrafamilial levels.

It is logical to conclude from the results of the causal modeling studies that serious antisocial behavior in adolescents is multidetermined and that treatment approaches must have the flexibility to address the multiple known determinants of such behavior. Indeed, there is a growing consensus among reviewers that the major limitation of most treatments for serious antisocial behavior is their failure to account for the multidetermined nature of such behavior and that effective treatments must have the capacity to intervene comprehensively, at individual, family, peer, school, and possibly even neighborhood levels (Borduin, 1994; Henggeler, 1989; Levesque, 1996; Melton and Pagliocca, 1992; Mulvey et al., 1993).

TREATMENT THEORY, CLINICAL FEATURES, AND PRINCIPLES OF MST

The theoretical foundation of MST draws upon the identified correlates/causes of serious antisocial behavior and Bronfenbrenner's (1979) social-ecological theory of behavior. Social-ecological theory views the child and family's school, work, peers, and community as interconnected systems with dynamic and reciprocal influences on the behavior of family members. Problem behavior can be maintained by problematic transactions within and/or between any one or combination of these systems. Thus, consistent with both the empirically established correlates/causes of youth criminality and with social-ecological theory, MST interventions target identified child and family problems within and between the multiple systems in which family members are embedded, and such interventions are delivered in the natural environment (home, school, neighborhood) to optimize ecological validity.

The overriding goals of MST are to empower parents with the skills and resources needed to independently address the inevitable difficulties that arise in raising adolescents and to empower adolescents to cope with familial and extrafamilial problems. Using well-validated treatment strategies derived from strategic family therapy, structural family therapy, behavioral parent training, and cognitive-behavioral therapy, MST directly addresses intrapersonal (e.g., cognitive), familial, and extrafamilial (i.e., peer, school, neighborhood) factors that are known to contribute to adolescent violent and serious antisocial behavior. Biological contributors to identified problems (e.g., major depression, attention-deficit/hyperactivity disorder) in family members are also identified, and, when appropriate, psychopharmacological treatment is integrated with psychosocial treatment. Because different contributing factors are relevant for different adolescents and families, MST interventions are individualized and highly flexible.

Although the exact nature and sequence of interventions in MST can vary widely from family to family, several types of interventions are commonly used with serious juvenile offenders and their parents. At the family level, MST interventions generally aim to remove barriers to effective parenting (e.g., parental substance abuse, parental psychopathology, low social support, high stress, marital conflict), to enhance parenting knowledge, and to promote affection and communication among family members. At the peer level, interventions frequently are designed to decrease affiliation with delinquent and drug-using peers and to increase affiliation with prosocial peers (e.g., through church youth groups, organized athletics, after-school activities). Such interventions are optimally conducted by the adolescent's parents, with the guidance of the therapist, and often consist of active support and encouragement of associations with nonproblem peers (e.g., providing transportation, increased privileges) and substantive discouragement of associations with deviant peers (e.g., applying significant sanctions). Likewise, under the guidance of the therapist, the parents often develop strategies to monitor and promote the adolescent's school performance and/or vocational functioning; interventions in this domain typically focus on establishing positive communication lines between parents and teachers and on restructuring after-school hours to promote academic efforts. Finally, in some cases, individual interventions are used with an adolescent or parent to modify the individual's social perspective-taking skills, problem-solving skills (e.g., learning to deal assertively with negative peer pressure), belief system, or motivational system.

MST is usually delivered by a master's-level therapist with a caseload of 4 to 8 families. The MST therapist is a generalist who directly provides most mental health services and coordinates access to other important services (e.g., medical, educational, recreational), always monitoring quality control. Although the therapist is available to the family 24 hours a day, 7 days a week, therapeutic intensity is titrated to clinical need; thus, the range of direct contact hours per family can vary considerably. In general, therapists spend more time with families in the initial weeks of therapy (daily, if indicated) and gradually taper off (as infrequently as once a week) during a 3- to 5-month course of treatment. Treatment fidelity is maintained by weekly group supervision meetings involving 3 to 4 therapists and a doctoral-level clinical supervisor (usually a child psychologist or child psychiatrist). During these meetings, the treatment team (i.e., therapists, supervisor, and, as needed, a consulting psychiatrist) review the goals and progress of each case to ensure the multisystemic focus of therapists' intervention strategies and to identify obstacles to success. Importantly, the treatment team accepts responsibility for engaging families in treatment and for effecting therapeutic change. Thus, when obstacles to successful engagement or to therapeutic change are identified, the team develops strategies to address those obstacles and to promote success.

The 9 treatment principles enumerated below serve as general guidelines for designing multisystemic interventions. Detailed descriptions of these principles, and examples that illustrate the translation of these principles into specific intervention strategies, are provided in a clinical volume (Henggeler and Borduin, 1990) and a treatment manual (Henggeler et al., 1998).

1. The primary purpose of assessment is to understand the "fit" between the identified problems and their broader systemic context.
2. Therapeutic contacts emphasize the positive and use systemic strengths as levers for change.
3. Interventions are designed to promote responsible behavior and decrease irresponsible behavior among family members.
4. Interventions are present-focused and action-oriented, targeting specific and well-defined problems.
5. Interventions target sequences of behavior within and between multiple systems that maintain the identified problems.
6. Interventions are developmentally appropriate and fit the developmental needs of the youth.
7. Interventions are designed to require daily or weekly effort by family members.
8. Intervention effectiveness is evaluated continuously from multiple perspectives with providers assuming accountability for overcoming barriers to successful outcomes.
9. Interventions are designed to promote treatment generalization and long-term maintenance of therapeutic change by empowering caregivers to address family members' needs across multiple systemic contexts.

ISSUES RELATED TO SUCCESSFUL IMPLEMENTATION OF MST PROGRAMS

MST programs for violent and other serious youthful offenders are typically implemented by public (mental health, juvenile justice, social welfare) or private service organizations to provide a community-based alternative to incarceration and other out-of-home placements. Although the preceding clinical elements are believed to be fundamental to the successful implementation of MST programs with serious juvenile offenders (see the following section on effectiveness), an MST program cannot be successful without several key administrative elements as well. As discussed elsewhere (Schoenwald and Henggeler, in press), a service organization (including key administrators, supervisors, and therapists) must be fully committed to the philosophical (e.g., definition of the mental health professional's role) and empirical (e.g., accountability for clinical outcomes) framework of the MST approach and should receive intensive training and ongoing consultation in the MST model. The MST program should have distinct, dedicated staff (i.e., 100% time MST therapists) and include a clinical supervisor who has credible authority regarding clinical decisions. Substantial changes in agency policies and in staff members' work routines are often required to implement successfully the clinical approach of MST, and concrete support should be evident from the administration of the service organization (e.g., implementing flexible working hours and compensatory time policies for staff, scheduling supervision and consultation times, providing highly competitive salaries and incentives).

Successful implementation of an MST program also requires initiative in developing and maintaining collaborative relationships with other agencies in the community (i.e., schools, juvenile justice, social welfare, mental health, and substance abuse) that are involved in the lives of serious juvenile offenders (Schoenwald and Henggeler, in press). Indeed, a strength of the MST approach is that it assumes accountability as the single point of responsibility for ensuring that the broad needs of serious juvenile offenders and their families are met. Thus, the main purpose of coordinating MST activities with those of other agencies is to produce favorable long-term clinical outcomes. Moreover, given that the funding mechanisms in many communities include disincentives for public agencies to use community-based services in lieu of out-of-home placements, an MST program is unlikely to attain a sufficient referral base and concomitant funding without first seeking the support and cooperation of key agencies and stakeholders in the community. One mechanism for funding used in MST programs at different sites across the nation has involved shifting local or state children's services monies allocated for residential treatment programs or other out-of-home placements (e.g., foster care) to the MST program.

EFFECTIVENESS OF MST WITH SERIOUS JUVENILE OFFENDERS

Clearly, for both ethical and pragmatic reasons, it is important that mental health services for serious juvenile offenders and their families be evaluated rigorously. Rigorous evaluation of outcomes produced by MST has been a high priority since the initial development of this treatment model in the late 1970s.

General Delinquency

The first MST outcome study (Henggeler et al., 1986) was conducted with inner-city juvenile offenders (N = 80) with arrest histories that included relatively serious violent and nonviolent crimes (mean = 2.1 arrests). Findings showed that MST was more effective than usual services in decreasing adolescent behavior problems, decreasing adolescent association with deviant peers, and improving family relations, especially family communication and affect. The favorable effects of MST in improving key correlates of antisocial behavior supported the viability of conducting further evaluations of MST with serious juvenile offenders.

Violent/Chronic Offenses

Two different randomized clinical trials have been conducted to evaluate the efficacy of MST with violent and chronic juvenile offenders. In the first study, Henggeler et al. (1992) compared MST and usual services (provided by a state agency) in the treatment of 84 serious juvenile offenders (54% violent offenders), who averaged 3.5 previous arrests and 9.5 weeks of prior incarceration. Findings at posttreatment showed that MST improved family and peer relations of the youths and their families. In addition, at a 59-week postreferral follow-up, youths who received MST had significantly fewer rearrests (means = 0.87 versus 1.52) and weeks incarcerated (means = 5.8 versus 16.2) than did youths who received usual services; the cost per youth for treatment in the MST group was also substantially lower than the average cost in the usual services group ($2,800 versus $16,300). Importantly, results from a 2.4-year follow-up (Henggeler et al., 1993) showed that MST doubled the survival rate (i.e., percentage of youths not arrested) of these serious juvenile offenders when compared with usual services.

In the most comprehensive and extensive evaluation of MST to date, Borduin et al. (1995) examined the long-term effects of MST versus individual therapy (IT) on violent offending and other criminal offending in 200 serious juvenile offenders, who averaged 4.2 previous arrests. Results from multiagent, multimethod assessment batteries conducted before and after treatment showed that MST was more effective than IT in improving key family correlates of antisocial behavior and in ameliorating adjustment problems in individual family members. Moreover, results from a 4-year follow-up of rearrest data showed that youths who received MST were significantly less likely to be rearrested than youths who received IT. Specifically, MST completers (n = 77) had lower recidivism rates (22.1%) than MST dropouts (46.6%; n = 15), IT completers (71.4%; n = 63), IT dropouts (71.4%; n = 21), or treatment refusers (87.5%; n = 24); MST dropouts also were at lower risk of arrest than IT dropouts or treatment refusers. Examination of recidivists from each group revealed that MST youths arrested during follow-up were arrested less often and for less serious crimes than IT youths arrested during follow-up. Significantly, MST youths also were less likely to be arrested for violent crimes (i.e., rape, attempted rape, sexual assault, aggravated assault, assault/battery) after treatment than were IT youths.

Substance Use and Abuse

Prior to the completion of the 2 MST trials with violent/chronic juvenile offenders (Borduin et al., 1995; Henggeler et al., 1992), Henggeler et al. (1991) examined the effects of MST on reductions in substance use and abuse in the offenders participating in these studies. Analyses of arrest data from the Borduin et al. (1995) sample indicated that youths who participated in MST had a significantly lower rate of substance-related arrests 4 years after treatment than did youths who participated in IT (i.e., 4% versus 16%). Similarly, analyses of self-report data from the Henggeler et al. (1992) sample showed that juvenile offenders in the MST condition reported significantly less soft drug use at posttreatment than did offenders who received usual services.

In a more recent study of substance-abusing/dependent juvenile offenders (N = 118), Henggeler et al. found that, in comparison with youths who received usual community services, youths who participated in MST reported less drug use, had fewer rearrests, and had spent fewer days in out-of-home placement (i.e., incarceration, residential treatment, inpatient treatment) at a 6-month follow-up (S.W. Henggeler, S.G. Pickrel, M.J. Brondino, unpublished, 1998). In a related study, Schoenwald et al. (1996) found that the incremental costs of MST (i.e., costs that were above and beyond the usual costs of services for substance-abusing/dependent juvenile offenders) were nearly offset by the savings incurred as a result of reductions in days of out-of-home placement during the first year after referral.

Current and Future Evaluations

The refinement of MST with violent and chronic juvenile offenders is a continuous, ongoing, and dynamic process (see Henggeler et al., 1998). Current projects are examining treatment processes and potential moderators of MST effectiveness in families of early adolescent violent offenders and are evaluating the dissemination of MST to various community settings serving violent and chronic adolescent offenders (e.g., Henggeler et al., 1997); a major task in our dissemination research is to evaluate those factors (e.g., therapist characteristics, supervisory behaviors, agency policies) that are linked with treatment adherence and with clinical outcomes. We are also planning to conduct a 10-year follow-up of the juvenile offenders (now in their 20s and early 30s) who participated in the Henggeler et al. (1992) and Borduin et al. (1995) randomized trials; a major component of the follow-up is an assessment of each participant's service utilization (mental health, juvenile justice, social welfare, education) during the follow-up period and a delineation of the costs of such services in order to evaluate the cost-effectiveness of MST.

Additional evaluations of MST are currently under way in an effort to adapt and extend the treatment model to other populations with serious clinical problems (e.g., youths presenting psychiatric emergencies such as suicidal behavior), to populations with different demographic characteristics (e.g., Hispanic-American gang members), and as an alternative to out-of-home placements (e.g., residential treatment). We are also currently evaluating the effectiveness of MST with child and adolescent sexual offenders. The foundation for this work is an earlier study (Borduin et al., 1990) that remains, to date, the only published randomized trial with juvenile sexual offenders; though modest in scope and size (i.e., N = 16), this study demonstrated that MST was relatively effective in reducing recidivism for both sexual offenses and nonsexual crimes at a 3-year follow-up.

CLINICAL IMPLICATIONS

The effectiveness of MST in reducing criminality and violence in serious juvenile offenders has important implications that can help guide the development of potentially more effective interventions for such youths. If, as suggested earlier, a major shortcoming of most interventions for treating serious antisocial behavior has been their neglect of the multiple determinants of such behavior, then the success of MST may be linked with its comprehensive and flexible nature; that is, the results of MST may be due to its explicit focus on ameliorating key social-ecological factors associated with serious antisocial behavior, including behavior problems, parental disturbance, problematic family relations, association with deviant peers, and poor school performance. In light of the multidetermined nature of adolescent antisocial behavior, it is unrealistic to expect even the best-conceived office-based treatments to be effective because of their relatively narrow focus.

A second implication of findings from our randomized clinical trials pertains to the accessibility and ecological validity of services. Traditionally, as Melton and Pagliocca (1992) emphasized, mental health services for serious juvenile offenders either have been inaccessible (i.e., office-based) or have provided interventions (e.g., residential treatment centers, wilderness programs, boot camps, incarceration) that have little bearing on the real-world environmental conditions that led to the youth's criminal behavior and to which the youth will eventually return. In contrast, MST is provided in natural community contexts (e.g., home, school, recreation center). The delivery of services in youths' natural environments enhances family cooperation, permits more accurate assessment of identified problems and of intervention results, and promotes long-term maintenance of therapeutic changes (Henggeler and Borduin, 1990). Likewise, other aspects of MST (e.g., intensive training and supervision of therapists, development of collaborative interagency relationships) may also contribute to the positive clinical outcomes that have been obtained with many youths and their families.

In conclusion, our work indicates that a comprehensive intervention, addressing the multiple determinants of antisocial behavior in youths' naturally occurring systems, can successfully reduce criminal activity and violent offending in serious juvenile offenders. Of course, extensive validation and replication are needed for even the most promising treatment approaches. Nevertheless, given the significant problems that violent adolescent offenders present for our society, as well as the questionable ethics of providing these adolescents with treatments that do not produce durable changes, it is time that priority be placed on the evaluation of promising treatment models such as MST.

REFERENCES

Bank L, Marlowe JH, Reid JB, Patterson GR, Weinrott MR (1991), A comparative evaluation of parent-training interventions for chronic delinquents. *J Abnorm Child Psychol* 19:15–33

Borduin CM (1994), Innovative models of treatment and service delivery in the juvenile justice system. *J Clin Child Psychol* 23(suppl):19–25

Borduin CM, Henggeler SW (1990), A multisystemic approach to the treatment of serious delinquent behavior. In: *Behavior Disorders of Adolescence: Research, Intervention, and Policy in Clinical and School Settings*, McMahon RJ, Peters R DeV, eds. New York: Plenum, pp 62–80

Borduin CM, Henggeler SW, Blaske DM, Stein R (1990), Multisystemic treatment of adolescent sexual offenders. *Int J Offender Ther Comp Criminol* 34:105–113

Borduin CM, Mann BJ, Cone LT et al. (1995), Multisystemic treatment of serious juvenile offenders: long-term prevention of criminality and violence. *J Consult Clin Psychol* 63:569–578

Borduin CM, Schaeffer CM (1998), Violent offending in adolescence: epidemiology, correlates, outcomes, and treatment. In: *Delinquent Violent Youth: Theory and Interventions*, Gullotta TP, Adams GR, Montemayor R, eds. Newbury Park, CA: Sage, pp 144–174

Bronfenbrenner U (1979), *The Ecology of Human Development: Experiments by Nature and Design*. Cambridge, MA: Harvard University Press

Elliott DS, Dunford FW, Huizinga D (1987), The identification and prediction of career offenders utilizing self-reported and official data. In: *Prevention of Delinquent Behavior*, Burchard JD, Burchard SN, eds. Newbury Park, CA: Sage, pp 90–121

Elliott DS, Huizinga D, Ageton SS (1985), *Explaining Delinquency and Drug Use*. Beverly Hills, CA: Sage

Farrington DP, Ohlin L, Wilson JQ (1986), *Understanding and Controlling Crime*. New York: Springer-Verlag

Federal Bureau of Investigation (1996), *Uniform Crime Reports*. Washington, DC: US Government Printing Office

Gottfredson GD (1989), The experiences of violent and serious victimization. In: *Pathways to Criminal Violence*, Weiner NA, Wolfgang ME, eds. Newbury Park, CA: Sage, pp 202–234

Henggeler SW (1989), *Delinquency in Adolescence*. Newbury Park, CA: Sage

Henggeler SW (1991), Multidimensional causal models of delinquent behavior and their implications for treatment. In: *Context and Development*, Cohen R, Siegel AW, eds. Hillsdale, NJ: Erlbaum, pp 211–231

Henggeler SW, Borduin CM (1990), *Family Therapy and Beyond: A Multisystemic Approach to Treating the Behavior Problems of Children and Adolescents*. Pacific Grove, CA: Brooks/Cole

Henggeler SW, Borduin CM, Melton GB et al. (1991), Effects of multisystemic therapy on drug use and abuse in serious juvenile offenders: a progress report from two outcome studies. *Fam Dynam Addict Q* 1:40–51

Henggeler SW, Melton GB, Brondino MJ, Scherer DG, Hanley JH (1997), Multisystemic therapy with violent and chronic juvenile offenders and their families: the role of treatment fidelity in successful dissemination. *J Consult Clin Psychol* 65:821–833

Henggeler SW, Melton GB, Smith LA (1992), Family preservation using multisystemic therapy: an effective alternative to incarcerating serious juvenile offenders. *J Consult Clin Psychol* 60:953–961

Henggeler SW, Melton GB, Smith LA, Schoenwald SK, Hanley JH (1993), Family preservation using multisystemic treatment: long-term follow-up to a clinical trial with serious juvenile offenders. *J Child Fam Stud* 2:283–293

Henggeler SW, Rodick JD, Borduin CM, Hanson CL, Watson SM, Urey JR (1986), Multisystemic treatment of juvenile offenders: effects on adolescent behavior and family interaction. *Dev Psychol* 22:132–141

Henggeler SW, Schoenwald SK, Borduin CM, Rowland MD, Cunningham PB (1998), *Multisystemic Treatment of Antisocial Behavior in Children and Adolescents*. New York: Guilford

Kazdin AE (1995), *Conduct Disorders in Childhood and Adolescence*, 2nd ed. Thousand Oaks, CA: Sage

Levesque RJR (1996), Is there still a place for violent youth in juvenile justice? *Aggression Violent Behav* 1:69–79

Lipsey MW (1992), The effects of treatment on juvenile delinquents: results from meta-analysis. Paper presented at the NIMH Meeting for Research to Prevent Youth Violence, Bethesda, MD, November

Loeber R, Farrington DP, Waschbusch DA (1998), Serious and violent juvenile offenders. In: *Serious and Violent Juvenile Offenders: Risk Factors and Successful Interventions*, Loeber R, Farrington DP, eds. Thousand Oaks, CA: Sage, pp 13–29

Melton GB, Lyons PM, Spaulding WJ (1998), *No Place to Go: The Civil Commitment of Minors*. Lincoln: University of Nebraska Press

Melton GB, Pagliocca PM (1992), Treatment in the juvenile justice system: directions for policy and practice. In: *Responding to the Mental Health Needs of Youth in the Juvenile Justice System*, Cocozza JJ, ed. Seattle: National Coalition for the Mentally Ill in the Criminal Justice System, pp 107–139

Miller TR, Cohen MA, Rossman SB (1993), Victim costs of violent crime and resulting injuries. *Health Aff* 12:186–197

Moffitt TE (1993), Adolescence-limited and life-course-persistent antisocial behavior: a developmental taxonomy. *Psychol Rev* 100:674–701

Mulvey EP, Arthur MA, Reppucci ND (1993), The prevention and treatment of juvenile delinquency: a review of the research. *Clin Psychol Rev* 13:133–167

Oswald DP, Singh NN (1996), Emerging trends in child and adolescent mental health services. In: *Advances in Clinical Child Psychology*, Ollendick TH, Prinz RJ, eds. New York: Plenum, pp 331–365

Schoenwald SK, Henggeler SW (in press), Services research and family based treatment. In: *Family Psychology Intervention Science*, Liddle H, Diamond G, Levant R, Bray J, eds. Washington, DC: American Psychological Association

Schoenwald SK, Ward DM, Henggeler SW, Pickrel SG, Patel H (1996), Multisystemic therapy treatment of substance abusing or dependent adolescent offenders: costs of reducing incarceration, inpatient, and residential treatment. *J Child Fam Stud* 5:431–444

Simcha-Fagan O, Schwartz JE (1986), Neighborhood and delinquency: an assessment of contextual effects. *Criminology* 24:667–703

Tate DC, Reppucci ND, Mulvey EP (1995), Violent juvenile delinquents: treatment effectiveness and implications for future action. *Am Psychol* 50:777–781

Thornberry TP, Huizinga D, Loeber R (1995), The prevention of serious delinquency and violence: implications from the program of research on the causes and correlates of delinquency. In: *A Sourcebook: Serious, Violent, and Chronic Juvenile Offenders*, Howell JC, Krisberg B, Hawkins JD, Wilson JJ, eds. Newbury Park, CA: Sage, pp 213–237

Weisz JR, Walter BR, Weiss B, Fernandez GA, Mikow VA (1990), Arrests among emotionally disturbed violent and assaultive individuals following minimal versus lengthy intervention in North Carolina's Willie M Program. *J Consult Clin Psychol* 58:720–728

Documentation of Child Physical Abuse: How Far Have We Come? Mary Ann P. Limbos, MD, MPH, Carol D. Berkowitz, MD

Objectives: To determine the effects of increased physician training and a structured clinical form on physician documentation of child physical abuse. *Design:* Retrospective chart review. *Participants:* Children evaluated in the pediatric emergency department in 1980 and 1995 who were given the diagnosis of physical abuse. *Measurements:* The unstructured pediatric emergency department form and the structured child abuse reporting form were reviewed for documentation of 20 items including history, physical examination, diagnostic procedures, and disposition. Data documented in 1980 were compared with that in 1995. *Results:* The only significant differences between 1980 and 1995 concerning documentation on the unstructured pediatric emergency department form were better recording in the latter year of Child Protective Services involvement and case disposition. Half or more of the records omitted documentation of at least one of the following: witness to injury, past injuries, description of size and/or color of injuries, illustration, and a genital exam. None of the records contained a developmental history. Significantly fewer skeletal surveys were obtained in 1995, although notation of the results was similar to 1980. For both years, the structured child abuse reporting form improved documentation of only two items: time of arrival to the pediatric emergency department and illustrations of injuries. *Conclusions:* Little improvement in physician documentation of child physical abuse was noted between 1980 and 1995 despite increased efforts to educate housestaff in the evaluation of child abuse during this time period. Although a structured form prompted physicians to document dates and times and to illustrate physical injuries on the diagram provided, it did not significantly improve documentation of other items. **Pediatrics** 1998;102:53–58

Abstracts selected by Michael J. Maloney, M.D., Assistant Editor.

[23]

Managing At-Risk Juvenile Offenders in the Community

Putting Evidence-Based Principles Into Practice

RANDY BORUM
University of South Florida

More than a half-million juveniles are under community supervision as a result of violent or delinquent behavior. Research has shown that treatment can reduce their risk of reoffending. This article reviews and distills the key lessons from hundreds of empirical studies and meta-analyses and applies them to practice. The author argues for conducting systematic and developmentally informed risk assessments, selectively assigning intensive intervention to the highest risk offenders, focusing on criminogenic treatment targets, using proven interventions and treatment strategies, and applying rigor in implementation and follow-up.

Keywords: *youth violence; risk assessment; juvenile delinquency; juvenile offenders; treatment; rehabilitation*

The justice system has long recognized that developmental differences between youth and adults affect offender needs, behavior, culpability, and amenability to treatment (McCord, Widom, & Crowell, 2001). Since at least the European period of enlightenment, young offenders have been regarded as a vulnerable population (Scott, 2000). Contemporary descriptions of juvenile offenders suggest that they continue to have special needs and vulnerabilities that may affect their treatment in and by the legal system (Kazdin, 2000). The rate of behavioral health—mental health and substance abuse—problems in this population is so high that they are regarded as the rule rather than the exception (Kazdin, 2000; Marsteller et al., 1997; Otto, Greenstein, Johnson, & Friedman, 1992; Policy Design Team, 1994; Shelton, 1998; Ulzen & Hamilton, 1998). Many juvenile perpetrators have also been victims of crime and violence (Finkelhor, & Hashima, 2001). A majority have experienced severe physical abuse or neglect by parents or caregivers (Hamilton, Falshaw, & Browne, 2002; Stouthamer-Loeber, Loeber, Homish, & Wei, 2001). Exposure to trauma is extraordinarily common (Cauffman, Feldman, Waterman, & Steiner, 1998; Steiner, Garcia, & Matthews, 1997). All of these adverse events also are occurring during the most formative years of development when their impact is likely to have the most profound and pervasive effect on lifelong adjustment and functioning.

In 1961, the President's Commission on Juvenile Delinquency and Youth Crime recognized that a large number of these vulnerable youth were routinely confined in detention facilities for relatively minor offenses (Gottfredson & Barton, 1993; Griffin & Torbet, 2002). They advocated for moving more delinquent youth into the community through legislation that ultimately became known as the Juvenile Justice and Delinquency Prevention Act of 1974. In the mid-1980s, however, there was a surge of youth violence and widespread prognostications about an emerging breed of juvenile superpredators that fueled public fear of juveniles and steered juvenile justice policy toward a more punitive, rather than rehabilitative, approach (Grisso, 1996; Grisso & Schwartz, 2000). Youths are regarded as more dangerous than ever before. According to results of a 1994 Gallup poll, Americans believe that juveniles are responsible for nearly half (43%) of all violent crime. Most reliable crime statistics, however, suggest the proportion actually is closer to 13%. Juveniles are believed to be responsible for much more violent crime than they actually commit; nevertheless, while young offenders are in the community, their risk must be managed. Adolescence is a peak risk period for initiating or participating in an act of serious violence (U.S. Department of Health and Human Services, 2001).

Although the absolute number of youth placed in detention is increasing, most—before and after adjudication—are still managed in the community. Indeed, the number of juveniles placed on community probation—including those charged with person offenses—has risen sharply (Gottfredson & Barton, 1993). Despite increased construction of juvenile prisons and detention facilities, probation remains the most common disposition, accounting for nearly two thirds of all adjudications (Puzzanchera, Stahl, Finnegan, Tierney, & Snyder, 2002). At any given time, even more juveniles are under supervision in the community while awaiting trial. Still others are monitored in community-based diversion programs. The result is that every year, professionals in juvenile justice and behavioral health are responsible for supervising and managing nearly a half a million youths who may be at risk for delinquency or violent offenses.

The good news is that treatment—particularly community-based treatment—is effective in reducing recidivism among juvenile offenders (Lipsey, 1999a, 1999b; Lipsey & Wilson, 1998). The challenge, though, is the fact that all interventions do not work equally well, and they tend to work best when they respond to the specific needs of the juvenile (Dowden & Andrews, 1999; Hoge, 2001; Lipsey & Wilson, 1998). Based on analyses of literally hundreds of research studies and program evaluations, several key discernible principles can be applied—individually and programmatically—to enhance the effectiveness of community supervision and treatment for juvenile offenders (Andrews et al., 1990; Dowden & Andrews, 1999; Griffin & Torbet, 2002; Hoge, 2001; Hoge & Andrews, 1996; Lipsey, 1995, 1999b). This article elucidates those evidence-based principles and provides guidance about how they can be applied to reduce recidivism among juvenile offenders in the community.

First, it is essential to identify the offender's risk and needs in developmental context. Second, the most intensive monitoring and supervision resources should be applied to the highest risk cases. Third, the community supervision professional must identify key criminogenic factors to target for intervention, then attempt to engage the offender in a collaborative treatment planning effort. Fourth, the planned interventions should be based on what has been proven to work and what will fit with the juvenile's existing capacities. Fifth, and finally, the plan should be implemented, monitored, and continually reassessed.

EVIDENCE-BASED PRINCIPLES FOR RISK MANAGEMENT WITH JUVENILE OFFENDERS

Conduct Systematic Assessment of Risk and Needs

The fields of criminology, psychology, sociology, and other behavioral sciences have accumulated more than 50 years worth of research identifying factors associated with increased risk of violent and delinquent offending in juveniles (Borum, 2000; Borum & Verhaagen, in press; Howell, 1997; Lipsey & Derzon, 1998). This research has been repeatedly summarized and synthesized through critical scholarly review articles and statistical meta-analyses (combining the results from multiple studies) (Hann & Borek, 2001; Hawkins et al., 1998, 2000). Yet, until recently, there have been very few attempts to make that information user friendly for professionals in juvenile justice and behavioral health or to apply that information to provide structure for offender assessments. Systematic assessment of risk and needs, however, provides the foundation for effective intervention.

Risk of reoffending is the result of dynamic and reciprocal interplay between factors that increase and those that decrease the likelihood of offending in the developing juvenile over time (Borum & Verhaagen, in press). If one's aim is to prevent recidivism, then it will be necessary to identify the historical, situational, and individual factors that increase (risk factors) and decrease (protective factors) reoffense risk.

Risk factors have been classified as broadly falling into two categories: static and dynamic. Static risk factors are those that are historical (e.g., early onset of violence) or dispositional (e.g., gender) in nature and that are unlikely to change over time. Dynamic factors are typically individual, social, or situational factors that often do change (e.g., attitudes, associates, high levels of stress) and, therefore, might be more amenable to modification through intervention (Borum, 2000). These have sometimes been referred to as "needs" factors (Hoge, 2001, 2002; Hoge & Andrews, 1996).

In contrast to the voluminous research on risk factors, there has been relatively little empirical study of protective factors for violence and antisocial behavior (McCord, Widom, & Crowell, 2001; U.S. Department of Health and Human Services, 2001). A protective factor is not simply the absence of a risk factor (e.g., no history of violence). Rather, it is the positive presence of some person, characteristic, or circumstance that can act to reduce the negative impact of one or more risk factors or otherwise directly buffer risk (Jessor, van den Bos, Vanderryn, Costa, & Turbin, 1995). Howell (1997) identified the following three classes of protective factors: (a) factors inherent in the individual, (b) factors related to the development of social bonding, and (c) healthy beliefs and clear standards for behavior.

Any risk assessment conducted with juvenile offenders carries the additional requirement of being developmentally informed (Borum & Verhaagen, in press; Hoge, 1999, 2001; Hoge & Andrews, 1996). Children and adolescents are different from adults in many ways, not just in age or size (Griffin & Torbet, 2002; McCord, Widom, & Crowell, 2001; Rosado, 2000). There are numerous reasons that assessing risk in juveniles is different than in adults: The base rates of violence are quite different; the risk factors are different; behavioral norms are different; individual factors are less stable; and psychosocial maturity is more central (Borum, 2000, 2002, in press; Borum & Verhaagen, in press). Even among youth, predictors of violent behavior also vary by developmental stages. For example, "during childhood, individual characteristics and family risk factors are most important. Later, during adolescence, peer group and school risk factors become important" (Howell, 1997, p. 164).

To develop an effective plan for managing a juvenile's risk for reoffending, it is critical to conduct a systematic assessment of risk, need, and protective factors (Borum, in press; Hoge, 2002; Hoge & Andrews, 1996). Unsystematic assessments often result in decisions that are inaccurate, inequitable, and lacking in accountability (Borum, in press; Hoge, 2002). One reason for these problems is that, without proper structure, evaluators tend to rely on factors that do not have a demonstrated relationship to violence recidivism and overlook some of the factors that do (Borum, 1996; Borum, Otto, & Golding, 1993; Cooper & Werner, 1990; Werner, Rose, Murdach, & Yesavage, 1989; Werner, Rose, & Yesavage, 1983). Wiebush, Baird, Krisberg, and Onek (1995) noted, "Historically, risk assessments and classifications have been informal, highly discretionary procedures carried out by individuals who have varying philosophies and different levels of experience and knowledge, and who use dissimilar criteria in the assessment process" (p. 173).

Although many jurisdictions have developed some type of assessment form or list of factors for juvenile classification decisions, these often are not comprehensive, not based on proven predictors, and do not generalize well beyond the locale for which they were developed (Hoge, 2001, 2002; Wiebush et al., 1995). Three recently developed instruments show tremendous promise for helping to structure assessments of risk and protective factors in juvenile offenders. The first two—the SAVRY (Structured Assessment of Violence Risk in Youth) and EARL (Early Assessment Risk List)—focus specifically on violence risk, whereas the third—the YLS/CMI (Youth Level of Service/Case Management Inventory) focuses more generally on delinquency recidivism.

The SAVRY and the EARL instruments both are based on Structured Professional Judgment (SPJ) risk-assessment model. In the SPJ model, an evaluator conducts a systematic assessment of predetermined risk factors that have demonstrated significant empirical relationships with criterion violence in prior research. Each risk factor is considered and coded for severity, but the ultimate determination of risk level is made according to the examiner's professional judgment—not based on a particular cutting score derived from summing the items.

In this way, the SPJ model draws on the strengths of both the clinical and actuarial approaches to decision making. The assessment is structured, systematic, empirically based, and yet sensitive to case-specific facts and situational influences. The research conducted to date suggests strongly that clinical risk judgments made using an SPJ instrument are much more accurate than those based on unaided clinical judgment and are likely to be as accurate as, or more accurate than, actuarial formulas (Borum & Douglas, in press).

SAVRY.[1] The SAVRY (Bartel, Borum, & Forth, 2000; Borum, Bartel, & Forth, 2001) is designed to focus specifically on violence risk in adolescents. The SAVRY protocol is composed of 24 risk items, divided into three categories (historical, individual, and social/contextual), and six protective items (see Table 1). The risk items each have a three-level coding structure (high,

TABLE 1
Items from the Structured Assessment of Violence Risk in Youth (SAVRY)

Historical risk factors:
- History of violence
- History of nonviolent offending
- Early initiation of violence
- Past supervision/intervention failures
- History of self-harm or suicide attempts
- Exposure to violence in the home
- Childhood history of maltreatment
- Parental/caregiver criminality
- Early caregiver disruption
- Poor school achievement

Social/contextual risk factors:
- Peer delinquency
- Peer rejection
- Stress and poor coping
- Poor parental management
- Lack of personal/social support
- Community disorganization

Individual/clinical risk factors:
- Negative attitudes
- Risk taking/impulsivity
- Substance-use difficulties
- Anger management problems
- Psychopathic traits
- Attention deficit/hyperactivity difficulties
- Poor compliance
- Low interest/commitment to school

Protective factors:
- Prosocial involvement
- Strong social support
- Strong attachments and bonds
- Positive attitude toward intervention and authority
- Strong commitment to school
- Resilient personality traits

moderate, and low) and the protective items have a two-level structure (present or absent). Specific coding guidelines are provided for each level. The identified risk factors all have been reviewed, analyzed, and well documented in the professional literature. The SAVRY has been translated into Dutch (by Henny Lodewijks) and Swedish (by Niklas Langstrom), and there are ongoing or completed projects in Canada, the Netherlands, Sweden, Singapore, Great Britain, Connecticut, and Nevada, with additional data being collected in at least a half dozen other jurisdictions.

Research conducted to date shows significant correlations between SAVRY scores and various measures of violence in juvenile justice and high-risk community-dwelling populations (Bartel, Forth, & Borum, 2001; Fitch, 2002; Catchpole & Gretton, in press; Lodewijks, 2002; McEachran, 2001). Using receiver operating characteristic analysis, which measures predictive accuracy in terms of relative improvement over chance, areas under the curve (AUCs) for the total score average about .74 to .80 across studies. Validity coefficients are generally as strong for females as for males, although much less research has been conducted with adolescent females (Fitch, 2002). What is, perhaps, of greatest interest is that the examiner judgments (summary risk rating), not made on the basis of any cutting score, consistently perform as well as, and often better than, the linear combination of the scores themselves. This finding has been evident in research on structured professional judgment tools and provides some of the first empirical evidence that clinical judgments—properly structured and based on sound assessments—can achieve levels of accuracy that rival that of any other known predictors while maintaining latitude for case-specific analysis.

EARL.[2] The EARL-20B (Early Assessment Risk List for Boys) (Augimeri, Koegl, Webster, & Levene, 2001) is an SPJ tool designed to aid evaluators in making judgments about future violence and antisocial behavior among boys under the age of 12—particularly those who exhibit behavioral problems and are considered to be at high risk. Like most of the adult instruments, the protocol contains 20 risk items, each of which is assigned a score of 0, 1, or 2, depending on the certainty and severity of the characteristic's presence in a given case. The 20 items are divided into three categories, including 6 family items (household circumstances, caregiver continuity, supports, stressors, parenting style, antisocial values and conduct), 12 child items (developmental problems; onset of behavioral difficulties; abuse/neglect/trauma; hyperactivity/impulsivity/attention deficits [HIA]; likeability; peer socialization; academic performance; neighborhood; authority contact; antisocial attitudes; antisocial behavior; and coping ability), and 2 responsivity items (family responsivity and child responsivity).

The authors have conducted a preliminary investigation with 378 boys and 69 girls in a court-based intervention program for young offenders. There was evidence of good interrater reliability (.80-.97) and validity with high scorers being much more likely than low scorers to have a subsequent criminal conviction after age 12 (Kogel, Augimeri, & Webster, 2000). The developers of this tool have created an analogous measure for assessing risk in young girls, called the EARL-21G. Although the domain names are the same, a few of the risk factors are different than on the version for boys. Results of a preliminary unpublished study also show promising psychometric characteristics (Levene et al., 2001).

YLS/CMI.[3] The YLS/CMI (Youth Level of Service/Case Management Inventory) is a tool for assessing risk, need, and protective factors that may relate to a juvenile's risk for general delinquent reoffending. This version represents an adaptation of the LSIR (Level of Service Inventory–Revised), an extensively researched commonly used risk assessment tool for adult offenders (Andrews & Bonta, 1995). Like its counterpart, the instrument is structured as a checklist of 42 items, grouped into eight domains (offense history, family circumstances/parenting, education, peer relations, substance abuse, leisure/recreation, personality/behavior, and attitudes). Items were selected based on their theoretical and empirical support in the literature. Importantly, the YLS/CMI also includes a comprehensive assessment of strengths.

The assessment model is similar in many ways to the SPJ model, but there are some distinctions. Each item is defined and assigned a risk level, but the item coding is somewhat less detailed than with most SPJ instruments. The other significant structural difference between the YLS/CMI and SPJ guides is that YLS/CMI scores are explicitly linked to decision making. In this way, it operates more like an formal actuarial tool (Grove & Meehl, 1996). Scores on the instrument are tallied, and the total score is matched to its corresponding percentile ranking based on norms from a juvenile sample. The manual suggests that certain score/percentile ranges should correspond to specified levels of relative risk and that those risk levels should guide the nature and intensity of supervision and intervention in the case. Existing research on the YLS/CMI is quite promising (Hoge & Andrews, 2002; Hoge, Andrews, & Leschied, 1996). With training, raters are able to score the items reliably and the scores themselves are significantly related to reoffending (Hoge & Andrews, 2002).

Apply Intensive Resources Selectively in High-Risk Cases

Historically, the development of probation or community supervision caseloads has carried the assumption that all juvenile offenders have an equal degree of risk and need. That is, a caseload of 50 kids is assumed to translate to 50 equal units of work. The reality is that juvenile offenders vary widely in the nature and degree of strengths, risks, and needs. Consequently, effective management requires different levels of contact and intervention (Hurst, 1999).

In nearly every system in which the issue has been studied, a relatively small proportion of juvenile offenders account for a majority of offenses. "For example, in Rochester, about 15% of high-risk youth accounted for 75% of all violent offenses committed by the entire sample from the time they were age 13 to when they were 17" (Howell, 1997, p. 163). That small group of high-rate offenders has been referred to as chronic juvenile offenders. Those who commit violent offenses are serious, violent chronic juvenile offenders (Krisberg, Neuenfeldt, Wiebush, & Rodriguez, 1994). They typically begin offending during childhood and continue both violent and nonviolent offenses throughout adolescence and into adulthood. They share many characteristics of those whom Terrie Moffitt called "life course persistent" offenders (Moffitt, 1993, 1997) and who Gerald Patterson called "early starters." They also tend to carry a substantial number of risk and need factors.

If it is true that 15% to 20% of juveniles commit 75% to 80% of juvenile offenses, does the equal-weighting model really make sense for caseload determination? Probably not. The American Probation and Parole Association suggested a different approach to load determination: one based on workload rather than caseload. This concept recognizes that cases of different intensity require a different amount of time to manage (Hurst, 1999). The serious, violent, and chronic—the high-rate offenders—require more contact and more intervention. Not only do they need more treatment, they also need different treatment. To be effective, interventions need to be individually targeted to the juvenile's particular risk/need factors (Krisberg et al., 1994). Altschuler and Armstrong (1991) concluded that "high rate offenders often exhibit a qualitatively different response to traditional treatment and are uniquely resistant to conventional intervention strategies" (p. 80). Trying to do one-size-fits-all supervision or giving equal units of attention to vastly different offenders results in very poor use of resources and is largely ineffective in reducing recidivism.

The logical- and evidence-based alternative is to assign more intensive resources to higher risk cases. This is one of the central "what works" principles in correctional treatment (Andrews et al., 1990; Dowden & Andrews, 1999). Of course, this requires that a reliable risk assessment/classification system exists to identify the true high risk/need cases. When this is accomplished and properly implemented, however, intensive supervision for high-risk offenders, combined with evidence-based interventions matched to their needs, can substantially reduce recidivism and enhance effective use of existing resources (Altschuler, Armstrong, & MacKenzie, 1999; Krisberg et al., 1994). Even without a focus on evidence-based treatments, intensive supervision programs that properly target high-risk cases produce recidivism rates that are at least as low as for institutional commitment/ incarceration with traditional parole but carry only a third of the associated costs (Barton & Butts, 1990, 1991).

Matching intensity of service with risk and need is a core tenet of "state of the art" prevention programs (Griffin & Torbet, 2002; Wiebush, McNulty, & Le, 2000). The so-called Comprehensive Strategy for serious, violent, chronic offenders developed and evaluated by the Office of Juvenile Justice and Delinquency Prevention (OJJDP) places a strong emphasis on appropriately identifying a high-risk population (Howell, Krisberg, Hawkins, & Wilson, 1995). The 8% Solution pioneered in Orange County, California, is built on the understanding that 8% of the juvenile offenders in that county are responsible for more than half of the juvenile crime—a pattern typical for many jurisdictions (Schumaker & Kurz, 1999). Administering intensive monitoring and intervention for low-level, infrequent (including many of the adolescent limited) offenders wastes resources. Conversely, mandating minimal contact and intervention for serious, violent, chronic offenders not only is wasteful and ineffective, but it also places the community at greater risk.

Choose Criminogenic Targets for Intervention

Traditional treatments for children and adolescents typically are designed to improve some aspect of their psychological adjustment, not to prevent violent and delinquent behavior. It should not be surprising that early evaluations of the effectiveness of juvenile offender rehabilitation showed very little impact in reducing recidivism (Romig, 1978). Even contemporary studies show that interventions for juvenile delinquents show their greatest success in improvements on measures of psychological functioning. As a result of treatment, more than one in four young offenders show improvements in psychological outcomes (28%)—more than twice as many as show improvements in interpersonal adjustment (12%), the next most amenable outcome (Lipsey, 1992, 1995). Improving psychological functioning in young people is a positive thing—but those changes, broadly defined, are statistically unrelated to reductions in recidivism (Lipsey, 1992, 1995).

This does not imply that specific psychological symptoms or conditions never are proper targets for intervention. Indeed, in some cases they may be. Psychotic symptoms such as paranoid delusions or command hallucinations, for example, may place some young people at risk for acting on them in a way that might be causally related to their offending. Cornell and Bendek (Cornell, Benedek, & Benedek, 1987) have posited that there is a small subgroup of juvenile homicide offenders whose psychotic symptoms are linked to the murder they committed. Similarly, hyperactivity may be viewed as a psychological condition, but it is also linked directly to risk for violence and delinquency. Current research shows that hyperactive children show high rates of antisocial behavior and conduct problems in adolescence (Barkley, Fischer, Edelbrock, & Smallish, 1990; Hechtman, Weiss, Perlman, & Amsel, 1984; Klein & Mannuzza, 1991; Loeber, Green, Keenen, & Lahey, 1995; Mannuzza, Klein, Konig, & Giampino, 1989; Satterfield, Hoppe, & Schell, 1982). Hyperactive boys have even been shown to be significantly more violent than their nonhyperactive male siblings (Loney, Whaley-Klahn, Kosier, & Conboy, 1983). The relationship between hyperactivity and violence holds even in controlled, prospective studies. For example, Satterfield and Schell (1997) found that hyperactive youth had a significantly higher rate of arrest (46% vs. 11%) and incarceration (22% vs. 1%) than controls. They also had a higher rate of arrest specifically for violent crimes (34% vs. 9%). In light of this type of evidence, it would be imprudent not to address such a robust psychological risk factor. The guiding principle in selecting a behavior or symptom as a target for intervention, however, should be the extent to which it may increase risk for violent and delinquent behavior.

The primary goal of correctional treatment is to reduce the likelihood of reoffending. Interventions, therefore, should be designed to remediate or ameliorate the effects of factors and conditions that might increase risk for violence and/or delinquency. If done correctly, this integrates the dual functions of risk assessment and risk management (Borum & Verhaagen, in press). The assessment identifies factors from research and the juvenile's history that may increase and decrease the likelihood of offending. The key dynamic risk (or needs) factors from the assessment then become targets for intervention.

For example, research consistently supports the proposition that substance abuse is a risk factor for violent behavior (Loeber & Dishion, 1983; Loeber & Stouthamer-Loeber, 1987, 1998) and recidivism (Dembo et al., 1995). Conversely, treatment may reduce risk for delinquency and violence. In a sample of 1,167 adolescents from four U.S. cities (Chicago, Minneapolis, Pittsburgh, and Portland) who were participating in a community-based substance-abuse intervention program, involvement in treatment was substantially related to lower risk of recidivism. The improvement was even more pronounced when combined with supervision. The proportion of youth reporting drug-related criminal activity fell from 68% to 27% among those under supervision of the criminal justice system and from 49% to 22% for those not under supervision (Farabee, Shen, Hser, Grella, & Anglin, 2001).

Arguing that treatment targets should be selected on the basis of their known association with recidivism may seem self-evident. It is quite common, however, for juvenile offender treatment programs to focus on issues that would seem to be helpful but that are actually unrelated to offense risk. Table 2 draws on a meta-analysis by Dowden and Andrews (1999) to show a listing of the most frequent criminogenic (or offense enhancing) and noncriminogenic factors targeted in juvenile offender programs, along with the correlation between that factor and the effect size of the intervention in reducing recidivism. They found that programs focusing primarily on criminogenic factors showed much larger effect sizes in reducing reoffending than those that did not (.22 vs. –.01) It is important to note that

TABLE 2
Treatment Targets and Their Effect on Reducing Recidivism

Description	*Effect Size (r)*
Criminogenic	
Family supervision	.35
Family affection	.33
Barriers to treatment	.30
Self-control	.29
Anger/antisocial feelings	.28
Vocational skills and job	.26
Academic	.23
Prosocial model	.19
Antisocial attitudes	.13
Reduce antisocial peers	.11
Noncriminogenic	
Increase conventional ambition	.00
Physical activity	–.03
Respect antisocial thinking	–.05
Vague emotional/personal problems	–.06
Target self-esteem	–.09
Family, Other	–.11
Increase cohesive antisocial peers	–.12
Fear of official punishment	–.18

SOURCE: Adapted from Dowden and Andrews (1999).

some dynamic factors such as improving self-esteem or inducing fear of official punishment (as is often the focus of scared-straight or shock incarceration programs) actually have negative correlations with effect size. That is, targeting these factors tends to increase, rather than decrease, reoffending. Effective intervention with serious juvenile offenders requires reliance on this "need principle" (Andrews et al., 1990) in selecting known risk factors as targets for intervention.

Do What Works

It can no longer be said that "nothing works" in correctional treatment of juvenile offenders (Cullen & Gendreau, 1989; Lipsey, 1999a; Tate, Reppucci, & Mulvey, 1995; Whitehead & Lab, 1989). Based on a meta-analysis of approximately 400 studies on treatment of juvenile delinquency, Lipsey (1995) found a positive and significant effect for treatment in reducing general delinquent recidivism, by an average of approximately 10%. Treatment is even effective with the most serious young offenders. Lipsey and Wilson (1998) synthesized the results of approximately 200 experimental or quasi-experimental studies in a meta-analysis that included only serious and violent juvenile offenders and found an average significant reduction of 6%, with somewhat larger effects for community-based programs than for institutional programs.

Although average reductions of 6% to 10% represent a substantial number of prevented crimes, those seemingly modest numbers mask the important fact that there is enormous variability in the effectiveness of different programs. In Dowden and Andrews's (1999) meta-analysis of what works in young offender treatment, the effect sizes among the 134 studies ranged from –.43 to +.83; in practical terms—from shockingly detrimental to remarkably effective. Some popular and widely implemented programs (e.g., D.A.R.E. and peer-led programs) have been evaluated and have been shown not to work. As with targeting noncriminogenic factors, some well-intended programs, such as waiver to adult court, even produce higher rates of recidivism (U.S. Department of Health and Human Services, 2001).

One of the most surprising of these findings to many is that, in general, interventions that aggregate high-risk youth—even in therapeutic or treatment-oriented settings—tend to be ineffective. Moreover, there is good evidence to suggest that these programs may even increase a youth's risk for recidivism and that this effect may be particularly pronounced for youth with initially low levels of delinquency. That is, the least serious kids suffer the most (Dishion, Capaldi, Spracklen, & Li, 1995; Dishion, Eddy, Haas, Li, & Spracklen, 1997; Dishion, McCord, & Poulin, 1999; Elliott & Menard, 1996; Poulin, Dishion, & Burraston, 2001). With this kind of striking variability among programs, it is a wonder that when the effects of all forms of treatment are combined to calculate an average effect, the net result is even in the positive—much less significantly positive—direction.

The reason, of course, is that there are effective programs that offset the impact of those that do not work. Although treatments for juvenile delinquents, overall, reduce delinquency by about 10%, the most successful programs typically show reductions in the range of 20% to 30% (Lipsey, 1995, 1999a). Those programs (Howell, 1997),

> typically focused on changing overt behavior through structured training or behavior modification interventions designed to improve interpersonal relations, self-control, school achievement, and specific job skills. . . . [They] were characterized by multimodal services, more intensive services (contact hours, duration, and intensity), and services more closely monitored by research teams, which resulted in better implementation. (p. 170)

These types of programs also tend to be effective for serious and violent juvenile offenders in noninstitutional settings. Individual counseling, an exception, does not appear to have a strong effect on delinquency generally, but does appear to be effective with serious offenders—reducing recidivism by a little more than 40% (Lipsey, 1992, 1995). The other two treatment modalities showing consistently positive effects were interpersonal skills and behavioral programs—each of which reduced recidivism by about 40% (approximately a 20 percentage point decrease) (Lipsey, 1992, 1995).

What are the characteristics of the most effective programs? A review by Garrett (1985) found the greatest treatment effects for three general categories of intervention: (a) social learning approaches, (b) family therapy, and (c) cognitive approaches. Focusing only on recidivism as an outcome of interest, Izzo and Ross (1990) analyzed the results of 46 studies, focusing particularly on whether the intervention was based on some theory or conceptual model. What they found was that interventions based on some theoretical principle or model were, on average, 5 times more effective in reducing recidivism than those that did not, although no particular theory showed significantly better effects than any other. In addition, interventions that included a cognitive component were more than twice as effective as those that did not. In analyzing these studies, the authors defined cognitive component rather broadly to include problem solving, negotiation skills training, interpersonal skills training, rational emotive therapy, role playing and modeling, or cognitive behavior modification.

There is additional evidence that focusing on thinking and behavior is a critical combination. In an early review by Ross and Fabiano (1985), 94% (15/16) of programs that included a cognitive component were found to be effective, compared to 29% (10/34) of programs that did not include a cognitive component. More recently, results from an examination of 69 studies were reviewed as part of the Correctional Drug Abuse Treatment Effectiveness (CDATE) Project (Pearson, Lipton, Cleland, & Yee, 2002). The researchers found that cognitive-behavioral programs generally showed stronger effects in reducing recidivism than pure behavior modification strategies. The conclusion was that

> cognitive behavioral treatment can reduce recidivism by significant amounts. This was found to be true for the overall collection of cognitive-behavioral studies and also for the subcategory of social skills development training and cognitive skills training. On the other hand, the CDATE meta-analyses, like that of Whitehead and Lab (1989), did not allow us to reject the null hypothesis for contingency contracting, token economies, and other standard behavior modification as effective in reducing recidivism. (pp. 490-491)

Similarly, but more specifically to young offenders, a meta-analytic review of cognitive-behavioral rehabilitation programs for offenders, conducted by Lipsey, Chapman, and Landenberger (2001) found that "[cognitive behavioral] demonstration programs with juveniles both on probation/parole and in custodial institutions produced sizable reductions in recidivism, with treated offenders showing only one-third to two-thirds the recidivism rates of untreated controls" (p. 155). Regarding specific cognitive treatment targets, research by Kenneth Dodge and colleagues (Dodge, 1991; Dodge, Petit, McClaskey, & Brown, 1986) suggested that two very promising deficits for intervention are (a) social perceptions (social cognition)—particularly the tendency to misperceive hostility in others' intentions—and (b) problem solving—enhancing the ability to generate nonaggressive solutions to interpersonal conflicts.

Given the variability in program effectiveness, it will pay significant dividends—in program costs and in offense reduction—to apply what is already known about what works and what does not in treatment and program planning (Borum & Verhaagen, in press). Although literally hundreds of offender treatment programs exist, very few have been systematically evaluated to determine whether they are effective. Even many of those that have been evaluated have not been evaluated very well. To address this gap in our knowledge of evidence-based programs for preventing youth violence, in 1996, Del Elliott and his colleagues from the Center for the Study and Prevention Violence embarked on a project to identify best-practice programs that been subjected to a solid experimental evaluation, that had been replicated, where significant effects were found in reducing violence and those effects were sustained for at least a year (Mihalic, Irwin, Elliott, Fagan, & Hansen, 2001). The product of this effort was the designation of 10 blueprint programs. These are all programs that have been proven to work and several of them—particularly Multisystemic Therapy, Functional Family Therapy, and Aggression Replacement Training—are beginning to be implemented in juvenile justice systems throughout the United States. Using what is known about what works will lead to better use of resources and greater reductions in recidivism.

Implement, Follow Up, and Modify

At both a programmatic and at a case level, the implementation and follow-up of a proposed intervention is where many failures occur. Even the best evidence-based programs will not be effective if they are not properly implemented and monitored. Indeed, Lipsey's meta-analyses (1995, 1999a) showed that program success was strongly related to whether the intervention was fully implemented and whether its fidelity was strictly monitored.

As one example, results from a four-site (Boston, Memphis, Newark, and Detroit) evaluation (Fagan, 1990) of intensive supervision for violent juvenile offenders found that

> where the program design was well-implemented and its underlying theoretical principles were in strong evidence, *significantly lower recidivism rates* for violent, serious, and total crimes were observed. . . . In Boston, where implementation of the experimental program was strongest, youths consistently had lower recidivism scores than controls. Most percentage differences exceeded 25 percent and several were over 100 percent lower. (p. 260)

In addition to program-level implementation issues, with individual juvenile offenders it is critical to conduct regular reassessments of risk and need (Borum & Verhaagen, in press). As noted above, one of the developmental differences between juvenile and adult offenders is that juveniles are "moving targets" (Borum, 2000, in press; Grisso, 1998). Adolescence is a time when major life changes are occurring—cognitively, biologically, socially, and emotionally. Identity and, by inference, personality, is not fully formed and its behavioral manifestations are much less stable than in adults. Because juveniles are developing and changing, it is particularly important to ensure that mechanisms are in place to ensure that treatment needs and risk factors are reassessed and that intervention plans are modified accordingly (Borum, in press; Borum & Verhaagen, in press).

CONCLUSION

Over the past 50 years, social scientists have amassed an enormous amount of evidence about predictors, patterns, and pathways of serious juvenile offending. During that same period, hundreds and perhaps thousands of programs have been developed and implemented with the goal of reducing violence risk in young offenders. Relatively few of those programs, however, are based on the existing research knowledge and even fewer have been rigorously evaluated to determine whether they are effective. One lesson we have learned, though, is that good intentions and good ideas are not sufficient to produce a successful intervention. Some factors assumed to predict violence, turned out, when examined, not even to be statistically related. Interventions assumed to reduce reoffending, did not, and in some cases they made kids worse.

With increasing economic and policy pressures to do more good with less money, our choices are perhaps more important than ever before. If we are to make the best use of scarce resources, we should invest in what works. We know that treatment—even with serious, violent offenders—can work and can save money. But to do it right, we must apply existing research to policy and practice. The principles discussed in this article are evidence based in the truest sense. They are founded on the results of hundreds of research studies and they point consistently in the same direction.

Serious, chronic juvenile offenders, almost by definition, have very high rates of recidivism; typically about two thirds reoffend over the course of a year. It is possible, though, to manage most of these cases in the community with success rates that are at least as good—probably better—than with institutional confinement. The key is to adequately assess the offender's risks, needs, and strengths; to choose treatment targets that are related to offense risk; and apply proven interventions—especially those that are theoretically grounded and that use cognitive behavioral methods—to address those problems. And if we reserve intensive interventions—both monitoring and treatment—for the highest risk cases but apply it there with rigor and fidelity, we will prevent much more overall crime and violence. The verdict is in: Evidence-based intervention works.

NOTES

1. More information on the SAVRY can be found on the Web at www.fmhi.usf.edu/mhlp/savry/statement.htm. Copies of the SAVRY can be ordered from Specialized Training Services, 9606 Tierra Grande, Suite 105, San Diego, CA. 92126; (800) 848-1226. Web: www.specializedtraining.com.

2. Copies of the EARL-20B and EARL-21G can be ordered from Earlscourt Child and Family Centre, 46 St. Clair Gardens, Toronto, Ontario, Canada M6E 3V4; (416) 654-8981; e-mail: mailus@earlscourt.on.ca; Web: www.earlscourt.on.ca.

3. Copies of the YLSI/CMI can be ordered from Multi-health Systems, P.O. Box 950, North Tonawanda, NY 14120-0950; (800) 456-3003; e-mail: customerservice@mhs.com; Web: www.mhs.com.

REFERENCES

Altschuler, D. M., & Armstrong, T. L. (1991). Intensive aftercare for the high-risk juvenile parolee: Issues and approaches in reintegration and community supervision. In T. Armstrong (Ed.), *Intensive interventions with high-risk youths: Promising approaches in juvenile probation and parole* (pp. 45-84). Monsey, NY: Criminal Justice Press.

Altschuler, D., Armstrong, T., & MacKenzie, D. (1999, July). Reintegration, supervised release, and intensive aftercare. *Bulletin*. Washington, DC: Office of Juvenile Justice and Delinquency Prevention.

Andrews, D., & Bonta, J. (1995). *Level of Service Inventory–Revised*. Toronto, Canada: Multi-Health Systems.

Andrews, D. A., Zinger, I., Hoge, R. D., Bonta, J., Gendreau, P., & Cullen, F. T. (1990). Does correctional treatment work? A clinically-relevant and psychologically-informed meta-analysis. *Criminology, 28*(3), 369-404.

Atkins, D. L., Pumariega, A. J., Montgomery, L., Rogers, K., Nybro, C., Jeffers, G., & Sease, F. (1999). Mental health and incarcerated youth. I: Prevalence and nature of psychopathology. *Journal of Child and Family Studies, 8*, 193-204.

Augimeri, L., Webster, C., Koegl, C., & Levene, K. (2001). Early Assessment Risk List for Boys: EARL-20B, Version 2 [Computer software]. Toronto, Canada: Earlscourt Child and Family Centre.

Barkley, R., Fischer, M., Edelbrock, C., & Smallish, L. (1990). The adolescent outcome of hyperactive children diagnosed by research criteria: I. An 8 year prospective follow-up study. *Journal of the American Academy of Child and Adolescent Psychiatry, 29*, 546-557.

Bartel, P., Borum, R., & Forth, A. (2000). *Structured Assessment for Violence Risk in Youth (SAVRY)* (Consultation Ed.). Tampa, FL: Louis de la Parte Florida Mental Health Institute, University of South Florida.

Bartel, P., Forth, A., & Borum, R. (2001). *Development and validation of the Structured Assessment for Violence Risk in Youth (SAVRY)*. Manuscript in preparation.

Barton, W. H., & Butts, J. A. (1990). Viable options: Intensive supervision programs for juvenile delinquents. *Crime and Delinquency, 36*, 238-255.

Barton, W. H., & Butts, J. A. (1991). Intensive supervision alternatives for adjudicated juveniles. In T. Armstrong (Ed.), *Intensive interventions with high-risk youths: Promising approaches in juvenile probation and parole* (pp. 317-340). New York: Criminal Justice Press.

Borum, R. (1996). Improving the clinical practice of violence risk assessment: Technology, guidelines and training. *American Psychologist, 51*, 945-956.

Borum, R. (2000). Assessing violence risk among youth. *Journal of Clinical Psychology, 56*, 1263-1288.

Borum, R. (2002, March). *Why is assessing violence risk in juveniles different than in adults?* Paper presented at the biennial conference of the American Psychology-Law Society, Austin, TX.

Borum, R. (in press). Assessing risk for violence among juvenile offenders. In S. Sparta & G. Koocher (Eds.), *The forensic assessment of children and adolescents: Issues and applications*. New York: Oxford University Press.

Borum, R., Bartel, P., & Forth, A. (2001). *Manual for the Structured Assessment for Violence Risk in Youth (SAVRY)* (Consultation Ed.). Tampa: University of South Florida.

Borum, R. & Douglas, K. (in press). New directions in violence risk assessment. *Psychiatric Times*.

Borum, R., Otto, R., & Golding, S. (1993). Improving clinical judgment and decision making in forensic evaluation. *Journal of Psychiatry and Law, 21*, 35-76.

Borum, R., & Verhaagen, D. (in press). *A practical guide to assessing and managing violence risk in juveniles*. New York: Guilford.

Catchpole, R. E. H., & Gretton, H. M. (in press). The predictive validity of risk assessment with violent young offenders: A one-year examination of criminal outcome. *Criminal Justice and Behavior.*

Cauffman, E., Feldman, S., Waterman, J., & Steiner, H. (1998). Posttraumatic stress disorder among female juvenile offenders. *Journal of the American Academy of Child and Adolescent Psychiatry, 37*(11), 1209-1216.

Cooper, R., & Werner, P. (1990). Predicting violence in newly admitted inmates: A lens model analysis of staff decision making. *Criminal Justice and Behavior, 17*, 431-447.

Cornell, D., Benedek, E., & Benedek, D. (1987). Juvenile homicide: Prior adjustment and a proposed typology. *American Journal of Orthopsychiatry, 57*, 383-393.

Cullen, F. T., & Gendreau, P. (1989). The effectiveness of correctional rehabilitation: Reconsidering the "nothing works" debate. In L. Goodstein & D. MacKenzie (Eds.), *The American prison: Issues in research and policy.* New York: Plenum.

Dembo, R., Turner, G., Chin Sue, C., Schmeidler, J., Borden, P., & Manning, D. (1995). Predictors of recidivism to a juvenile assessment center. *International Journal of the Addictions, 30*, 1425-1452.

Dishion, T. J., Capaldi, D. M., Spracklen, K. M., & Li, F. (1995). Peer ecology of male adolescent drug use. *Development and Psychopathology, 7*, 803-824.

Dishion, T. J., Eddy, J. M., Haas, E., Li, F., & Spracklen, K. (1997). Friendships and violent behavior during adolescence. *Social Development, 6*, 207-223.

Dishion, T. J., McCord, J., & Poulin, F. (1999). When interventions harm: Peer groups and problem behavior. *American Psychologist, 54*, 755-764.

Dodge, K. (1991). The structure and function of reactive and proactive aggression. In D. Pepler & K. Rubin (Eds.), *The development and treatment of childhood aggression.* Hillsdale, NJ: Erlbaum.

Dodge, K., Petit, G., McClaskey, C., & Brown, M. (1986). Social competence in children. *Monograph on Social Research in Child Development, 51*, Series No. 213.

Dowden, C., & Andrews, D. (1999). What works in young offender treatment: A meta-analysis. *FORUM on Corrections Research, 11*(2), 21-24.

Elliott, D. S., & Menard, S. (1996). Delinquent friends and delinquent behavior: Temporal and developmental patterns. In J. D. Hawkins (Ed.), *Current theories of crime and deviance* (pp. 28-67). Thousand Oaks, CA: Sage.

Fagan, J. (1990). Treatment and re-integration of violent juvenile offenders: Experimental results. *Justice Quarterly, 7*, 233-263.

Farabee, D., Shen, H., Hser, Y. I., Grella, C. E., & Anglin, M. D. (2001). The effect of drug treatment on criminal behavior among adolescents in DATOS-A. *Journal of Adolescent Research, 16*, 679-696.

Finkelhor, D., & Hashima, P. (2001). The victimization of children and youth: A comprehensive overview. In S. White (Ed.), *Handbook of youth and justice* (pp. 49-78). Newell, MA: Kluwer Plenum.

Fitch, D. (2002). *Analysis of common risk factors for violent behavior in Native American adolescents referred for residential treatment.* Unpublished doctoral dissertation, Department of Counselor Education, Texas Southern University.

Garrett, C. J. (1985). Effects of residential treatment of adjudicated delinquents: A meta-analysis. *Journal of Research in Crime and Delinquency, 22*(2), 287-308.

Gottfredson, D. C., & Barton, W. H. (1993). Deinstitutionalization of juvenile offenders. *Criminology, 31*(4), 591-611.

Griffin, P., & Torbet, P. (2002). *Desktop guide to good juvenile probation practice*. National Center for Juvenile Justice, Pittsburgh, PA [producer]. Washington, DC: Office of Juvenile Justice and Delinquency Prevention.

Grisso, T. (1996). Society's retributive response to juvenile violence: A developmental perspective. *Law and Human Behavior, 20*, 229-247.

Grisso, T. (1998). *Forensic evaluation of juveniles*. Sarasota, FL: Professional Resource Press.

Grisso, T., & Schwartz, R. (Eds.). (2000). *Youth on trial: A developmental perspective on juvenile justice*. Chicago: University of Chicago Press.

Grove, W., & Meehl, P. (1996). Comparative efficiency of informal (subjective, impressionistic) and formal (mechanical, algorithmic) prediction procedures: The clinical-statistical controversy. *Psychology, Public Policy and Law, 2*, 293-323.

Hamilton, C., Falshaw, L., & Browne, K. (2002). The link between recurrent maltreatment and offending behaviour. *International Journal of Offender Therapy & Comparative Criminology, 46*, 75-94.

Hann, D. A., & Borek, N. (2001). Taking stock of risk factors for child/youth externalizing behavior problems. Bethesda, MD: National Institute of Mental Health.

Hawkins, J., Herrenkohl, T., Farrington, D., Brewer, D., Catalano, R., & Harachi, T. (1998). A review of predictors of youth violence. In R. Loeber & D. Farrington (Eds.), *Serious and violent juvenile offenders: Risk factors and successful interventions* (pp. 106-146). Thousand Oaks, CA: Sage.

Hawkins, J., Herrenkohl, T., Farrington, D., Brewer, D., Catalano, R., Harachi, T., et al. (2000, April). Predictors of youth violence. *Bulletin*. Washington, DC: Office of Juvenile Justice and Delinquency Prevention.

Hechtman, L., Weiss, G., Perlman, T., & Amsel, R. (1984). Hyperactives as young adults: Initial predictors of adult outcome. *Journal of the American Academy of Child Psychiatry, 23*, 250-260.

Hoge, R. (1999). *Assessing adolescents in educational, counseling and other settings*. Mahwah, NJ: Erlbaum.

Hoge, R. (2001). *The juvenile offender: Theory, research and applications*. Norwell, MA: Kluwer Plenum.

Hoge, R. (2002). Standardized instruments for assessing risk and need in youthful offenders. *Criminal Justice and Behavior, 29*, 380-396.

Hoge, R., & Andrews, D. (1996). *Assessing the youthful offender: Issues and techniques*. New York: Plenum.

Hoge, R., & Andrews, D. (2002). *The youth level of service/case management inventory manual and scoring key*. Toronto, Canada: Multi-Health Systems.

Hoge, R. D., Andrews, D. A., & Leschied, A. (1996). An investigation of risk and protective factors in a sample of youthful offenders. *Journal of Child Psychology and Psychiatry, 37*, 419-424.

Howell, J. (1997). *Juvenile justice and youth violence.* Thousand Oaks, CA: Sage.

Howell, J., Krisberg, B., Hawkins, J., & Wilson, J. (1995). *Sourcebook on serious, violent, and chronic juvenile offenders.* Thousand Oaks, CA: Sage.

Hurst, H., III. (1999, November). Workload measurement for juvenile justice system personnel: Practices and needs. *Bulletin.* Washington, DC: Department of Justice, Office of Justice Programs, Office of Juvenile Justice and Delinquency Prevention.

Izzo, R., & Ross, R. (1990). A meta-analysis of rehabilitation programs for juvenile delinquents: A brief report. *Criminal Justice and Behavior, 17*, 134-142.

Jessor, R., van den Bos, J., Vanderryn, J., Costa, F., & Turbin, M. (1995). Protective factors in adolescent problem behavior: Moderator effects and developmental change. *Developmental Psychology, 31*, 923-933.

Kazdin, A. (2000). Adolescent development, mental disorders, and decision making of delinquent youths. In T Grisso & R. Schwartz (Eds.), *Youth on trial: A developmental perspective on juvenile justice* (pp. 33-65). Chicago: University of Chicago Press.

Klein, R., & Mannuzza, S. (1991). Long-term outcome of hyperactive children: A review. *Journal of the American Academy of Child and Adolescent Psychiatry, 30*, 383-387.

Koegl, C., Augimeri, L., & Webster, C. (2000). *Very young offenders: Risk factors and outcome.* Paper presented at the 2000 biennial conference of the American Psychology-Law Society, New Orleans, LA.

Krisberg, B., Neuenfeldt, D., Wiebush, R., & Rodriguez, O. (1994). *Juvenile intensive supervision: Planning guide.* Washington, DC: Office of Juvenile Justice and Delinquency Prevention.

Levene, K., Augimeri, L., Pepler, D., Walsh, M., Webster, C., & Koegl, C. (2001). Early Assessment Risk List for Girls: EARL-21G, Version 1, Consultation Edition [Computer software]. Toronto, Canada: Earlscourt Child and Family Centre.

Lipsey, M. (1992). Juvenile delinquency treatment: A meta-analytic inquiry into the variability of effects. In T. D. Cook, H. Cooper, D. S. Cordray, H. Hartmann, L. V. Hedges, R. J. Light, et al. (Eds.), *Meta-analysis for explanation: A casebook.* New York: Russell Sage.

Lipsey, M. (1995). What do we learn from 400 research studies on the effectiveness of treatment with juvenile delinquents? In J. McGuire (Ed.), *What works? Reducing reoffending* (pp. 63-78). New York: John Wiley.

Lipsey, M. (1999a). Can intervention rehabilitate serious delinquents? *Annals of the American Academy of Political and Social Science, 564*, 142-166.

Lipsey, M. (1999b). Can rehabilitative programs reduce the recidivism of juvenile offenders? An inquiry into the effectiveness of practical programs. *Virginia Journal of Social Policy & the Law, 6*(3), 101-129.

Lipsey, M., Chapman, G., & Landenberger, N. (2001). Cognitive-behavioral programs for offenders. *Annals for the American Academy of Political and Social Science, 578*, 144-157.

Lipsey, M., & Derzon, J. (1998). Predictors of violent or serious delinquency in adolescence and early adulthood: A synthesis of longitudinal research. In R. Loeber

& D. P. Farrington (Eds.), *Serious and violent juvenile offenders: Risk factors and successful interventions* (pp. 86-105). Thousand Oaks, CA: Sage.

Lipsey, M., & Wilson, D. (1998). Effective intervention for serious juvenile offenders: A synthesis of research. In R. Loeber & D. P. Farrington (Eds.), *Serious and violent juvenile offenders: Risk factors and successful interventions* (pp. 313-345). Thousand Oaks, CA: Sage.

Lodewijks, H. (2002, July). *The reliability and predictive validity of the SAVRY (Structured Assessment of Violence Risk in Youth) in a Dutch population of male adolescent delinquents.* Paper presented at the XXVIIth International Congress on Law and Mental Health: Amsterdam, Netherlands.

Loeber, R., & Dishion, T. (1983). Early predictors of male delinquency: A review. *Psychological Bulletin, 94,* 68-99.

Loeber, R., Green, S., Keenen, K., & Lahey, B. (1995). Which boys will fare worse? Early predictors of the onset of conduct disorder in a six-year longitudinal study. *Journal of the American Academy of Child and Adolescent Psychiatry, 34,* 499-509.

Loeber, R., & Stouthamer-Loeber, M. (1998). Development of juvenile aggression and violence: Some common misperceptions and controversies. *American Psychologist, 53,* 242-259.

Loeber, R., & Stouthamer-Loeber, M. (1987). Prediction. In H. C. Quay (Ed.), *Handbook of juvenile delinquency* (pp. 325-382). New York: John Wiley.

Loney, J., Whaley-Klahn, M., Kosier, T., & Conboy, J. (1983). Hyperactive boys and their brothers at age 21: Predictors of aggressive and antisocial outcomes. In K. van Dusen & S. Mednick (Eds.), *Prospective studies of crime and delinquency* (pp. 181-207). Boston: Kluwer-Nijhoff.

Mannuzza, S., Klein, R., Konig, P., & Giampino, T. (1989). Hyperactive boys almost grown up: IV. Criminality and its relationship to psychiatric status. *Archives of General Psychiatry, 46,* 1073-1079.

Marsteller, F., Brogan, D., Smith, I., Ash, P., Daniels, D., Rolka, D., et al. (1997). *The prevalence of substance use disorders among juveniles admitted to regional youth detention centers operated by the Georgia Department of Children and Youth Services.* CSAT Final Report. Retrieved from http://www.behav.com/projects/CSATFinalReport.html

McCord, J., Widom, C. S., & Crowell, N. A. (Eds.) (2001). *Juvenile crime, juvenile justice.* Washington, DC: National Academy Press.

McEachran, A. (2001). *The predictive validity of the PCL-YV and the SAVRY in a population of adolescent offenders.* Unpublished master's thesis, Simon Fraser University, Burnaby, British Columbia.

Mihalic, S., Irwin, K., Elliott, D., Fagan, A., & Hansen, D. (2001, July). Blueprints for violence prevention. *Bulletin.* Washington, DC: Office of Juvenile Justice and Delinquency Prevention.

Moffitt, T. (1993). "Life course persistent" and "adolescence limited" antisocial behavior: A developmental taxonomy. *Psychological Review, 100,* 674-701.

Moffitt, T. (1997). Adolescence-limited and life-course-persistent offending: A complementary pair of developmental theories. In T. Thornberry (Ed.), *Developmen-*

tal theories of crime and delinquency (pp. 11-54). New Brunswick, NJ: Transaction.

Otto, R., Greenstein, J., Johnson, M., & Friedman, R. (1992). Prevalence of mental disorders among youth in the juvenile justice system. In J. Cocozza (Ed.), *Responding to the mental health needs of youth in the juvenile justice system* (pp. 7-48). Seattle, WA: National Coalition for the Mentally Ill in the Criminal Justice System.

Pearson, F., Lipton, D., Cleland, C., & Yee, D. (2002). The effects of behavioral/cognitive-behavioral programs on recidivism. *Crime & Delinquency, 48*, 476-496.

Policy Design Team. (1994). *Mental health needs of youth in Virginia's juvenile detention centers*. Richmond, VA: Department of Criminal Justice Services.

Poulin, F., Dishion, T., & Burraston, B. (2001). 3-year iatrogenic effects associated with aggregating high-risk adolescents in cognitive-behavioral preventive interventions. *Applied Developmental Science, 5*, 214-224.

Puzzanchera, C., Stahl, A., Finnegan, T., Tierney, N., & Snyder, H. (2002). *Juvenile Court Statistics 1999*. Washington, DC: Office of Juvenile Justice and Delinquency Prevention.

Romig, D. (1978). *Justice for our children: An examination of juvenile delinquent rehabilitation programs*. Lexington, MA: Lexington Books.

Rosado, L. (Ed.). (2000). *Kids are different: How knowledge of adolescent development theory can aid decision-making in court*. Washington, DC: American Bar Association Juvenile Justice Center.

Ross, R. R., & Fabiano, E. (1985). *Time to think: A cognitive model of delinquency prevention and offender rehabilitation*. Johnson City, TN: Institute of Social Sciences and Arts.

Satterfield, J., Hoppe, C., & Schell, A. (1982). A prospective study of delinquency in 110 adolescent boys with attention-deficit disorder and 88 normal adolescent boys. *American Journal of Psychiatry, 139*, 795-798.

Satterfield, J., & Schell, A. (1997). A prospective study of hyperactive boys with conduct problems and normal boys: Adolescent and adult criminality. *Journal of the American Academy of Child and Adolescent Psychiatry, 36*, 1726-1735.

Schumaker, M., & Kurz, G. (1999). *The 8% solution: Preventing serious, repeat juvenile crime*. Thousand Oaks, CA: Sage.

Scott, E. (2000). Criminal responsibility in adolescence: Lessons from developmental psychology, (pp.291-324). In T Grisso & R. Schwartz (Eds.), *Youth on trial: A developmental perspective on juvenile justice*. Chicago: University of Chicago Press.

Shaffer, D., Fisher, P., Dulcan, M. K., Davies, M., Piacentini, J., Schwab-Stone, M. E., et al. (1996). The NIMH Diagnostic Interview Schedule for Children, version 2.3 (DISC 2.3): Description, acceptability, prevalence rates and performance in the MECA study. methods for the epidemiology of child and adolescent mental disorders study. *Journal of the American Academy of Child and Adolescent Psychiatry, 35*, 865-877.

Shelton, D. (1998). *Estimates of emotional disorder in detained and committed youth in the Maryland juvenile justice system.* Report to the Maryland Juvenile Justice Advisory Council.

Steiner, H., Garcia, I., & Matthews, Z. (1997). Posttraumatic Stress disorder in incarcerated juvenile delinquents. *Journal of the American Academy of Child and Adolescent Psychiatry, 36*(3), 357-365.

Stouthamer-Loeber, M., Loeber, R., Homish, L., & Wei, E. (2001). Maltreatment of boys and the development of disruptive and delinquent behavior. *Development & Psychopathology, 13*, 941-955.

Tate, D. C., Reppucci, N. D., & Mulvey, E. (1995). Violent juvenile delinquents: Treatment efficacy and implications for future action. *American Psychologist, 50*, 777-785.

Ulzen, T., & Hamilton, H. (1998). The nature and characteristics of psychiatric comorbidity in incarcerated adolescents. *Canadian Journal of Psychiatry, 43*(1), 57-63.

U.S. Department of Health and Human Services. (2001). *Youth violence: A report of the Surgeon General.* Rockville, MD: U.S. Department of Health and Human Services, Substance Abuse and Mental Health Services Administration, Center for Mental Health Services, National Institutes of Health, National Institute of Mental Health. Retrieved from www.surgeongeneral.gov/library/youthviolence

Werner, P., Rose, T., Murdach, A., & Yesavage, J. (1989). Social workers' decision making about the violent client. *Social Work Research and Abstracts, 25*(3), 17-20.

Werner, P., Rose, T., & Yesavage, J. (1983). Reliability, accuracy and decision making strategy in clinical predictions of imminent dangerousness. *Journal of Consulting and Clinical Psychology, 51*, 815-825.

Whitehead, J. T., & Lab, S. P. (1989). A meta-analysis of juvenile correctional treatment. *Journal of Research in Crime and Delinquency, 26*(3), 276-295.

Wiebush, R., Baird, C., Krisberg, B., & Onek, D. (1995). Risk assessment and classification for serious, violent, and chronic juvenile offenders. In J. Howell, B. Krisberg, J. Hawkins, & J. Wilson (Eds.), *A sourcebook: Serious, violent and chronic juvenile offenders* (pp. 171-212). Thousand Oaks, CA: Sage.

Wiebush, R., McNulty, B., & Le, T. (2000, July). Implementation of the Intensive Community-Based Aftercare Program. *Bulletin.* Washington, DC: U.S. Department of Justice, Office of Justice Programs, Office of Juvenile Justice and Delinquency Prevention.

Randy Borum is a board-certified (ABPP) forensic psychologist and associate professor in the Department of Mental Health Law and Policy at the University of South Florida. He is author/coauthor of more than 80 professional publications and currently serves as a senior consultant to the U.S. Secret Service in the National Threat Assessment Center, Advisory Board member for the FBI's Behavioral Science Unit, and a senior research scientist in the James and Jennifer Harrell Center for the Study of Family Violence. He is currently president of the American Academy of Forensic Psychology.

Part V
Forensic Practice: Professional And Ethical Issues

[24]

The Practice of Forensic Psychology

A Look Toward the Future in Light of the Past

Randy K. Otto *University of South Florida*
Kirk Heilbrun *MCP Hahnemahn University*

In a 1987 American Psychologist *article, Tom Grisso summarized the state of forensic psychological assessment, noted its limitations and potential, and offered suggestions for researchers and practitioners interested in contributing to its future. Since that time, there have been many important developments in the field of forensic psychology, as well as in clinical psychology more generally, some of which were anticipated and recommended by Grisso, and some of which were not. Forensic psychology is now at a crossroads, and the specialty must make an effort to respond to current challenges if it is to aid in the administration of justice by assisting legal decision makers. The need to distinguish between and identify levels of forensic knowledge and practice, establish guidelines for practice, educate legal consumers, and devote more attention to treatment issues in forensic contexts is highlighted.*

During its 50-year existence, the field of forensic psychology has gone through considerable change. Although psychologists provided some clinical services in correctional, delinquency, and other forensic settings toward the end of the 19th century, service provision by psychologists in forensic settings was not significant until after the Second World War, when clinical psychology became clearly established as a profession and practice area. Beginning in the 1950s and continuing to the present, clinical and counseling psychologists have become integral to the provision of assessment and therapeutic services in correctional, delinquency, and other forensic settings.

Psychologists have provided therapeutic services in what could be described as forensic settings (e.g., juvenile justice programs, correctional institutions, and noncorrectional settings in which therapy services are provided to forensic populations such as abuse and crime victims) since the profession of clinical psychology was established. Indeed, it can be argued that some forensic institutional settings provided the first opportunities for clinical psychologists to provide assessment and therapeutic services (e.g., see Travis, 1908, for a description of psychology's contributions to the juvenile justice system at the beginning of the 20th century). In contrast, *forensic psychological assessment* (for the purposes of this article, defined as the psychological assessment of persons for the purpose of assisting the legal fact finder[1]) is a relatively new specialty of clinical psychology. Although there is some evidence that turn-of-the-century legal decision makers were willing to consider the input of psychologists in some select legal matters (see Wrightsman, 2001, for a review of this history), forensic psychologists were not fully welcome in the courts until much later. Indeed, a 40-year-old case (*Jenkins v. U.S.*, 1962), in which a federal appellate court ruled that (a) psychologists with appropriate training and expertise were qualified to offer expert testimony on matters of mental disorder and (b) possession of a medical degree was not necessary for such testimony, is uniformly identified as a watershed case with respect to the participation of psychologists in the legal arena. Since that time, psychologists have become involved in the legal decision-making process in increasing numbers, leading some to refer to the field of forensic psychological assessment as a "cottage industry" (Grisso, 1987, p. 831).

Data that shed some light on the volume of forensic evaluations conducted annually are sparse and limited to criminal forensic evaluation. For example, Bonnie and Grisso (2000) reported that approximately 60,000 criminal defendants are evaluated each year for competence to stand trial. Stephen Hart (personal communication, January 23, 2001) stated that between 60,000 and 80,000 evaluations in which the Psychopathy Checklist—Revised (Hare, 1991) is used are conducted each year. Data providing insight into the numbers of civil forensic evaluations and other types of criminal forensic evaluations performed each year are un-

Randy K. Otto, Department of Mental Health Law and Policy, Florida Mental Health Institute, University of South Florida; Kirk Heilbrun, Department of Clinical and Health Psychology, MCP Hahnemahn University.

We acknowledge the helpful comments of Tom Grisso, who reviewed an earlier version of this article.

Correspondence concerning this article should be addressed to Randy K. Otto, Department of Mental Health Law and Policy, Florida Mental Health Institute, University of South Florida, 13301 Bruce B. Downs Boulevard, Tampa, FL 33612-3899. E-mail: otto@mirage.fmhi.usf.edu

[1] This definition incorporates evaluations done by mental health professionals in which the only purpose is to assist the legal decision maker (e.g., a court-ordered evaluation of competence to stand trial), as well as evaluations requested by an attorney, the results of which will be presented into evidence only at that attorney's discretion. If such results are presented, then certainly one purpose of presenting them would involve assisting the legal decision maker, but another purpose would involve presenting these results as clearly as possible, which, from the attorney's perspective, would presumably help that attorney argue his or her case more effectively.

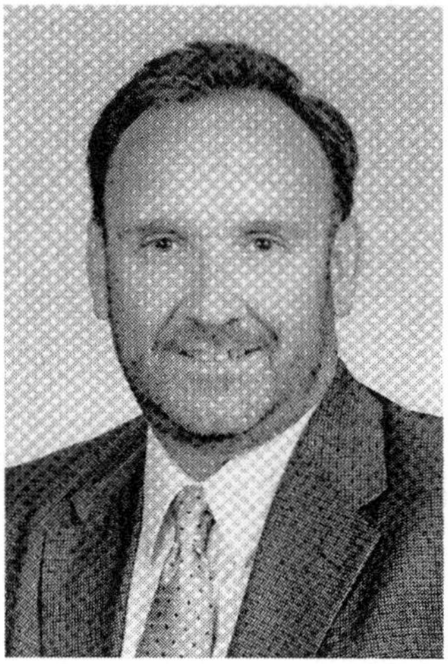

Randy K. Otto

available, but it seems reasonable to assume that literally hundreds of thousands of forensic evaluations are conducted annually by psychologists and other mental health professionals. And although it is also difficult to determine the number of psychologists providing treatment in what could be considered forensic settings, their prevalence in juvenile justice programs, correctional institutions, and noncorrectional settings in which therapy services are provided to forensic populations (e.g., abuse and crime victims) makes clear that forensic psychologists have established themselves as treatment providers, too.

Measures of Progress and Development in the Field

The growth of a profession and specialty area can be measured in a number of ways, such as with the development of professional organizations, outlets for dissemination of research and practice findings, practice standards, and processes that certify competence and advanced abilities. As reviewed below, using any of these yardsticks, one can see the specialty area of clinical forensic psychology has matured considerably in the past 25 years.

Professional Organizations

Contributing to and reflecting the growth and development of forensic psychology has been the establishment of professional organizations composed of psychologists and affiliated professionals who are interested in this specialty area. Some organizations (e.g., see Appendix) restrict membership to psychologists and focus on the applications of clinical psychology to law (e.g., the American Academy of Forensic Psychology, the American Association of Correctional Psychologists, the American College of Forensic Psychology), whereas other organizations are interdisciplinary and focus on the broad interface between psychology and law (e.g., the American Psychology–Law Society, which is Division 41 of the American Psychological Association [APA]). Additionally, a number of other interdisciplinary organizations do not simply focus on interactions between psychology and the legal system but on social, medical, forensic, and biological sciences and the legal system as well (e.g., the American Academy of Forensic Sciences). The American Psychology–Law Society, with a membership of nearly 3,000, is the largest, oldest, and probably the most influential organization in the psychology and law area (see Grisso, 1991, for a detailed description of the history and development of the organization).

Together, these organizations represent a body of professionals interested in the interface between clinical psychology and law. They sponsor professional and scientific meetings, their memberships collaborate with relevant legal organizations, they recognize achievement in the field, and they publish scientific journals and book series.

Publications

Perhaps the best indicator of the tremendous growth in the area of forensic psychological assessment is the proliferation of books and periodicals devoted to psychology and law and to forensic clinical psychology more specifically. As recently as 1980, only a few scientific journals primarily addressed psychology and law issues. At present, however, a large number of journals are devoted to law–psychology issues (e.g., *Law and Human Behavior*, *American Journal of Forensic Psychology*, *Behavioral Sciences and the Law*, *Criminal Justice and Behavior*, *Journal of Forensic Psychology Practice*, *Journal of Threat Assessment*). In addition to these psychology- and law-focused journals, a number of other scientific periodicals are more interdisciplinary in nature and are clearly relevant to forensic clinical psychologists (e.g., *Journal of Forensic Sciences*, *Journal of Psychiatry and Law*, *International Journal of Law and Psychiatry*, *Journal of the American Academy of Psychiatry and Law*, *American Journal of Forensic Psychiatry*). Also, an increasing number of books are devoted to forensic psychology and related concerns.

According to Grisso (1987), prior to the 1970s, there was a dearth of literature on forensic psychological assessment, and the 1970s saw the publication of a few books and monographs devoted to forensic assessment issues (e.g., McGarry, 1971; Megargee & Bohn, 1979; Ziskin, 1975). In the 1980s, the number of such publications increased and included a number of textbooks primarily or fully devoted to forensic psychology (e.g., Blau, 1984; Cooke, 1980; Ewing, 1985; Grisso, 1981, 1986; Melton, Petrila, Poythress, & Slobogin, 1987; Monahan, 1980; Roesch & Golding, 1980; Rogers, 1987a). More recently, a new era has begun in the forensic psychological assessment arena, with some classic books undergoing revision (e.g., Grisso, in press; Melton, Petrila, Poythress, & Slobogin, 1997; Rogers, 1997) and representing, in the words of Grisso (1987), "the development of a formal body of specialized knowledge called 'psycholegal assessment' . . . or 'forensic psy-

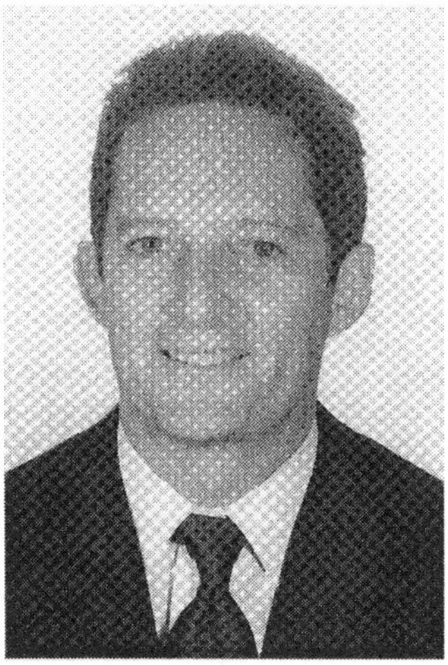

Kirk Heilbrun

chological assessment'" (p. 831), or, more broadly, "forensic mental health assessment" (Heilbrun, 2001).

Practice Standards

Another hallmark of a substantive specialty area or area of concentration is the development of a consensus regarding acceptable practice. Of considerable interest and importance to the development of forensic psychology and its identity as a unique area has been the development of forensic practice standards over the past 10 years. Two different types of standards have been developed: general practice guidelines and specific practice standards.

Specialty guidelines for forensic psychologists. In 1991, the American Academy of Forensic Psychology (an affiliate of the American Board of Forensic Psychology) and the American Psychology–Law Society published the Specialty Guidelines for Forensic Psychologists (SGFP; Committee on Ethical Guidelines for Forensic Psychologists, 1991). The primary goal of the SGFP is to improve the quality of forensic psychological services by providing guidance to psychologists delivering services to courts, members of the bar, litigants, and persons housed in forensic, delinquency, or correctional facilities. The SGFP are general in nature and scope but provide forensic psychologists with considerable direction in (a) identifying competent forensic practice; (b) practicing responsibly; (c) establishing relationships with parties involved in assessment, treatment, or consultation; and (d) identifying issues related to privacy, confidentiality, and privilege of services and communications.

APA practice guidelines. During the 1990s, APA promulgated two sets of guidelines relevant to forensic practice. In 1994, the Council of Representatives of APA adopted as policy the Guidelines for Child Custody Evaluations in Divorce Proceedings, the goal of which is to "promote proficiency in using psychological expertise in child custody evaluations" (APA, 1994, p. 677). In contrast to custody evaluation guidelines published by other organizations (e.g., see American Academy of Child and Adolescent Psychiatry, 1997; Association of Family and Conciliation Courts, n.d.), the APA guidelines focus less on the substantive task of child custody evaluation and more on the format and process of the evaluation. Reviewed in these guidelines, which are described in their introduction as aspirational and neither exhaustive nor mandatory, are the goals of the evaluation, the role and orientation of the examiner, the need for competence and ability in the examiner, confidentiality, record keeping, informed consent, data interpretation, and financial arrangements. Although these guidelines indeed provide some direction for psychologists conducting child custody evaluations, they do not necessarily set a standard of care, and they have been criticized by some as lacking substance (Otto, Buffington, & Edens, in press).

In 1998, APA's Council of Representatives adopted the Guidelines for Psychological Evaluations in Child Protection Matters (APA Committee on Professional Practice and Standards, 1998; APACOPP). The child protection guidelines are similar to the child custody evaluation guidelines in many ways. For example, the child protection evaluation guidelines are also aspirational. They are neither mandatory nor exhaustive, and their goal is to "facilitate the continued systematic development of the professional and help to assure a high level of practice by psychologists" (APACOPP, 1998, p. 2). Additionally, the guidelines are primarily concerned with the form and structure of the evaluation, and they provide considerably less direction for conducting the evaluation itself. Issues such as the purpose of the evaluation, role definition, evaluator competence, informed consent, confidentiality, record keeping, financial arrangements, and the structure of the evaluation are described in considerable detail.

Certification and Recognition of Advanced Practice

Mechanisms to identify advanced competence are frequently seen in established areas of practice. Further evidence of the maturation of forensic psychology as a field is provided by two relatively recent developments: certification for forensic practice and recognition of advanced forensic competence.

State-sponsored credentialing. In an attempt to provide some quality assurance in the area of criminal forensic evaluation, a number of states have adopted credentialing or certification programs for psychologists and other mental health professionals who assess criminal defendants to determine their competence to proceed in the criminal process or their mental state at the time of the offense. Presently, at least nine states require certification of some type (Farkas, DeLeon, & Newman, 1997), although the nature and extent of the credentialing process vary considerably across jurisdictions.

Board certification. Certification of competence in forensic psychology is accomplished on a national level in the United States through specialized board certification or diplomate status granted by a number of professional boards, with differing functions and practices. Some boards are discipline-bound and are specific to the practice of forensic psychology. Other boards are interdisciplinary and technique focused, insofar as they are concerned with a specific type of forensic practice (e.g., disability evaluation, child custody evaluation, evaluation and treatment of traumatic stress). Finally, at least one board is interdisciplinary and devoted to credentialing an array of forensic professionals (e.g., psychologists, handwriting experts, polygraphers, dentists, ballistics professionals) in general forensic practice. The issue of board certification, including recent developments, is discussed in more detail later in this article.

Contemporary Developments of Significance

There have been a number of important developments in the areas of forensic psychology and clinical psychology more generally since Grisso's 1987 article describing the state of forensic psychological assessment, some of which were anticipated by Grisso and some of which were not. Here we discuss these developments and their implications for the practice of forensic psychology.

Development of Specialty Training Programs

During the past 20 years, the field has witnessed an expansion in the opportunities for didactic training and supervised experience in forensic psychology at the graduate school, predoctoral, internship, and postdoctoral levels. There has been a steady increase in the number of doctoral programs in clinical and counseling psychology that feature at least one course or offer at least one practicum experience in forensic psychology. The number of predoctoral clinical internships offering supervised experience in forensic practice has also increased. However, despite the increase in formal forensic training of any kind offered by predoctoral and internship training sites, still relatively few doctoral programs have an emphasis in forensic training, and specialty forensic internship training in programs accredited by the Association of Psychology Postdoctoral and Internship Centers is available only at a limited number of sites (for a more comprehensive listing and description, see American Psychology–Law Society Careers and Training Committee, 1998; Cruise, 2001; Van Zelfde & Otto, 1997).

Somewhat more advanced in the development of forensic specialty training are postdoctoral fellowships. A total of 11 forensic postdoctoral fellowships were recently cited as available in the United States (Bersoff et al., 1997; Cruise, 2001), and, undoubtedly, other postdoctoral fellowships offer a significant amount of forensic training (for a detailed discussion of forensic training at all levels, see Tomkins, 1990). It is important that training opportunities expand in forensic psychology at the predoctoral through fellowship levels during the coming decade. Such development may be facilitated by APA's designation of forensic psychology as a practice specialty, which is discussed in the next section.

APA Specialization in Forensic Psychology

APA has historically designated four areas of specialty practice: clinical, counseling, school, and industrial–organizational. In the early 1990s, it was decided that additional areas of specialty practice in psychology would be considered, and APA formed the Committee for the Recognition of Specialties and Proficiencies in Professional Psychology (CRSPPP). Those within any specialty or proficiency in psychology could petition CRSPPP for recognition of *specialty* status—involving a greater degree of depth and breadth, more intensive training requirements, and greater development as a distinct area—or *proficiency* status—involving narrower and more specific skills (e.g., treatment of substance abuse)—for their area of expertise. However, under the rules established by APA for this process, an area cannot be both a specialty and a proficiency.

Psychologists within a number of areas have petitioned CRSPPP for specialty status for their area; if approved, a petition is voted on by APA's Council of Representatives. Areas with approval from both CRSPPP and the Council of Representatives that are now officially APA specialties include three traditional specialties—clinical, counseling, and school—as well as behavioral, child clinical, clinical neuropsychology, clinical health, and psychoanalysis. In September 2000, a petition for recognition of forensic psychology as a specialty was submitted by two important organizations in the area: the APA law and psychology division (the American Psychology–Law Society, Division 41) and the American Board of Professional Psychology specialty board in the area (the American Board of Forensic Psychology). Before this collaboration was finalized, however, psychologists practicing in the area went through a nearly four-year process involving vigorous debate about the nature and definition of forensic psychology, the appropriateness of APA specialization given the development of the field, the implications for training, and the potential impact on nonclinical areas of law and psychology (e.g., social, cognitive, developmental, and experimental). It was ultimately decided that the petition for specialization should define forensic psychology narrowly, to include the primarily clinical aspects of forensic assessment, treatment, and consultation. It was also clear from this debate that the area of law and psychology is unusual, if not unique, in the combination of areas of psychology that psychologists attracted to the application of their research and practice in legal contexts embrace: Preserving the combination of these areas is quite important to the larger field.

After public inspection of and comment on the petition, the Council of Representatives voted in August 2001 to recognize forensic psychology as a specialty (see the minutes of the Council of Representatives meeting, Section IX, Subsection B, at http://members.apa.org/governance/crminutes-aug01.html). Recognition of forensic psychology as an APA specialty could have several implications.

First, the applied area of forensic psychology, which has grown significantly during the past 20 years, may continue to grow even more rapidly with the increased exposure that will result from specialty status. Second, as a mainstream APA specialty, it should be clearer to psychologists in other areas and to applied psychologists who do forensic work that a recognized field associated with a body of knowledge and standards of practice should be learned and respected when practicing in forensic contexts. Third, the accreditation of specialty training programs in forensic psychology may occur sooner than it otherwise might have. It is expected that such accreditation would occur first at the postdoctoral level, as much of the specialty training in forensic psychology currently occurs following completion of the doctorate. The process of accreditation should encourage postdoctoral programs to become somewhat more uniform, incorporating the relevant body of knowledge and practice standards into their training but providing flexibility to consider the particular focus (e.g., criminal vs. civil, adult vs. child or family) of the program.

Instrument Development

Grisso (1987) identified both economic and legal factors that discouraged research and innovation in the area of forensic psychological assessment and warned of the negative consequences the field and its professionals might experience in the absence of such ongoing research and development. Indeed, Grisso (1987) saw research-based knowledge and expertise as one important way that forensic psychologists could distinguish themselves from other disciplines (e.g., psychiatrists and social workers) and provide a product that would not be limited by some of the problems with forensic assessment more generally (for an elaboration of these problems, see, e.g., Grisso, 1987; Ziskin, 1995). Whether researchers were specifically responding to Grisso's call remains unclear, but the number of commercially available psychological instruments that have clear forensic applications has increased dramatically.

Types of assessment instruments used in forensic settings. Heilbrun, Rogers, and Otto (in press) proposed a typology of assessment instruments used in forensic evaluation. As first defined and conceptualized by Grisso (1986), *forensic assessment instruments* are measures that are directly relevant to a specific legal standard and reflect and focus on specific capacities, abilities, or knowledge that are embodied by the law. Tests designed to assess a criminal defendant's competence to stand trial or an older person's ability to manage legal, financial, and health care matters are examples of such instruments. Problems in operationalizing the law that are related to psycholegal capacities, changes in the law over time, and jurisdictional variations in the law can make developing such instruments difficult (Douglas, Otto, & Borum, in press).

Forensically relevant instruments can be distinguished from forensic assessment instruments in that they do not assess or focus on specific legal standards and the associated functional capacities of the examinee, but, rather, they address clinical constructs that are often pertinent to evaluating persons in the legal system. Because these instruments are used to assess clinical constructs rather than legal constructs, problems with definitional ambiguity and idiographic influences are minimized. Examples of these instruments and techniques include those used to assess malingering and response style more generally, recidivism or violence risk, and psychopathy. Well-validated, forensically relevant instruments provide a good balance between clinical confidence and legal relevance; the constructs they assess can be rigorously tested; and their applicability and relevance to forensic assessment and decision making can also be examined.

Most commonly used in forensic evaluations are *clinical measures and assessment techniques*. These are the psychological tests and measures developed for assessment, diagnosis, and treatment planning with clinical populations in therapeutic contexts. Examples include instruments used to assess psychopathology, intelligence, personality, and academic achievement. Many clinical measures are the product of careful development, benefit from a considerable research base, and have been well validated. Although these instruments may assist in understanding the examinee in the context of a particular legal issue, they typically assess constructs (e.g., intelligence, depression, academic abilities, anxiety level) that are considerably removed from the specific question before the legal decision maker (Heilbrun et al., in press). As such, they require the examiner to exercise a greater level of inference to move from the construct assessed to the issue before the court (Otto, Edens, & Barcus, 2000). Related to this, Rogers (1987b) observed the peculiar circumstance in which psychologists conducting forensic evaluations find themselves: The best-validated assessment instruments are often those which are least relevant to the legal issue(s).

The explosion of forensic assessment instruments and forensically relevant instruments. The first forensic instrument—a checklist of criteria for competency to stand trial—was published in 1965 by a psychiatrist, Ames Robey. After its publication, a number of other forensic assessment instruments were developed during the 1970s, all of which were devoted to the assessment of criminal defendants (for a review and discussion, see Heilbrun et al., in press). During the 1980s, a number of other forensic assessment instruments and forensically relevant instruments were published, and their scope and focus expanded as they began to address issues in addition to defendants' competence to stand trial. Grisso first published a book describing the Miranda waiver assessment instruments in 1981, and instruments for use in child custody assessments were published by Bricklin (1984) and Gordon and Peek (1989) in the 1980s. However, the few forensic assessment instruments and forensically relevant instruments that were developed prior to 1990 typically suffered from one or more shortcomings, including (a) lack of complete test manuals describing test development, test use, and test characteristics; (b) lack of adequate data regarding instrument reliability, validity, and psychometric properties; (c) lack of appropriate norms; and (d) lack of commercial publication, resulting in difficulty obtaining and using the instruments (Heilbrun et al., in press; Poythress et al., 1999).

More forensic assessment instruments and forensically relevant instruments have been published in the past 10 years than in the preceding 40. Heilbrun et al. (in press) identified a minimum of 33 assessment instruments and techniques that had been developed and promulgated for use in forensic evaluations during the 1990s, whereas a total of 10 such instruments were developed prior to 1990. Otto (1999) hypothesized that the proliferation of these tests and measures might be partly a function of managed care and changes in reimbursement for mental health services. He suggested that as reimbursement for therapy and therapy-related assessment has become more restricted as a result of managed care, test publishers confronted with decreasing sales of clinical assessment instruments (i.e., tests of intelligence, psychopathology, personality, and academic achievement) have come to see forensic assessment as an untapped market that is less vulnerable to the economic pressures associated with managed care. Additionally, he offered that the recent proliferation of commercially published forensic instruments might reflect, in part, the increasing economic sophistication and motivation of those responsible for developing these instruments.

In addition to an increase in the sheer number of instruments and assessment techniques available for use in forensic settings, a change in the process by which they are developed and published has occurred. Early forensic instruments were not commercially published, and psychologists interested in using them had to obtain a copy of the instruments and determine how to use them on the basis of published research. While some instruments gained recognition in the field and other researchers investigated their reliability and validity (see, e.g., the research regarding the Competence Screening Test; Lipsitt, Lelos, & McGarry, 1971), others fell by the wayside and became little more than footnotes in journal articles and book chapters (e.g., Robey's checklist; Robey, 1965).

More recently, forensic assessment instruments and forensically relevant instruments have been developed and published in two different ways. Some measures have been commercially published and made available for use in clinical forensic evaluations after their designs were reviewed and refined, their reliability and validity were researched and subjected to peer review, and normative data were collected (Heilbrun et al., in press). It is this methodical and scientific approach that Grisso (1987) argued was necessary in his review of the field.

By contrast, a number of forensic instruments have been published and promulgated for use in forensic evaluations after only preliminary research and development (for a more detailed discussion of this issue, see Heilbrun et al., in press; Otto et al., 2000). For example, some instruments used now do not yet have comprehensive test manuals as required by the *Standards for Educational and Psychological Testing* (American Educational Research Association, APA, & National Council on Measurement in Education, 1999; e.g., Rapid Risk Assessment for Sex Offender Recidivism, R. K. Hanson, 1997; Minnesota Sex Offender Screening Tool—Revised, Epperson, Kaul, & Hesselton, 1998; Static-99, K. Hanson & Thornton, 2000). Some instruments are used that have limited sample sizes and lack appropriate cross-validation (e.g., Minnesota Sex Offender Screening Tool—Revised, Epperson et al., 1998). Some instruments use manuals that are incomplete and do not provide even the most basic information about the psychometric properties of the tests (e.g., Parent Awareness of Skills Survey, Bricklin, 1990; Parent Perception of Child Profile, Bricklin & Elliott, 1991). Other instruments have been published and used with limited research data and prior to any formal peer review (e.g., Malingering Probability Scale, Silverton & Gruber, 1998; Parent Perception of Child Profile, Bricklin & Elliott, 1991; Parent Awareness of Skills Survey, Bricklin, 1990).

Organized psychology's response. In an unfortunate recent trend, some forensic assessment instruments and forensically relevant instruments have been developed and introduced for use in clinical decision making without adequate research and development. This trend is inconsistent with what Grisso (1987) believed was necessary with respect to instrument development. It also threatens the credibility of forensic psychology in the courts, as legal decision makers who subject these newer techniques to evidentiary review under Frye (*Frye v. U.S.*, 1923) or Daubert (*Daubert v. Merrell Dow Pharmaceuticals, Inc.*, 1993) may conclude that forensic psychologists are willing to use unvalidated approaches. Of perhaps greater concern is that the safeguards that should minimize misuse of these instruments have failed to do so. The *Standards for Educational and Psychological Testing* (American Educational Research Association, APA, & National Council on Measurement in Education, 1999), the Specialty Guidelines for Forensic Psychologists (Committee on Ethical Guidelines for Forensic Psychologists, 1991), and forensic assessment guidelines promulgated by professionals in the field (for a summary of recommendations, see Heilbrun, 1992; Heilbrun et al., in press; Otto et al., 2000) are apparently insufficient to dissuade some forensic psychologists from using inadequate assessment techniques. This situation must be addressed immediately, or forensic psychology will risk its reputation in the courtroom, particularly as legal decision makers become more knowledgeable about the science of assessment (also see below for a discussion of the increasing sophistication of the legal community). As the field continues to mature, it is clear that it will be important to educate a larger number of consumers of forensic psychology about general principles and specific examples of what constitutes reasonable, empirically supported practice in this area.

Impact of Managed Care on Forensic Practice

Few are unaware of the impact of managed care on the delivery of health care services and the incomes of health care providers in the late 20th century. Mental health and medical professionals report that both the quality of their professional lives and the quality of patient care have been negatively affected by changes in third-party reimbursement for services associated with managed care. Indeed, some authors have attributed increased rates of physicians applying for disability, in part, to the impact of managed care on health care providers (Wall & Appelbaum, 1998).[2]

Otto (1998) cited some anecdotal evidence in support of his suggestion that increasing numbers of psychologists and psychiatrists were entering the forensic arena and abandoning traditional therapeutic practice, in part because of economic pressures associated with managed care. Administrators of institutions that historically have experienced problems hiring and retaining staff and have sometimes operated as training and licensing grounds for newly minted psychologists (e.g., forensic hospitals, prisons, jails, community mental health centers) now enjoy having large numbers of experienced applicants competing for positions that sometimes in the past have gone unfilled. Thus, the public forensic sector may be an indirect beneficiary of the managed care movement in the United States today.

Anecdotal reports by psychologists enrolled in continuing education workshops devoted to forensic topics also provide some support for the claim that there is some movement of psychologists into the forensic arena from more traditional psychological practice areas, as does the increasing number of continuing education workshops devoted to forensic practice. Some of the advertisements associated with continuing education materials and workshops provide telling evidence. In an advertisement for a manual on how to establish a forensic practice, a psychologist from the southwest reports that he or she turns down forensic referrals on a regular basis, attorneys regularly pay fees to psychologists of hundreds of dollars per hour, and transitioning into forensic practice will free psychologists from managed care and allow them to control the insurance companies that once controlled them. In its announcement for newly established forensic workshops, the Prescribing Psychologists Register offers that "forensic and psychopharmacology training are the newest ways to enhance private practice" and "court testimony regarding forensic issues for psychologists has long been recognized as a means to avoid the HMO fee structure" (Prescribing Psychologists Register, n.d., p. 2). Another advertisement invites psychologists, psychiatrists, neurologists, and other medical professionals with the "HMO blues" to attend a one-day forensic practice workshop that will prepare them to enter the lucrative forensic arena. A careful review of the promotional materials indicates that the majority of the workshop is devoted to the business side of forensic practice (e.g., generating referrals, billing), whereas a minority of time is spent on substantive forensic practice issues.

That some psychologists are motivated to enter the forensic arena because of economic concerns is not, in itself, problematic. Those psychologists who actively seek to increase their forensic knowledge, skills, and abilities through continuing education, supervision, and other methods are to be commended and supported. However, it becomes problematic when some psychologists, in response to financial concerns, enter and practice in the forensic arena unprepared. Psychological expertise, forensic or otherwise, is not developed overnight. By its very nature, forensic work is likely to be subjected to a greater degree of scrutiny than are other kinds of psychological services, and there is some support for the claim that this is occurring over time.

Grisso (1987) suggested that the quality of forensic evaluations could also be improved by increased knowledge and sophistication on the part of legal consumers (i.e., attorneys and judges). If forensic psychologists and other mental health professionals fail to monitor themselves and to practice in a professional and an appropriate way, Grisso argued, judges and attorneys educated about appropriate forensic standards and practice might take matters into their own hands to ensure that self-proclaimed experts using substandard techniques and providing uninformed opinions are not allowed to enter the courtroom. Although no empirical evidence supports this claim, anecdotal accounts suggest that the bar is becoming more knowledgeable about forensic practice as a result of efforts devoted to training.

For example, the American Academy of Forensic Psychology has established a program whereby academy fellows (all of whom hold a diploma in forensic psychology from the American Board of Forensic Psychology) provide, free of charge, one-day training programs for judges and attorneys on forensic practice standards and specific areas of interest. The American Bar Association Juvenile Justice Center, the Juvenile Law Center, and the Youth Law Center—with funding from the John D. and Catherine T. MacArthur Foundation—developed a six-volume curriculum that educates attorneys, judges, and other court officials about relevant forensic practice standards and appropriate use of mental health professionals in juvenile justice proceedings. Training programs featuring *Understanding Adolescents: A Juvenile Court Training Curriculum* (Rosado, 2000) have been conducted in Florida, California, Illinois, Virginia, Pennsylvania, Indiana, New Jersey, Tennessee, Texas, and Nevada.[3] Further, psychologists and psychiatrists who testify in civil commitment hearings for sex offenders (i.e., sexually violent predator proceedings) regularly attest to the sophistication and competence of attorneys representing the state and respondents in these newly developed proceedings, and they often find themselves sitting next to attorneys involved in these proceedings at continuing education workshops.

If such efforts continue and expand, forensic psychologists and other mental health professionals practicing in the legal arena should expect that the gatekeepers who control their involvement in legal proceedings will become increasingly knowledgeable and sophisticated over time. As such, forensic psychologists must assume the responsibility to ensure appropriate practice. If they do not, others

[2] It is interesting to note that although some see forensic work as a safe harbor in which professionals can protect themselves from managed care, there is some evidence that managed care may be making inroads into the provision of forensic services, too (e.g., see Packer, 1998; Petrila, 1999).

[3] For more information about this curriculum, go to http://www.jlc.org.

will do so for them—but not until after forensic psychologists have harmed the reputation of the field, as some anecdotal accounts indicate has already occurred.[4]

Development of Practice Standards

As reviewed above, a number of standards and guidelines relevant to forensic psychology practice have been published in the past decade. However, there are no practice guidelines for the large majority of forensic psychology pursuits. With the exception of those for custody, abuse, and neglect evaluations, no consensus guidelines for any other type of forensic evaluations performed by forensic psychologists exist.[5] Similarly, no psychological practice guidelines are devoted to the provision of treatment in forensic settings. Such standards or guidelines can prove valuable to forensic psychologists and legal consumers alike, to the extent that they identify a valid and defensible approach to practice.

Of course, development of practice guidelines or standards is only appropriate when a professional consensus, based on scientific knowledge and clinical experience, can be reached. Surveys of forensic practice reveal considerable variability among forensic psychologists in their practice approaches. In a detailed summary of such research to date, Nicholson and Norwood (2000) provided a strong argument that substantial improvement is needed in the practice of forensic assessment. For example, six studies conducted between 1994 and 1998 (Heilbrun & Collins, 1995; Heilbrun, Rosenfeld, Warren, & Collins, 1994; Nicholson, LaFortune, Norwood, & Roach, 1995; Otto, Barnes, & Jacobson, 1996; Robbins, Waters, & Herbert, 1997; Skeem & Golding, 1998) revealed a wide range of characteristics for the criminal forensic evaluations completed in five states.

On the positive side, essential elements such as citing the source of authority for the evaluation (e.g., a court order) and documenting the delivery of the informed consent and notification of purpose prior to beginning the evaluation were completed with a high degree of frequency. Psycholegal abilities related to the capacities to understand one's legal situation and to assist counsel in one's own defense, which are important components of competence to stand trial, were also frequently described in reports. Less encouraging, however, were the findings that examiners seldom cited the use of any third-party information beyond the arrest report and mental health history (and even those were cited in a minority of reports, according to some studies; e.g., Nicholson & Norwood, 2000). Moreover, examiners often used psychological tests that were not relevant or not psychometrically sound, and they often failed to provide sufficient detail in their reports to allow the reader to understand the findings or follow the reasoning that led to their conclusions. On the basis of their review of the literature, Nicholson and Norwood (2000) concluded, "the practice of forensic assessment falls far short of its promise" (p. 40).

Given the development and state of the art of forensic psychology, it is clear that a consensus cannot not be reached in all areas of forensic practice. However, in certain broad areas, formal standards could be developed for the practice of forensic mental health assessment (e.g., see Heilbrun, 2001; Melton et al., 1997); such standards could be set forth in more specific areas (e.g., evaluation of criminal competencies) as well. It is incumbent on the leading professional organizations (e.g., American Academy of Forensic Psychology, American Psychology–Law Society) to initiate the development of such standards, perhaps in concert with related organizations (e.g., American Academy of Psychiatry and Law, American Bar Association).

Credentialing and Certification

The history of credentialing in forensic psychology is brief, and the credentialing has occurred in two forms: (a) state credentialing of psychologists (and other mental health professionals) who are deemed qualified to conduct forensic evaluations in criminal contexts (also see above) and (b) a more generic forensic credentialing by the American Board of Forensic Psychology (Otto, Heilbrun, & Grisso, 1990). More recently, however, a number of additional credentialing boards and bodies have developed that grant fellow or diplomate status. These boards credential (a) generic forensic evaluation for professionals in a variety of disciplines, (b) the practice of forensic psychology more specifically, or (c) specific areas of forensic practice for professionals in a variety of disciplines (e.g., child custody, traumatic stress).

State credentialing. At least nine states have credentialing or certification programs for psychologists and other mental health professionals who assess criminal defendants to determine their competence to proceed in the criminal process or their mental state at the time of the offense (Farkas, DeLeon, & Newman, 1997). The requirements for certification vary considerably. For example, all of the nine states require attendance at a state-sponsored training program, but only six require potential examiners to pass an examination for certification. In some states, certification is only required if the examiner wishes to be appointed and reimbursed by the court, although examiners are permitted to become involved in criminal cases without state certification when retained by one of the parties (i.e., the defense or the prosecutor). The Massachusetts credentialing program may be the most extensive, requiring mental health professionals to visit different forensic sites, perform several evaluations under supervision, and submit

[4] Although numerous examples are available, a good example of inadequate practice comes from Randy K. Otto's involvement in a sexually violent predator commitment proceeding. A psychologist with little forensic experience predating his involvement in this case administered the Violence Risk Appraisal Guide (VRAG; Quinsey, Harris, Rice, & Cormier, 1998) to the person subject to commitment. A review of the psychologist's scoring of the VRAG indicated that he gave the respondent scores on some items that were impossible to obtain.

[5] Of course, we are aware that other disciplines have developed guidelines relevant to forensic practice (e.g., American Academy of Psychiatry and Law, American Academy of Child and Adolescent Psychiatry).

work samples for review (Fein et al., 1991; Otto et al., 1990).

Preliminary data indicate that training and certification programs may be successful in improving the quality of forensic practice by psychologists and other mental health professionals. Melton, Weithorn, and Slobogin (1985) reported that professionals completing a Virginia training program were more knowledgeable than those who had not about issues relevant to forensic evaluation, and judges were satisfied with their work product. Otto and Peters (1990) and Poythress (1990) reported similar findings in their respective analyses of the Florida and Alabama training programs: Professionals completing forensic training were more knowledgeable about the law and clinical issues relevant to forensic evaluation than were those who did not. Finally, data reported by Otto et al. (1996) provide additional support for the potential value of such programs. They found that reports completed by mental health professionals who attended the (nonmandatory) Florida training program were more likely than those who did not attend to meet evaluation requirements set out in the Florida Statutes and Rules of Criminal Procedure.

Despite these encouraging findings, a number of caveats are indicated. First, state-sponsored credentialing, by way of either state statutes or regulations, has been limited to criminal forensic evaluation, and it is generic to all mental health professionals rather than specific to psychologists. Second, empirical support for the utility of credentialing programs is preliminary, and the value of these programs should be studied more thoroughly. These training and credentialing programs likely increase the cost of services (e.g., costs of training, increased cost of evaluations that can only be conducted by a limited pool of examiners), so it is important to establish that the programs result in better services. If they do not, then the need for credentialing or a revision of the credentialing process would require reconsideration.

Board certification. Since the late 1970s, forensic psychologists have been able to demonstrate advanced knowledge, competence, and ability by obtaining board certification. Initially, board certification in forensic practice was only offered by the American Board of Forensic Psychology, an affiliate of the American Board of Professional Psychology since the mid-1980s. More recently, however, a large number of boards have been developed that grant "board certification," "diplomate" status, "fellow" status, or other titles and purport to identify credential holders as having advanced forensic knowledge, competence, skills, and abilities.

Some of the newly developed boards are associated with larger multidisciplinary organizations and certify practitioners ranging from ballistic experts to handwriting analysts (e.g., see the American Board of Psychological Specialties [ABPS] affiliated with the American College and Board of Forensic Examiners). Others certify or credential a variety of professionals in a particular technique or practice. For example, the Professional Academy of Custody Evaluators offers certification to a variety of mental health professionals. The American Academy of Experts in Traumatic Stress board certifies mental health professionals in 12 different subject areas, including forensic traumatology, pain management, illness trauma, school crisis response, emergency crisis response, bereavement trauma, and motor vehicle trauma. ABPS is a recently developed board affiliated with the American College and Board of Forensic Examiners, an interdisciplinary college and board that is less than 10 years old. ABPS grants board certification in 20 specialties, including areas such as forensic psychoanalysis, behavioral science, forensic psychology, forensic clinical psychology, psychotherapy, and psychopharmacology. The most recently developed title that can be gained by the aspiring forensic clinician is *board-certified, diplomate fellow in forensic sciences*. This credential is offered by the Prescribing Psychologists Register, a group that offers continuing education and board certification in psychopharmacology and other areas (Prescribing Psychologists Register, n.d.).

Criteria used by the various boards to grant the relevant credentials or titles vary dramatically. Some boards appear to be little more than vanity boards that offer checkbook credentials, whereas other boards make significant attempts to verify the applicant's education, training, skills, knowledge, and practice abilities. For example, criteria used by the American Board of Forensic Psychology—the oldest board that certifies advanced forensic psychology practice—include professional education and licensure, professional experience and supervision, and demonstrated competence as determined by a review of written work products and oral examination. To be eligible for the American Board of Forensic Psychology's title of diplomate, candidates must (a) hold a doctoral degree from an appropriately accredited institution, (b) be licensed to practice psychology, (c) have received formal training that provides a basis for their work in forensic psychology, and (d) have completed 1,000 hours of practice in forensic psychology over a minimum period of at least five years, four of which must be postdoctoral. Once these criteria have been met, the candidate must submit two written work products for review. Candidates who pass this step then complete a three-hour oral examination on their written work products and their broad knowledge of forensic psychology. No grandfathering or other waivers of examination requirements are or ever have been used by the American Board of Forensic Psychology.

By contrast, a number of newer boards appear to provide a title or credential based on minimal criteria, typically evidence of an appropriate degree (e.g., a doctoral degree in psychology) in combination with some experiential requirement (e.g., having practiced in the field for a certain number of years). Another board grants its diploma after the applicant has completed continuing education workshops offered by an affiliate organization. Few of the more recently developed boards appear to require a review and examination by which the skills, knowledge, and abilities of the candidate are considered in a meaningful way. Many newer boards also take advantage of the benefits associated with offering liberal grandfather periods, whereby applicants who apply for board status before a certain date do so with the promise of avoiding more rigorous requirements that the board indicates will be imposed on later applicants. The practice of repeatedly extending grandfathering privileges suggests that the purpose of these periods is to stimulate enlistment early on and earn associated income, and it raises questions about the boards' stated intent to adopt more rigorous criteria at some point in the future.

Although the development of such vanity boards did not garner much attention at first, they have been the subject of criticism more recently. Golding (1999) offered a critical analysis of one board in particular and raised concerns regarding the impact of the credentials offered by vanity boards on the quality of expert psychological testimony delivered to the courts and on the reputation of forensic psychology. Although Golding questioned the ability of judges, attorneys, and juries to distinguish between legitimate boards and vanity boards, some evidence shows that both the bar and the general public are taking notice. In a *Wall Street Journal* article, MacDonald (1999) raised questions about the legitimacy of the American Board of Forensic Examiners and the American College of Forensic Examiners after describing the qualification procedures and providing samples of items reported to have been taken from the groups' ethics test. One true–false item purportedly read, "In giving testimony at a deposition it is appropriate to engage in shouting matches or arguments with abusive attorneys" (p. B1). Questions about the legitimacy of the American Board of Forensic Examiners and the American College of Forensic Examiners were also raised in an article published in the *American Bar Association Journal* entitled "Expertise to Go" (Hansen, 2000). Additionally, anecdotal accounts suggest that psychologists holding vanity credentials are, on occasion, being subjected to embarrassing and damaging cross-examinations regarding the real meaning of their credentials.

Some critics of board certification note that there is no empirical support for the claim that board-certified psychologists are more competent or knowledgeable than their non–board-certified counterparts (e.g., see Ziskin, 1995). It is more accurate to conclude that there is no evidence either way, because this remains an unstudied question.

A number of important issues remain with respect to board certification. Perhaps most important is the distinction between boards that identify professionals who have advanced forensic knowledge, skills, and ability (as assessed by a review of credentials, substantive knowledge, and work product) and boards that simply provide the credential holder with the mantle of expertise without any substantive, rigorous examination. Golding (1999) suggested that the only way to protect the legal consumer from misleading credentials is through education, as legislative or professional initiatives against such enterprises are less likely to have any impact.

Also important is evidence that persons holding credentials from legitimate boards have knowledge, skills, or abilities that those without the credentials do not. It would be helpful to have such evidence, although it seems likely that any board that requires a rigorous examination of these areas is likely to certify a more consistently competent group than will a board that does not. If psychologists certified by a particular board do not, as a group, practice at a higher level of competence than do their non–board-certified counterparts, then, at a minimum, the meaning of this board certification should be made clear to legal consumers. At that point, the respective board might wish to reconsider the meanings of its credentials and its certification and review processes.

The Absence of a Treatment Focus

The absence of a clear treatment emphasis within the forensic psychology specialty area is also significant. In contrast to forensic psychological assessment, in which developments have occurred at a rapid pace, there is little to say about research or training programs devoted to treating forensic populations or others involved with the legal system in some way (Borum & Otto, 2000).[6] The relative paucity of forensic treatment literature might be explained by the claim that treatment is treatment, regardless of the context in which it takes place. On the basis of this position, there is no need for a unique forensic treatment literature, because treatment research and practice with other populations is just as relevant. However, it is clear that some issues are overrepresented in (or even unique to) treatment of forensic populations and are part of legal decisions that are made about these populations.[7] There are a number of examples of such treatment issues, such as determining (a) the treatment amenability of juveniles as part of the legal decision to transfer a youth from juvenile to criminal court; (b) whether an individual found not guilty by reason of insanity has progressed sufficiently in treatment to justify conditional release into the community; (c) the likely length of treatment necessary for an individual to recover from a traumatic experience as part of a personal injury case; (d) whether legal coercion enhances treatment compliance and overall effectiveness for individuals on parole; (e) effective treatment strategies for addressing deficits that have resulted in a defendant's adjudication as incompetent to proceed and the relation of the duration of such treatment to deficit reduction, to better inform the decision about when a defendant may be unrestorably incompetent; and (f) the efficacy and effectiveness of violence risk reduction interventions in the context of outpatient commitment, civil commitment release decision

[6] Some might suggest that the arrival of therapeutic jurisprudence constitutes a major development in treatment of forensic populations. We see this as more significantly affecting the legal system and its operation than the provision of forensic psychological services.

[7] The considerations of both population (to whom treatment services are delivered) and purpose (whether a legal decision will be part of the reason for describing or delivering the services) are important in our conceptualization of forensic treatment. Under this conceptualization, we regard group therapy delivered to prison inmates as falling more under the purview of clinical psychology or correctional psychology, as there is no legal decision clearly linked to the delivery of this service. However, we see the delivery of group therapy in a forensic hospital for the purpose of restoring trial competency as falling within the realm of forensic psychology as described in this article.

making, and associated malpractice litigation. Relatively little research and scholarly attention has been paid to these aspects of forensic psychology when contrasted with the attention given to forensic assessment. Although this may be changing somewhat (e.g., see Hodgins, 2000), it will be important for the field of forensic psychology to greatly expand its efforts in the next decade to consider treatment-related questions that are part of legal decisions.

Future Directions: Developing Forensic Psychology in the Next Decade

One of the important priorities for forensic psychology, if it is to continue to develop and grow as a field, is to become more mainstream. There presently appears to be a gap between a relatively small group of forensic specialists (active in such organizations as the American Psychology–Law Society and the American Academy of Forensic Psychology) and a much larger group of psychologists who provide occasional forensic services or provide such services only within a circumscribed area (e.g., child custody evaluation). There are also the *accidental experts*—those who provide clinical services and are unexpectedly asked by a client's attorney to offer an expert opinion about that client in litigation—and the *economically driven experts*—those who have entered forensic practice to compensate for diminished fee-for-service practice opportunities. Unless forensic psychology can (a) acknowledge the reality that forensic practice is being performed at a variety of levels and for different reasons and (b) provide a plan that will help to ensure that such practice is well-informed and competent, then the field will continue to suffer the problems described in this article. Despite important developments on a variety of fronts, wide-scale practice has significant flaws.

It will be important to undertake this process with various participants and stakeholders in forensic psychological assessment. The enhanced integration of forensic psychology with the larger field should involve a variety of APA divisions (e.g., Developmental Psychology; Society for the Psychological Study of Social Issues; Society of Clinical Psychology; School Psychology; Counseling Psychology; Psychologists in Public Service; Military Psychology; Rehabilitation Psychology; Society for Community Research and Action: Division of Community Psychology; Mental Retardation and Developmental Disabilities; Society for the Psychology of Women; Child, Youth, and Family Services; Health Psychology; Clinical Neuropsychology; Psychologists in Independent Practice; Family Psychology; Society for the Psychological Study of Lesbian, Gay, and Bisexual Issues; Society for the Psychological Study of Ethnic Minority Issues; Addictions; and the Society for the Psychological Study of Men and Masculinity). Some of these divisions include current or developing APA applied specializations; it will be important to have the involvement of psychologists within all specializations that include psychological assessment and treatment in legal contexts as a significant part of their work. The integration of specialties recognized by the American Board of Professional Psychology will also be important. Such broad involvement of individuals, divisions, societies, and interest groups within psychology will be enormously challenging, but it is probably the most effective approach to ensuring the meaningful integration of forensic psychology into the larger field.

We propose a three-part strategy. This plan could reasonably be implemented (at least in part) during the coming decade. The strategy relies on implementation by diverse constituencies across applied psychology who share a professional interest in psychological assessment in forensic contexts. The first part of the three-part strategy involves updating the Specialty Guidelines for Forensic Psychologists (Committee on Ethical Guidelines for Forensic Psychologists, 1991) and developing and disseminating practice standards in a variety of areas within forensic psychology. The second part is conceptualizing the training of practicing psychologists on three levels within forensic psychology, modeled on the types identified at the Villanova Conference on the state of the larger field of law and psychology (Bersoff et al., 1997): the *legally informed* clinician,[8] the *proficient* clinician,[9] and the *specialist* clinician.[10] The third part of the strategy is intensifying training efforts directed toward consumers of forensic psychology, including judges, attorneys, mental health administrators, and policymakers, and better informing the general public about the nature of forensic psychology. Each of these steps should be accompanied by research efforts to determine their impact and effectiveness.

The field has taken some important steps toward the development of practice guidelines that are both broad (e.g., the Specialty Guidelines for Forensic Psychologists; Committee on Ethical Guidelines for Forensic Psychologists, 1991) and more specific (e.g., the Guidelines for Child Custody Evaluations in Divorce Proceedings; APA, 1994). However, several additional steps should be taken in the foreseeable future. First, the Specialty Guidelines for Forensic Psychologists should be revised, and psychologists within the field should consider whether a broad set of practice guidelines applicable to all aspects of forensic psychological assessment and treatment is needed in light of this revision. Second, psychologists within the field should identify more specific areas of practice in addition

[8] The legally informed clinician would have a basic education in law relevant to professional practice, including information about confidentiality, privileged communication, and responses to subpoenas for clinical records and personal notes. The legally informed clinician would also have an awareness of the distinction between therapeutic and forensic roles.

[9] The proficient clinician would have midlevel expertise obtained through formal coursework, professional continuing education, or both, as well as supervised experience in forensic psychology. Such knowledge would include relevant law, procedures, and ethics applicable to the kinds of forensic practice in which the person will be engaged.

[10] The specialist clinician would have the highest level of expertise, obtained through formal training in forensic psychology at the graduate and postdoctoral fellowship levels; would need an intensive and in-depth understanding of relevant law and legal procedures; would typically become board certified in forensic psychology through the American Board of Professional Psychology; and would have expertise in a range of forensic procedures and issues.

to child custody and dependency evaluations and develop practice guidelines associated with each. When such development would be premature because of the current level of knowledge in the area, this information should be disseminated to the field and accompanied by suggestions for research and development that would, when implemented, allow the development of area-specific practice guidelines in the future. Such practice guidelines could be disseminated to graduate programs, internships, and fellowships, as well as to practicing psychologists and consumers of forensic psychology. They could serve as a useful marker of the field's progress, a helpful training heuristic, and a mechanism for shaping forensic practice generally.

Our second proposed remedy involves the wider dissemination of relevant information about forensic psychology at the graduate training, internship, and fellowship levels, with the goal of providing the legally informed, proficient, or specialist clinician with the necessary information to allow him or her to function effectively within that level.[11] This would help realize the related goals of ensuring that practicing psychologists (a) recognize that there are such levels and (b) know what is necessary to achieve competence at each level. Presumably, it would also discourage the "accidental" practice of forensic psychology. Psychologists motivated to increase their forensic practice by health market considerations would not be discouraged from doing so, provided that they had invested the necessary time and energy to become competent to practice at the appropriate level. One of the effective means of disseminating such information at the professional level is state-level training or training and certification in forensic psychology. It seems premature to recommend either model specifically. Given the relatively small number of states in which either model is currently in place and the limited available data on outcome, we do not yet know what works best. However, there is enough evidence to encourage the establishment of one model or the other to promote the competent public practice of forensic psychology.

Finally, we underscore Grisso's (1987) call for enhanced training of consumers of forensic psychology—attorneys and judges—and broaden that to encompass mental health administrators, policymakers, and the general public. This past decade has witnessed increased collaboration between attorneys and psychologists, exemplified by conferences such as those jointly sponsored by APA and the American Bar Association. Foundation-sponsored development of model curricula for the training of attorneys and judges has been implemented on a national level (Rosado, 2000). The American Academy of Forensic Psychology has, for a number of years, sponsored a lecture presented to forensic mental health administrators attending the annual conference of the National Association of State Mental Health Program Directors' Forensic Division. *American Psychologist* has published articles on areas of great interest to society that are both methodologically sophisticated and legally germane (e.g., see Mulvey & Cauffman, 2001, on the topic of the limits of prediction in the context of school violence). Efforts such as these should be intensified, as the field of forensic psychology provides consumers with information about broad developments, as well as very specific findings, and the tools, standards, and guidelines to promote competent practice.

The impact of these three activities over the next decade will be significantly strengthened by research conducted to identify needs, monitor implementation, and measure results. Psychology as a field has developed by making research-driven advances integral to its core. As forensic psychology assumes a more mainstream position within the larger field, it must continue to be guided by research findings relevant to its development.

Summary and Conclusions

Forensic psychology practice continues to grow rapidly. The past 25 years have seen the establishment of a specialty area that is reflected in the development of professional organizations, publications, and emerging practice standards and the recognition of competent and advanced practice. In his 1987 review of the area, Grisso indicated that forensic psychology was at an important crossroads. This is true today as well, although progress has been made since 1987. But recent economic pressures, particularly, have strengthened the temptation to practice forensic psychology in a way that does not incorporate the relevant empirical data and standards of practice that have emerged during the past decade. This temptation must be resisted if forensic psychology is to develop and continue to enjoy acceptance by legal consumers.

[11] This updates the call made by Poythress (1979) over 20 years ago for training in forensic psychology at the graduate level. Given the increased number of areas within professional psychology that are now designated APA specialties, it would probably be helpful for graduate training programs to provide a course in specializations in psychology.

REFERENCES

American Academy of Child and Adolescent Psychiatry. (1997). Practice parameters for child custody evaluation. *Journal of the American Academy of Child and Adolescent Psychiatry, 36,* 57S–68S.

American Educational Research Association, American Psychological Association, & National Council on Measurement in Education. (1999). *Standards for educational and psychological testing* (3rd ed.). Washington, DC: American Educational Research Association.

American Psychological Association. (1994). Guidelines for child custody evaluations in divorce proceedings. *American Psychologist, 49,* 677–680.

American Psychological Association Committee on Professional Practice and Standards. (1998). *Guidelines for psychological evaluations in child protection matters.* Washington, DC: American Psychological Association.

American Psychology–Law Society Careers and Training Committee. (1998). *Careers and training in psychology and law* [brochure]. Lincoln, NE: American Psychology–Law Society.

Association of Family and Conciliation Courts. (n.d.). *Model standards of practice for child custody evaluation.* Madison, WI: Author.

Bersoff, D., Goodman-Delahunty, J., Grisso, T., Hans, V., Poythress, N. G., & Roesch, R. (1997). Training in law and psychology: Models from the Villanova Conference. *American Psychologist, 52,* 1301–1310.

Blau, T. (1984). *The psychologist as expert witness.* New York: Wiley.

Bonnie, R., & Grisso, T. (2000). Adjudicative competence and youthful offenders. In T. Grisso & R. Schwartz (Eds.), *Youth on trial* (pp. 73–103). Chicago: University of Chicago Press.

Borum, R., & Otto, R. (2000). Advances in forensic assessment and treatment. *Law and Human Behavior, 24,* 1–7.

Bricklin, B. (1984). *Bricklin Perceptual Scales manual.* Furlong, PA: Village.

Bricklin, B. (1990). *Perception of Relationships Test manual.* Furlong, PA: Village.

Bricklin, B., & Elliott, G. (1991). *Parent Perception of Child manual.* Doylestown, PA: Village.

Committee on Ethical Guidelines for Forensic Psychologists. (1991). Specialty guidelines for forensic psychologists. *Law and Human Behavior, 15,* 655–665.

Cooke, G. (1980). *The role of the forensic psychologist.* Springfield, IL: Charles C Thomas.

Cruise, K. R. (2001). *Resource directory of forensic psychology predcotoral internship training programs.* Lincoln, NE: American Psychology–Law Society and the American Academy of Forensic Psychology.

Daubert vs. Merrell Dow Pharmaceuticals, Inc., 113 S. Ct. 2786 (1993).

Douglas, K., Otto, R., & Borum, R. (in press). Research in clinical forensic psychology. In J. Schinka (Ed.), *Research in psychology, handbook of psychology.* New York: Wiley.

Epperson, D., Kaul, J., & Hesselton, D. (1998, September). *Final report on the development of the Minnesota Sex Offender Screening Tool—Revised.* Paper presented at the Annual Meeting of the Association for the Treatment of Sexual Abusers, Vancouver, British Columbia, Canada.

Ewing, C. P. (1985). *Psychology, psychiatry, and the law: A clinical and forensic handbook.* Sarasota, FL: Professional Resource Press.

Farkas, G., DeLeon, P., & Newman, R. (1997). Sanity examiner certification: An evolving national agenda. *Professional Psychology: Research and Practice, 28,* 73–76.

Fein, R., Appelbaum, K., Barnum, R., Baxter, P., Grisso, T., & Leavitt, N. (1991). The designated forensic professional program: A state government–university partnership to improve forensic mental health services. *Journal of Mental Health Administration, 18,* 223–230.

Frye v. United States, 293 F. 1013 (DC Cir. 1923).

Golding, S. (1999, August). *The voir dire of forensic experts: Issues of qualification and training.* Paper presented at the 107th Annual Convention of the American Psychological Association, Boston, MA.

Gordon, R., & Peek, L. (1989). *The custody quotient: Research manual.* Dallas, TX: Wilmington Institute.

Grisso, T. (1981). *Juveniles' waiver of Miranda rights: Legal and psychological competence.* New York: Plenum.

Grisso, T. (1986). *Evaluating competencies.* New York: Plenum.

Grisso, T. (1987). The economic and scientific future of forensic psychological assessment. *American Psychologist, 9,* 831–839.

Grisso, T. (1991). A developmental history of the American Psychology–Law Society. *Law and Human Behavior, 15,* 213–231.

Grisso, T. (in press). *Evaluating competencies: Forensic assessments and instruments* (2nd ed.). New York: Kluwer/Plenum.

Hansen, M. (2000, February). Expertise to go. *American Bar Association Journal, 86,* 44–52.

Hanson, R. K., & Thornton, D. (2000). Improving risk assessment of sex offenders: A comparison of three actuarial scales. *Law and Human Behavior, 24,* 119–136.

Hanson, R. K. (1997). *The development of a brief actuarial risk scale for sexual offense recidivism* (User Report No. 1997-04). Ottawa, Ontario, Canada: Department of the Solicitor General of Canada.

Hare, R. (1991). *Manual for the Psychopathy Checklist–Revised.* North Tonawanda, New York: Multi-Health Systems.

Heilbrun, K. (1992). The role of psychological testing in forensic assessment. *Law and Human Behavior, 16,* 257–272.

Heilbrun, K. (2001). *Principles of forensic mental health assessment.* New York: Kluwer/Plenum.

Heilbrun, K., & Collins, S. (1995). Evaluations of trial competency and mental state at the time of the offense: Report characteristics. *Professional Psychology: Research and Practice, 26,* 61–67.

Heilbrun, K., Rogers, R., & Otto, R. K. (in press). Forensic assessment: Current status and future directions. In J. R. P. Ogloff (Ed.), *Psychology and law: Reviewing the discipline.* New York: Kluwer/Plenum.

Heilbrun, K., Rosenfeld, B., Warren, J., & Collins, S. (1994). The use of third-party information in forensic assessments: A two-state comparison. *Bulletin of the American Academy of Psychiatry and the Law, 22,* 399–406.

Hodgins, S. (Ed). (2000). *Violence among the mentally ill: Effective treatments and management strategies.* Boston: Kluwer Academic.

Jenkins v. U.S., 307 F.2d 637 (1962).

Lipsitt, P., Lelos, D., & McGarry, A. L. (1971). Competency for trial: A screening instrument. *American Journal of Psychiatry, 128,* 105–109.

MacDonald, E. (1999, February 8). The making of an expert witness: It's in the credentials. *Wall Street Journal,* pp. B1, B4.

McGarry, A. (1971). *Competency to stand trial and mental illness.* Rockville, MD: Department of Health, Education, and Welfare.

Megargee, E. I., & Bohn, M. (1979). *Classifying criminal offenders: A new system based on the MMPI.* Thousand Oaks, CA: Sage.

Melton, G. B., Petrila, J., Poythress, N., & Slobogin, C. (1987). *Psychological evaluations for the courts.* New York: Guilford Press.

Melton, G. B., Petrila, J., Poythress, N., & Slobogin, C. (1997). *Psychological evaluations for the courts* (2nd ed.). New York: Guilford Press.

Melton, G., Weithorn, L., & Slobogin, C. (1985). *Community mental health centers and the courts.* Lincoln, NE: University of Nebraska Press.

Monahan, J. (1980). *Who is the client? The ethics of psychological intervention in the criminal justice system.* Washington, DC: American Psychological Association.

Mulvey, E., & Cauffman, E. (2001). The inherent limits of predicting school violence. *American Psychologist, 56,* 797–802.

Nicholson, R., LaFortune, K., Norwood, S., & Roach, R. (1995, August). *Quality of pretrial competency evaluations in Oklahoma: Report content and consumer satisfaction.* Paper presented at the 103rd Annual Convention of the American Psychological Association, New York, NY.

Nicholson, R., & Norwood, S. (2000). The quality of forensic psychological assessments, reports, and testimony: Acknowledging the gap between promise and practice. *Law and Human Behavior, 24,* 9–44.

Otto, R. K. (1998). The rain of managed care and the perceived oasis of forensic psychology. *Bulletin of the American Academy of Forensic Psychology, 19*(1), 1–3, 9.

Otto, R. K. (1999, February). *The future of forensic psychology.* Address presented to the Department of Psychology, Sam Houston State University, Huntsville, TX.

Otto, R. K., Barnes, G., & Jacobson, K. (1996, March). *The content and quality of criminal forensic evaluations in Florida.* Paper presented at the Biennial Meeting of the American Psychology–Law Society, Hilton Head, SC.

Otto, R. K., Buffington, J., & Edens, J. (in press). Child custody evaluation: Research and practice. In I. Weiner (Ed.), *Encyclopedia of psychology.* New York: Wiley.

Otto, R. K., Edens, J., & Barcus, E. (2000). The use of psychological testing in child custody evaluations. *Family and Conciliation Courts Review, 38,* 312–340.

Otto, R., Heilbrun, K., & Grisso, T. (1990). Training and credentialing in forensic psychology. *Behavioral Sciences and the Law, 8,* 217–231.

Otto, R., & Peters, R. (1990, March). *The Florida forensic evaluator training program.* Paper presented at the Biennial Meeting of the American Psychology–Law Society, Williamsburg, VA.

Packer, I. (1998). Privatized managed care and forensic mental health services. *Journal of the American Academy of Psychiatry and Law, 28,* 123–129.

Petrila, J. (1999, October). *Emerging issues in managed care and delivery of forensic services.* Paper presented at the annual meeting of the National Association of State Mental Health Program Directors–Forensic Division, Tarrytown, NY.

Poythress, N. (1979). A proposal for training in forensic psychology. *American Psychologist, 34,* 612–621.

Poythress, N. (1990, March). *The Alabama forensic evaluator training program.* Paper presented at the Biennial Meeting of the American Psychology–Law Society, Williamsburg, VA.

Poythress, N., Nicholson, R., Otto, R., Edens, J., Bonnie, R., Monahan, J., & Hoge, S. K. (1999). *Professional manual for the MacArthur Competence Assessment Tool–Criminal Adjudication.* Odessa, FL: Psychological Assessment Resources.

Prescribing Psychologists Register. (n.d.). *The Prescriber, Special Edition.*

Quinsey, V., Harris, G., Rice, M., & Cormier, C. (1998). *Violent offenders: Appraising and managing risk.* Washington, DC: American Psychological Association.

Robbins, E., Waters, J., & Herbert, P. (1997). Competency to stand trial evaluations: A study of actual practice in two states. *Journal of the American Academy of Psychiatry and Law, 25,* 469–483.

Robey, A. (1965). Criteria for competency to stand trial: A checklist for psychiatrists. *American Journal of Psychiatry, 122,* 616–622.

Roesch, R., & Golding, S. L. (1980). *Competency to stand trial.* Champaign-Urbana, IL: University of Illinois Press.

Rogers, R. (1987a). *Clinical assessment of malingering and deception.* New York: Guilford Press.

Rogers, R. (1987b). Ethical dilemmas in forensic evaluations. *Behavioral Sciences and the Law, 5,* 149–160

Rogers, R. (1997). *Clinical assessment of malingering and deception* (2nd ed.). New York: Guilford Press.

Rosado, L. (Ed.). (2000). *Understanding adolescents: A juvenile court training curriculum.* Washington, DC: American Bar Association Juvenile Justice Center, Juvenile Law Center, Youth Law Center.

Silverton, L., & Gruber, C. (1998). *Manual for the Malingering Probability Scale.* Los Angeles, CA: Western Psychological Services.

Skeem, J., & Golding, S. (1998). Community examiners' evaluations of competence to stand trial: Common problems and suggestions for improvement. *Professional Psychology: Research and Practice, 29,* 357–367.

Tomkins, A. (Ed.). (1990). Behavioral sciences and the law, training and career options [Special issue]. *Behavioral Sciences and the Law, 8*(3).

Travis, T. (1908). *The young malefactor.* New York: Crowell.

Van Zelfde, G., & Otto, R. (1997). *Directory of practicum, internship, and fellowship training opportunities in clinical–forensic psychology.* Pittsburgh, PA: American Academy of Forensic Psychology.

Wall, B. W., & Appelbaum, K. L. (1998). Disabled doctors: The insurance industry seeks a second opinion. *Journal of the American Academy of Psychiatry and Law, 26,* 7–20.

Wrightsman, L. (2001). *Forensic psychology.* Belmont, CA: Wadsworth.

Ziskin, J. (1975). *Coping with psychiatric and psychological testimony.* Los Angeles: Law & Psychology Press.

Ziskin, J. (1995). *Coping with psychiatric and psychological testimony* (5th ed.). Los Angeles: Law & Psychology Press.

[25]

Training in Law and Psychology

Models From the Villanova Conference

Donald N. Bersoff — *Villanova Law School and Allegheny University of the Health Sciences*
Jane Goodman-Delahunty — *JAMS/ENDISPUTE*
J. Thomas Grisso — *University of Massachusetts Medical School*
Valerie P. Hans — *University of Delaware*
Norman G. Poythress, Jr. — *Florida Mental Health Institute*
Ronald G. Roesch — *Simon Fraser University*

Although the domain of law and psychology is a burgeoning and popular field of study, there has never been a concerted effort to evaluate current training models or to develop newer, more effective ones. Forty-eight invited participants attended a national conference held at Villanova Law School to remedy this deficiency. Working groups addressed issues of education and training for the undergraduate level; for doctoral-level programs in law and social science; for forensic clinical training; for joint-degree (JD/PhD–PsyD) programs; for those in practica, internships, and postdoctoral programs; and for continuing education. This article delineates levels and models of training in each of these areas.

The scientific and professional domain of law and psychology is currently enjoying immense popularity. For the first 50 years of its existence, however, law and psychology led a dismal, dispirited life. Hugo Munsterberg's (1908) attempt to bring experimental psychology into the courtroom early in this century was a miserable failure (Wigmore, 1909). The legal-realism movement, which challenged the fiction that law was based solely on rules and precedent, led to a brief period in the 1920s of interdisciplinary cooperation between law professors and social scientists, but it finally succumbed to a lingering death (Loh, 1981; Schlegel, 1979). It took *Brown v. Board of Education* (1954) 30 years later to stimulate a buoyant resurgence of vitality to the law–psychology enterprise. In that landmark decision, holding that separate but equal public schools violated the Constitutional rights of African American children, the Supreme Court cited the works of social scientists in what is perhaps the law's most famous footnote. As an eminent legal scholar and jury researcher declared at the time, "undoubtedly this is a high point in the periodic flirtation between law and social science" (Kalven, 1958, p. 94). But the works cited in *Brown v. Board of Education* were themselves severely criticized (Cahn, 1955; Tomkins & Oursland, 1991; Van den Haag, 1960). Like most dalliances in the 1960s, the affiliation between law and psychology did not flower into a mature relationship.

Although there continues to be some disagreement about whether a successful rapprochement is possible between law and psychology (compare Hafemeister, Ogloff, & Small, 1990; Saks, 1989; see Bersoff, in press, generally), there is sound evidence that in the past 20 years, law and psychology have evoked renewed optimism that supports the conclusion that as we tread expectantly toward the millennium, there is a great deal of interest in this burgeoning amalgam of interdisciplinary science and practice.

Determinants of Optimism and Concern

There are now more than 2,000 members of the American Psychology–Law Society (APLS; Division 41 of the American Psychological Association [APA]), with a strong and vital student section. There are at least four highly regarded joint programs that award law degrees and doctorates in psychology. The Law and Society Association and the American Academy and American Board of Forensic Psychology are energetic and growing organizations. *Law and Human Behavior*, *Behavioral Sciences and the Law*, and *Criminal Justice and Behavior*, among

Donald N. Bersoff, Villanova Law School, and Department of Clinical and Health Psychology, Allegheny University of the Health Sciences; Jane Goodman-Delahunty, JAMS/ENDISPUTE, San Diego, CA; J. Thomas Grisso, Department of Psychiatry, University of Massachusetts Medical School; Valerie P. Hans, Department of Psychology, University of Delaware; Norman G. Poythress, Jr., Florida Mental Health Institute, Tampa; Ronald G. Roesch, Department of Psychology, Simon Fraser University, Burnaby, British Columbia, Canada.

The first author assumed overall responsibility for the article. All other authors contributed equally, and their names are arranged alphabetically merely for the sake of convention.

Correspondence concerning this article should be addressed to Donald N. Bersoff, Villanova Law School, Garey Hall, Villanova, PA 19085. Electronic mail may be sent via Internet to bersoffd@law.vill.edu.

other important periodicals in the field, were joined in 1995 by *Psychology, Public Policy, and Law*, an APA-published, law school-sponsored journal. Not to be outpaced by technology, there is now a Psych–Law Listserv on the Internet that, despite some dross, has become a rich source of opinion, resources, and comment. In the mid-1990s, of the 11 elected members of the APA Board of Directors, 2 had dual degrees in law and psychology. Five prominent members of the Federal Judicial Center, the research arm of the federal courts, also have dual degrees. A significant number of highly regarded law schools have psychologists as members of their tenured, full-time faculty or have granted them joint appointments (Melton, Monahan, & Saks, 1987). Two *Master Lecture Series* presented during APA conventions in the last 15 years have been devoted exclusively to law and psychology (Sales & VandenBos, 1994; Schierer & Hammonds, 1983). Undergraduate offerings on the topic are often the most popular courses in psychology departments, and continuing education workshops in forensic psychology are almost always oversubscribed. The field has been able to attract several well-known, thoughtful, and prolific law professors. And, law and psychology have been the subject of two major and scholarly reviews of the field's contributions to science (Monahan & Loftus, 1982; Tapp, 1976).

Despite its cyclical nature and "manic–depressive quality" (Kalven, 1958, p. 95), the connections among law, the social sciences, and mental health practice have served to stimulate not only experimentalists like Munsterberg but clinicians as noteworthy as Freud (1906/1959). The result has been the development of three somewhat orthogonal lines of scholarship and training. There are those whose interests are devoted to exploring empirically how the law works—sort of a social science of law. Correspondingly, there are those whose interests are focused on understanding and analyzing the ways in which the law defines and regulates the activities of psychologists, whether in research or clinical practice. And, there are those who seek to influence the development of social policy by bringing to bear social science data on legal issues that are essentially empirical in nature (Grisso, Sales, & Bayless, 1982).

In U.S. courtrooms, psychology is still seen as a mysterious, inexact discipline (Berger, 1994; *Berger v. Board of Psychologist Examiners*, 1975; Goodman-Delahunty, in press), populated by hired guns who will switch sides and proffer opinions for the right fee and greatest notoriety (Bersoff, 1995a). Some of the most hotly contested issues in psychology are being fought out in the courtroom arena. New, often unvalidated "psychological" syndromes seem to proliferate every day (Freckleton, 1994; McCord, 1987; Morse, 1995). We are just beginning to understand the extent of the relationship between violence and mental illness (Monahan & Steadman, 1994), and we still have not reached agreement as to whether memories are false, uncovered, or repressed (APA Working Group, 1996; Pope & Brown, 1996). The Supreme Court, despite the best efforts of psycholegal scholars, remains naive, if not downright hostile, to the application of social science research to empirically based constitutional questions (Bersoff & Glass, 1995; Saks & Baron, 1980; Tremper, 1987).

It is very relevant that this is also a time of ferment, turmoil, and anxiety in the education and training of future scholars, practitioners, and researchers in law and psychology, with a host of unresolved issues that are directly related to teaching and training. At the undergraduate level, there is little consensus as to the subject matter that should be taught and whether the thrust ought to be on the relationship of psychology to law or to the broad-based study of law as a social instrument. At the graduate level, proponents are faced with bearing the burden to prove to financially anxious administrators that their programs are justified from economic and scholarly perspectives. Even more problematic, it is quite possible that funding for graduate students, who are accustomed to tuition waivers and stipends, will be drastically reduced or even eliminated before this decade ends. In an era of budget tightening and politicization of science, no one can predict the fates of the National Institutes of Health or the National Science Foundation and the grants they provide. Practicum sites and institutions providing pre- and postdoctoral internships are reducing the number of slots for training.

Students who wish to pursue research must be trained in two disciplines, which raises the question of whether there is enough time in graduate school to accomplish that goal. There is little like-mindedness about what should be taught in law-oriented, social science programs, perhaps because there has been little field-wide discussion about what to teach and the field has been slow to expand beyond the borders of eyewitness identification and jury behavior (Saks, 1986).

With regard to the training of forensic practitioners, who must also learn two epistemological systems, there is little agreement about the primary focus of training. Some proponents believe that the curriculum should concentrate on educating students to be social scientists and researchers, with practical forensic training postponed until the postdoctoral years. Others assert with equal vigor that the paramount concern at the graduate level is educating applied professionals to perform clinical functions. There is greater agreement, however, that training should include predoctoral practica and internship experiences, but there is less consensus about postdoctoral internships or residencies. Even if there were agreement, there are relatively few postdoctoral facilities available. It is unclear what the impact will be of the APA's creation of identifiable specialties and proficiencies on forensic psychology and of the newly adopted movement to accredit postdoctoral programs and forensic facilities.

The lengthiest forms of graduate training are joint-degree programs that culminate in attaining the Juris Doctor (JD) in law and the doctorate in psychology. Although we are now in the third decade of such training, there is still sharp disagreement about the worth of joint programs and whether the contributions they make are justified by their costs, both temporal and financial (Bersoff, in press; Freeman & Roesch, 1992; Melton, 1987b).

Relatively neglected in the consideration of law and psychology training is the role of continuing education. Currently, most clinicians who provide forensic services are not trained to do so in graduate school but in weekend or one-day seminars and workshops. Yet, there is little regulation of these experiences or scrutiny of the credentials of those who provide them. Most continuing education training is by psychologists for psychologists, which neglects members of the legal profession. The vast majority of lawyers are fundamentally ignorant about basic mental health principles, the vagaries of diagnosis, the limits of assessment data, and the principles of science and research design. Teaching judges and lawyers is crucial, but it has been perhaps the least successful of our efforts at continuing education.

Origins, Issues, and Goals of the Villanova Conference

By the mid-1990s, it seemed time to address the several serious issues concerning the nature and direction of law and psychology as a transdisciplinary, practical, and research enterprise. Beyond reflecting on the history of law and psychology and its current status, it seemed appropriate to develop models of training from undergraduate through postdoctoral education and to create more regular and formal means to disseminate knowledge about training.

These were the purposes of the National Invitational Conference on Education and Training in Law and Psychology held from May 25–28, 1995, at Villanova Law School in suburban Philadelphia. Now more popularly known as the "Villanova Conference," it was attended by 48 invited participants who were primarily identified with one of six major areas: (a) undergraduate education; (b) graduate social science programs; (c) graduate forensic programs; (d) practical training, including predoctoral practica, internships, and postdoctoral experiences; (e) joint-degree programs; and (f) continuing education. Students' issues were integrated into these six.[1] The conference was funded by APA, APLS, the American Academy of Forensic Psychology, the Florida Mental Health Institute, and Villanova Law School. It was organized by a steering committee comprised of the authors of this article, with Donald N. Bersoff as chair.

Outcomes and Emerging Models

In his keynote address initiating the proceedings, Bersoff (1995b) asked conference participants to focus on several overarching questions. The predominant concern was whether the field can develop models of training and, concomitantly, means for evaluating what educators in law and psychology do all along the training continuum. As a subset of that fundamental issue, he set out more practical goals: (a) identify those aspects of education and training that worked well in the past or were current successes; (b) identify ongoing problems that remained unresolved; (c) develop strategies for addressing those problems; (d) focus on and describe those strategies with the most potential for being practical, implementable, and effective; and (e) recommend possible model curricula, programs, and levels of training.

One of the criteria for selecting attendees to the Villanova Conference was an interest and involvement in one of the content areas to be discussed at the conference. There were, thus, six working groups, each identified with education and training at the undergraduate through postdoctoral and continuing education levels and committed to addressing the substantive issues delineated in the keynote address. Each of these groups made material contributions to the success of the conference. What follows is the substance of their deliberations.

Undergraduate Education[2]

Undergraduate education in psychology and law is not only valuable in fleshing out the content areas of psychology, but it has a useful place in the undergraduate curriculum generally because it contributes to several goals of a liberal education. The field offers an array of topics that touch on highly significant and relevant issues that students will encounter in their lives and that are intrinsically fascinating. Furthermore, it nurtures critical thinking, acknowledges the role of personal values, develops sensitivity to ethical principles, and adds to increasing opportunities for interdisciplinary training, both didactic and practical.

There is evidence, in fact, that the number of undergraduate courses in psychology and law has been rising (Ogloff, Tomkins, & Bersoff, 1996). Many conference participants reported that the introductory psychology and law course was one of the most popular classes at their colleges and universities. One survey of the 25 highest ranking psychology departments revealed that 15 (60%) of these eminent programs offered at least one undergraduate psychology and law course and 4 of the 25 (16%) offered two or more courses (Wrightsman et al., 1997). A survey, however, of 10 highly rated liberal arts colleges indicated that just 2 included a law and psychology course in their curriculum (Wrightsman et al., 1997). Thus, it can be concluded that the representation of the field at the undergraduate level is uneven, that student demand for the subject matter generally exceeds availability, and that more should be done to improve undergraduate offerings in psychology and law. A central issue for this group at the conference was to consider ways of expanding relevant offerings.

Within psychology departments, the key point of entry is the introductory course, where students gain their initial exposure to psychology and to potential careers.

[1] Another area, the place of psychology and social science in the law school curriculum, was not fully realized and is not discussed in this article.

[2] The working group on undergraduate education included Solomon Fulero, Edith Greene, Valerie P. Hans, Michael Nietzel, Mark Small, and Lawrence Wrightsman, who served as chair.

For students to seriously consider law and social science (legal psychology) or forensic psychology as an undergraduate specialization and a legitimate career option, the most effective place to begin is in their first course in psychology. A review of several dozen textbooks in introductory psychology revealed that there is some coverage of topics directly related to psychology and law, particularly with regard to memory, lie detection, and insanity (Fulero, 1996; Ogloff et al., 1996). No textbooks that were reviewed, however, included a separate chapter devoted to the field (Fulero, 1996).

Given the growth of psychology and law, it is unfortunate that its coverage is sparser than warranted. Because it merits expansion, the working group recommended that psychologists encourage textbook authors and publishers to include legal psychology in their introductory texts. To help those teaching general psychology courses, who would tend to be unfamiliar with the major issues and findings in psychology and law, it is also recommended that experts help develop multimedia materials, bibliographies, sample lectures, and other materials to be included in such a course.

The place that undergraduate students are most likely to encounter law and psychology is in an advanced survey course. But even here, the field could benefit by additional resources that would widen the range of topics that could be taught. There are a number of comprehensive textbooks in psychology and law, some with teacher's manuals. APLS's Training and Career Committee recently published the *Handbook of Teaching Materials for Undergraduate Legal Psychology Courses* (Greene, 1996), which contains an excellent compilation of demonstration materials, Internet resources, and an annotated bibliography of films and videotapes. One of the more exciting proposals emanating from the conference was the development of a series of videotapes in which well-known experts in particular law–psychology specialties would appear, present didactic material, and demonstrate fundamental techniques.

The single survey course represents the most frequent option that psychology departments now use to introduce students to law and psychology, but for departments serious about this popular enterprise, it is possible to develop a specialization track within a psychology major or even an independent major in law and psychology. In these specialized programs, the survey course would be complemented by an upper level seminar on more specific topics or by special sections in standard courses that highlight law and psychology. An undergraduate track would include the basic foundation courses; the survey course in law and psychology; courses in the psychology of law enforcement, criminology, and forensic psychology; and a multidisciplinary social science and justice seminar. A capstone experience, such as a practicum, supervised research project, or honors thesis, would complete the track or major. Given financial realities, it may be desirable to use distance-learning technology to bring together a consortium of universities and colleges to offer a psychology and law major to students at several institutions.

Finally, it may be possible to increase the role of psychology and law in the numerous interdisciplinary criminal justice and legal studies programs at colleges and universities. More than 1,000 programs offer undergraduate training in criminal justice (Wallace, 1990), and increasing numbers are starting or expanding interdisciplinary legal studies programs (American Bar Association [ABA] Commission on College and University Legal Studies, 1996). Despite their growth and popularity, psychologists have played a minimal role in these programs, demonstrated by the present sociological, theoretical, and research emphases in many of them. Establishing a psychology–law specialty within criminal justice and legal studies programs would develop and enrich the field, broaden its base, and enhance the number and diversity of new entrants to law and psychology.

Graduate Social Science and Law Programs[3]

Within the broad spectrum that encompasses law and psychology, relatively little attention has been paid to nonclinical or social science training at the graduate level (Ogloff, 1990; Ogloff et al., 1996). Because many important areas of law fall outside the traditional bounds of the clinical psychology–law interface (Ogloff, 1990; Roesch, 1990), it is important to develop programs to train legal psychologists to work more comprehensively. Yet, few such programs exist; indeed, for most departments, education is limited to one or two courses in social science and the law.

The objectives of a doctoral-level legal psychology program would be to educate future scholars to generate and apply social science and legal knowledge to legal problems. Career options for legal psychologists are diverse. Training may facilitate careers in academia, public service, and the private sector. Some of the substantive areas of application include the following: (a) policy development, analysis, and evaluation; (b) training of law enforcement personnel, lawyers, and judges; (c) assessment of court functioning and administrative processes; (d) mediation and dispute resolution; (e) case and jury consultation; (f) employment on legislative committee staffs; (g) service as an expert witness; and (h) social science research.

Conference participants did not endorse a single model of training to accomplish these objectives. Given the present state of university resources, the highly idiosyncratic interests of department faculty, and the cold fact that most departments have only one, if any, faculty member interested in social science applications to law, it would be unrealistic to agree on and implement a single model. The members of this working group attempted to address

[3] The working group on graduate social science education included Bette Bottoms, Brian Cutler, Ronald Dillehay, Jane Goodman-Delahunty, Jeffrey Haugaard, Trudi Kirk, Roy Malpass, Michelle McCauley, Barry Ruback, Alan Tomkins, Richard Wiener, Brian Wilcox, and James Ogloff, who served as chair.

and perhaps correct these problems. To further these goals, one of its aims was to identify the knowledge base, skills, and experience necessary to train students to become legal psychologists. The five areas detailed below may be identified as crucial for the psycholegal scholar.

Substantive psychology. Law and social science programs must ensure that students have a core knowledge of basic areas of psychology (e.g., developmental, cognitive, abnormal, ethical, and professional issues). Beyond these core courses, students should have an understanding of social and cultural influences and the implications of these influences for their work because of the role that these scholars will play in conducting social policy research and in developing social policy itself.

Research design and statistics. Because one of the assets of legal psychologists is their ability to use psychological methodology and statistical analysis to address legal questions, training programs need to ensure that students have a core knowledge of experimental and quasi-experimental methods, both in the laboratory and in the field and across methodological approaches (e.g., naturalistic observation, survey research, case studies, program evaluation). Similarly, students should become sophisticated in both basic (e.g., multivariate analysis) and innovative (e.g., meta-analysis, hierarchical linear modeling) statistical procedures.

Legal knowledge. Melton (1987a) urged that psychologists interested in applying their knowledge to the law "focus on 'thinking like a lawyer' and becoming a comfortable guest, if not an insider, in the legal community" (p. 293). With these attributes, psychologists are better able to design ecologically valid, legally relevant research; frame their results so that they are useful to lawyers; more easily disseminate their work to judges, legislators, and lawyers; and increase their credibility as experts.

To accomplish these goals, the working group recommended that students learn the basic tools of law (e.g., legal processes, evidence), sources of law (e.g., common law, statutory law, constitutional law, administrative law), and the core substance of law itself (e.g., civil, criminal). This knowledge can be obtained in a number of ways. It can be gathered initially at the undergraduate level (see above); in interdisciplinary, law-related courses at the graduate level; and in law schools that offer a yearlong Master of Legal Studies to those who have already established themselves in another profession.

Substantive legal psychology. In addition to basic education in law and psychology, it is recommended that students complete integrative foundation courses in law and psychology. These courses should expose students to contemporary original research in legal psychology, original legal materials like statutes and cases, and a historical and contemporary appreciation of how social science evidence is used in law. The list of topics in such courses would vary but would likely include information on eyewitness testimony, jury decision making, procedural justice, expert testimony, the standards for admitting scientific evidence, competency and responsibility in criminal law, civil commitment, unlawful discrimination, mental health and educational services, criminal justice, domestic violence and abuse, law enforcement, and professional regulation and ethics.

Scholarship and training. Finally, students should participate in developing and conducting original research and scholarship, which culminates in a doctoral dissertation that is relevant to law and psychology. To ensure that students gain experience and expertise in disseminating knowledge, they should present at professional meetings such as the biennial meeting of APLS, teach undergraduates, conduct workshops, and publish their research. It would be especially helpful if in addition to didactic work, opportunities were provided for students to gain appropriate real-life experience in legislative, administrative, and judicial settings.

There is an abundance of untapped and underexamined areas of research open to psycholegal scholars interested in social science applications to the law. However, there are not enough well-trained researchers to tread these exciting paths.

Graduate Forensic Psychology Programs[4]

Until recently, course work in forensic psychology was not a component of most graduate clinical psychology programs. This may be changing, perhaps in response to the recognition that a growing number of clinicians are engaged in forensic practice and research. Nevertheless, any model of forensic training must take into account that students in professional training programs already have a heavy course load and that the majority of clinical programs lack the critical mass of faculty and finances to offer forensic courses on a regular basis, much less a specialty track. As a result, and because approaches for providing forensic training can take many forms (Melton, 1987b; Roesch, Grisso, & Poythress, 1986), this working group, like its social science counterpart, rejected the idea of developing absolute standards of training and focused instead on developing basic options that graduate departments could offer to those interested in careers in forensic practice. These options fit neatly within a three-level hierarchy of skills, knowledges, and abilities that are applicable to forensic psychology.

Entry level—the legally informed clinician. Beyond general clinical training, all professional psychologists would receive basic education in law as it applies to professional practice, including information about confidentiality and privileged communications, and appropriate procedures for responding to subpoenas for clinical records and personal notes. Some of this forensic content can be introduced in many, if not all, required clinical courses, especially those on assessment, intervention, and ethics. Ethics courses would include discussion not only of the APA's ethical code of conduct (APA, 1992) and other policy documents but of the Specialty Guidelines

[4] The working group on forensic training included Diane Follingstad, Phyllis Hofnung, Richard Rogers, and Ronald Roesch, who served as chair.

for Forensic Psychologists (Committee on Ethical Guidelines for Forensic Psychologists, 1991) as well.

Dissemination of other important didactic content would require the periodic offering of an overview course in mental health law. Such a course would provide a basic understanding of the theoretical and practical differences between law and psychology, fundamental knowledge of how the civil and criminal justice systems operate, a primer on how to find and read the law, and advanced consideration of ethical issues that are unique to forensic practice. This minimal level of law-related training is essential because

> it would be a mistake . . . to believe that only those psychologists who identify themselves as *forensic mental health professionals* will find themselves involved with the law. Every psychologist is a potential expert witness, and each must be prepared to interact with the legal system. (Bersoff, 1995a, p. 416)

Proficiency level. Psychologists attaining this mid-level expertise may be trained through general professional programs, with an emphasis on forensics; training programs offering a "concentration" in forensic psychology; or, for already trained clinicians, through extensive continuing education or postdoctoral programs. The modal model would probably be the concentration.

Although not a formal track, a concentration is envisioned as an opportunity for a graduate program to offer course work, practica, and research experiences within forensic psychology. Beyond course work that would focus on didactics, students concentrating on forensics would receive practical training in court clinics, forensic hospitals, juvenile facilities, public defenders' offices, or workers' compensation clinics. There would be greater exposure, compared with entry-level students, to legal concepts and to training in testifying as an expert witness, consulting with legal counsel, and performing forensic evaluations related to their clinical specialties (e.g., family therapists might learn to do child custody evaluations). Students in this concentration would most likely do their dissertation research on forensic topics.

Another option within the proficiency level is the forensic minor. This would be a formal program in which courses are offered on a regular basis and students completing all requirements would receive a certificate or some other formal recognition of their accomplishment. The training itself would at least be as comprehensive as in the concentration option. At least two, if not three, faculty members would be required so that enough courses could be offered and the requirements completed in a reasonable period of time.

Specialty level. Those professional psychologists wishing to attain the highest level of training would almost assuredly be educated in programs dedicated to producing forensic psychologists. These programs would have an integrated, carefully developed sequence of training with an identifiable, experienced forensic faculty with recognized credentials. Beyond intensive and in-depth understanding of case law and extensive training in forensic skills, the forensic specialist would work with a variety of populations (e.g., children, victims of sex offenders, sex offenders and other criminal defendants, elderly adults, and those for whom civil commitment is sought).

These options coincide serendipitously with correlative events within APA. In February 1995, APA created a Commission for the Recognition of Specialties and Proficiencies in Professional Psychology (CRSPPP), whose role is to recommend approval or disapproval of petitions from organizations requesting APA to recognize a professional specialty or proficiency. CRSPPP defines a *proficiency* as "a circumscribed activity in the general practice of professional psychology" (Joint Interim Committee for the Identification and Recognition of Specialties and Proficiencies, 1995a, p. 1). A *specialty* is "a defined area of psychological practice which requires advanced knowledge and skills required through an organized sequence of education and training . . . subsequent to the acquisition of core scientific and professional foundations of psychology" (Joint Interim Committee for the Identification and Recognition of Specialties and Proficiencies, 1995b, p. 2). Clearly, forensic psychology is eligible for denomination as a proficiency and a specialty.

Although "in forensic psychology, there is yet no generally accepted and well-codified training model" (Freeman & Roesch, 1992, p. 568), there is a growing consensus that the vitality and future growth of forensic psychology rests on its ability to apply the scientist–practitioner model to psycholegal questions (Heilbrun, 1990; Roesch, 1990). In any event, forensic psychology should fare well in an increasingly competitive and skeptical marketplace. More and more of its instruments and procedures have withstood empirical scrutiny (e.g., Grisso, 1986; Monahan & Steadman, 1994; Roesch, Ogloff, & Golding, 1993; Rogers, 1995), and it is not beholden to the vagaries of managed mental health care.

Practical Training[5]

As we have described, each of the career paths for forensic clinicians would begin with formal preparation in graduate courses that provide the conceptual bases for forensic practice and an appreciation for how the law affects clinical practice. This class work should be augmented by, at least for those at the proficiency and specialty levels, supervised, real-world experience that may include practica, predoctoral internships, and postdoctoral forensic fellowships or residencies. One of the most important goals of the practical-training working group was to discover the extent of the development of these training facilities.

Predoctoral forensic practica. The working group sent a mail survey to 151 APA-accredited graduate training programs in clinical psychology, of which 71 responded (47%). Of those 71, 61 (86%) reported at least one practicum placement at which students receive supervised clinical forensic experience, usually in assess-

[5] The working group on practical training included Allen Brown, Kirk Heilbrun, Steven Norton, Norman G. Poythress, Jr., Gail Vant Zelfde, and J. Thomas Grisso, who served as chair.

ment. These 61 programs identified over 200 settings in which students could obtain some supervised clinical forensic training. These settings include state civil or forensic hospitals, special units of county or community hospitals, county jails and juvenile detention facilities, state or federal prisons, state juvenile justice agencies, local private practice groups, community mental health centers (CMHCs), and intradepartmental or university clinics. The sites most commonly identified by the survey respondents were CMHCs (74%), state civil hospitals (56%), state forensic hospitals (44%), and private practice groups (43%).

The precise nature of the training opportunities depend on the site in which the function is performed. Practicum students at forensic units, for example, perform assessments of competence to stand trial, insanity, and risk for violence. At state hospitals, they are more likely to perform assessments for civil commitment, guardianship, and capacity to consent to treatment. For those at CMHCs, students are more likely to be involved with child abuse and neglect, child custody, and civil commitment.

Predoctoral internships. The working group sent a mail survey to the 259 programs identified by the *APPIC Directory: Internship and Postdoctoral Programs in Professional Psychology* (Association of Psychology and Postdoctoral Internship Centers [APPIC], 1995) as offering major (i.e., students spend about 50% of their time) or minor (i.e., students spend about 25% of their time) forensic rotations, of which 79 responded (31%). Of those 79, 9 reported they no longer provide any significant forensic training. Of the remaining 70 sites, 38 (54%) offer major forensic rotations, and 15 of these offer both major and minor rotations.

Sites offering major forensic rotations report an average of 4.64 intern positions but with 3.45 actually available and filled. These sites primarily offer inpatient experiences with adult criminal forensic populations. Fewer (although almost half) offer either a corrections–prison experience or outpatient experience. Fewer than 15% offer training in a court clinic or a juvenile residential setting.

Sites offering minor rotations are more likely to offer outpatient placements, experience with child and family forensic issues, forensic neuropsychology, and juvenile court experience, with less emphasis on working with adult criminal clients. Both major and minor rotation settings commonly offer forensic seminars and other pedagogical training.

Postdoctoral fellowships–residencies. In contrast to predoctoral training experiences, the number of postdoctoral forensic psychology training programs is small. There appear to be 10 such programs in the United States (an additional 1 is to begin in 1997), with most of them evolving in the 1990s (see the Appendix). These programs have developed in relative isolation from each other and are highly selective. A mail and telephone survey to all of these programs indicated that each admits only one or two fellows annually. The programs are located in diverse sites, including forensic hospitals, medical schools, and correctional facilities. They all provide clinical forensic experience supervised by clinicians who specialize in forensic psychology. The focus is on assessment more than treatment and with criminal populations more than civil and family cases. Stipends range from $22,000–30,000 for a full year.

Given the small number of programs and the competition for limited slots, the purpose of postdoctoral forensic psychology training programs is to produce the future leaders in forensic psychology. They should be prepared to model the most advanced skills and ethical integrity, to teach and train others, and to produce new concepts, knowledge, and technology.

The working group strongly recommended that postdoctoral training programs in forensic psychology form a network within which information could be disseminated. It would be helpful to collect didactic course descriptions, syllabi, and other curricular information. This information would be particularly useful as APA begins to accredit postdoctoral programs in psychology.

Joint-Degree Programs[6]

One of the first tasks of this working group was to define the nature and aims of joint-degree programs. Joint programs are those that meet the following criteria (see also Bersoff, in press): (a) Students are enrolled simultaneously in a JD program at an accredited law school and a doctoral program (PhD–PsyD) in psychology, (b) the program is led by an individual designated as its administrative head, and (c) the program contains an identifiable and integrative law and psychology curriculum in addition to ensuring that students complete all formal requirements toward both degrees. As defined, these programs are differentiated from dual-degree programs in which students are allowed to enroll for both degrees but the universities that offer them take a predominantly laissez-faire attitude toward integration. In such dual-degree programs, students are primarily, if not solely, responsible for arranging the curriculum and integrating what they have learned.

There are only four programs in North America currently meeting the definition of a joint program (although each site may have its distinct nomenclature). There is the real possibility that two more such programs may emerge in the near future.[7] The current programs are at the University of Nebraska, the University of Arizona, Allegheny University of the Health Sciences–Villanova Law School, and Widener University.

The four programs vary in the kinds of lawyer–psychologists they produce. Some prepare researchers who concentrate primarily in social, developmental, or experimental psychology; some prepare students primarily for health and mental health policy positions; some

[6] The working group on joint-degree programs included Donald N. Bersoff, James Cassidy, Amiram Elwork, Stephen Penrod, and Bruce D. Sales, who served as chair.

[7] As this article went to press, the Pacific Graduate School of Psychology and Golden Gate University Law School announced they had accepted students in a fifth joint program, directed by Bruce Bongar.

are devoted to practitioners who concentrate their efforts in clinical psychology; and some have several purposes.

> Although the specific training goals of the programs vary, they share the common goal of training scholars and practitioners interested in research and policy careers who will produce theoretically and methodologically sophisticated research integrating the psychology, law, and policy interface. (Ogloff et al., 1996, p. 217)

"They intend to produce lawyer–psychologists who can bring the information base, research methods, and concerns of psychology to bear upon questions of law and policy" (Roesch et al., 1986, p. 89).

Despite their lofty aims, competitiveness, and prestige, joint programs remain controversial. The uniqueness of their training permits graduates of these programs to pursue careers that singly trained graduates would find difficult to enter. But the program requires a great deal of time and effort as well as the payment of tuition to two schools. Some of the law school requirements, such as courses in tax and trusts and estates, may be seen as wasteful. For students whose goals for forensic practice are clear, it may be more efficient to enroll in doctoral programs in which the aims and curricula are designed to produce forensic clinicians, as we have described above.

It was clear to the working group on joint programs that attention should be paid to two issues. First, there is no coordination of the efforts of the directors of these programs or a means of regular communication. To that end, the four directors formed the Council of Graduate Programs in Psychology and Law, to which other directors of graduate social science programs in law and psychology are invited. The group plans to meet at least annually and to eventually develop a model curriculum in psycholegal studies.

Second, although one can denominate the benefits and costs of joint-degree training, its worth is still unproven. It has been 25 years since the first joint program was developed, and our profession still has "no empirical evidence that full training in any two disciplines produces more insightful contributions to society" (Roesch et al., 1986, p. 100) than single-degree training. The working group agreed that we need to evaluate these programs.

Nevertheless, students and graduates of these program concur, at least as measured by the only survey of these populations, that although they are "time-consuming, expensive, and sometimes lacking precise definition, . . . joint degree . . . law/psychology programs provide unique insights, skills, and opportunities for its [sic] participants" (Hafemeister et al., 1990). They remain the most "direct route to achieving law/psychology integration" (Tomkins & Ogloff, 1990, p. 208).

Continuing and Cooperative Education[8]

Although continuing education in law and psychology has an ongoing impact on the training of a large number of psychologists, it has not enjoyed a prominent position within this specialty. Nevertheless, it fills a unique place in training forensic psychologists. Continuing education courses address topics in greater depth than there is time for in the undergraduate and graduate curricula and may, at times, address issues that are not included in these curricula. It usually attracts those who are already licensed professionals and, as a result, can apply their experience to forensic issues. Finally, advanced levels of training may be focused on the most sophisticated and theoretical issues that forensic psychologists will face.

The working group delineated five goals of continuing education: (a) improve standards of forensic practice and ethical decision making, (b) improve and update knowledge in specific content areas, (c) provide paths for the improvement of forensic skills, (d) provide opportunities for interdisciplinary interchange, and (e) stimulate research and the dissemination of new knowledge.

Current continuing education efforts, however, are not entirely and uniformly successful. Often those who provide workshops do not inform participants about the level of sophistication of their offerings. Their quality is uneven, and there is a dearth of measures for evaluating the success of workshops and seminars. Some fail to bridge the gap between research and practice. Many are not adequately accessible in terms of cost, location, and time.

In that light, the working group offered several recommendations for improving continuing education. First, it would be helpful to delineate three levels of training (basic, specialty, and advanced), develop their respective definitions, and apply them to course offerings. Second, the field should consider a credentialing process for providers of forensic continuing education. Third, course leaders should address ethnic, cultural, linguistic, and gender differences in forensic practice, and the leaders themselves should represent more diverse and underrepresented groups. Fourth, alternative forms of offerings should be considered, particularly summer institutes that would include real practical experience and case supervision.

A final recommendation, perhaps the most noteworthy of all, is to make continuing education more multidisciplinary and interactive. In fact, one of the outgrowths of the Villanova Conference was the development and implementation of a conference offering continuing education credits for psychologists and lawyers jointly sponsored by the APA and the ABA's Section on Family Law. The conference was held in April 1997 in Los Angeles. Its focus was on children and divorce, with several crucial topics presented and discussed by lawyers, psychologists, and those with combined training in both. A similar conference is planned with the ABA's Section on Criminal Law.

The concept of collaborative interdisciplinary meetings such as these should be reinforced. Psychologists and lawyers alike talk primarily to their own colleagues. Both professions tend to be ignorant about the serious issues that confront each of them. Joint meetings can become a model for chipping away at the formidable barriers that imprison each profession in its own stereo-

[8] The working group on continuing education included William Foote, Bruce Frumkin, Patricia Griffin, Gary Hawk, Ira Packer, and Gregory Van Rybroek, who served as chair.

types. Perhaps not only can both professions educate themselves and each other, but we can learn to alter our respective perceptions that all lawyers are "sharks" and all psychologists "hired guns."

Conclusion

Our personal vision for the Villanova Conference was the history-making Boulder Conference (Raimy, 1950), at which was developed the scientist–practitioner model of professional education in clinical psychology, a model that continues to have a major impact on that field. We have hopes that the Villanova Conference will have a similar influence on education and training in law and psychology for the first half of the 21st century. It took four years to obtain the imprimatur of the APA to cosponsor the conference, to raise the money to fund it, to select and invite participants to it, and to structure it so that it would have the greatest possibility for success. The conference was perhaps the only time in the next several decades that the field will be able to gather together, formulate ideas, and translate those ideas into implementable plans. We would like those who follow us to read the record of the conference proceedings in 2050 and say that its participants provided definitive models for education and training in law and psychology that survived for five decades. We hope that readers will be stimulated to contribute to this goal by developing and disseminating creative models of education and training.

REFERENCES

American Bar Association Commission on College and University Legal Studies. (1996). *Directory of undergraduate programs of legal studies, law and society, etc.* (4th ed.). Chicago: Author.

American Psychological Association. (1992). Ethical principles of psychologists and code of conduct. *American Psychologist, 47,* 1597–1611.

American Psychological Association Working Group. (1996). *Working group on investigation of memories of childhood abuse: Final report* (Available from the American Psychological Association, 750 First Street, NE, Washington, DC 20002-4242). Washington, DC: Author.

Association of Psychology and Postdoctoral Internship Centers. (1995). *APPIC directory: Internship and postdoctoral programs in professional psychology* (24th ed.). Washington, DC: Author.

Berger, M. A. (1994). Procedural paradigms for applying the Daubert test. *Minnesota Law Review, 78,* 1345–1385.

Berger v. Board of Psychologist Examiners. 521 F.2d 1056 (D.C. Cir. 1975).

Bersoff, D. N. (1995a). *Ethical conflicts in psychology.* Washington, DC: American Psychological Association.

Bersoff, D. N. (1995b, May). *Facts, faults, and fantasies.* Keynote address presented at the National Invitational Conference on Education and Training in Law and Psychology, Villanova, PA.

Bersoff, D. N. (in press). Preparing for two cultures: Education and training in law and psychology. In R. Roesch & S. D. Hart (Eds.), *Psychology and law: The state of the discipline.* New York: Plenum.

Bersoff, D. N., & Glass, D. J. (1995). The not-so "Weisman": The Supreme Court's continuing misuse of social science research. *University of Chicago Law School Roundtable, 2,* 279–302.

Brown v. Board of Education, 347 U.S. 483 (1954).

Cahn, E. (1955). Jurisprudence. *New York University Law Review, 30,* 150–169.

Committee on Ethical Guidelines for Forensic Psychologists. (1991). Specialty guidelines for forensic psychologists. *Law and Human Behavior, 15,* 655–665.

Freckleton, I. (1994). When plight makes right—the forensic abuse syndrome. *Criminal Law Journal, 18,* 29–49.

Freeman, R. J., & Roesch, R. (1992). Psycholegal education: Training for form and function. In D. K. Kagehiro & W. S. Laufer (Eds.), *Handbook of psychology and law* (pp. 567–576). New York: Springer-Verlag.

Freud, S. (1959). Psycho-analysis and the ascertaining of truth in courts of law. In E. Jones (Ed.), *Collected papers of Sigmund Freud* (Vol. 2, pp. 13–24). New York: Basic Books. (Original work published 1906)

Fulero, S. F. (1996, March). *Integration of legal psychology into the introductory psychology course: Legal psychology made "legit."* Paper presented at the biennial meeting of the American Psychology-Law Society, Hilton Head, SC.

Goodman-Delahunty, J. (in press). Forensic psychological expertise in the wake of Daubert. *Law and Human Behavior, 21.*

Greene, E. (1996). *Handbook of teaching materials for undergraduate legal psychology course* (Available from the American Psychology-Law Society, c/o American Psychological Association, 750 First Street, NE, Washington, DC 20002-4242). Washington, DC: American Psychology–Law Society.

Grisso, T. (1986). *Evaluating competencies: Forensic assessments and instruments.* New York: Plenum.

Grisso, T., Sales, B. D., & Bayless, S. (1982). Law-related courses and programs in graduate psychology departments. *American Psychologist, 37,* 267–278.

Hafemeister, T. L., Ogloff, J. R. P., & Small, M. A. (1990). Training and careers in law and psychology: The perspectives of students and graduates of dual degree programs. *Behavioral Sciences and the Law, 8,* 263–283.

Heilbrun, K. (1990). Response style, third-party information, and competence to stand trial: Research issues in practice. *Law and Human Behavior, 14,* 193–196.

Joint Interim Committee for the Identification and Recognition of Specialties and Proficiencies. (1995a). *Principles for the recognition of proficiencies in psychology* (Available from the American Psychological Association, 750 First Street, NE, Washington, DC 20002-4242). Washington, DC: American Psychological Association.

Joint Interim Committee for the Identification and Recognition of Specialties and Proficiencies. (1995b). *Principles for the recognition of specialties in psychology* (Available from the American Psychological Association, 750 First Street, NE, Washington, DC 20002-4242). Washington, DC: American Psychological Association.

Kalven, H. (1958). Some comments on the Law and Behavioral Science Project at the University of Pennsylvania. *Journal of Legal Education, 11,* 94–99.

Loh, W. (1981). Psycholegal research: Past and present. *Michigan Law Review, 79,* 659–707.

McCord, D. (1987). Syndromes, profiles and other mental exotica: A new approach to the admissibility of nontraditional psychological evidence in criminal cases. *Oregon Law Review, 66,* 19–107.

Melton, G. B. (1987a). Guidelines for effective diffusion of child development research in the legal system. In G. B. Melton (Ed.), *Reforming the law: Impact of child development research* (pp. 280–300). New York: Guilford Press.

Melton, G. B. (1987b). Training in psychology and law. In I. B. Weiner & A. K. Hess (Eds.), *Handbook of forensic psychology* (pp. 681–697). New York: Wiley.

Melton, G. B., Monahan, J., & Saks, M. J. (1987). Psychologists as law professors. *American Psychologist, 42,* 502–509.

Monahan, J., & Loftus, E. (1982). The psychology of law. In M. L. Rozenzweig & L. W. Porter (Eds.), *Annual review of psychology* (Vol. 33, pp. 441–475). Palo Alto, CA: Annual Reviews.

Monahan, J., & Steadman, H. J. (Eds.). (1994). *Violence and mental disorder: Developments in risk assessment.* Chicago: University of Chicago Press.

Morse, S. J. (1995, Winter/Spring). The "new syndrome excuse syndrome." *Criminal Justice Ethics, 14,* 3–15.

Munsterberg, H. (1908). *On the witness stand: Essays on psychology and crime.* New York: Doubleday.

Ogloff, J. R. P. (1990). Law and psychology in Canada: The need for training and research. *Canadian Psychology, 31,* 61–73.

Ogloff, J. R. P., Tomkins, A. J., & Bersoff, D. N. (1996). Education and training in law/criminal justice: Historical foundations, present structures, and future developments. *Criminal Justice and Behavior, 23,* 200–235.

Pope, K. S., & Brown, L. S. (1996). *Recovered memories of abuse.* Washington, DC: American Psychological Association.

Raimy, V. (1950). *Training in clinical psychology.* Englewood Cliffs, NJ: Prentice Hall.

Roesch, R. (1990). From the editor. *Law and Human Behavior, 14,* 1–3.

Roesch, R., Grisso, T., & Poythress, N. G. (1986). Training programs, courses, and workshops in psychology and law. In M. F. Kaplan (Ed.), *The impact of social psychology on procedural justice* (pp. 83–108). Springfield, IL: Charles C Thomas.

Roesch, R., Ogloff, J. R. P., & Golding, S. L. (1993). Competency to stand trial: Legal and clinical issues. *Applied and Preventive Psychology, 2,* 43–51.

Rogers, R. (1995). *Diagnostic and structured interviewing: A handbook for psychologists.* Odessa, FL: Psychological Assessment Resources.

Saks, M. J. (1986). The law does not live by eyewitness testimony alone. *Law and Human Behavior, 10,* 279–280.

Saks, M. J. (1989). Legal policy analysis and evaluation. *American Psychologist, 44,* 1110–1117.

Saks, M. J., & Baron, C. (1980). *The use/nonuse/misuse of applied social research in the courts.* Cambridge, MA: Abt Books.

Sales, B. D., & VandenBos, G. R. (Eds.). (1994). *Psychology in litigation and legislation.* Washington, DC: American Psychological Association.

Schierer, C. J., & Hammonds, B. J. (Eds.). (1983). *The master lecture series: Vol. 2. Psychology and the law.* Washington, DC: American Psychological Association.

Schlegel, J. (1979). American legal realism and empirical social science: From the Yale experience. *Buffalo Law Review, 28,* 459–586.

Tapp, J. L. (1976). Psychology and law: An overture. In M. L. Rosenzweig & L. W. Porter (Eds.), *Annual review of psychology* (Vol. 27, pp. 359–404). Palo Alto, CA: Annual Reviews.

Tomkins, A. J., & Ogloff, J. R. P. (1990). Training and career options in psychology and law. *Behavioral Sciences and the Law, 8,* 205–216.

Tomkins, A. J., & Oursland, K. (1991). Social and social scientific perspectives in judicial interpretations of the Constitution: A historical view and an overview. *Law and Human Behavior, 15,* 101–120.

Tremper, C. R. (1987). Organized psychology's efforts to influence judicial policymaking. *American Psychologist, 42,* 496–501.

Van den Haag, E. (1960). Social science testimony in the desegregation cases: A reply to Professor Kenneth Clark. *Villanova Law Review, 6,* 69–79.

Wallace, D. H. (1990). Training in law and behavioral sciences: Issues from the criminal justice perspective. *Behavioral Sciences and the Law, 8,* 249–262.

Wigmore, J. (1909). Professor Munsterberg and the psychology of testimony: Being the report of the case of *Cokestone v. Munsterberg. Illinois Law Review, 3,* 399–445.

Wrightsman, L. S., Fulero, S. F., Greene, E., Hans, V., Nietzel, M. T., & Small, M. A. (1997). Undergraduate education in legal psychology. In D. N. Bersoff (Ed.), *Education and training in law and psychology.* Manuscript in preparation.

[26]

Irreconcilable Conflict Between Therapeutic and Forensic Roles

Stuart A. Greenberg
University of Washington

Daniel W. Shuman
Southern Methodist University

Despite being contrary to good patient care and existing clinical and forensic practice guidelines, some therapists nevertheless engage in dual clinical and forensic roles. Perhaps because an injured litigant seeking treatment is required to engage in 2 distinct roles (litigant and patient), care providers may be tempted to meet both sets of that person's needs. Through the presentation of 10 principles that underlie why combining these roles is conflicting and problematical, the authors stress the importance of avoiding such conflicts, avoiding the threat to the efficacy of therapy, avoiding the threat to the accuracy of judicial determinations, and avoiding deception when providing testimony.

With increasing frequency, psychologists, psychiatrists, and other mental health professionals are participating as forensic experts in litigation on behalf of their patients. Factors such as tightened insurance reimbursement rules, a growing market for forensic mental health professionals, and zealous patient advocacy by therapists have combined to induce many therapists, including those who once zealously avoided the judicial system, to appear, often willingly, as forensic expert witnesses on behalf of their patients. Although therapists' concerns for their patients and for their own employment is understandable, this practice constitutes engaging in dual-role relationships and often leads to bad results for patients, courts, and clinicians.

Although there are explicit ethical precepts about psychologists and psychiatrists engaging in these conflicting roles, they have not eliminated this conduct. One important factor contributing to this continued conduct is that psychologists and psychiatrists have not understood why these ethical precepts exist and how they affect the behavior of even the most competent therapists. When the reasons for the ethical precepts are understood, it is clear why no psychologist, psychiatrist, or other mental health professional is immune from the concerns that underlie them.

This article contrasts the role of therapeutic clinician as care provider and the role of forensic evaluator as expert to the court, acknowledges the temptation to engage in these two roles in the same matter, explains the inherent problems and argues strongly against doing so, and discusses the ethical precepts that discourage the undertaking of the dual roles, as well as the legal and professional responses to this dilemma. The specific problem addressed here is that of the psychologist or psychiatrist who provides clinical assessment or therapy to a patient–litigant and who concurrently or subsequently attempts to serve as a forensic expert for that patient in civil litigation.

Expert persons may testify as fact witnesses as well as either of two types of expert witnesses: treating experts and forensic experts. No special expertise beyond the ability to tell the court what is known from first-hand observation is required to be a fact witness. Being an expert person, however, does not preclude one from simply providing to the court first-hand observations in the role of a fact witness. What distinguishes expert witnesses from fact witnesses is that expert witness have relevant specialized knowledge beyond that of the average person that may qualify them to provide opinions, as well as facts, to aid the court in reaching a just conclusion. Psychologists and psychiatrists who provide patient care can usually qualify to testify as treating experts, in that they have the specialized knowledge, not possessed by most individuals, to offer a clinical diagnosis and prognosis. However, a role conflict arises when a treating therapist also attempts to testify as a forensic expert addressing the psycholegal issues in the case (e.g., testamentary capacity, proximate cause of injury, parental capacity).

Although in the preceding description the therapeutic relationship occurs first and the forensic role second, there are parallel concerns with the reverse sequence (i.e., the subsequent provision of therapy by a psychologist or psychiatrist who previously provided a forensic assessment of that litigant). There are also similar concerns about the treating therapist's role in criminal litigation. However, this article will only address civil litigation because the concerns and considerations arising in criminal litigation are somewhat different, such as therapy provided under court order and the provision of therapy and evaluation in forensic hospitals pending criminal responsibility or competency to stand trial determinations.

Role Conflict

In most jurisdictions, a properly qualified therapist testifies as a fact witness for some purposes, as he or she is expected to

---

STUART A. GREENBERG is a diplomate in forensic psychology, ABPP; is in the full-time private practice of forensic psychology in Seattle, Washington; and is on the adjunct faculty of the University of Washington, Department of Psychiatry and Behavioral Sciences. His private practice specializes in civil forensic psychology, primarily personal injury and employment litigation. He frequently lectures on these topics, on forensic roles and ethics, and on the forensic uses of the Minnesota Multiphasic Personality Inventory.

DANIEL W. SHUMAN is a professor of law at Southern Methodist University School of Law in Dallas, Texas, and an adjunct professor of psychiatry at the University of Texas Health Science Center at Dallas. His work addresses ethical, evidentiary, liability, and mental health law policy issues.

His work on this article was supported by a grant from the M.D. Anderson Foundation.

CORRESPONDENCE CONCERNING THIS ARTICLE should be addressed to Stuart A. Greenberg, 720 Olive Way, Suite 605, Seattle, Washington 98101-1853. Electronic mail may be sent via the Internet to stuartg@u.washington.edu.

testify to information learned first hand in therapy, and as an expert witness for some purposes, as he or she is permitted to testify to opinions about mental disorder that a layperson would not be permitted to offer. Thus, a therapist may, if requested to do so by a patient or ordered to do so by a court, properly testify to facts, observations, and clinical opinions for which the therapy process provides a trustworthy basis. This testimony may include the history as provided by a patient; the clinical diagnosis; the care provided to a patient; the patient's response to that treatment; the patient's prognosis; the mood, cognitions, or behavior of the patient at particular times; and any other statements that the patient made in treatment. A therapist may properly testify, for example, that Ms. Jones reported the history of a motor vehicle accident (MVA) 2 weeks prior to the start of therapy and that the therapist observed the patient to be bruised, bandaged, tearful, and extremely anxious. The therapist may properly testify that he or she observed, and that Ms. Jones reported, symptoms that led to a diagnosis of posttraumatic stress disorder (PTSD). The therapist may also describe the particular type of treatment used, the patient's response to that treatment, and her prognosis. The therapist may properly testify that the primary focus for the therapy was the MVA, or the PTSD secondary to the MVA. The therapist may even properly testify that, for treatment purposes, the operating assumption was that the MVA rather than her impending divorce or recent job termination or the death of a family member was what caused the patient's distress.

To be admissible, an expert opinion must be reliable and valid to a reasonable degree of scientific certainty (a metric for scrutinizing the certainty of expert testimony as a condition of its admissibility). It is improper for the therapist to offer an expert opinion that the MVA was the proximate cause of her impairments rather than the divorce, job termination, or bereavement. This is true for two reasons. First, the type and amount of data routinely observed in therapy is rarely adequate to form a proper foundation to determine the psycholegal (as opposed to the clinically assumed) cause of the litigant's impairment, nor is therapy usually adequate to rule out other potential causes. Second, such testimony engages the therapist in conflicting roles with the patient. Common examples of this role conflict occur when a patient's therapist testifies to the psycholegal issues that arise in competency, personal injury, worker's compensation, and custody litigation.

These concerns do not apply when the treating expert witness stays within the boundaries of facts and opinions that can be reliably known by the treating professional. Indeed, the treating therapist can be compelled to testify to information perceived during the therapeutic process and to opinions previously formed for the purpose of therapy but cannot be compelled to do a forensic examination or analysis (Shuman, 1983). Clinical, ethical, and legal concerns arise when the treating expert offers psycholegal assessment—an assessment for which the treating expert does not have adequate professional basis, for which there are inherent role conflicts, and for which there will almost certainly be negative implications for continued therapy.

The temptation to use therapists as forensic experts falls on fertile ground because clinical psychology and psychiatry graduate students often do not receive adequate training in forensic ethics. Although graduate training in ethics has vastly improved in general, most graduate ethics courses teach clinicians in training about the dual roles that most often get therapists in difficulties: mainly, sexual and other nonprofessional relationships with patients. The legal arena is sufficiently foreign to most academicians and their students that ethics training primarily focuses on licensing laws and ethical codes for general practice. For example, few psychologists receive training in the Specialty Guidelines for Forensic Psychologists (Committee on Ethical Guidelines for Forensic Psychologists, 1991) because few see themselves as forensic psychologists. When these clinicians eventually testify in court, they see themselves as benignly telling the court about their patients and perhaps even benevolently testifying on behalf of their patients. Therapists are not typically trained to know that the rules of procedure, rules of evidence, and the standard of proof is different for court room testimony than for clinical practice.

The temptation to use therapists as forensic experts on behalf of patient–litigants exists because of erroneous beliefs about efficiency, candor, neutrality, and expertise. Using a therapist to provide forensic assessment appears efficient because the therapist has already spent time with the patient and knows much about him or her that others are yet to learn and not without substantial expenditures of time and money for an additional evaluation. A therapist appears to gain candid information from a patient–litigant because of the patient's assumed incentive to be candid with the therapist to receive effective treatment. Although litigants may learn much about themselves as a consequence of receiving thorough forensic evaluations (Finn & Tonsager, 1996), the same treatment incentive does not exist in a forensic examination. Thus, the facts forming the basis for a therapist's opinion may initially appear more accurate and complete than the facts that could be gathered in a separate forensic assessment.

In addition, a therapist does not appear to be the attorney's hired gun who came into the case solely to assist in advancing or defeating a legal claim or defense. Thus, a therapist's forensic assessment may appear more neutral and less immediately subject to financial incentives to reach a particular result than does a separate forensic evaluation. And, it is sometimes assumed that if a therapist has the expertise to be trusted to treat the condition for which a patient seeks compensation, surely the therapist has the expertise to testify about it. Indeed, in many ways it would appear from this analysis that one would have to be foolish not to have therapists also testify as forensic experts. Nevertheless, examining the differences between the therapeutic and forensic relationships, process, and expertise reveals that such foolishness is the mirror image of sensibility.

Ten Differences Between Therapeutic and Forensic Relationships

As can be seen from Table 1, the therapeutic and forensic roles demand different and inconsistent orientations and procedures (adapted from Greenberg & Moreland, 1995). The superficial and perilous appeal of using a therapist as a forensic examiner is debunked by examining the conceptual and practical differences between the therapist–patient relationship and the forensic examiner–litigant relationship.

The first and perhaps most crucial difference between the

Table 1
Ten Differences Between Therapeutic and Forensic Relationships

		Care provision	Forensic evaluation
1.	Whose client is patient/litigant?	The mental health practitioner	The attorney
2.	The relational privilege that governs disclosure in each relationship	Therapist–patient privilege	Attorney-client and attorney work-product privilege
3.	The cognitive set and evaluative attitude of each expert	Supportive, accepting, empathic	Neutral, objective, detached
4.	The differing areas of competency of each expert	Therapy techniques for treatment of the impairment	Forensic evaluation techniques relevant to the legal claim
5.	The nature of the hypotheses tested by each expert	Diagnostic criteria for the purpose of therapy	Psychologal criteria for purpose of legal adjudication
6.	The scrutiny applied to the information utilized in the process and the role of historical truth	Mostly based on information from the person being treated with little scrutiny of that information by the therapist	Litigant information supplemented with that of collateral sources and scrutinized by the evaluator and the court
7.	The amount and control of structure in each relationship	Patient structured and relatively less structured than forensic evaluation	Evaluator structured and relatively more structured than therapy
8.	The nature and degree of "adversarialness" in each relationship	A helping relationship; rarely adversarial	An evaluative relationship; frequently adversarial
9.	The goal of the professional in each relationship	Therapist attempts to benefit the patient by working within the therapeutic relationship	Evaluator advocates for the results and implications of the evaluation for the benefit of the court
10.	The impact on each relationship of critical judgment by the expert	The basis of the relationship is the therapeutic alliance and critical judgment is likely to impair that alliance	The basis of the relationship is evaluative and critical judgment is unlikely to cause serious emotional harm

roles is the identification of whose client the patient–litigant is. As implied by the name, the patient–litigant has two roles, one as therapy patient and another as plaintiff in the legal process. The patient–litigant is the client of the therapist for the purposes of treatment. The patient–litigant is as well the client of the attorney for guidance and representation through the legal system.

The nature of each relationship and the person who chooses to create it differs for therapy and forensic evaluation. The therapist is ultimately answerable to the client, who decides whether to use the services of a particular therapist; the forensic evaluator is ultimately answerable to the attorney, or the court in the case of a court-appointed expert, who decides whether to use the services of a particular forensic evaluator. The patient retains the therapist for treatment. The attorney (or the court) retains the forensic evaluator for litigation. This arrangement allows for the relationship that is most straightforward and free of conflict of interest. It best protects the parties' interests as well as the integrity of the therapist and the forensic evaluator.

Second, the legal protection against compelled disclosure of the contents of a therapist–patient relationship is governed by the therapist–patient privilege and can usually only be waived by the patient or by court order. Society seeks to further the goal of treatment through recognition of a privilege for confidential communications between a therapist and patient in most jurisdictions under a physician, psychiatrist, psychologist, or psychotherapist–patient privilege (Shuman & Weiner, 1987).

Legal protection against compelled disclosure of the contents of the forensic evaluator–litigant relationship is governed by the attorney–client and attorney–work-product privileges. Because the purpose of a forensic relationship is litigation, not treatment nor even diagnosis for the purpose of planning treatment, communications between a forensic examiner and a litigant are not protected under a physician–, psychiatrist–, psychologist–, or psychotherapist–patient privilege. The forensic evaluator, however, having been retained by the attorney, is acting as an agent of the attorney in evaluating the party or parties in the legal matter. This legal agency status puts the forensic evaluator under the umbrella of the attorney–client privilege and usually protects privileged information until such time that the evaluator is declared to be a witness at trial. Until that time, most states, especially in civil matters, allow the attorney to prevent access to that attorney's retained expert by opposing counsel, thus best protecting the party's interest should the evaluator's independent opinion not favor the party of the attorney who has retained him or her. Because it would not be a therapeutic relationship, no such potential protection is available if the forensic evaluator were to be retained directly by the party, thereby creating the onus of one's own expert who was hired to evaluate some potential merit to the case instead being used to discredit the retaining side. Because parties, through their attorneys, need to be able to evaluate the merits of their case candidly without such jeopardy, the attorney–work-product privilege covers such trial-preparation use of experts retained by counsel.

The main practice point to be made here is that the logic, the legal basis, and the rules governing the privilege that applies to care providers are substantially different from those that apply to forensic evaluators. Given this, the duty to inform forensic examinees of the potential lack of privilege and the intended use of the examination product is embodied in case law (*Estelle v. Smith,* 1981) and the Specialty Guidelines for Forensic Psychologists (SGFP) adopted by the American Psychology–Law Society (APA Division 41) and the American Board of Forensic

Psychology in 1991. The Specialty Guidelines state the following:

> Forensic psychologists have an obligation to ensure that prospective clients are informed of their legal rights with respect to the anticipated forensic service, of the purposes of any evaluation, of the nature of procedures to be employed, of the intended uses of any product of their services, and of the party who has employed the forensic psychologist. (Committee on Ethical Guidelines for Forensic Psychologists, 1991, p. 659)

The third difference is evident in the evaluative attitude of each of the experts. The therapist is a care provider and usually supportive, accepting, and empathic; the forensic evaluator is an assessor and usually neutral, objective, and detached as to the forensic issues. A forensic evaluator's task is to gain an empathic understanding of the person but to remain dispassionate as to the psycholegal issues being evaluated. For therapists, empathy and sympathy—generating a desire to help—usually go hand-in-hand. For forensic evaluators, the task is a dispassionate assessment of the psycholegal issues.

Fourth, to perform his or her task, a therapist must be competent in the clinical assessment and treatment of the patient's impairment. In contrast, a forensic evaluator must be competent in forensic evaluation procedures and psycholegal issues relevant to the case. A therapist must be familiar with the literature on diagnoses and treatment interventions, knowing from among which diagnostic categories and treatment interventions the patient's difficulties would be best identified and treated. The forensic evaluator must know the basic law as it relates to the assessment of the particular impairment claimed.

Fifth, a therapist then uses this expertise to test rival diagnostic hypotheses to ascertain which therapeutic intervention is most likely to be effective. For example, a therapeutic diagnostic question might be whether a patient is a better candidate for insight-oriented psychotherapy, systematic desensitization, or psychopharmacologic intervention. A forensic evaluator must know the relevant law and how it relates to a particular psychological assessment. A forensic evaluator then uses this expertise to test a very different set of rival psycholegal hypotheses that are generated by the elements of the law applicable to the legal case being adjudicated. A psycholegal question might be whether an impairment in the plaintiff's functioning would not have occurred but for the death of the plaintiff's child that was allegedly caused by the defendant. Another forensic question might be whether the proximate cause of a plaintiff's impairment is a discriminatory promotional practice, a hostile work environment, quid pro quo sexual harassment, or management retaliation for having filed a complaint.

The sixth difference is the degree of scrutiny to which information from the patient–litigant is subjected. Historical truth plays a different role in each relationship. At least with competent adults, therapy is primarily based on information from the person being treated, information that may be somewhat incomplete, grossly biased, or honestly misperceived. Even when the therapist does seek collateral information from outside of therapy, such as when treating children and incompetent adults, the purpose of the information gathering is to further treatment, not in the pursuit of validating historical truth. In most instances, it is not realistic, nor is it typically the standard of care, to expect a therapist to be an investigator to validate the historical truth of what a patient discusses in therapy. Indeed, trying to do so by contacting family members, friends, or coworkers and by requesting corroborating documentation may frustrate therapy even if the patient has signed a release of information. Further, this corroboration is usually unnecessary. Effective therapy can usually proceed even in the face of substantial historical inaccuracy. For example, a patient's impaired self-esteem, body image, and sexual interest might be effectively treated regardless of the fact that her reported memory of having been sexually abused early in childhood by her maternal uncle was inaccurate and that she was actually abused by her paternal uncle. Similarly, a fear of small places can be effectively treated even if the cause was having been locked in a closet by an angry spouse or parent and not by being trapped in a faulty elevator. Depression from poor work performance, excessive and losing gambling, almost being caught defrauding an employer, and having to resign can be treated even if the reason for the depression conveyed to the therapist by the patient is that he or she was the victim of an incompetent and unfair supervisor.

The more important question for most psychotherapeutic techniques is how a patient perceives or feels about the world—what is real to that patient—not factual or historical truth (Wesson, 1985). Even for those therapeutic techniques that involve confrontation and challenge of a patient's conceptions of events, therapists rarely conduct factual investigations into circumstances surrounding patient claims in therapy. Thus, the historical truth of matters raised during therapy cannot, simply on that basis alone, be considered valid and reliable for legal purposes. This is not a criticism of therapy. This approach to psychotherapy makes sense given its temporal framework. If a patient report or a diagnostic hypothesis is not borne out, it can be revised in later sessions. This approach to therapy, which is informed and educated but still somewhat trial-and-error, typically does no harm unless the patient is in a high-risk situation, such as being suicidal or in an abusive environment.

In contrast, the role of a forensic examiner is, among other things, to offer opinions regarding historical truth and the validity of the psychological aspects of a litigant's claims. The accuracy of this assessment is almost always more critical in a forensic context than it is in psychotherapy. A competent forensic evaluation almost always includes verification of the litigant's accuracy against other information sources about the events in question. These sources may include collateral interviews with coworkers, neighbors, family members, emergency room personnel, or a child's teacher or pediatrician and a review of documents such as police reports, school records, military records, medical records, personnel files, athletic team attendance, credit card bills, check stubs, changes in one's resume, depositions, witness statements, and any other possible sources of information about the litigant's pre- and postincident thoughts, emotions, and behaviors. However, therapists do face a dilemma regarding the historical accuracy of the information provided by the patient, depending on how they or their patients act on that information. This is illustrated by a case in which a therapist was successfully sued for slander by a father who was identified through memories recovered in therapy as allegedly having abused the therapist's patient as a child every Friday evening. The father offered employment records at the therapist's trial that revealed that he had worked for the railroad and had been working out of town every Friday evening in question (Blow, 1995).

Seventh, the need for historical accuracy in forensic evaluations leads to a need for completeness in the information acquired and for structure in the assessment process to accomplish that goal. Therapeutic evaluation, in comparison, is relatively less complete and less structured than a forensic evaluation. Moreover, a patient provides more structure to a therapeutic evaluation than does a litigant to a forensic evaluation. Ideally, a patient and therapist work collaboratively to define the goals of a therapeutic interaction and a time frame within which to realize them. The time frame and goals of a forensic evaluation are defined by the legal rules that govern the proceeding, and once these are determined, the forensic evaluator and litigant are usually constrained to operate within them. To make maximum use of the time available, forensic evaluators usually conduct highly structured assessments using structured interviews supplemented with a battery of psychological tests and forensically oriented history and impairment questionnaires. Certainly the plaintiff is encouraged to describe the events in question, but it is the forensic evaluator's task to establish a preincident baseline of functioning, a complete description of the incidents alleged in the legal complaint, the subsequent areas of resilience and impairment of the plaintiff's functioning, the proximate cause of any impairment, and the likely future functioning of the plaintiff, if necessary, ameliorated or enhanced by any needed therapy.

Eighth, although some patients will resist discussing emotionally laden information, the psychotherapeutic process is rarely adversarial in the attempt to reveal that information. Forensic evaluation, although not necessarily unfriendly or hostile, is nonetheless adversarial in that the forensic evaluator seeks information that both supports and refutes the litigant's legal assertions. This struggle for information is also handled quite differently by each expert: The therapist exercises therapeutic judgment about pressing a patient to discuss troubling material, whereas a forensic evaluator will routinely seek information from other sources if the litigant will not provide it or to corroborate it when the litigant does provide information. In the extreme, when presented with excessive underreporting or overreporting of critical information, the forensic evaluator might even decide that the litigant is dissembling.

Ninth, consider the goals of each of these relationships. Therapy is intended to aid the person being treated. A therapist–patient relationship is predicated on principles of beneficence and nonmaleficence—doing good and avoiding harm. A therapist attempts to intervene in a way that will improve or enhance the quality of the person's life. Effective treatment for a patient is the reason and the principal defining force for the therapeutic relationship. According to the Hippocratic oath, "Into whatever house I enter, I will do so to help the sick, keeping myself free from all intentional wrong-doing and harm. . . ." Similarly, according to the ethical principles of psychologists, "Psychologists seek to contribute to the welfare of those with whom they interact professionally. . . . [They attempt] to perform their roles in a responsible fashion that avoids or minimizes harm" (APA, 1992, p. 1600).

Forensic examiners strive to gather and present objective information that may ultimately aid a trier of fact (i.e., judge or jury) to reach a just solution to a legal conflict. A forensic examiner is obligated to be neutral, independent, and honest, without becoming invested in the legal outcome. A forensic evaluator advocates for the findings of the evaluation, whatever those findings turn out to be. Thus, the results of a forensic examination may well be detrimental to the legal position of an examinee (American Psychiatric Association, 1984) and contrary to basic therapeutic principles.

Tenth, the patient–litigant is likely to feel differently about expert opinions rendered by therapists than those rendered by forensic experts. Consider the role of judgment in therapeutic relationships. There is a robust, positive relationship between the success of the therapist–patient alliance and success in therapy (Horvath & Luborsky, 1993). To develop a positive therapist–patient alliance, a therapist must suspend judgment of the patient so that the therapist can enter and understand the private perceptual world of the patient without doing anything that would substantially threaten that relationship. Indeed, some believe that even a posttherapy disturbance of this therapeutic alliance may cause serious harm to a patient; hence many advocate substantial limitations on personal relationships between former patients and their therapists.

In contrast, the role of a forensic examiner is to assess, to judge, and to report that finding to a third party (attorney, judge, or jury) who will use that information in an adversarial setting. To assess, a forensic examiner must be detached, maybe even skeptical, and must carefully question what the litigant presents. Because a forensic psychologist or psychiatrist has not engaged in a helping relationship with the litigant, it is less likely that his or her judgment-laden testimony would cause serious or lasting emotional harm to the litigant than would that of the psychologist or psychiatrist who has occupied a therapeutic role.

Waiving the Dual-Role Conflict

These role differences are not merely artificial distinctions but are substantial differences that make inherently good sense. Unless these distinctions are respected, not only are both the therapeutic and forensic endeavors jeopardized for the patient–litigant but as well the rights of all parties who are affected by this erroneous and conflictual choice. Unlike some conflicts of interest, this role conflict is not one that the plaintiff can waive, because it is not the exclusive province of the plaintiff's side of the case. The conflict affects not only the plaintiff but also the defense and the court. This conflict not only poses therapeutic risks to the patient–litigant but also risks of inaccuracy and lack of objectivity to the court's process and to all of the litigants.

Existing Professional Guidelines

On the basis of these concerns, both psychological and psychiatric organizations have sought to limit these situations when dual functions are performed by a single psychologist or psychiatrist. In increasing detail and specificity, professional organizations have discouraged psychologists and psychiatrists from engaging in conflicting dual professional roles with patient–litigants. As the Ethical Guidelines for the Practice of Forensic

Psychiatry, adopted by the American Academy of Psychiatry and the Law (AAPL) in 1989, note:

> A treating psychiatrist should generally avoid agreeing to be an expert witness or to perform an evaluation of his patient for legal purposes because a forensic evaluation usually requires that other people be interviewed and testimony may adversely affect the therapeutic relationship.

In a very similar vein, the Specialty Guidelines for Forensic Psychologists indicate the following:

> Forensic psychologists avoid providing professional services to parties in a legal proceeding with whom they have personal or professional relationships that are inconsistent with the anticipated relationship.
>
> When it is necessary to provide both evaluation and treatment services to a party in a legal proceeding (as may be the case in small forensic hospital settings or small communities), the forensic psychologist takes reasonable steps to minimize the potential negative effects of these circumstances on the rights of the party, confidentiality, and the process of treatment and evaluation. (Committee on Ethical Guidelines for Forensic Psychologists, 1991, p. 659)

The Committee on Psychiatry and Law of the Group for the Advancement of Psychiatry (GAP, 1991) concluded in 1991 that "While, in some areas of the country with limited number of mental health practitioners, the therapist may have the role of forensic expert thrust upon him, ordinarily, it is wise to avoid mixing the therapeutic and forensic roles" (p. 44). Similarly, the Ethical Principles of Psychologists and Code of Conduct of the American Psychological Association (APA, 1992) admonishes that "In most circumstances, psychologists avoid performing multiple and potentially conflicting roles in forensic matters" (p. 1610). Finally, the most recent and the most specific of these codes, the American Psychological Association's (1994) guidelines for conducting child custody evaluations, concluded the following:

> Psychologists generally avoid conducting a child custody evaluation in a case in which the psychologist served in a therapeutic role for the child or his or her immediate family or has had other involvement that may compromise the psychologist's objectivity. This should not, however, preclude the psychologist from testifying in the case as a fact witness concerning treatment of the child. In addition, during the course of a child custody evaluation, a psychologist does not accept any of the involved participants in the evaluation as a therapy client. Therapeutic contact with the child or involved participants following a child custody evaluation is undertaken with caution.
>
> A psychologist asked to testify regarding a therapy client who is involved in a child custody case is aware of the limitations and possible biases inherent in such a role and the possible impact on the ongoing therapeutic relationship. Although the court may require the psychologist to testify as a fact witness regarding factual information he or she became aware of in a professional relationship with a client, that psychologist should decline the role of an expert witness who gives a professional opinion regarding custody and visitation issues (see Ethical Standard 7.03) unless so ordered by the court. (p. 678)

The Legal Perspective

Although there are explicit ethical precepts addressing this dual role, there are no reported judicial decisions to date that address the exclusion of a forensic assessment by a psychologist or psychiatrist who served as a litigant's therapist. Courts may not see this as an issue of competence or qualification, but instead, at most, as one of weight or credibility. Thus, the therapist would be permitted to testify and the ethical precept could be used to challenge credibility. Some courts may not recognize the role conflicts or not see them as important; other courts may see them but are too concerned with efficiency to give them great weight.

Although even the clear ethical conflict may not yet persuade a court to exclude the testimony of a therapist who offers a forensic assessment, the effect of this departure from professional standards on the perceived credibility of the witness may persuade attorneys to resist this two-for-one strategy. Deviating from the ethical codes or practice guidelines of one's profession is an appropriate and effective basis for impeaching a witness and the explicit ethical and specialty guidelines that address this problem simplify this task for the cross-examining attorney.

Similarly, under both the test of "general acceptance" in the relevant professional community of *Frye v. United States* (1923) and the "good grounds given what is known" test of *Daubert v. Merrell Dow Pharmaceuticals* (1993), forensic assessment by a patient's therapist does not generally provide a reliable basis for a forensic assessment and therefore should be avoided by the ethical psychologist and viewed skeptically by the courts. Expert witnesses are held highly accountable for the accuracy of their opinions through the rules of evidence; the rigors of deposition, voir dire, cross-examination; and the testimony of opposing experts. Courts now scrutinize the admissibility of expert opinion testimony on the basis of the quality of the science that underlies the testimony (Shuman, 1994). The Supreme Court's decision in *Daubert* (1993) requires federal courts to make a "preliminary assessment of whether the reasoning or methodology underlying the testimony is scientifically valid and whether that reasoning properly can be applied to the facts in issue" (p. 592). This decision is part of a trend in both state and federal courts toward a more demanding level of scrutiny requiring scientific support or validation for the assertions made by mental health professionals in forensic settings. This trend (e.g., *State v. Russel,* 1994) is even seen in states that have chosen to apply the "general acceptance in the relevant professional community" test (*Frye,* 1923) instead of the test in *Daubert.* Psychologists and psychiatrists should expect courts to demand evidence of the research that supports their opinions and that supports the data acquisition methods on which opinions are based. A forensic evaluation must be based on information that is more complete and more accurate than that typically obtained as part of therapy.

To date, society has taken a largely laissez-faire, market orientation to psychotherapy. Most successful malpractice claims against mental health professionals have involved sex with patients, drug interactions, failure to warn or protect, and suicide (Smith, 1991). However, engaging in dual roles raises the potential for a lawsuit against a therapist by a patient alleging lack of informed consent. This could be claimed by a disgruntled patient–litigant who expected the therapist to be as successful and partisan an expert witness as he or she was a therapist. The argument would follow that the therapist should have reasonably known that the patient would be less likely to disclose certain information knowing that a third person would be made aware of, and potentially use, the information to the detriment of the discloser and, therefore, the therapist should have warned the patient of that potential consequence not just before the therapist changed roles but also before therapy (and the disclosures) even began. It is similarly likely that most people would choose to disclose more information with less self-censorship in psychotherapy than in forensic examinations. Once this information has been disclosed in therapy, and the therapy process then becomes the basis for forensic testimony by the therapist, this then places the otherwise innocuous information into a different context and makes it more likely that this disclosure will be used to the detriment of the patient (Shuman & Weiner, 1987).

Where Then Should the Line Be Drawn?

As stated earlier, psychologists and psychiatrists may appropriately testify as treating experts (subject to privilege, confidentiality, and qualifications) without risk of conflict on matters of the reported history as provided by the patient; mental status; the clinical diagnosis; the care provided to the patient and the patient's response to it; the patient's prognosis; the mood, cognitions, or behavior of the patient; and any other relevant statements that the patient made in treatment. These matters, presented in the manner of descriptive "occurrences" and not psycholegal opinions, do not raise issues of judgment, foundation, or historical truth. Therapists do not ordinarily have the requisite database to testify appropriately about psycholegal issues of causation (i.e., the relationship of a specific act to claimant's current condition) or capacity (i.e., the relationship of diagnosis or mental status to legally defined standards of functional capacity). These matters raise problems of judgment, foundation, and historical truth that are problematic for treating experts.

When faced with issues that seem to fall between these guideposts, it is useful to ask whether each opinion is one that could or should have been reached in therapy. Thus, if the legal system did not exist, would therapists be expected to reach these sorts of conclusions on their own? Would doing so ordinarily be considered an aspect of the therapy process? In doing so, would the opinion be considered exploratory, tentative, and speculative, or instead as providing an adequate basis for guiding legal action outside of therapy? Is the therapist generating hypotheses to facilitate treatment or is he or she reasonably scientifically certain that this opinion is accurate? Is it based on something substantially more than, "My patient said so," "My patient would have no reason to lie," or "My patient would not lie to me"?

Conclusion

Psychologists, psychiatrists, and other mental health professionals have given and received criticism about the use of expert witnesses whose partisanship appears to overwhelm their professionalism. Engaging in conflicting therapeutic and forensic relationships exacerbates the danger that experts will be more concerned with case outcome than the accuracy of their testimony. Therapists are usually highly invested in the welfare of their patients and rightfully concerned that publicly offering some candid opinions about their patient's deficits could seriously impair their patient's trust in them. They are often unfamiliar with the relevant law and the psycholegal issues it raises. They are often unaware of much of the factual information in the case, and much of what they know comes solely from the patient and is often uncorroborated. What they do know, they know primarily, if not solely, from their patient's point of view. They are usually sympathetic to their patient's plight, and they usually want their patient to prevail.

By failing to recognize the inherent limitations of their work as therapists, as well as the conflicting therapeutic and forensic roles, psychologists, psychiatrists, and other mental health professionals risk harm to their profession, their patients, and the courts. Although therapists frequently enter the forensic arena in their efforts to help, these efforts may not only put therapists in ethical difficulty but may also neutralize the impact both of their testimony and their work as therapists. Therapists need to acknowledge the limits of what they can accurately and reliably say on the basis of therapeutic relationships. Although it is difficult, when asked psycholegal questions, therapists must be willing to testify "I cannot answer that question given my role in this case," "I do not have an adequate professional basis to answer that question," "I did not conduct the kind of evaluation necessary to reliably answer that question." "I can only tell you what I observed," or "I can only tell you what my patient told me." No matter how laudable their motives might be, therapists who venture beyond these limits and into the arena of psycholegal opinion are deceiving themselves and others. Engaging in an irreconcilable role conflict and lacking an adequate professional basis for their testimony, they can be neither neutral, objective, nor impartial.

References

American Academy of Psychiatry and the Law. (1989). Ethical guidelines for the practice of forensic psychiatry. In *Membership directory of American Academy of Psychiatry and the Law* (pp. x–xiii). Bloomfield, CT: Author.

American Psychological Association. (1992). Ethical principles of psychologists and code of conduct. *American Psychologist, 47*, 1597–1611.

American Psychological Association. (1994). Guidelines for child custody evaluations in divorce proceedings. *American Psychologist, 49*, 677–680.

American Psychiatric Association. (1984). *Psychiatry in the sentencing process: A report of the task force on the role of psychiatry in the sentencing process.* Washington, DC: Author.

Blow, S. (1995, January 11). Slander case shakes family. *Dallas Morning News*, p. 25a.

Committee on Ethical Guidelines for Forensic Psychologists. (1991). Specialty guidelines for forensic psychologists. *Law and Human Behavior, 15*, 655–665.

Committee on Psychiatry and Law, Group for the Advancement of Psychiatry. (1991). *The mental health professional and the legal system* (Rep. No. 131). New York: Brunner/Mazel.

Daubert v. Merrell Dow Pharmaceuticals, Inc., 405 U.S. 597 (1993).

Estelle v. Smith, 451 U.S. 454 (1981).

Finn, S. E., and Tonsager, M. E. (1996). *Therapeutic assessment: Using psychological testing to help clients change.* Manuscript in preparation.

Frye v. United States, 293 F. 1013 (D.C. Cir. 1923).

Greenberg, S. A., & Moreland, K. (1995). *Forensic evaluations and forensic applications of the MMPI/MMPI-2.* Unpublished manuscript, University of Minnesota, Department of Continuing Education and Conference Services, Minneapolis, and The American Academy of Forensic Psychology.

Horvath, A. O., & Luborsky, L. (1993). The role of the therapeutic alliance in psychotherapy. *Journal of Consulting and Clinical Psychology, 61,* 561–573.

Shuman, D. W. (1983). Testimonial compulsion: The involuntary medical expert witness. *Journal of Legal Medicine, 4,* 419–446.

Shuman, D. W. (1994). *Psychiatric and psychological evidence* (2nd ed.). Colorado Springs, CO: Shepherds/McGraw-Hill.

Shuman, D. W., & Weiner, M. F. (1987). *The psychotherapist–patient privilege: A critical examination.* Springfield, IL: Thomas.

Smith, S. R. (1991). Mental health malpractice in the 1990's. *Hous. L. Rev., 28,* 209–283.

State v. Russel, 882 P.2d 747 (Wash. 1994).

Wesson, M. (1985). Historical truth, narrative truth, and expert testimony, *Wash. L. Rev., 60,* 331–354.

Received October 2, 1995
Revision received February 22, 1996
Accepted May 20, 1996 ■

[27]

The Quality of Forensic Psychological Assessments, Reports, and Testimony: Acknowledging the Gap Between Promise and Practice

Robert A. Nicholson[1] and Steve Norwood[2]

During the past decade, the field of forensic psychological assessment entered a period of standard setting, reflected in the publication of specialty guidelines for practice and in the proliferation of educational opportunities, training programs, and credentialing and certification procedures for forensic examiners. Representing significant efforts to advance the quality of psychological assessments in legal contexts, these developments foreshadow the promise of forensic assessment. During this same time period, new evidence emerged regarding the quality of forensic practice. This article reviews this evidence and evaluates current practice against the promise of forensic assessment. Forensic reports appear to be of higher quality than those described by commentators in the 1970s and early 1980s; nevertheless, the level of practice falls far short of professional aspirations for the field. The review identifies significant areas of weakness that demand the attention of professional organizations, accrediting agencies, educators, lawmakers, practitioners, and consumers.

The truth is what is, not what should be.
—Lenny Bruce

The recent development and publication of professionally sanctioned and proposed guidelines for forensic practice (Committee on Ethical Guidelines for Forensic Psychologists, 1991; Committee on Professional Practice and Standards, 1994, 1995; Golding, 1990; Grisso, 1990; Heilbrun, 1992, 1995; Jenkins & Howell, 1994), and the introduction of training programs and certification procedures for forensic examiners in some jurisdictions (e.g., Fein, Appelbaum, Barnum, Baxter, Grisso, & Leavitt, 1991; Melton, Weithorn, & Slobogin, 1985; Peters & Otto, 1990; Poythress, 1990), represent significant efforts to advance the overall quality of psychological assessments in legal contexts, including the reports and expert testimony provided to legal decision makers. Collectively, these efforts seek to establish a forensic

[1]University of Tulsa, Tulsa, Oklahoma.
[2]Oklahoma Department of Mental Health and Substance Abuse Services.

practice in which reports and testimony reflect high-quality clinical assessment, document the examiner's adherence to the legal and ethical contours of the evaluation, focus on relevant legal questions and criteria, describe the factual and clinical material that led to the opinions expressed, and communicate findings in language that is comprehensible to persons not trained as mental health professionals (see Melton et al., 1985). These efforts to create guidelines and standards for practice, develop training programs, and establish certification procedures reflect the maturing of the discipline, and they foreshadow the promise of forensic psychological assessment. In short, such developments point to what should be, not necessarily what is.

Evaluating the state of the discipline of forensic assessment during a particular time period is not an easy task. Systematic investigations of the practices of forensic examiners or the content and quality of forensic reports and testimony have rarely been undertaken (for exceptions, see Melton et al., 1985; Petrella & Poythress, 1983). Apart from conceptually driven criticisms targeting the insufficiency and intrusiveness of mental health expert opinions in legal contexts (e.g., Morse, 1978) and frontal assaults on the empirical foundations of psychology and psychiatry (e.g., Faust & Ziskin, 1988; Ziskin, 1970, 1995), early critiques of mental health experts' reports and testimony relied heavily on a few studies in which report quality was a secondary issue (e.g., Geller & Lister, 1978; Hess & Thomas, 1963; Roesch & Golding, 1977; Vann, 1965) or, more often, on anecdotal accounts of the content of experts' reports or their courtroom testimony. Certainly, examples of poor practice abound (see Poythress, 1979, for some memorable descriptions). I once reviewed a transcript in which the following exchange between expert and attorney was recorded (I am not making this up):

Doctor: Memory loss may be an early sign of psychosis.
Attorney: What questions did you ask to assess memory loss?
Doctor: I don't remember.

Such bits of anecdotal evidence, at once amusing and disconcerting, give no indication of customary standards, nor do they delimit the boundaries of poor or incompetent practice. Recently, however, a body of research evidence has emerged that provides information on key characteristics of forensic evaluations, including data that address the content and quality of the reports submitted to legal decision makers. This research speaks to "what is" in the field, permitting an empirical evaluation of the correspondence between the promise and the practice of forensic psychological assessment.

Forensic assessment differs substantially from traditional clinical assessment on a number of dimensions, including the goals, scope, and product of the evaluation; the role of the examiner; and the nature of the relationship between examiner and examinee (see Melton, Petrila, Poythress, & Slobogin, 1997). Several characteristics of forensic evaluations and reports are of particular importance in assessing the quality of forensic practice. Did the examiner adhere to the ethical demands of forensic assessment (e.g., by providing notification to the examinee regarding the purposes of the evaluation and any limitations on confidentiality) and document that adherence in the report? What types and sources of data did the examiner use? In particular, did the examiner use standard psychological tests selectively and appropriately? Forensic assessment instruments? Also, to what extent did the examiner endeavor to collect and incorporate information from third parties? Did the examiner offer an opinion on the ultimate legal issue? Did the examiner describe the clinical facts and reasoning underlying his or her opinion (e.g., in the form of data on the defendant's mental status, legally relevant functional abilities, and the relationship between them)?

The use of standard psychological instruments by clinical psychologists in non-forensic settings has been surveyed repeatedly since the mid-1970s (e.g., Brown & McGuire, 1976; Lubin, Larsen, Matarazzo, & Seever, 1985; Piotrowski, 1999; Piotrowski, Belter, & Keller, 1998; Piotrowski & Keller, 1978, 1989, 1992; Piotrowski, Sherry, & Keller, 1985; Sweeney, Clarkin, & Fitzgibbon, 1987; Watkins, Campbell, Nieberding, & Hallmark, 1995). However, relatively little attention has been given to the use of such instruments in forensic contexts until recently (e.g., Heilbrun, 1992; Lees-Haley, 1992). Indeed, only one relevant study (Keilin & Bloom, 1986), a survey of test use in child custody evaluations, was conducted prior to 1990. The more recent surveys have focused on particular types of forensic assessments, including criminal forensic (Borum & Grisso, 1995), child custody (Ackerman & Ackerman, 1997; LaFortune & Carpenter, 1996), and emotional injury (Boccaccini & Brodsky, 1999) evaluations, or on use of a particular instrument or class of instruments in forensic contexts (e.g., Lees-Haley, Smith, Williams, & Dunn, 1995; Piotrowski, 1996). The frequency with which psychological measures are incorporated into test batteries for various kinds of forensic assessments has important implications for evolving standards of practice and for psycholegal research. The appropriate role of psychological testing in forensic assessment remains unclear, although recent guidelines have underscored the forensic examiner's obligation to incorporate clinical instruments selectively, based on their relevance to the legal question at issue (Committee on Ethical Guidelines for Forensic Psychologists, 1991; Heilbrun, 1992, 1995).

The development of psycholegal measures or forensic assessment instruments (FAIs) with demonstrated reliability and validity represents a significant contribution of psychological science to forensic assessment. As Grisso (1987) noted, "Operationalization, standardization, and quantification have always distinguished psychology from other mental health professions in their contributions to assessment" (p. 835). By focusing on legally relevant functional abilities, psycholegal measures can structure forensic evaluations, improve communication with members of the legal profession, and increase the relevance of oral and written expert testimony (e.g., see Elwork, 1984; Grisso, 1986, esp. chapters 1–3). Arguably, then, use of FAIs can enhance the overall quality of evaluations conducted in legal contexts (Skeem & Golding, 1998).

The collection of third-party information (e.g., from review of medical, criminal justice, educational, and employment records; from interviews with or review of statements by witnesses, relatives, and victims) is a central characteristic of forensic assessment that distinguishes it from traditional therapeutic assessment (Heilbrun, Warren, Rosenfeld, & Collins, 1994; Melton et al., 1997). Because of the incentives for examinees to distort their responses to interview questions or test items, information from third parties can be essential in corroborating or disconfirming hypotheses generated from the traditional sources (Heilbrun, 1992; Melton et al., 1997). For example, in their informative discussion of strategies for improving clinical judgment in forensic evaluations, Borum, Otto, and Golding (1993) described a hypothetical personal injury case and argued, "Numerous third-party contacts are also indicated to best develop a picture of the examinee's adjustment across different situations and further address the issue of dissimulation" (p. 43).

The question whether mental health professionals should offer opinions concerning dispositive facts at issue before the court (i.e., Was the defendant insane at the time of the crime? Is the defendant incompetent to stand trial?) has been a point of continuing controversy and debate (Golding, 1990). Because ultimate decisions necessarily involve questions of morality and justice that lie outside the mental health professional's domain of expertise, some scholars have argued that psychologists (or other experts) should not answer the ultimate legal-question (e.g., Melton et al., 1997); others, however, have challenged that view (e.g., Rogers & Ewing, 1989). In any case, as Skeem and Golding (1998) have noted, providing an opinion on the ultimate legal issue is the least important part of the forensic examiner's role; rather, the examiner's principal role is to describe the examinee's capacities and deficits relevant to the legal issue at hand, along with the examiner's inferences and reasoning regarding the causes of the observed deficits. Moreover, because court decisions are often based on reports submitted by mental health experts rather than courtroom testimony, failure to include the aformentioned data and reasoning in a report should be viewed as a fundamental flaw (see Skeem & Golding, 1998).

Recent investigations of the practice of forensic assessment have relied on two methods of data collection. Some investigators have surveyed practitioners to obtain descriptions of their assessment practices, or consumers to assay their use of and satisfaction with assessments by mental health professionals. Other investigators have obtained sanitized copies of forensic reports and coded their content, including the types of information sought and obtained during the assessments. Both of these approaches permit some statements about the quality of forensic psychological assessment as currently practiced.

In the presentation that follows, evidence is reviewed for two domains of practice, criminal forensic evaluations (adjudicative competence, criminal responsibility) and child custody evaluations. In each domain, findings from surveys of mental health practitioners are described first, followed by results from studies involving direct examination of the content of forensic reports when these were available. Finally, information regarding consumers' perceptions of and satisfaction with forensic evaluations is reported.

CRIMINAL FORENSIC EVALUATIONS

Surveys of Mental Health Practitioners

Borum and Grisso (1995) surveyed experienced forensic psychologists and psychiatrists regarding perceived importance and use of psychological tests and

FAIs in evaluations of competency to stand trial (adjudicative competence, or AC) and criminal responsibility (CR). For present purposes, we will focus on the responses of the forensic psychologists who participated in the study. This group of respondents averaged about 20 years of experience in forensic evaluation and devoted almost one-half of their practice to that endeavor; more than 70% were diplomates of the American Board of Forensic Psychology (ABFP).[3] Thus, the Borum and Grisso (1995) data reflect the opinions of leading practitioners who have devoted a considerable portion of their professional lives to forensic work and have achieved special stature in the field.

Of the psychologists who participated in the AC survey ($n = 57$), more than one-half deemed psychological testing essential (22%) or recommended (29%). In addition, all of the respondents indicated that they used psychological tests in at least some AC evaluations, with 56% of respondents reporting use of such tests "almost always" (in more than 80% of their cases) or "frequently" (in 41–80% of their cases). The tests most likely to be used at least frequently were objective personality tests (reported by 56% of the sample), especially the MMPI/MMPI-2, followed by intellectual/cognitive tests (reported by 41% of the sample), especially the WAIS-R. In contrast, much smaller percentages of respondents indicated such rates of projective (14% of the sample) and neuropsychological (20% of the sample) test use in AC evaluations.

Reported use of FAIs in AC evaluations exhibited greater variability, approximating a bimodal distribution. Although 40% of the sample reportedly used such measures almost always or frequently, almost half (49%) indicated that they "rarely" (1–10% of their cases) or "never" used such measures. Of the specific forensic measures mentioned, the Competency Assessment Instrument (CAI; Laboratory of Community Psychiatry, 1974) and Competency Screening Test (CST; Laboratory of Community Psychiatry, 1974; Lipsitt, Lelos, & McGarry, 1971) were by far the most commonly cited.

Of the psychologists who responded to the CR survey ($n = 53$), more than two-thirds considered psychological testing to be essential (29%) or recommended (39%). Furthermore, 68% of the sample reportedly incorporated psychological testing into CR evaluations almost always or frequently, and all of the respondents reported use of psychological tests in some CR evaluations. Again, objective personality tests and intellectual/cognitive tests were the types that appeared to be used most often; these two types of tests were reportedly used at least frequently by 60% and 44% of the sample, respectively. As with AC evaluations, the MMPI/MMPI-2 and WAIS-R were the specific clinical measures cited most often by respondents. In contrast to the reported use of objective personality and intellectual/cognitive tests in CR evaluations, fewer than 25% of respondents endorsed a comparable frequency of test use for either projective or neuropsychological tests. Use

[3]National board certification in forensic psychology has been available since 1978, when the American Board of Forensic Psychology (ABFP) and the American Academy of Forensic Psychology (AAFP) were established. A diploma awarded by the ABFP confers membership in the AAFP and represents the highest level of credentialing in forensic psychology (Otto et al., 1990). The diploma recognizes the diplomate's forensic experience (minimum of 1000 hours within 5 years, 4 years which must be postdoctoral), training (minimum of 200 hours of supervision), and proficiency (based on submitted professional work samples and an oral examination).

of FAIs was similarly infrequent; only one-quarter of the sample (24%) reported that they used forensic instruments almost always or frequently, whereas two-thirds of the sample (66%) never or rarely used such measures. Of the specific FAIs cited by respondents, the Rogers Criminal Responsibility Assessment Scales (R-CRAS; Rogers, 1984) was the measure named most often.

Borum and Grisso (1996) subsequently summarized respondents' opinions regarding the key components of criminal forensic evaluations. For AC evaluations, a majority of psychologists rated as "essential" a number of report ingredients: (1) identification of defendant and evaluation methods, including basic identifying information, list of data sources, and a description given to the defendant concerning the purposes of the evaluation; (2) clinical data, such as psychiatric history, information from a formal mental status examination, and current use of psychotropic medication; and (3) psycholegal data elements, including understanding of charges/penalties, understanding of possible pleas, appreciation of consequences of a guilty plea and accepting a plea bargain, understanding of the roles of trial participants, ability to communicate with legal counsel, ability to consider advice of counsel, capacity for self-control, and ability to make decisions (process information) without distortion due to mental illness. Among the "opinion" elements surveyed, those deemed "important" centered on description of deficits in functional abilities relevant to AC, the presence or absence of mental illness/mental retardation (MI/MR), and the expert's reasoning regarding the relationship between MI/MR and the observed deficits in psycholegal abilities. Also judged "important" was a description of the situational circumstances in which the defendant's deficits might be more or less likely to compromise his or her participation. Notably, offering an ultimate opinion about AC was seen as "essential" by about 50% of the sample but "contraindicated" by more than 10%. Furthermore, including a defendant's view of the offense was seen as "contraindicated" by 53% of those surveyed.

In addition to the clinical data noted for AC evaluations, psychologists regarded several clinical data elements as "essential" for CR evaluations: information from past mental health records (including prior psychiatric diagnoses), information about the presence/absence of substance abuse, and police information about the defendant's behavior at the time of the alleged offense. In addition, the defendant's description of events surrounding the time of the alleged offense was considered essential, and information from witnesses or other collateral sources nearly reached consensus as essential. Of the opinion elements surveyed, the presence/absence of MI/MR, the relationship between MI/MR and capacities relevant for CR, and an explanation of the expert's reasoning regarding the latter relationship were deemed essential. There was less consensus regarding provision of an ultimate opinion about CR; fewer than one-half of the respondents considered such opinions as essential and almost one-fifth characterized that element as contraindicated.

Borum and Grisso (1995, 1996) argued against reflexive application of the findings from their survey to questions of standards of practice. Nevertheless, the opinions of experienced forensic experts regarding the content of AC and CR evaluations constitute an important source of information for furthering the development of formal and recognized standards of practice. Moreover, the opinions summarized in their survey provide a backdrop against which to evaluate findings from recent investigations that have attempted to characterize the content of AC and CR reports.

Studies of the Content of Forensic Reports

Six studies have examined the content of criminal forensic reports in six states, Florida (Heilbrun & Collins, 1995; Otto, Barnes, & Jacobson, 1996), Nebraska (Robbins, Waters, & Herbert, 1997), New Jersey (Robbins et al., 1997), Oklahoma (Nicholson, LaFortune, Norwood, & Roach, 1995), Virginia (Heilbrun et al., 1994), and Utah (Skeem, Golding, Cohn, & Berge, 1998). The organizational systems for pretrial forensic services in these states include four of the six system types identified in a nationwide survey of forensic program directors and other state forensic mental health personnel (Grisso, Cocozza, Steadman, Fisher, & Greer, 1994). Not represented in the research base are studies from jurisdictions with *traditional* and *modified-traditional* systems. Under the traditional model, pretrial assessments are typically conducted by a small number of practitioners (employees of the state department of mental health) in an inpatient setting (e.g., the state's forensic unit). The modified-traditional model uses outpatient assessment by practitioners who are employees of the state department of mental health; these assessments are conducted in one or two settings with statewide catchment areas (typically state mental hospitals).

Two of the states examined in this body of research, Florida and New Jersey, use a *private practitioner* system, characterized by reliance on outpatient assessments conducted by mental health professionals in private practice. Oklahoma and Virginia also use a type of outpatient system termed *community-based.* In *community-based* systems, most pretrial evaluations are performed locally by public sector clinicians employed by state departments of mental health. One notable difference in the systems represented here is that Virginia provides pretrial assessments of both AC and CR, whereas Oklahoma provides for AC evaluations only. Nebraska uses a third kind of system for delivery of pretrial services, referred to as *mixed.* Such a system typically involves a combination of either the private practitioner or community-based model with the traditional model. Thus, evaluations are conducted in roughly equal proportions on an inpatient basis in a hospital with statewide catchment and on an outpatient basis by local evaluators. The pretrial forensic service delivery system in Utah was placed in a residual category, *unclassified,* under the Grisso et al. (1994) typology. Skeem et al. (1998) obtained a sample of reports from the largest jurisdiction in the state, and they characterized that system as one that uses both private and public sector clinicians to perform two independent assessments of adjudicative competence for each defendant court-ordered to undergo evaluation.

The absence of data from traditional and modified-traditional system types in the extant research base is unfortunate. Such systems are relatively more centralized than others and, rightly or wrongly, have prompted fewer concerns about quality control than decentralized systems. Furthermore, some have suggested that centralized systems are likely to produce evaluations and reports that are less variable in content and quality (even if they are not of higher quality overall) than reports generated in decentralized systems (Grisso et al., 1994; Poythress, Otto, & Heilbrun, 1991). At least one recent investigation (Edens, Poythress, Nicholson, & Otto, 1999) found that system type and forensic examiner etraining did not affect the degree of impairment in competence-related functional abilities exhibited by incompetent defendants; however, the latter investigation did not directly examine variability in report content or quality.

Table 1 presents descriptive information for the six studies. Five of the studies (Hebrun & Collins, 1995; Nicholson et al., 1995; Otto et al., 1996; Robbins et al., 1997; Skeem et al., 1998) relied on trained raters to code the content of criminal forensic evaluations; one study (Heilbrun et al., 1994) used a summary information sheet completed for the state department of mental health by an examiner at the time a forensic report was submitted to the appropriate parties. As the table shows, in four of six states doctoral level psychologists accounted for more of the evaluations than any other professional group, with percentages ranging from almost 50% to 80% of the evaluations across studies. One exception to this pattern arose in New

Table 1. Characteristics of Studies that Examined the Content of Criminal Forensic Reports

	State						
Characteristic	FL	FL	NE	NJ	OK	UT	VA
No. of reports	277	205	16	50	362	100	316
No. of defendants	277	89	NR	NR	349	50	NR
No. of examiners	76	107	9	7	46	18	NR
Education of examiner (% of reports)							
Psychologist	58	53	NR[a]	0	48	80	48
Psychiatrist	18	47	NR	100	36	14	37
Other	24[b]	0	NR	0	16[c]	6[d]	15[e]
Site of evaluation (% of reports)							
Hospital	60	0	44	100	26	9	43
Community	40	100	56	0	74	91	57
Legal issues (% of reports)							
AC	71	65	87	88	100	99	23
CR	1	6	0	0	0	0	11
Both	18	28	13	8	0	0	66
Other[f]	10	0	0	4	0	1	0

Note. Studies providing these data were, from left to right by state, Heilbrun & Collins (1995), Otto et al. (1996), Robbins et al. (1997), Robbins et al. (1997), Nicholson et al. (1995), Skeem et al. (1998), and Heilbrun et al. (1994). Studies from Florida sampled community-based reports for incompetent/insane defendants only. NR indicates that the information was not reported in the study. AC = Adjudicative competence. CR = Criminal responsibility.

[a]Data for Nebraska were reported as percentages of examiners; three (33%) examiners were psychologists, five (56%) were psychiatrists, and one (11%) was a neurologist. The proportion of forensic reports attributable to psychologists could have ranged from 19% (assuming that each psychologist did one evaluation) to 63% (assuming that each nonpsychologist did one evaluation).

[b]Most evaluations performed by M.A.-level staff psychologists at state hospital.

[c]Evaluations performed by JD/LCSW (5% of total), and by M.A.-level and bachelor's-level staff at CMHCs.

[d]Evaluations performed by a doctoral-level social worker.

[e]Education of examiner not specified.

[f]Refers to reports in which neither AC nor CR was addressed. In some cases no legal issue was discernible, and in other cases, legal issues other than AC or CR were addressed (e.g., civil commitment) even though the report was used to hospitalize the defendant as incompetent to proceed to adjudication.

Jersey, where all of the reports were submitted by psychiatrists. A possible exception also emerged in Nebraska. Although the percentage of reports submitted by different professional groups could not be determined, 33% of the evaluators were psychologists.[4]

Table 1 also shows that a majority of the reports (56%–91%) in Nebraska, Oklahoma, Virginia, Utah, and one of the Florida studies were generated by community-based (outpatient) evaluations. The percentage of community-based evaluations was smaller in the first Florida study (Heilbrun & Collins, 1995) because the authors purposefully sampled hospital-based assessments of competence restoration in addition to initial evaluations. Finally, all of the New Jersey reports examined by Robbins et al. (1997) were obtained from hospital-based evaluations. The absence of community-based assessments in the New Jersey sample appears highly unusual, given the state's use of a private practitioner model for the conduct of pretrial assessments. Although some states with such systems have inpatient assessment as a secondary "back-up" option, Grisso et al. (1994) reported that only 2% of all pretrial forensic evaluations from private practitioner states were conducted in an inpatient setting.

At least 89% of the reports in each study addressed the issue of adjudicative competence. As can be seen in the table, the percentages of reports addressing criminal responsibility were more variable, ranging from 0% in Oklahoma and Utah to 77% in Virginia. Curiously, 9% of the reports in the first Florida study (24% of the community-based reports from that study) addressed a variety of legal issues but not AC, even though the reports were used to hospitalize defendants as incompetent to proceed. In addition, small percentages of reports from that study (1%), and from the studies in New Jersey (4%) and Utah (1%) did not mention the legal issue that ostensibly provided the focus of evaluation.

Table 2 summarizes information regarding the general characteristics of the forensic reports examined in these studies, including data on examiners' adherence to the ethical dictates of forensic assessment. As the table shows, many reports failed to document the examiner's notification to the defendant regarding the purpose of the evaluation and the associated limits on confidentiality. For example, only about one-third of community-based reports in Florida (30% and 37% in the two studies) mentioned notification. This practice was even more rare in Oklahoma; fewer than 5% of both community-based and hospital-based reports documented notification of the defendant.

The table also shows that the overwhelming majority of reports from each state included an ultimate opinion about AC; that is, most reports included a statement to the effect that in the opinion of the evaluator the defendant was competent or incompetent. Indeed, even the comparatively low percentages reported for the second Florida study (82%) and for the Utah study (71%) are somewhat misleading in this regard. For example, Otto et al. (1996) reported that ultimate issue opinions were "offered indirectly" in an additional 17% of the Florida

[4]The 16 reports in the Nebraska sample were submitted by nine examiners. Arguably, the percentage of reports by psychologists could range from 19% (if each psychologist performed only one evaluation) to 63% (if each nonpsychologist performed only one evaluation).

Table 2. General Characteristics of Criminal Forensic Reports

Characteristic	State					
	FL (*n* = 277)	FL (*n* = 205)	NE (*n* = 16)	NJ (*n* = 50)	OK (*n* = 362)	UT (*n* = 100)
Court order cited (%)	98/91	NR	NR	NR	99/72	NR
Notification documented (%)	97/30	37	NR	NR	4/4	NR
Information sources noted (%)	NR[a]	78[b]	NR[c]	NR	85/87	NR[d]
Ultimate opinion provided (%)						
AC	99/95	82[e]	88	96	100/99	71[f]
CR	—/47	41	—	—	—/—	—
Average length (pages)	3.9/3.9	3.5	NR	NR	1.2/2.8	NR

Note. Studies providing these data were, from left to right by state, Heilbrun & Collins (1995), Otto et al. (1996), Robbins et al. (1997), Robbins et al. (1997), Nicholson et al. (1995), and Skeem et al. (1998). Studies from Florida sampled community-based reports for incompetent/insane defendants only. Multiple values for the first Florida and Oklahoma studies reflect findings for hospital—and community—based evaluations, respectively. NR indicates that the information was not reported in the study; dashes indicate that the characteristic is not applicable. AC = Adjudicative competence. CR = Criminal responsibility.
[a]Findings were reported for individual sources but not for "any" source. However, the authors noted that "virtually all" of the reports in both hospital and community settings included a clinical interview, implying that at least one source of information could be inferred for almost all of the reports.
[b]In view of other findings reported for this study (e.g., 97% of all evaluations included a clinical interview), the figure reported here must refer to specific listing of sources in reports.
[c]Findings were reported for individual sources but not for "any" source.
[d]Ultimate opinions were offered "indirectly" in an additional 17% of the reports.
[e]Opinions on competence were "easily inferred" from all reports.

reports. Similarly, Skeem et al. (1998) indicated that opinions about overall competence were "easily inferred" from all of the Utah reports. In contrast to the findings for AC, ultimate opinions about CR (e.g., a statement that in the examiner's opinion the defendant was sane or insane at the time of the offense) were provided in fewer than one-half (41–47%) of the reports that included CR as a referral issue. If any report in which the examiner declined to offer an opinion due to insufficient information is excluded from consideration, the percentage of CR reports with an ultimate opinion rises to 66%, still substantially lower than the rate observed among AC evaluations. Unfortunately, only the Florida studies provided comparative data from different kinds of criminal forensic evaluations.

Heilbrun and Collins (1995) argued that the average length of the reports in their study (almost four single-spaced pages for both community-based and hospital-based reports) suggested that the examiners were documenting their evaluations and not simply providing a conclusory opinion. By way of contrast, the reports in Oklahoma were much briefer, especially those submitted from the hospital setting, where 80% of the reports were a single page. Such brevity assuredly limits the information provided to the courts, and increases the likelihood that poorly substantiated conclusions were offered. Nevertheless, longer reports are not necessarily better reports. Stronger inferences about the quality of forensic reports can be drawn from a detailed examination and analysis of their content, to which we now turn.

Table 3 summarizes the assessment methods used to obtain information from the defendant in criminal forensic evaluations. As the table shows, a clinical interview and mental status examination were fundamental components of the criminal

Table 3. Methods Used to Gather Information from Defendants as Cited in Criminal Forensic Reports

	State					
Method	FL (n = 277)	FL (n = 205)	NE (n = 16)	NJ (n = 50)	OK (n = 362)	UT (n = 100)
Interview (%)	>95/>95[a]	97	100[b]		85/85	NR
Mental status exam (%)	63/60	93	NR		80/62	45
Psychological tests (%)	13/41[c]	30[d]	12–23[e]		9/9	69
Competency measures (%)	NR	17[f]	5		0/9	25

Note. Studies providing these data were, from left to right by state, Heilbrun & Collins (1995), Otto et al. (1996), Robbins et al. (1997), Robbins et al. (1997), Nicholson et al. (1995), and Skeem et al. (1998). Studies in Florida sampled community-based reports for incompetent/insane defendants only. Multiple values reported for the first Florida and Oklahoma studies reflect findings for hospital- and community-based evaluations, respectively. NR indicates that the information was not reported in the study.

[a]"Virtually all" of the reports in both hospital and community settings included a clinical interview.

[b]"For the types of tests and procedures used, 11 reports used more than one procedure outside of the interview . . ." The preceding quotation implies that an interview was used in every case; hence, the percentage reported here is 100. Because Robbins et al. (1997) did not separate the findings for NE and NJ reports, the data are reported here in a single column for the "pooled" NE/NJ sample of reports.

[c]Percentages of reports by psychologists. For assessment of trial competency in the community, the rate of test usage by psychologists was 47%, and for the assessment of both trial competency and mental state at the time of the offense, the rate was 57%.

[d]Data were not reported separately for forensic measures and standard clinical instruments; hence, the percentage reported here reflects usage of either type of measure.

[e]The description of psychological test use in the NE/NJ sample of reports was ambiguous; the values reported here reflect minimum and maximum percentages of reports that used psychological tests based on different assumptions about administration of multiple tests in an evaluation.

[f]The percentage reported here includes "other forensic instruments" that may not be measures of competency to standard trial.

forensic evaluations examined in these studies. In contrast, use of psychological testing exhibited considerable variability across jurisdictions. Fewer than 10% of reports in Oklahoma but almost 70% of reports in Utah referenced such testing, with the rate in Florida falling between these extremes. The rate of testing in the combined sample of evaluations from Nebraska and New Jersey is not entirely clear from the text of the article, but it falls toward the lower end of the range observed in the other studies.

The tremendous variability in the use of psychological testing across studies is intriguing and warrants investigation. Variation in examiner characteristics (e.g., professional degree, training in assessment) might explain some of the observed differences. For example, in the combined Nebraska–New Jersey sample, psychiatrists were responsible for at least 83% of the evaluationss, whereas in Utah, psychologists were responsible for 80% of the evaluations. Under such circumstances, one would expect psychological testing to be noted much more often in the Utah sample of reports than in the Nebraska–New Jersey sample, just as the data reported in Table 3 demonstrate. Nevertheless, other findings presented in the table suggest that the prediction of psychological test use is not so straightforward. For example, the relatively low rates of psychological testing in criminal forensic evaluations in Florida and Oklahoma cannot be explained by the presence of nonpsychologists among the forensic examiners. The findings reported for Florida were extracted from a subset of evaluations conducted by psychologists (Heilbrun & Collins, 1995;

Otto et al., 1996), and the Oklahoma findings did not vary when the analysis was limited to reports submitted by psychologists (Nicholson et al., 1995). Thus, the anomalous finding that future research should endeavor to explore and explain is the much higher rate of psychological testing in AC evaluations in Utah.

In Florida, Utah, and Oklahoma, the most commonly used tests were measures of intellectual functioning, with the WAIS-R being cited most often. In Florida and especially Utah, personality tests (most often the MMPI or MMPI-2), neuropsychological screening measures, and even projective measures were also cited with some frequency. In the combined Nebraska–New Jersey sample, neuropsychological screening measures and measures of intellectual functioning were more common than other types of psychological testing. The specific intelligence and objective personality measures used most frequently in these reports (MMPI/MMPI-2, WAIS-R) were consistent with those nominated most often by respondents to the Borum and Grisso (1995) survey (see also Lees-Haley, 1992).

The practitioner survey and studies of report content also produced convergent results with regard to use of projective tests and with regard to the use of testing in different kinds of criminal forensic evaluations (AC vs. CR evaluations). Fewer than 1 in 10 experienced forensic psychologists endorsed routine use of projective techniques in AC evaluations, and only 1 in 5 did so for CR evaluations. Although studies of report content appeared to yield higher estimates of projective test use, such estimates may be misleading if they fail to take into account the nesting of reports within evaluators. Thus, Heilbrun and Collins (1995) argued that some projective measures (e.g., Rorschach) were cited frequently in Florida reports not because they were used occasionally by a large numberf evaluators, but rather because they were used consistently by a few evaluators. Hence, the reported test use for those measures did not reflect general trends in the Florida system, but rather the personal preferences of individual examiners. These same investigations in Florida also illuminated the role of psychological testing in different kinds of criminal forensic evaluations. Consistent with experienced forensic psychologists' perceptions of the relative importance of testing in AC and CR evaluations (Borum & Grisso, 1995), Heilbrun and Collins (1995) found that psychological testing was more common in reports that addressed both issues than in reports that addressed competency alone.

Earlier, Borum and Grisso (1995) observed that their survey findings did not support a standard requiring psychological testing in every criminal forensic evaluation. Nevertheless, they noted that reported test use was common enough among experienced forensic evaluators to be considered the norm rather than the exception, suggesting perhaps that psychologists ought to be held accountable to explain why they did not use psychological testing in an AC or CR evaluation. Such a suggestion may be premature in the absence of evidence regarding how psychological testing was used in evaluations conducted by these experienced examiners. Against such a benchmark, Utah evaluators would rarely be called to account because their reports reflected an even higher rate of testing than that endorsed by the respondents to the Borum and Grisso (1995) survey. However, Skeem et al. (1998) observed that most (70%) of the relevant reports in their study failed to articulate any relationship between test findings and competence. In addition, the relationships described in the remaining 30% of the reports were limited to vague assertions regarding a link between symptomatology identified by testing and general impairment in competence. Of the various types of tests described in those reports, intelligence test findings were only sometimes tied to competence judgments, and projective, personality, and neuropsychological test results were almost never or rarely related to competence. Robbins et al. (1997) reported similar deficiencies in the sample of reports from Nebraska and New Jersey. For example, they observed that more than one-half of the Nebraska–New Jersey reports "did not discuss the types of tests and/or procedures used" (Robbins et al., 1997, p. 476). More importantly, of the reports that did mention tests or procedures, "most of them did not discuss how the results identified any deficits in functional abilities" (Robbins et al., 1997, p. 477). The patterns observed by Skeem et al. (1998) and Robbins et al. (1997) suggest that the examiners may not have had a clear rationale for selection and administration of the psychological tests cited in these reports. Exploration of examiners' uses of psychological testing in criminal forensic evaluations in other jurisdictions is necessary to assess the generality of these findings and refine suggestions regarding guidelines and possible standards for psychological test use in such evaluations.

Table 3 also documents the frequency with which competency assessment instruments were cited in reports. As the table shows, findings from such measures were cited in a small minority of reports from each of the states, ranging from lows of under 5% in the combined sample of Nebraska–New Jersey reports and 7% in Oklahoma (hospital and community reports combined) to a high of only 25% in Utah. Comparison of these data with the survey findings reported by Borum and Grisso (1995) is instructive: Competency assessment instruments were reportedly used at least "frequently" by 40% of the sample of experienced forensic psychologists. Although 36% of the respondents indicated that they never used competency assesment instruments, Borum and Grisso (1995) concluded that the rate of endorsement was undoubtedly higher than in the mid-1980s and that acceptance and use of these measures was increasing.

Table 4 summarizes findings regarding examiners' use of information from third parties, data thought to be of central importance in forensic assessment. As the top half of the table shows, review of the arrest or offense report, which is not only fundamental to assessment of CR but has been termed the "backbone" of competence assessment as well (Skeem et al., 1998), was the most frequently observed type of record review in these criminal forensic evaluations. Nevertheless, use of the arrest report exhibited substantial variability across studies, ranging from 40% to 87% of community-based reports and from 68% to 96% of hospital-based reports.

Review of prior mental health records was also an important component of the pretrial criminal forensic evaluations in these studies, second only to review of the arrest/offense report in terms of observed frequencies. However, citation of prior mental health records was the norm rather than the exception only for hospital-based reports in Florida (86%). At the other extreme, this source of information was noted in fewer than 3% of reports in Oklahoma. In the remaining settings, documentation of the use of prior mental health records was observed in about one-third to one-half of the reports.

Table 4. Use of Third Party Information in Criminal Forensic Reports

Type of Information	State				
	FL	FL	OK	VA	UT
Review of records					
Arrest/offense report	96/49	40	NR[a]	65	68/87
Prior mental health	86/40	37	0/4	37	35/50
Victim or witness	1/2	1–2[b]	NR	NR	18/36
Current jail	NR	24	1/13	NR	NR
Prior criminal justice	NR	8	1/<1	8	NR
Collateral interviews					
Attorneys	NR	8	0/5	NR	9
Hospital staff	70/4	0	NR	NR	NR
Jail personnel	1/17	14–19[c]	0/4	NR	7
Relative	NR	9	0/9	NR	22

Note. Studies providing these data were, from left to right by state, Heilbrun & Collins (1995), Otto et al. (1996), Nicholson et al. (1995), Heilbrun et al. (1994), and Skeem et al. (1998). Although Robbins et al. (1997) reported findings for the citation of "any" third-party information in their sample of forensic reports, they did not report findings for specific types of third-party information. Hence, Robbins et al. (1997) is not included in the table. Studies in Florida sampled community-based reports for incompetent/ insane defendants only. Multiple values reported for the first Florida, Oklahoma, and Virginia studies reflect findings for hospital- and community-based evaluations, respectively. NR indicates that the information was not reported in the study.

[a]In Oklahoma, an information sheet, which lists the charge and provides basic data regarding the alleged offense (e.g., approximate time, location, witnesses), typically accompanies the court order for pretrial competence assessment. Examiners presumably review this information, although they rarely cite it in reports submitted to the court.

[b]The reported percentage reflects citation of interviews with victims or other witnesses, rather than review of statements by victims or witnesses. Because such statements are often incorporated into or appended to arrest reports in Florida (R. Otto, personal communication, March 29, 1999), the percentage of criminal forensic reports using this type of third-party information is probably comparable to that listed for arrest report (i.e., about 40%).

[c]Findings were reported separately for medical staff and detention officers. The reported values reflect minimum and maximum percentages.

Victim or witness statements appeared to be used rarely in reports from Florida, but were sometimes used in evaluations in Virginia, being cited in about one-third of the community-based reports and in almost one-fifth of the hospital-based reports in that state. Current jail records were sometimes used in community-based evaluations in Florida and Oklahoma, but use of prior criminal justice records was rare in all three of the settings that provided such information.

Several factors likely contribute to the observed variability in the use of third-party records across settings and states. First, as Heilbrun et al. (1994) noted, an "accessibility effect" is probably at work. Information that is more readily obtainable, for whatever reason (e.g., agency regulation, statutory directive), is more likely to be incorporated into an evaluation and later cited in a report to the court. Second, the importance of third-party reports and reviews of records varies as a function of the legal issue(s) being evaluated (e.g., competency, criminal responsibility, or both) as well as the specifics of the case (e.g., suspected malingering). For example, evaluations of both adjudicative competence and mental state at the time of the offense would be expected to include more sources and types of information than assessments of competence alone. Thus, the greater frequency of combined evaluations in Virginia would promote the increased use of victim and witness statements relative to assessments conducted in other states. Third, differences in forensic training and in the personal preferences and habits of evaluators may contribute to observed differences in report characteristics. The absence of a single reference to review of mental health records in hospital-based assessments in Oklahoma is clearly at odds with the "accessibility effect" and can better be accounted for by reference to evaluator training and preferences. Finally, in some cases, the observed variability across reports may be attributed more to differences in local procedures and associated documentation practices than to differences in the behavior being documented. For example, Otto (personal communication, March 29, 1999) noted that victim or witness statements in Florida are typically incorporated into or appended to the arrest report. That being the case, Florida evaluators who cite review of the arrest report as a source of information for their evaluations may not perceive the need to document a separate review of victim and/or witness statements. Therefore, although the findings reported in the third row of the table suggest a discrepancy between evaluators in Virginia and Florida with regard to review of victim and witness statements, it is quite possible that such information is incorporated into pretrial evaluations at comparable rates in the two jurisdictions.

The lower half of Table 4 provides information on the use of another type of third-party information: collateral interviews. With one exception, collateral interviews were used infrequently in all four studies that provided such information. For example, contact with attorneys was cited in no more than 9% of the reports from any state. This is surprising given that the attorney should be able to provide important information regarding the difficulties he or she has experienced in working with the defendant, examples of the defendant's putative psychological problems, as well as the anticipated demands of the particular legal case at hand. Also surprising is the infrequency with which the reports listed interviews with jail personnel as a source of information. For community-based evaluators in particular, contacts with medical staff and detention officers at the jail can provide useful information about the defendant's behavior over a longer period of time and outside the context of the evaluation itself. The one exception to the generally low rate of collateral interviews was not surprising: A majority of hospital-based evaluations of competence restoration in Florida cited interviews with other hospital staff.

Table 5 provides data on the extent to which examiners addressed the functional objective in forensic assessment (see Grisso, 1986, 1988) by noting defendants' relevant psycholegal abilities. In interpreting the findings, careful attention must be given to the coding schemes that were used because these varied somewhat across studies. Interpreted properly, the data presented in the table suggest that specification of competence domains by statute or rules of procedure may have an impact on report content, but only a limited one. Such statutes can probably increase the frequency with which the components of competence are cited by evaluators in their reports to the court, but they probably cannot guarantee that the targeted psycholegal abilities will be discussed in more than a conclusory fashion, as the following examples from studies in Florida and Oklahoma show.

Florida Rules of Criminal Procedure identify six domains to be considered in evaluating competence (the first six functional abilities listed in Table 5). As the

Table 5. Description of Defendants' Psycholegal Abilities in Criminal Forensic Reports

	State					
Psycholegal ability	FL	FL	NE	NJ	OK	UT
AC Reports (No.)	239	192	16	50	362	100
Appreciate charge (%)	98/81	91	NR	NR	71/64	85
Appreciate penalty (%)	98/72	79	NR	NR	17/43	77
Understand legal process (%)	98/76	85	NR	NR	12/32	73
Control behavior in court (%)	98/61	76	NR	NR	5/9	31
Testify relevantly (%)	95/64	77	NR	NR	NR	24
Able to disclose to attorney (%)[a]	98/73	90	44	22	3/33	70
Relationship with attorney (%)	NR	NR	NR	NR	5/36	49
Understand plea bargaining (%)	NR	11	NR	NR	3/22	26–41[b]
Appreciate legal options (%)	NR	NR	NR	NR	NR	53
Exercise reasoned choice (%)	NR	NR	NR	NR	NR	37
CR Reports (No.)	51	71	—	—	—	—
Knowledge of act (%)	—/41	NR	—	—	—	—
Knowledge of consequences (%)	—/27	NR	—	—	—	—
Knowledge of wrongfulness (%)	—/29	NR	—	—	—	—

Note. Studies providing these data were, from left to right by state, Heilbrun & Collins (1995), Otto et al. (1996), Robbins et al. (1997), Robbins et al. (1997), Nicholson et al. (1995), and Skeem et al. (1998). In each study, data were reliably coded directly from forensic reports. Studies in Florida sampled community-based reports for incompetent/insane defendants only. Multiple values reported for the first Florida and Oklahoma studies reflect findings for hospital- and community-based evaluations, respectively. NR indicates that the information was not reported in the study; dashes indicate that the characteristic is not applicable. AC = Adjudicative competence. CR = Criminal responsibility.

[a]According to Florida Rules of Criminal Procedure, one of six domains to be considered in assessing competence. Described as ability to disclose relevant information to the defense attorney by Heilbrun & Collins (1995) and as ability to work with his/her attorney by Otto et al. (1996).

[b]Findings reported for understanding of the rights waived as a result of plea bargaining and understanding of the mechanics of a plea bargain.

table shows, a majority of both hospital- and community-based reports addressed these legally relevant abilities. For community-based reports, the percentages were even higher in the Otto et al. (1996) study than in the earlier Heilbrun and Collins (1995) investigation. Moreover, the citation rate for these six abilities in Florida reports was comparable to or higher than the citation rate for those same abilities in reports submitted by evaluators in Utah or Oklahoma. However, the percentages reported for the Florida studies may be misleading. Heilbrun and Collins (1995) reported the frequency with which each psycholegal ability was "directly discussed" (p. 65) but did not examine whether the legal criteria were described in "appropriate detail" (p. 67). Furthermore, the values reported for the Otto et al. (1996) study refer to the percentages of reports in which the examiner addressed the psycholegal abilities with a conclusory statement. If describing functional abilities in appropriate detail requires evaluators to provide examples and a description of the defendant's capacity or impairment, the rates obtained by Otto et al. (1996) were substantially lower, ranging from 36% for defendant's capacity to testify and understanding of possible penalties to 53% for defendant's capacity to work with the attorney.

A similar phenomenon occurs in Oklahoma, where the statute requires an examiner to answer two questions related to a defendant's functional abilities. The first concerns the defendant's ability "to appreciate the nature of the charges" and the second concerns the ability "to consult with his lawyer and rationally assist in the preparation of his defense." Each of these questions was answered in virtually all of the Oklahoma reports (98% overall). However, examiners typically did not provide a description of the defendant's functional abilities relevant to the two statutory questions. Of the seven domains examined by Nicholson et al. (1995), only knowledge of the charge, which is closely related to the first statutory question, was described in a majority of the reports (66% overall). The remaining components of competence were described occasionally at best. Indeed, the next most frequently described component, knowledge of the penalty, was included in just more than one-third of the reports (36% overall).

As the foregoing examples demonstrate, statutory or other specification of competence domains may fail to advance the quality of the information provided to the courts. Moreover, it is important to consider whether such specification has unintended adverse effects by fostering less adequate consideration of psycholegal abilities not incorporated into the statute or rules of procedure. Unfortunately, evidence bearing on the question of adverse effects is mixed and does not permit a firm conclusion at present. On one hand, data presented by Otto et al. (1996) suggest the possibility of such adverse effects. In order to enhance comparability of their findings with those from other jurisdictions, the authors coded a seventh domain, understanding of plea bargaining, which is not covered by Florida's Rules of Criminal Procedure. As Table 5 shows, community-based evaluators in Florida rarely (11%) mentioned this component of competence in their reports. Indeed, they mentioned it less often than evaluators in Utah and community-based evaluators in Oklahoma. On the other hand, Robbins et al. (1997) provided evidence that argues against such negative effects. One-half of the reports in their study included a description of at least one relevant functional ability that was not contained in the criteria set forth by New Jersey statute, the controlling case in Nebraska, or the 13 components of competence from the CAI. In other words, the Nebraska and New Jersey examiners did not limit the information they provided to the courts as a result of statute, case law, or other specification of criteria for AC. Furthermore, Robbins et al. (1997) discovered only two (3%) reports that contained information about an irrelevant functional ability. At the same time, it should be noted that Nebraska and New Jersey evaluators did not appear to exhibit a higher level of performance overall than evaluators from other jurisdictions. For example, Robbins et al. (1997) indicated that the New Jersey evaluators covered all of the statutory criteria for competence in about one-half of the reports.

One additional pattern can be discerned from the data reported for AC studies in the upper portion of Table 5. To the extent that the competency reports from these five states provide information about defendants' legally relevant functional abilities, they focused on foundational abilities encompassed by Bonnie's (1993) concept of competence to assist counsel rather than abilities related to decisional competence. For example, reports from Utah were more likely to include descriptions of the defendant's appreciation of the charges and penalties, understanding of legal proceedings and the roles of courtroom personnel, and ability to disclose information to an attorney. They were less likely to include appreciation of legal options, understanding of plea bargaining, and capacity for reasoned choice

(Skeem & Golding, 1998). Similarly, in reports from Florida and Oklahoma, information about the defendant's understanding of plea bargaining was cited in fewer reports than were the foundational abilities.[5] Robbins et al. (1997) did not provide a detailed description of their findings , as evidenced by the number of "not reported" symbols in the two middle columns of Table 5. However, Robbins et al. did observe that the four most frequently cited abilities were consistent across both the Nebraska and New Jersey samples. All four were foundational abilities and almost identical to those cited in the reports form Utah: appreciation of the charge, appreciation of the penalties, understanding of the roles of various courtroom participants, and quality of relating to the attorney (Robbins et al., 1997, p. 476).

The bottom portion of Table 5 presents information about the content of CR reports. Unfortunately, only one study (Heilbrun & Collins, 1995) examined the content of forensic reports to determine whether the evaluators addressed relevant components of the CR construct. The relevant standard for insanity in Florida at the time of the study was the M'Naughten standard. Of the 51 reports of community-based evaluations from Florida that included an assessment of criminal responsibility, fewer than one-half (41%) addressed the question of whether the defendant knew what he or she was doing at the time of the alleged offense. Even fewer reports addressed the defendant's knowledge of the consequences (27%) or the wrongfulness (29%) of his or her actions. Otto et al. (1996) examined 71 reports in which criminal responsibility was an issue. Although the authors did not provide data on the components of criminal responsibility evaluations, they observed that opinions about mental state at the time of the offense were based primarily on the defendant's narrative. Opinions were derived from other accounts (e.g., victim, witness, police) in fewer than 10% of the reports.

The direct assessment of legally relevant functional abilities in a pretrial population must be accompanied by systematic efforts to assess possible causes of any observed impairments in functioning that emerge. In Grisso's (1986, 1988) terminology, this task constitutes the causal objective of competence assessment, the process of endeavoring to draw causal inferences to explain observed impairment in legally relevant functional ability. For example, in the context of AC, poor performance on an FAI could occur for a number of reasons: (1) ignorance of the legal system that is easily remediated; (2) purposeful fabrication or exaggeration of symptoms of mental disorder or cognitive impairment; (3) a lack of cooperation with the assessment process; or (4) genuine mental disorder or deficits in cognitive and intellectual functioning that compromise the individual's ability to function in the context of the legal proceedings.

Table 6 provides data from three studies (Nicholson et al., 1995; Otto et al., 1996; Robbins et al., 1997) that examined the frequency with which criminal forensic reports contained descriptions of defendants' mental status, symptomatology, and

[5]It is possible that the infrequent citation of the functional ability "understanding of plea bargaining" in Florida reports is simply a manifestation of this tendency in all of the jurisdictions studied for evaluators to focus on fundamental competence to assist counsel abilities rather than decisional competence abilities. If so, then the low citation frequency should not be imbued with special significance, and my earlier speculations about the possible impact of statutory specificity on report content were off the mark.

Table 6. Description of Defendants' Mental Status Characteristics in Criminal Forensic Reports

	State			
Mental status characteristic	FL (n = 205)	NE (n = 16)	NJ (n = 50)	OK (n = 362)
Orientation	71	NR	NR	0/43
Attention/concentration	39	NR	NR	0/40
Memory	51	NR	NR	3/38
Thought processes	59	NR	NR	10/48
Psychotic symptoms	68–71[a]	NR	NR	14/54
Suicidal/homicidal ideation	47	NR	NR	13/39
Intellectual functioning	51	NR	NR	11/27
Diagnosis	51	81	98	NR
Current treatment	45	NR	NR	NR
Response style	50	NR	NR	NR

Note. Studies providing these data were, from left to right by state, Otto et al. (1996), Robbins et al. (1997), Robbins et al. (1997), and Nicholson et al. (1995). In each study, data were reliably coded directly from forensic reports. Otto et al. (1996) sampled community-based reports for incompetent/insane defendants only. Multiple values reported for the Oklahoma study reflect findings for hospital- and community-based evaluations, respectively. NR indicates that the information was not reported in the study.

[a]Findings for hallucinations and delusions, respectively.

psychiatric diagnosis, issues particularly relevant for drawing inferences about the causes of observed functional impairment. Skeem et al. (1998) also investigated these aspects of report content, but did not report findings in a way that allowed us to incorporate the data into Table 6. As the data presented in the table suggest, evaluators in both Florida and Oklahoma appear to be more consistent in describing defendants' mental status characteristics than in describing (as opposed to merely citing) competence criteria. Nevertheless, even on this dimension, a substantial percentage of the reports in both states could be judged inadequate. In Florida, two characteristics, orientation and psychotic symptoms, were described in at least 70% of the reports, but most were described in only about one-half of the reports. In Oklahoma, no aspects of the defendants' mental status were described in a majority of the reports, although among outpatient reports, the presence or absence of psychotic symptoms was noted in about one-half of the reports. Mental status characteristics of the defendants being assessed received only occasional mention in this sample of Oklahoma reports (ranging from 23% to 43% of hospital- and community-based reports combined). As the middle columns of Table 6 reveal, Robbins et al. (1997) did not provide information regarding the frequency with which criminal forensic reports in Nebraska and New Jersey describe various aspects of the defendant's mental status, including symptoms of severe psychopathology. However, the samples of reports studied by Robbins et al. (1997) were much more likely to include a formal psychiatric diagnosis than were reports sampled elsewhere. Indeed, 98% of the New Jersey reports and 81% of the Nebraska reports contained diagnostic information. Furthermore, Skeem et al. (1998) were complimentary of the performance of the Utah evaluators in this domain. For example, they noted that examiners in Utah generally did a respectable job of documenting their diagnostic opinions; two-thirds of the reports (67%) cited many of the symptoms that formed the basis for the diagnosis offered.

A further consideration in evaluating the quality of forensic reports is the extent to which a report describes the reasoning that underlies an examiner's opinion. For example, in a high-quality report of a pretrial competence evaluation, the examiner should articulate the relationship between observed impairment in particular psycholegal abilities and symptoms of psychopathology or limited intellectual functioning (Skeem & Golding, 1998). To address this aspect of report quality, Skeem et al. (1998) characterized the description of the relationship between these two classes of variables in their sample of reports from Utah. The analysis revealed that reports often provided no description of the relationship between impaired competence ability and psychopathology. In contrast, substantiated relationships, in which examiners provided specific descriptions of how psychopathology compromised psycholegal abilities, were rarely observed. Skeem et al. (1998) concluded that the reports demonstrated a general failure to provide an explanation of the relationship between psychopathology and impairment in psycholegal ability. Because the foregoing analysis was limited to reports in which defendants' competence abilities were described as impaired, Skeem et al. (1998) also investigated whether examiners who judged defendants to be competent supported those opinions by describing defendants' competence-related abilities. Analysis revealed that only 59% of the reports provided specific descriptions of defendants' psycholegal abilities.

Nicholson et al. (1995) also explored this dimension of report quality by determining how often reports from Oklahoma provided data or reasoning to support examiners' answers to the statutory questions described previously. They found that 63% of the reports provided appropriate data or reasoning to support the examiners' answers to the first statutory question (appreciation of the nature of the charge). However, answers to the second statutory question (consult with lawyer and rationally assist) were accompanied by supporting data or a rationale in only about one-half (51%) of the reports. Furthermore, it should be noted that Nicholson et al. (1995) adopted a much lower threshold for this aspect of report quality than did Skeem et al. (1998). Indeed, few if any of the Oklahoma reports would meet the "substantiated relationship" standard applied by the latter authors.

Previously, it was noted that the NE and NJ evaluators described by Robbins et al. (1997) did not perform up to expectations with regard to establishing a link between impaired performance on psychological tests and impairment in competence-related functional capacities. A similar pattern was observed with regard to the relationship among diagnosis, symptoms of psychopathology, and functional capacities in legal contexts. Although Robbins et al. (1997) again failed to describe their analyses and findings in detail, they nevertheless noted that only 27% of the combined sample of reports from Nebraska and New Jersey described the link between particular symptoms of psychopathology and impairment in specific functional capacities.

Surveys of Legal Consumers

Although some earlier investigations examined the issue of consumer satisfaction with criminal forensic reports (e.g., Melton et al., 1985), more recent investigations of this issue are generally lacking. LaFortune and Nicholson (1995) surveyed 256 members of the legal profession from the two most populous counties in Oklahoma to assess their satisfaction with pretrial competency reports and solicit their perceptions of the system in general, and the content and quality of reports in particular. Completed, usable surveys were obtained from 93 attorneys and 17 judges for a response rate of 43%. Respondents were an experienced group, averaging almost 11 years ($SD = 8.3$) in the practice of law. Consistent with the analysis of the content of Oklahoma reports (Nicholson et al., 1995), respondents rated community-based reports higher than hospital-based reports in overall quality. They also rated community-based reports higher on several dimensions related to quality, including timeliness, familiarity with legal criteria, use of understandable language, explanation of the factual basis for the opinions offered, and usefulness in decision making. Notably, for both community- and hospital-based reports, the dimension that received the lowest ratings was "explanation of the factual basis for opinions."

To explore further the attorneys' and judges' opinions about the content of the reports, respondents were asked to indicate, using 5-point Likert scales (1 = never, 5 = always), the frequency with which reports described any of 14 aspects of psycholegal ability or mental status relevant to competency, as well as the extent to which the reports should provide such descriptions. According to respondents, 9 of the 14 characteristics, including planning of legal strategy, understanding of plea bargaining, understanding of attorney–client privilege, and capacity to testify relevantly, were mentioned "rarely" to "sometimes" in competency reports. Only five defendant characteristics were mentioned more than "sometimes" in reports (appreciation of the charge, understanding of courtroom procedure, capacity to disclose pertinent facts, quality of relationship with attorney, thought disorder), and of these, only appreciation of the charge was rated as being mentioned more than "often" in the reports. Respondents opined that each characteristic should receive more frequent mention in competency reports. However, with the exception of appreciation of the charge (mention of which is required by statute), no single characteristic was thought to require mention in every report (as would be indicated by an average rating of "always").

An appropriate summary of the survey's findings was provided by approximately 50% of the sample who responded to open-ended questions regarding the adequacy of pretrial competency reports. In general, the attorneys and judges who responded did not appear to be satisfied with the degree of specificity contained in the mental health professionals' answers to the statutory questions regarding competence. The respondents complained that little attempt was made to individualize cases, and that reports should provide more extensive descriptions of defendants' background and history, psycholegal abilities (especially with regard to assisting an attorney), and psychiatric condition, as well as specific reasons for the expert's opinions.

CHILD CUSTODY EVALUATIONS

Surveys of Mental Health Practitioners

Until recently, the primary source of information about normative practices in child custody assessment was an often-cited survey by Keilin and Bloom (1986), who solicited opinions from 302 practitioners in the United States and Canada, with the western region of the United States being markedly overrepresented. The response rate for their survey is sometimes described as 63%, yielding a sample of 190 respondents (e.g., Ackerman, 1995; Grisso, 1990b; Otto & Collins, 1995), but this number included responses from individuals who declined to participate (n = 39) and from those who lacked experience with child custody evaluations (n = 69). Hence, usable responses were obtained from only 82 practitioners (35% of those with relevant experience). Of the latter group, the majority (n = 64, or 78%) were doctoral level psychologists. On average, respondents had 16 years of clinical experience and had conducted more than 150 child custody assessments.

Keilin and Bloom (1986) reported that the average custody evaluation took almost 19 hours to complete. All of the respondents reported that they conducted individual interviews with each parent, and almost all conducted individual interviews with each child. Use of psychological testing in custody evaluations was common; 75.6% of respondents reported testing of parents and 74.4% reported testing of children. For testing of parents, the instruments most frequently cited were the MMPI (cited by 71% of the respondents who reported using it in 88% of their cases), Rorschach (42% reported using it in 67% of their cases), Thematic Apperception Test (TAT; 38% reported using it in 67% of their cases), and the Wechsler Adult Intelligence Scale (WAIS; 29% of respondents; 67% of their cases). A considerably wider range of measures was cited for testing of children and adolescents. The most common measures were an individually administered intelligence test (45% of respondents reported using one such measure in 85% of their cases), the TAT or Children's Apperception Test (CAT; 39% of respondents in 75% of the cases), miscellaneous projective drawings (33% of respondents in 86% of the cases), Rorschach (29% of respondents in 78% of the cases), Bender–Gestalt (23% of respondents in 81% of the cases), an achievement test such as the Wide Range Achievement Test (WRAT; 21% of respondents in 76% of the cases), and the Draw-a-Person technique (20% of respondents in 79% of the cases). With regard to other methods of data collection, about 70% of the respondents reportedly observed an interaction between each parent and each child. Notably, only half observed interactions between the parents or sought information from third parties such as friends and relatives. Finally, fewer than one-third of the respondents made school or home visits.

More recently, Ackerman and Ackerman (1997) conducted a national survey of 800 psychologists engaged in child custody assessment, obtaining usable responses from 201 (25%). On average, these doctoral level psychologists had 19 years of clinical experience and had conducted 215 child custody evaluations. Estimates of the time required for conducting a child custody assessment averaged almost 30 hours, a substantial increase from that reported by Keilin and Bloom (1986). This overall difference apparently can be attributed to increases in the amount of time involved in reviewing materials and writing reports. Thus, the amount of time devoted to interviewing and testing was not markedly discrepant from that reported a decade earlier. In addition to individual interviews with each parent and child, psychological testing was the norm in these custody evaluations: 96.5% of respondents reported testing of parents and 90.5% reported testing of children. For assessing parents, the instruments most frequently cited were the MMPI or MMPI-2 (cited by 92% of the respondents who reported using it in 91% of their cases), Rorschach (48% reported using it in 64% of their cases), WAIS-R (43% of respondents in 49% of their cases), and MCMI II or MCMI III (34% of respondents in 73% of their cases). Notably, the Ackerman–Schoendorf Parent Evaluation of Custody Tests (ASPECT; Ackerman & Schoendorf, 1992) was ranked seventh, cited by 11% of respondents who used it in 89% of their evaluations. For testing children and adolescents, the most common measures were an individually administered intelligence test (58% of respondents reportedsing one such measure in 45% of their cases), TAT or CAT (37% of respondents in 53% of their cases), Bricklin Perceptual Scales (BPS; Bricklin, 1984a; 35% of respondents in 66% of their cases), sentence completion tasks (29% of respondents in 76% of their cases), an achievement test (28% of respondents in 56% of their cases), Rorschach (27% of respondents in 48% of their cases), miscellaneous projective drawings (24% of respondents in 72% of the cases), and the MMPI-A (20% of respondents in 49% of the cases). Ackerman and Ackerman (1997) noted that the most significant change in testing of children was the increased usage of the BPS, now the third most frequently used measure. They also noted that the ASPECT was the most commonly used custody measure with adults.

Respondents to the Ackerman and Ackerman (1997) survey were unanimous in expressing a preference for arrangements that placed them in a neutral role with regard to the proceedings, either because they were retained by both parties or by order of the court. Almost two-thirds of the psychologists (65%) endorsed the view that it was appropriate for them to answer the ultimate legal question, whereas only one-fifth (21%) opined that it would be inappropriate to do so. Interestingly, 6% indicated that they did not know what the term meant.

Concurrently with the survey by the Ackermans, LaFortune (1997) surveyed 268 mental health professionals from five states (Georgia, Nebraska, New York, North Carolina, and Oklahoma) who claimed child custody evaluation as an area of competence. The survey included questions designed to address attitudes toward and perceptions of the custody evaluation process, as well as assessment procedures, time involvement, fee structure, and report content. Completed, usable surveys were obtained from 141 professionals for a response rate of 53%. Of the respondents, 90% were licensed psychologists. The median number of child custody evaluations completed by respondents during their careers was 24.5. The respondents strongly endorsed the view that experts should be retained at the court's request so that their relationship with the litigating parties involved was a neutral one, a finding consistent with that reported by Ackerman and Ackerman (1997). In addition, they opined that the increased likelihood of being sued for malpractice was the greatest source of dissatisfaction in performing custody evaluations.

Respondents to the LaFortune (1997) survey almost always used interviews with each parent, interviews with children, and observations of parent–child interaction in conducting the evaluations. In addition, they often administered the MMPI-2, interviewed significant others, and reviewed school records. Interviews with informants, parenting scales, structured diagnostic interviews, and drawing tests were sometimes used. The reported frequency of use of measures of intellectual and cognitive functioning was in the rarely to sometimes range; however, projective tests, such as the Rorschach and TAT, were administered rarely.

In contrast to the previously described surveys, LaFortune (1997) also asked participants to characterize the content of their psychological reports. Thus, 93% of the respondents claimed to comply strictly with the practice of naming all of the procedures and tests used in the assessment. In addition, 94% indicated that they frequently or always gave examples of behavior or responses or descriptions of parents' strengths and weaknesses as factual bases for their conclusions. The clinicians also claimed that they frequently provided information regarding factors that might affect the validity of their findings. However, there was considerable variability with regard to the frequency with which they reportedly submitted clear recommendations about the ultimate legal issue. Nevertheless, only 15% of the respondents indicated that they never made such recommendations.

In sum, three surveys conducted since the late 1980s point to a common core in the practice of custody evaluation. Individual interviews of all parties, observation of interactions between each parent and the child(ren), and administration of a battery of psychological tests constitute the central components of the prototypic evaluation, and the great majority of custody evaluators indicated that they incorporated these components into their evaluations on a consistent basis. There was somewhat greater variability with regard to other components of the evaluation, such as contacts with collaterals, and with regard to the specific psychological tests administered. Interestingly, the two recent surveys, which were conducted at approximately the same time, suggested different patterns of psychological test usage. Respondents to LaFortune's (1997) survey apparently administered intelligence tests and projective techniques much less frequently than did respondents to the survey by Ackerman and Ackerman (1997).[6] However, for both groups the MMPI-2 was by far the most commonly used test with adults.

The three surveys also provide evidence suggestive of a shift in practice with regard to the selection of assessment instruments. Respondents to the Keilin and Bloom (1986) survey did not cite any of the measures described by Grisso (1986; 1990) as relevant to the assessment of parenting capacity or custody. A few (3–6%) of the respondents to the Ackerman and Ackerman (1997) survey reported that they incorporated some of the relevant measures—the Child Behavior Checklist (CBCL; Achenbach, 1978; Achenbach & Edelbrock, 1979), the Connors Rating Scales (CRS; Connors, 1969), and the Child Abuse Potential Inventory (CAP; Milner, 1986)—into their assessments. In addition, two newer measures relevant to the assessment of parenting skills—the Parent–Child Relationship Inventory

[6]The differences in reported test usage by respondents to the Ackerman and LaFortune surveys may be attributable to differences in sample characteristics. Respondents to the Ackerman survey had considerably more experience in child custody assessment than did respondents to the LaFortune survey. The greater experience of the Ackerman respondents is probably associated with other relevant characteristics such as probability of membership in an organization of child custody evaluators. If the Ackerman respondents were more likely to be familiar with measures specifically developed for use in custody evaluations, such as the ASPECT, it could account for the increased use of intellectual and projective measures. As noted elsewhere (Nicholson, 1999), examiners who use the ASPECT are likely to administer the entire gamut of standard clinical tests and techniques in order to respond to the items on the custody measure.

(PCRI; Gerard, 1994) and the Parenting Stress Index (PSI; Abidin, 1990)—were endorsed by somewhat larger percentages of respondents to the Ackermans' survey: 11% & 9%, respectively. Finally, respondents to both of the recent surveys (Ackerman & Ackerman, 1997; LaFortune, 1997) reported the use of instruments specifically developed for child custody evaluation—the BPS and the ASPECT. Indeed, among respondents to the Ackermans' survey, the BPS was the most common custody measure used with children and the ASPECT was the most common custody measure used with parents, cited by 35% and 11% of evaluators, respectively. However, because published reviews have identified numerous and substantial deficiencies in the last two instruments (e.g., see Arditti, 1995; Hagin, 1992; Heinz & Grisso, 1996; Melton, 1995; Melton et al., 1997; Nicholson, 1999), their endorsement by custody evaluators does not necessarily translate into improvements in professional practice.

At present, our knowledge of normative practices in the area of child custody assessment is limited to the information gleaned from these surveys. Although such information has the potential to enlighten us regarding current practice and possible standards, it must be acknowledged that we do not know whether these examiners actually do what they say they do when conducting a custody evaluation. Unfortunately, no studies have obtained copies of custody reports and coded their content. In the absence of such data, we cannot assess the accuracy of the survey findings, nor can we gauge the overall quality of work in the area. The next stage of research should therefore be directed toward examination of the content and quality of child custody reports submitted to the courts in various jurisdictions.

Surveys of Legal Consumers

An earlier survey of judges' perceptions of expert testimony revealed greater dissatisfaction with the work of mental health professionals in the area of child custody than in other domains such as competency to stand trial, insanity, or civil commitment (Melton et al., 1985). More recently, Lafortune (1997; see also LaFortune & Carpenter, 1996) assayed consumer satisfaction with child custody evaluations in a survey of members of the Family Law Section of the Oklahoma Bar Association. Of 235 members surveyed, completed questionnaires were returned by 162, for a response rate of 69%. Participants were an experienced group and reported having practiced family law for an average of more than 13 years ($M = 13.5$, $SD = 9.9$).

Fewer than 15% of the respondents expressed satisfaction with the present procedural system for divorce and custody cases, at least in part because of the common perception, endorsed by 78% of respondents, that divorce cases took too long to be resolved. Indeed, almost 45% of those queried agreed that divorce cases could best be handled in a nonadversarial setting. Furthermore, two-thirds (67%) agreed that when an expert is needed, the court should appoint one. The latter opinions may derive from the perception that experts tend to be biased. Respondents estimated that experts favored the party that hired them in more than 60% of cases. There was considerable disagreement with regard to ultimate issue testimony. Just more than one-half of the sample (51%) agreed that experts should be allowed to answer the ultimate legal question, whereas almost two-fifths (38%) disagreed with that view. Somewhat more consensus was reached with regard to whether experts should be able to say which of the parties was the better parent; 76% agreed and only 12% disagreed with such a statement.

Respondents were asked to indicate their endorsement of specific kinds of health professionals as experts in child custody cases. To do so, they rated each of five health professions (psychologist, psychiatrist, licensed social worker, licensed professional counselor, physician) on a 5-point scale, with 1 = strongly dislike and 5 = strongly prefer. Psychologists were endorsed (given ratings of 4 or 5) by more than four-fifths (82%) of the sample, whereas psychiatrists received the endorsements of less than one-half (49%) of the sample. The lowest rates of endorsement were for licensed clinical social workers (19%) and physicians (7%). Concern about bias on the part of experts is reflected in the respondents' ratings of the characteristics most valued in a child custody expert: (1) being unbiased and (2) being competent at providing an accurate and fair picture while staying within the limitations of scientific procedure were endorsed as important or very important by almost 97% of the sample. In contrast, only 28% thought it important for the expert to make a strong stand "almost as an advocate." Furthermore, fewer than one-third (31%) of respondents thought that it was important or very important that the expert conducted research or published in the area. Despite the attorneys' preference for unbiased experts and the opinion of more than three-fifths (62%) of the sample that multiple experts were confusing to the court, the most frequently endorsed reason for when an expert should be used was a pragmatic one: Almost three-fourths (74%) of the sample endorsed use of an expert "to balance testimony of opposing side's expert." Only a minority of respondents (27%) felt that experts should be used frequently or routinely.

The attorneys' perceptions of the quality of the work provided by experts in child custody cases was generally positive. The overwhelming majority of respondents provided positive ratings for experts' knowledge of relevant areas (81%), professional behavior (75%), and quality of evaluations (72%). In addition, three-fifths of the sample (61%) provided positive ratings of the quality of experts' in-court testimony. The lowest rate of endorsement was for quality of reports submitted to the court; only one-half of the respondents (50%) gave positive ratings of report quality.

One of the interesting findings from the survey involved correlations between attorneys' years of experience and perceptions of the nature of the proceedings in general, the quality of experts' work, and the procedures used by experts in conducting custody evaluations. Attorneys with more years of experience were less likely to endorse the use of court-appointed experts, a nonadversarial setting for resolution of divorce cases, and the view that lawyers needed more psychological training. Attorneys with more experience also rated the quality of reports higher. Surprisingly, attorneys' years of experience also correlated positively with their perceptions of the frequency with which the Rorschach and TAT were used, but negatively with perceptions of frequency with which interviews of parent and child were used in custody evaluations.

Given the sharp criticisms leveled by scholars at the quality of mental health experts' work in custody cases (e.g., Melton et al., 1997), the generally positive ratings of report quality by the attorneys who responded to LaFortune's (1997) survey were unexpected.[7] Because the perspective of those who labor in the trenches is necessarily more pragmatic, attorneys may apply different criteria in evaluating report quality than legal and mental health scholars. Regardless, the fact that attorneys with more years of experience provided higher ratings of quality yet perceived experts as more often using measures of questionable validity underscores the limitations of consumer satisfaction as a gold standard for guiding professional development. These findings also point, once again, to the need for research that directly examines the content and quality of experts' reports and in-court testimony. Even if the ratings are accepted at face value, there is clearly room for improvement in the quality of experts' work in the area, particularly with regard to written information and oral testimony provided to the courts. Note also that younger attorneys were more reform-oriented and dissatisfied with the present system, and they gave lower ratings of report quality, suggesting that opportunities for change will present themselves in the near future.

THE GAP BETWEEN PROMISE AND PRACTICE

Professional developments since the late 1980s—publication of the Specialty Guidelines (Committee on Ethical Guidelines for Forensic Psychologists, 1991), convocation of the Villanova Conference (Bersoff, Goodman-Delahunty, Grisso, Hans, Poythress, & Roesch, 1997), and the creation of training and certification programs in a number of states (e.g., Fein et al., 1991; Melton et al., 1985; Otto, Heilbrun, & Grisso, 1990; Peters & Otto, 1990; Poythress, 1990)—augur well for the future of our discipline. The field of forensic psychology has entered a period of standard-setting, and the American Psychology–Law Society/Division 41 and the American Academy of Forensic Psychology have been actively engaged in efforts to elevate the quality of psychological services rendered to the courts. However, recent investigations paint a less than flattering portrait of current practices in forensic assessment. Although the quality of forensic reports appears improved relative to earlier characterizations (e.g., Elwork, 1984; Grisso, 1986; Melton et al., 1985; Roesch & Golding, 1980), significant deficiencies remain. In my opinion, analyses of report content and surveys of legal consumers indicate that the current practices of forensic psychologists fall far short of the professional aspirations set forth in the Specialty Guidelines.

Previously, Roesch and Golding (1980) described reports of forensic evaluations as "most frequently stereotyped in form, often containing only summary conclusions (defendant is competent) or relatively abstract psychiatric phraseology (defendant showed evidence of persecutory delusions)" (p. 83), a characterization later echoed by Melton et al. (1985). The studies summarized previously suggest that this description may no longer be accurate. There was little evidence that reports were stereotyped in form, apart from the similarities introduced by statutory specification of questions to be answered by the evaluator and, in Oklahoma, the

[7]The findings are also at odds with a previous survey of judges in Virginia in which only 37.5% of the respondents considered a report or testimony from mental health professionals to be "essential" or "useful most of the time" in child custody cases (Melton et al., 1985).

habits of a handful of evaluators who provided only yes or no answers to those statutory questions. Furthermore, the average length of the reports across settings indicates that most reports contained more than summary conclusions. Although the studies that directly examined report quality did not include a rating for excessive mental health jargon, a survey of attorneys and judges yielded positive ratings for community-based reports on the characteristic "uses understandable language" (LaFortune & Nicholson, 1995).[8]

Other criticisms previously leveled at the work of mental health experts—specifically, charges of ignorance and irrelevance (Grisso, 1986)—also appear less appropriate when applied to more recent pretrial criminal forensic reports. There was little evidence that examiners confused one legal standard with another (e.g., conflating criteria for mental state at the time of the offense with those for AC) or that they confused legal and psychological or psychiatric concepts with one another (e.g., equating incompetence with psychosis). Thus, when specific psychole-gal abilities were described in the reports, they were typically relevant to the legal issue in question. One possible exception to this generally positive characterization should be noted. Heilbrun and Collins (1995) reported that almost 25% of community-based reports in their study addressed questions other than AC, yet the reports served as the basis for hospitalizing defendants as incompetent to proceed. Because this peculiarity may reflect the courts' misuse of evaluations conducted for other purposes, the finding cannot be attributed unequivocally to examiner ignorance and irrelevance without additional information. Nevertheless, forensic examiners have an obligation to prevent such misuse of the findings from an evaluation.

However, several of the earlier criticisms (Elwork, 1984; Grisso, 1986) again proved accurate, even when applied to samples of recent forensic evaluations. Although examiners in the recent samples appeared knowledgeable of the appropriate legal criteria, they nevertheless did not use the assessment methods and procedures with the strongest evidence of reliability and validity, nor did they select the most relevant methods for the task at hand. The clinical interview was probably the key source of information used in pretrial assessments. The more reliable and valid structured diagnostic interviews were rarely mentioned, and only a small minority of reports cited the use of one or more of the available FAIs, some of which have substantial empirical evidence to support their reliability and validity (Grisso, 1986, 1992; Heinz & Grisso, 1996; Nicholson & Kugler, 1991; Nicholson, 1999). Standard psychological tests were administered as often or more often than FAIs in each of the settings that provided information on both types of measure, despite the fact that the predictive validity of FAIs is substantially greater than that of traditional clinical measures in the legal context (see, e.g., Nicholson & Kugler, 1991). In addition, important sources of third-party information, such as defense attorneys and jail personnel, were underused. In short, the methods of assessment used in pretrial evaluations render the reports vulnerable to charges of unreliability and invalidity (Elwork, 1984), although perhaps in milder form.

[8]Two early studies of the quality of forensic evaluations also found that legal professionals provided favorable ratings of the clarity of the language contained in pretrial reports (Melton et al., 1985; Petrella & Poythress, 1983). Those studies did involve direct ratings of reports submitted by mental health professionals, but relied on small samples of raters and/or reports.

Even though clinical measures have less predictive power than FAIs in legal contexts, it may nevertheless be appropriate to use one or more clinical measures in a forensic evaluation. For example, such measures might be useful in the detection of malingering or other forms of response distortion, in attempts to corroborate the presence of severe mental disorder, or in the assessment of cognitive impairment that would explain an observed deficit in functional capacity, to name just a few. However, it is the responsibility of the forensic psychologist to select the appropriate measures and provide the needed rationale that would justify their use. Unfortunately, recent research in the context of criminal forensic assessment revealed that evaluators rarely attempted to establish the relationship of a particular test to the legal issue being evaluated or to a psychological construct that underlies the legal issue. In many cases psychological tests were administered but not discussed in the report that was submitted to the court. The most plausible explanation for such a pattern is that the examiners did not have a clear rationale for test selection and use in the forensic context in the first place.

Borum and Grisso (1995) argued that despite considerable division among experienced forensic psychologists with regard to the selection and use of FAIs, the overall trend is clearly in the direction of increasing use of the various legally relevant measures. Such a trend may be apparent among experienced, credentialed examiners, but it has not yet become evident in the practices of forensic examiners generally. As the recent studies of report content revealed, competency assessment instruments were cited in fewer than one in eight reports overall across three states. If forensic examiners are to incorporate instruments into their evaluations selectively, based not only on the usual reliability and validity considerations but also on the relevance of those instruments to the psycholegal issues being assessed (e.g., see Committee on Ethical Guidelines for Forensic Psychologists, 1991; Heilbrun, 1992, 1995), the relatively limited use of forensic assessment instruments, at least with regard to the assessment of adjudicative competence, must be considered a cause for continuing concern. This deficiency is all the more glaring in view of the availability of "second generation" competency assessment instruments, including newly-introduced measures such as the MacArthur Competence Assessment Tool—Criminal Adjudication (MacCAT-CA; Hoge, Bonnie, Poythress, & Monahan, 1999; Otto, Poythress, Nicholson, Edens, Monahan, Bonnie, Hoge, & Eisenberg, 1998; Poythress, Nicholson, Otto, Edens, Bonnie, Monahan, & Hoge, 1999) and substantially revised and expanded versions of previously developed assessment instruments such as the Interdisciplinary Fitness Interview–Revised (IFI-R; Golding, 1993).

One possible explanation for the apparent differences in use of FAIs between experienced, credentialed forensic psychologists and "occasional experts" is the different methodologies involved in assessing use frequency (i.e., survey vs. content coding of reports). That is, the difference might in fact be artifactual. There is a need for research designed to redress this deficiency in the literature by assaying the content of reports submitted by ABFP diplomates, and then comparing it with the content of reports submitted by less-experienced and/or noncredentialed forensic examiners. Of course, such comparisons would probably need to incorporate control over case complexity. If diplomates typically became involved in more complicated cases than nondiplomates, then differences between groups in the types and sources of information obtained could be attributed to differences in case complexity, not to differences in expertise. Comparisons controlling for case complexity would provide stronger evidence of a relationship between credentialing and professional experience on one hand and the quality of forensic reports on the other. In addition, follow-up research is needed to explore examiners' reasons for not incorporating one or more FAIs into pretrial assessments (e.g., Schreiber, 1978). Currently, it is unclear whether forensic practitioners who serve as "occasional experts" are unaware of the relevant literature on FAIs or whether they chose to ignore the research evidence for other reasons.[9]

The complaint that mental health professionals intrude on the province and authority of the court (Elwork, 1984; Grisso, 1986) is closely tied to concerns about ultimate issue testimony. In the jurisdictions studied, virtually all of the pretrial competency reports included an opinion on the ultimate legal issue, and about one-half of the criminal responsibility reports included such an opinion (although information on the latter was available only for Florida). Arguably, whether an ultimate opinion is viewed as intrusive depends on the adequacy of the examiner's description of the evidence and reasoning that underlies the opinion. Thus, complaints about intrusiveness are also closely related to charges of insufficiency and incredibility (Grisso, 1986). A majority of the competency reports in each jurisdiction cited at least one relevant psycholegal ability. However, the reports tended to emphasize foundational abilities (Bonnie, 1992, 1993), whereas abilities associated with decisional competence were cited infrequently. Furthermore, a substantial percentage of the reports that dealt with CR did not address the components of the relevant legal standard for insanity (in Florida, the M'Naughten standard), and in most reports, the defendant's account of the alleged offense was the basis for the opinion rendered. Thus, serious questions can be raised about the adequacy of the descriptions of defendants' legally relevant functional abilities and, in turn, the adequacy of the evidence on which exam-

[9]One of the reviewers of this manuscript made the astute observation that it is sometimes difficult to know what examiners mean when they either acknowledge or deny use of an FAI. For example, some FAIs, such as the Competency Assessment Instrument (CAI; Laboratory of Community Psychiatry, 1974), have had an obvious impact on the field in terms of identifying domains of legally relevant functional abilities that should be explored by an examiner during the course of competence assessment. These same psycholegal domains may also be used by the examiner to structure his or her description of the defendant's legally relevant functional abilities in a report to the court. If an examiner uses the CAI in this manner but chooses not to use the form that was developed for rating each of the components of competence, is the examiner using an FAI? As the reviewer noted, if the examiner indicates that he or she does not use the CAI, that answer is partly true and partly misleading. My preference for dealing with this issue in future surveys of mental health practitioners and in future investigations of the content of criminal forensic reports would be to treat the reviewer's description of examiner behavior as indicating use of "an FAI" but not "the CAI." Although the examiner's behavior may reflect conscientious application of the identified domains of competence in order to enhance the relevance of an evaluation, such behaviors are not the same as using the CAI. The CAI is not simply a list of content areas, each accompanied by a scale for rating degree of impairment. Rather, the CAI includes a handbook (Laboratory of Community Psychiatry, 1974) that provides the following: (1) definitions of the content domains to be explored during the competence assessment; (2) recommended questions to direct inquiry into and permit assessment of each of the aforementioned content domains; and (3) clinical case vignettes to illustrate the application of the rating form to real-world phenomena. Similarly, I would not consider an examiner's efforts to organize an evaluation around the psycholegal and psychopathological content domains described by Golding (1993) as indicating use of "the IFI-R," although I would probably consider the examiner's behavior as indicating use of "an FAI." In any case, the moral is that readers should guard against overinterpretation of the findings reported regarding the use of FAIs in the conduct of forensic psychological assessments.

iners' opinions were based. Descriptions of relevant components of mental status and psychiatric symptoms were generally more comprehensive than descriptions of psycholegal abilities. Nevertheless, substantial percentages of reports omitted reference to key aspects of mental status functioning and symptomatology. More importantly, the links between observed deficits in psycholegal abilities and cognitive impairment or symptoms of mental disorder were poorly articulated, if at all. In the absence of an adequate explication of the relationship between psychopathology or mental retardation and impairment in the individual's psycholegal abilities, the opinions offered in most of these reports could indeed be considered intrusive. When evaluated against the early anecdotal evidence on which many criticisms of forensic assessment and expert testimony rested, problems of insufficiency and intrusiveness have probably diminished. However, the magnitude of these deficiencies remains considerable, more so in light of the aspirations described in the Specialty Guidelines.

Elwork (1984) argued that mental health professionals could maximize the impact of forensic assessment and testimony by becoming more sensitive to procedural issues, especially those that involved legal and ethical obligations, in addition to addressing the substantive issues summarized previously. Unfortunately, the reports examined in these studies fared poorly on at least one index of adherence to the ethical contours of forensic evaluation. With the exception of the sample of inpatient reports from Florida, a majority of reports in the various settings failed to document the examiner's notification to the defendant regarding the purposes of the evaluation and limitations to confidentiality. For example, only about one-third of community-based reports from Florida included such documentation. The findings from Oklahoma were even more distressing in this regard, as only 4% of either community- or hospital-based reports documented notification. By way of contrast, disclosure to the defendant of the purposes of a criminal forensic evaluation was deemed "essential" (required by professional standards) by almost 67% and "recommended" (characteristic of more sophisticated reports) by an additional 28% of the psychologists surveyed by Borum and Grisso (1996). Similarly, informing the defendant about the limitations on confidentiality and privilege in forensic evaluations was judged to be "essential" by almost 60% of psychologists who responded, and "recommended" by almost 32% of the sample. A related issue is that examiners in some jurisdictions, such as Florida and Virginia, must address both adjudicative competence and criminal responsibility. Such circumstances complicate the examiner's ethical responsibility to protect the defendant's right against self-incrimination, underscoring the importance of giving the defendant notice and then documenting that notice in the report.[10]

[10]In both states, statements from the defendant regarding the offense are to be excluded from competency reports, and reports addressing mental state at the time of the offense are to be used only after the defense has given notice of intent to use an insanity defense. In Virginia, a full report on mental state at the time of the offense is submitted only to the defense attorney and is protected by attorney–client privilege. The court and the prosecuting attorney initially receive a summary of the findings and are later provided with a copy of the full report only after defense counsel gives notice of an intent to use the defense of insanity (see Melton et al., 1985, Appendix E). In Florida, when both issues are to be addressed, defendants are presumably given a comprehensive warning regarding the nature of the evaluation and the limitations to confidentiality. If statements from the defendant about the alleged offense cannot be used in a competency report, then the section on mental state at the time of the offense should contain only a summary of the findings.

As yet, no studies have scrutinized the content and quality of reports from other domains of forensic assessment, such as child custody or personal injury, perhaps because of the greater difficulty in obtaining samples of reports addressing these issues. Samples of criminal forensic reports are relatively easier to obtain because of the existence of state organizational systems for delivery of pretrial forensic assessment services. In contrast, personal injury and child custody assessments are virtually always undertaken by private practitioners; hence, there is no central repository or even a handful of repositories of the reports submitted to the courts. The lack of research examining reports from these other domains is unfortunate because findings from pretrial evaluations may not generalize to the other kinds of assessments. However, it seems highly unlikely that other kinds of evaluations would be markedly superior to pretrial evaluations. Formal training opportunities have been more readily available in the criminal domain than in areas such as child custody and personal injury. In addition, most criminal forensic evaluations are performed under the auspices of a state department of mental health, and there is likely to be more oversight of such evaluations than those performed for private attorneys on a fee-for-service basis. Regardless, there is a pressing need for research that examines the content and quality of forensic reports from these other domains. The potential impact of a similar set of studies of reports generated by child custody, personal injury, or other forensic evaluations is considerable. Perhaps reasonable samples of custody or personal injury reports could be obtained by undertaking cooperative investigations with the relevant sections of state bar associations (e.g., for custody reports, the Family Law Section of the state bar).

If the truth is what is, not what should be, we must acknowledge that the practice of forensic psychological assessment falls far short of its promise. This will come as no surprise to anyone who works in the area and follows the literature, but at least now the conclusion is based on systematic investigation rather than anecdotal accounts. Furthermore, the findings from recent studies are no cause for panic. Although I have tended to emphasize where current practice falls short, there are also some bright spots in the literature, not the least of which is the fact that a large percentage of the reports examined in the studies represent improvements over the characterizations of the 1970s and 1980s. We also now know more about the nature of the deficiencies and the specific areas where improvement is needed (see also Skeem & Golding, 1998). Moreover, the AP-LS (Grisso, 1991) and AAFP have taken important steps to improve the quality of forensic work by developing guidelines for practice, by providing and promoting educational and training opportunities, and by fostering the creation and continuation of credentialing and certification procedures. It is certainly too early to assess the impact of some of those efforts (e.g., the Villanova Conference, Bersoff et al., 1997), and probably premature to assess the impact of the Specialty Guidelines, as some of the data reported in these recent studies of forensic practice were gathered concurrently with circulation and publication of those guidelines. Nevertheless, the available evidence reveals significant deficiencies in the reports of forensic evaluations submitted to the courts. In order to advance the quality of forensic psychological assessments and communications to the courts, careful evaluation of current training and credentialing programs and thorough investigation of state organizational systems for delivery of forensic services must be undertaken. Information gleaned from empirical investigation must be supplemented by the generation and evaluation of new strategies for bridging the gap between current practices and the emerging promise of forensic psychological assessment.

REFERENCES

Abidin, R. R. (1990). *Parenting Stress Index* (3rd ed.). Odessa, FL: Psychological Assessment Resources.

Achenbach, T. (1978). The Child Behavior Profile–I. *Journal of Consulting and Clinical Psychology, 46,* 478–488.

Achenbach, T., & Edelbrock, C. (1979). The Child Behavior Profile–II. *Journal of Consulting and Clinical Psychology, 47,* 223–233.

Ackerman, M. J. (1995). *Clinician's guide to child custody evaluations.* New York: Wiley.

Ackerman, M. J., & Ackerman, M. C. (1997). Custody evaluation practices: A survey of experienced professionals (revisited). *Professional Psychology: Research and Practice, 28,* 137–145.

Ackerman, M. J., & Schoendorf, K. (1992). *The Ackerman–Schoendorf Parent Evaluation of Custody Tests (ASPECT).* Los Angeles: Western Psychological Services.

Arditti, J. A. (1995). Review of the Ackerman–Schoendorf Scales for Parent Evaluation of Custody. In J. C. Conoley & J. C. Impara (Eds.), *Mental measurements yearbook* (12th ed.) (pp. 20–22).

Bersoff, D. N., Goodman-Delahunty, J., Grisso, T., Hans, V. P., Poythress, N. G., & Roesch, R. G. (1997). Training in law and psychology: Models from the Villanova conference. *American Psychologist, 52,* 1301–1310.

Boccaccini, M. T., & Brodsky, S. L. (1999). Diagnostic test usage by forensic psychologists in emotional injury cases. *Professional Psychology: Research and Practice, 30,* 253–259.

Bonnie, R. J. (1992). The competence of criminal defendants: A theoretical reformulation. *Behavioral Sciences and the Law, 10,* 291–316.

Bonnie, R. J. (1993). The competence of criminal defendants: Beyond *Dusky* and *Drope. University of Miami Law Review, 47,* 539–601.

Bonnie, R. J., Hoge, S. K., Monahan, J., Poythress, N., Eisenberg, M., & Feucht-Haviar, T. (1997). The MacArthur Adjudicative Competence Study: A comparison of criteria for assessing the competence of criminal defendants. *Journal of the American Academy of Psychiatry and the Law, 25,* 249–259.

Borum, R., & Grisso, T. (1995). Psychological test use in criminal forensic evaluations. *Professional Psychology: Research and Practice, 26,* 465–473.

Borum, R., & Grisso, T. (1996). Establishing standards for criminal forensic reports: An empirical analysis. *Bulletin of the American Academy of Psychiatry and Law, 24,* 297–317.

Borum, R., Otto, R., & Golding, S. (1993). Improving clinical judgment and decision making in forensic evaluation. *Journal of Psychiatry and Law, 21,* 35–76.

Brown, W. R., & McGuire, J. M. (1976). Current psychological assessment practices. *Professional Psychology, 7,* 475–484.

Committee on Ethical Guidelines for Forensic Psychologists. (1991). Specialty guidelines for forensic psychologists. *Law and Human Behavior, 15,* 655–665.

Committee on Professional Practice and Standards. (1994). Guidelines for child custody evaluations in divorce proceedings. *American Psychologist, 49,* 677–680.

Committee on Professional Practice and Standards. (1995). Twenty-four questions (and answers) about professional practice in the area of child abuse. *Professional Psychology: Research and Practice, 26,* 377–385.

Edens, J. F., Poythress, N. G., Nicholson, R. A., & Otto, R. K. (1999). Effects of state organizational structure and forensic examiner training on pre-trial competence assessments. *Journal of Behavioral Health Services and Research, 26,* 140–150.

Elwork, A. (1984). Psycholegal assessment, diagnosis, and testimony: A new beginning. *Law and Human Behavior, 8,* 197–203.

Faust, D. & Ziskin, J. (1988). The expert witness in psychology and psychiatry. *Science, 241,* 31–35.

Fein, R, Appelbaum, K., Barnum, R., Baxter, P., Grisso, T., & Leavitt, N. (1991). The designated forensic professional program: A state government–university partnership to improve forensic mental health services. *Journal of Mental Health Administration, 18,* 223–230.

Geller, J., & Lister, E. (1978). The process of criminal commitment for pre-trial psychiatric examination: An evaluation. *American Journal of Psychiatry, 135,* 53–63.

Gerard, A. B. (1994). *Parent–Child Relationship Inventory (PCRI) Manual.* Los Angeles: Western Psychological Services.

Golding, S. L. (1990). Mental health professionals and the courts: The ethics of expertise. *International Journal of Law and Psychiatry, 13,* 281–307.

Golding, S. L. (1993). Interdisciplinary Fitness Interview–Revised: Training manual. Unpublished manuscript.

Grisso, T. (1986). *Evaluating competencies: Forensic assessments and instruments.* New York: Plenum.

Grisso, T. (1987). The economic and scientific future of forensic psychological assessment. *American Psychologist, 42,* 831–839.

Grisso, T. (1988). *Competency to stand trial evaluations: A manual for practice.* Sarasota, FL: Professional Resource Exchange.

Grisso, T. (1990a). Forensic evaluations and the fourth estate. *Forensic Reports, 3,* 427–437.

Grisso, T. (1990b). Evolving guidelines for divorce custody evaluations. *Family and Conciliation Courts Review, 28,* 35–41.

Grisso, T., Cocozza, J. J., Steadman, H. J., Fisher, W. H., & Greer, A. (1994). The organization of pretrial forensic evaluation services: A national profile. *Law and Human Behavior, 18,* 377–393.

Hagin, R. A. (1992). Review of the Bricklin Perceptual Scales. In J. J. Kramer & J. C. Conoley (Eds.), *Mental measurements yearbook* (11th ed.) (pp. 117–118).

Heilbrun, K. (1990). Response style, situation, third-party information and competency to stand trial. *Law and Human Behavior, 14,* 193–196.

Heilbrun, K. (1992). The role of psychological testing in forensic assessment. *Law and Human Behavior, 16,* 321–334.

Heilbrun, K. (1995). Child custody evaluation: Critically assessing mental health experts and psychological tests. *Family Law Quarterly, 29,* 63–78.

Heilbrun, K., & Collins, S. (1995). Evaluations of trial competency and mental state at the time of the offense: Report characteristics. *Professional Psychology: Research and Practice, 26,* 61–67.

Heilbrun, K., Warren, J., Rosenfeld, B., & Collins, S. (1994). The use of third party information in forensic assessments: A two-state comparison. *Bulletin of the American Academy of Psychiatry and Law, 22,* 399–406.

Heinze, M. C., & Grisso, T. (1996). Review of instruments assessing parenting competencies used in childcustody evaluations. *Behavioral Sciences and the Law, 14,* 295–313.

Hess, J., & Thomas, H. (1963). Incompetence to stand trial: Procedures, results, and problems. *American Journal of Psychiatry, 119,* 713–720.

Hoge, S. K., Bonnie, R. J., Poythress, N. G., & Monahan, J. (1999). *The MacArthur Competence Assessment Tool—Criminal Adjudication (MacCAT-CA).* Odessa, FL: Psychological Assessment Resources.

Hoge, S. K., Bonnie, R. J., Poythress, N. G., Monahan, J., Eisenberg, M., & Feucht-Haviar, T. (1997). The MacArthur Adjudicative Competence Study: Development and validation of a research instrument. *Law and Human Behavior, 21,* 141–179.

Jenkins, P. H., & Howell, R. J. (1994). Child sexual abuse examinations: Proposed guidelines for a standard of care. *Bulletin of the American Academy of Psychiatry and Law, 22,* 5–17.

Keilin, W. G., & Bloom, L. J. (1986). Child custody evaluation practices: A survey of experienced professionals. *Professional Psychology: Research and Practice, 17,* 338–346.

Laboratory of Community Psychiatry (1974). *Competency to stand trial and mental illness.* New York: Jason Aronson.

LaFortune, K. A. (1997). *An investigation of mental health and legal professionals' activities, beliefs, and experiences in domestic court: An interdisciplinary survey.* Unpublished doctoral dissertation. University of Tulsa.

LaFortune, K. A., & Carpenter, B. N. (1996). Attorneys' perceptions of the usefulness of extrajudicial procedures and mental health evaluations in domestic court. Paper presented at the biennial convention of the American Psychology-Law Society, Hilton Head, SC.

LaFortune, K. A., & Nicholson, R. A. (1995). How adequate are Oklahoma's mental health evaluations for determining competency in criminal proceedings? The Bench and the Bar respond. *Journal of Psychiatry and Law, 23,* 231–262.

Lees-Haley, P. R. (1992). Psychodiagnostic test usage by forensic psychologists. *American Journal of Forensic Psychology, 10,* 25–30.

Lees-Haley, P. R., Smith, H. H., Williams, C. W., & Dunn, J. T. (1995). Forensic neuropsychological test usage: An empirical survey. *Archives of Clinical Neuropsychology, 11,* 45–51.

Lubin, B., Larsen, R. M., Matarazzo, J. D., & Seever, M. (1985). Psychological test usage patterns in five professional settings. *American Psychologist, 40,* 857–861.

Melton, G. B. (1995). Review of the Ackerman–Schoendorf Scales for Parent Evaluation of Custody. In J. C. Conoley & J. C. Impara (eds.), *Mental measurements yearbook* (12th ed.) (pp. 22–23).

Melton, G. B., Petrila, J., Poythress, N. G., & Slobogin, C. (1997). *Psychological evaluations for the courts: A handbook for mental health professionals and lawyers* (2nd ed.). New York: Guilford Press.

Melton, G. B., Weithorn, L. A., & Slobogin, C. (1985). *Community mental health centers and the courts: An evaluation of community-based forensic services.* University of Nebraska Press: Lincoln.

Milner, J. (1986). *The Child Abuse Potential Inventory Manual* (2nd ed.). Webster, NC: Psytec, Inc.

Morse, S. J. (1978). Law and mental health professionals: The limits of expertise. *Professional Psychology, 9,* 389–399.

Nicholson, R. A. (1999). Forensic assessment. In R. Roesch, S. Hart, & J. R. P. Ogloff (Eds.), *Psychology and law: The state of the discipline* (pp. 121–173). New York: Plenum.

Nicholson, R. A., LaFortune, K. A., Norwood, S., & Roach, R. L. (August, 1995). Quality of pretrial competency evaluations in Oklahoma: Report content and consumer satisfaction. Paper presented as part of a symposium, *Assessing the content and quality of forensic evaluations,* R. K. Otto, Chair, at the annual convention of the American Psychological Association, New York, NY.

Nicholson, R. A., Poythress, N. G., Edens, J., & Otto, R. K. (1999). Norms and interpretive guidelines for clinical use of the MacArthur Competence Assessment Tool–Criminal Adjudication (MacCAT-CA). Manuscript submitted for publication.

Otto, R. K., Barnes, G., & Jacobson, K. (March, 1996). The content and quality of criminal forensic evaluations in Florida. Paper presented at the biennial meeting of the American Psychology-Law Society, Hilton Head, SC.

Otto, R. K., & Collins, R. P. (1995). Use of the MMPI-2/MMPI-A in child custody evaluations. In Y. S. Ben-Porath, J. R. Graham, G. C. N. Hall, R. D. Hirschman, & M. S. Zaragoza (Eds.), *Forensic applications of the MMPI-2* (pp. 222–252). Thousand Oaks, CA: Sage.

Otto, R. K., Heilbrun, K., & Grisso, T. (1990). Training and credentialing in forensic psychology. *Behavioral Sciences and the Law, 8,* 217–231.

Otto, R. K., Poythress, N. G., Nicholson, R. A., Edens, J. F., Monahan, J., Bonnie, R., Hoge, S. K., & Eisenberg, M. (1998). Psychometric properties of the MacArthur Competence Assessment Tool–Criminal Adjudication (MacCAT-CA). *Psychological Assessment, 10,* 435–443.

Peters, R. H., & Otto, R. K. (March, 1990). The Florida Forensic Evaluator Training program. In R. K. Otto (Chair), State forensic evaluator training programs. Symposium presented at the biennial meeting of the American Psychology-Law Society, Williamsburg, VA.

Petrella, R. C. & Poythress, N. G. (1983). The quality of forensic evaluations: An interdisciplinary study. *Journal of Consulting and Clinical Psychology, 51,* 76–85.

Piotrowski, C., Belter, R. W., & Keller, J. W. (1998). The impact of "managed care" on the practice of psychological testing: Preliminary findings. *Journal of Personality Assessment, 70,* 441–447.

Piotrowski, C., & Keller, J. W. (1978). Psychological test usage in southeastern outpatient mental health facilities in 1975. *Professional Psychology, 9,* 63–67.

Piotrowski, C., & Keller, J. W. (1989). Psychological testing in outpatient mental health facilities: A national study. *Professional Psychology: Research and Practice, 20,* 423–425.

Piotrowski, C., & Keller, J. W. (1992). Psychological testing in applied settings: A literature review from 1982-1992. *Journal of Training and Practice in Professional Psychology, 6,* 74–82.

Piotrowski, C., Sherry, D., & Keller, J. W. (1985). Psychodiagnostic test usage: A survey of the Society for Personality Assessment. *Journal of Personality Assessment, 49,* 115–119.

Piotrowski, C. (1996). Use of the Rorschach in forensic practice. *Perceptual and Motor Skills, 82,* 254.

Piotrowski, C. (1999). Assessment practices in the era of managed care: Current status and future directions. *Journal of Clinical Psychology, 55,* 787–796.

Poythress, N. G. (1979). A proposal for training in forensic psychology. *American Psychologist, 34,* 612–621.

Poythress, N. G. (March, 1990). Forensic examiner training in Alabama. In R. K. Otto (Chair), State forensic evaluator training programs. Symposium presented at the biennial meeting of the American Psychology-Law Society, Williamsburg, VA.

Poythress, N. G., Nicholson, R., Otto, R. K., Edens, J. F., Bonnie, R. J., Monahan, J., & Hoge, S. K. (1999). *MacArthur Competence Assessment Tool–Criminal Adjudication (MacCAT-CA) Professional Manual.* Odessa, FL: Psychological Assessment Resources.

Poythress, N. G., Otto, R. K., & Heilbrun, K. (1991). Pretrial evaluations for criminal courts: Contemporary models for service delivery. *Journal of Mental Health Administration, 18,* 198–208.

Robbins, E., Waters, J., & Herbert, P. (1997). Competency to stand trial evaluations: A study of actual practice in two states. *Journal of the American Academy of Psychiatry and Law, 25,* 469–483.

Roesch, R., & Golding, S. L. (1977). *A systems analysis of competency to stand trial procedures: Implications for forensic services in North Carolina.* Urbana: University of Illinois.

Roesch, R., & Golding, S. L. (1980). *Competency to stand trial.* Urbana, Illinois: University of Illinois Press.

Rogers, R. (1984). *Rogers Criminal Responsibility Assessment Scales.* Odessa, FL: Psychological Assessment Resources.

Schreiber, J. (1978). Assessing competency to stand trial: A case study of technology diffusion in four states. *Bulletin of the American Academy of Psychiatry and Law, 6,* 439–457.

Shaffer, M. B. (1992). Review of the Bricklin Perceptual Scales. In J. J. Kramer & J. C. Conoley (Eds.), *Mental measurements yearbook* (11th ed.) (pp. 118–119).

Skeem, J. L., & Golding, S. L. (1998). Community examiners' evaluations of competence to stand trial: Common problems and suggestions for improvement. *Professional Psychology: Research and Practice, 29,* 357–367.

Skeem, J. L3., Golding, S. L., Cohn, N. B., & Berge, G. (1998). The logic and reliability of evaluations of competence to stand trial. *Law and Human Behavior, 22,* 519–547.

Sweeney, J. A., Clarkin, J. F., & Fitzgibbon, M. L. (1987). Current practice of psychological assessment. *Professional Psychology: Research a Practice, 18,* 377–380.

Vann, C. (1965). Pre-trial determination and judicial decision-making: An analysis of the use of psychiatric information in the administration of criminal justice. *University of Detroit Law Journal, 43,* 13–33.

Watkins, C. E., Campbell, V. L., Nieberding, R., & Hallmark, R. (1995). Contemporary practice of psychological assessment by clinical psychologists. *Professional Psychology: Research and Practice, 26,* 54–60.

Ziskin, J. (1970). *Coping with psychiatric and psychological testimony.* Marina Del Rey, CA: Law and Psychology Press.

Ziskin, J. (1975). *Coping with psychiatric and psychological testimony* (2nd ed.). Marina del Rey, CA: Law and Psychology Press.

Ziskin, J., & Faust, D. (1988). *Coping with psychiatric and psychological testimony* (4th ed.). Marina del Rey: Law and Psychology Press.

[28]

EMERGING ISSUES IN FORENSIC MENTAL HEALTH

John Petrila, J.D., LL.M.

Forensic mental health traditionally was considered the backwater of forensic practice. However, because of advances in knowledge regarding the core issues of capacity and risk, and because of changes in the location of forensic assessment and treatment, "forensic" issues now permeate mental health practice and policy. While these advances have been important, there are a number of new issues that will occupy the attention of practitioners, researchers, and policymakers in the future. This article explores these issues and their implications, including the need to better integrate treatment and risk; the need to address the emergence of special jurisdiction courts and their impact on systems design issues; the need to address the impact of conservative social policies, particularly in the areas of juvenile justice and sexual predator legislation; and the need to better understand the use of coercion in the context of community treatment.

KEY WORDS: forensics; risk assessment; mental health policy.

John Petrila is Chair and Professor, Department of Mental Health Law and Policy, Louis de la Parte Florida Mental Health Institute, University of South Florida, Tampa, Florida.

Address correspondence to John Petrila, J.D., LL.M., Department of Mental Health Law and Policy, Louis de la Parte Florida Mental Health Institute, University of South Florida, Tampa, FL 33612; e-mail: petrila@mirage.fmhi.usf.edu.

Thirty years ago, forensic mental health was a backwater, both intellectually and clinically. For example, Henry Steadman, reporting on insanity acquittals in New York, wrote "the current paucity of the type of data presented here relegates most debates on the insanity defense to little more than fodder for campus forensic societies (1)." While public safety and risk were at the heart of forensic practice, much as they are today, the primary activity was the prediction of risk in individual cases. Such predictions were made despite the fact that most evidence available at that time suggested that mental health professionals had little to offer on this topic (2,3). However, the legal system continued to insist on receiving the opinions of mental health professionals on the issue of future dangerousness, an opinion many were content to provide.

Treatment for individuals found not guilty by reason of insanity or not competent to stand trial was provided primarily in state maximum-security facilities. While a handful of court clinics provided competency assessments in some urban areas, many individuals referred for evaluation of competency to stand trial also spent lengthy periods in maximum-security settings solely for evaluation.(4,5,6).

This state of affairs has changed dramatically in the last 20 years, in three areas in particular. First, there have been changes in the location of assessment and treatment. Pretrial examinations are now done routinely in community settings, though the organization of such services varies from state to state (7). Individuals who enter the mental health system through the criminal courts also are now routinely treated not only in maximum-security institutions but also in a variety of institutional and community settings. As a result of this shift and the increased use of community settings for pretrial examinations, "forensic" patients now inhabit many treatment settings which not many years ago would have distanced themselves from such patients.

Second, there have been significant increases in our knowledge regarding the topics at the heart of forensic practice and application of that knowledge. For example, our understanding of the relationship between mental illness and violence has increased markedly (8). In addition, a number of assessment tools have been developed for use by forensic examiners, creating a foundation for the increased standardization of practice in a variety of critical areas, including though not limited to competency to stand trial (9,10); risk assessment (11,12,13); malingering (14); and psychopathology (15).

Third, practice and ethical standards have been developed to address the difficult issues that often arise in forensic practice (16). These efforts have been abetted by the development of organizations designed to create opportunities for academicians and practitioners interested in forensic issues to share information and experiences. Some of these organizations include the American Academy of Psychiatry and Law; the American Psychology-Law Society (Division 41 of the American Psychological Association); the International Association of Forensic Mental Health Services; and the American Academy of Forensic Psychology.

These changes, all important, have improved forensic practice. However, important challenges in forensic mental health and in the relationship between the criminal justice system and the mental health system still exist. It is useful occasionally to look ahead in an effort to anticipate what issues are likely to dominate the policy, practice and research agenda in the future.

This paper explores four issues that in the author's view are of overarching importance not only to those interested in forensic mental health but to those interested in behavioral health questions more broadly. These issues, which will largely define the agenda for forensic and general mental health in the coming decade include: 1) the need to integrate risk and treatment; 2) the need to understand and address the impact of the emergence of special courts such as drug courts and mental health courts on treatment and system planning; 3) the need to address assessment and treatment issues that continue to flow from the "criminalization" of the juvenile justice system and broader but related social policy trends; and 4) the need to better understand from a research, policy and practice perspective the use of coercion and mandates in the provision of community treatment for mental illnesses and substance abuse. As even this brief discussion will illustrate, "forensic mental health" today is far from a backwater. Rather, it now dominates much of the agenda for mental health policy and practice.

THE NEED TO BETTER INTEGRATE TREATMENT AND RISK

There is no question that there have been enormous strides in our understanding of the dynamic and static factors associated with potential risk. It is also clear that risk *assessment* can be performed in much more rigorous fashion than was the case several decades ago. In addition, there have been some (though fewer) improvements in formulating strategies for *managing* risk. Some of the most thoughtful suggestions have drawn on strategies used in other treatment settings, as illustrated by Dvoskin's and Steadman's report that intensive case management is an effective risk management tool (17). In addition, more coherent risk-assessment techniques also serve as a tool for risk management (18).

However, despite limited exceptions, there has been much less attention paid to the integration of treatment and risk reduction (19,20). For example, in defending hospitals in more than one-dozen class action right to treatment lawsuits, I have been struck repeatedly by the apparent lack of a relationship between risk factors (which were largely responsible in most cases for the person's hospitalization) and the treatment that is then prescribed for the individual. Typically, an admissions note reflects the circumstances that brought the person to a hospital, for example, an assault on another individual. Certain risk factors (use of alcohol or drugs, a history of violence toward a particular individual) might be described. However, few clinical records then describe why or how the specific treatment that follows (anger management group, for example) is expected to address specific risk factors presented by the individual in question. On discharge, there is also little discussion regarding the manner in which the treatment either addressed, or did not address, specific risk factors. This makes it difficult for another party, whether a judge or subsequent treatment provider, to gauge the impact of the treatment on the person's future risk.

Beyond anecdotal evidence, it also has been assumed that some categories of individuals are simply untreatable. This has been particularly true in the case of individuals labeled "psychopathic." In fact, it has been reported that treatment may *increase* rates of recidivism among some individuals who are psychopathic (21). The assumption of untreatability can be devastating, leading to shunting people away from treatment based on a label and perhaps creating barriers to research that might otherwise explore the impact of treatment on such individuals (22).

A more recent report challenges these assumptions and illustrates the importance of examining the impact of treatment on the reduction of risk even when it has been assumed that such treatment is ineffective. Skeem and her colleagues report that civil psychiatric patients who had scored highly on the Screening Version of the Psychopathy Checklist (a version of the PCL designed to measure psychopathy in noncriminal settings) (23) may become less violent after receiving adequate outpatient treatment (24). While this is a single study, it should lead to additional research into the question of the efficacy of treatment for those labeled psychopaths. In addition, it points to the continuing need to examine treatment interventions that target dynamic and contextual risk factors and to then translate that knowledge into clinical practice.

The field has made great strides in the area of risk assessment. Integration of treatment strategies with our growing knowledge of risk factors will be one of the core issues of the next decade.

THE EMERGENCE OF SPECIAL JURISDICTION COURTS AND ITS LONG-TERM IMPLICATIONS

The courts, both civil and criminal, play an important and growing role in allocating health and human services. This gate-keeping role has evolved in recent years because of the volume of people entering the criminal justice system with mental health and/or substance abuse disorders: The United States Department of Justice estimated in 1999 that approximately 700,000 people with major mental disorders enter the criminal justice system each year (25). One response has been the creation of diversion programs, often utilizing specially trained law enforcement officers, to divert people into treatment *before* they are booked into the criminal justice system.

Another response, important here, has been the creation of special-jurisdiction courts designed to enable certain categories of defendants to gain access to treatment. Special-jurisdiction courts have been defined as "forums of highly limited jurisdiction to which all of the cases of a particular type are introduced (26)." Special-jurisdiction courts, including business courts, drug courts, and juvenile courts exist in many countries (27).

Perhaps the prototypical example of a therapeutically-oriented court is the traditional juvenile court. More recently and in response to the number of individuals entering the criminal justice system with mental disorders, a number of jurisdictions also have created drug courts and mental health courts. These courts are explicitly therapeutic in approach (28). Today there are nearly 1,000 drug courts either in operation or being planned, a remarkable number given that the first drug court was established in 1989. These courts were established both to reduce recidivism by placing the defendant in supervised treatment and to reduce court dockets swollen by the tougher sentencing laws for drug offenses adopted by the federal government and most states in the 1980s and early 1990s (29). A typical drug court accepts individuals charged with felonies and uses punishment as a tool in causing the person to adhere to treatment (30).

In contrast, mental health courts have developed more recently (following the establishment of a mental health court in Broward County Florida in 1997) and it is estimated that at present there are approximately 30 mental health courts in the United States. While there is no "typical" mental health court, most accept misdemeanor cases rather than felonies; the focus is on gaining access to treatment for the individual; and the courts vary in their use of punishment as a sanction for noncompliance with treatment (31).

These courts have important implications for treatment planning and for treatment system design. First, such courts place judges squarely in the center of treatment planning. While the court itself serves primarily as a gate into treatment, the manner in which individual cases are resolved and the explicitly therapeutic orientation of these courts means that the judge (and lawyers) play much different roles than those played in a traditional, adversarial process.

In addition, the emergence of these courts suggests something important about the manner in which treatment system planning occurs today: Increasingly, system design occurs in localities, rather than at the state or federal level. In part, this is because in many states the authority of the state mental health agency has been eroded (32). In part, however, it is because the issues that led to the creation of these courts (e.g., inadequate psychiatric emergency services, an increased volume of individuals with mental disorders entering the criminal courts; the "revolving door" defendant with mental illness) have the most significant impact at a local level. This has led recently to efforts at systems design that involve not only mental health administrators and policymakers, but local judges, jail administrators, law enforcement officials and others who traditionally did not play such a role when the locus of planning was the state or federal government.

Not all judges are comfortable with this new role, nor are all judges competent in this new role. However, the fact that judges are now involved not only in individual decisions that allocate health resources but are involved in system design as well is a significant change for the court systems but also for the mental health and human services systems which must accommodate themselves to this change.

THE NEED TO ADDRESS ASSESSMENT AND TREATMENT ISSUES FLOWING FROM THE "CRIMINALIZATION" OF JUVENILE JUSTICE AND OTHER SOCIAL POLICY TRENDS

One of the most striking features of American jurisprudential policy in the 1990s was the broad retreat from the rehabilitative philosophy that had anchored the juvenile justice system since the end of the 19th century. One commentator wrote "as the juvenile court approaches its

100th birthday . . . its future is less secure than an any point in its history" because of "historic increases in juvenile homicides" and other violent crimes (33).

While the rise in violent crime in the early 1990s that sparked these changes proved temporary (with juvenile crime dropping dramatically from 1995–1997) (34) state and federal legislators responded by making it easier to waive juveniles to adult court, imposed increased levels of punishment, and sanctioned an increased use of detention. In addition, the use of formal competency to proceed standards became increasingly common in delinquency proceedings, in part because of the growing legalization of juvenile court processes that began with the United States Supreme Court decision in *Gault* in 1967 (35). In *Gault*, the Supreme Court ruled that certain procedural protections available to adult criminal defendants had to be made available to defendants in juvenile court. The Court intended to reform the juvenile process because of abuses that had occurred in the very informal atmosphere of traditional juvenile court; the result, ironically, has been a juvenile court process increasingly resembling adult criminal court, while the rehabilitative spirit that long animated juvenile court under siege.

The more punitive approach to juvenile justice took place against a backdrop of increasingly conservative policies on crime and public safety. The growing use of "sexual predator" legislation is another example of this trend. Such legislation permits the indefinite confinement of individuals at the end of their prison terms based on a finding that they present a continuing danger to others because of a sexual disorder. The legislation constitutes a use of the state's civil commitment authority and has been upheld against legal challenge (36). The result, in at least some states, has been the creation of large psychiatric institutions to hold such individuals. The difficulty for state administrators is that individuals confined to these institutions must prove they no longer represent a public risk; this means inevitably that it is difficult to maintain a flow of patients through such institutions because more people will be deemed eligible for admission than discharge.

Assessment Issues

These trends raise difficult assessment and treatment issues that will be part of the "forensic mental health" agenda over the next few years. In the area of assessment, there are significant issues regarding the "fit" between the legal standards that have been established and the clinical tools used to provide the legal system with the information it requires. For example, those states that have created a "competency to proceed" standard in delinquency proceedings generally rely on the legal standard for adult competency to stand trial, despite many compelling arguments that standards for juvenile competency should recognize the developmental differences between juveniles and adults (37,38). In addition, the one study into the characteristics of juveniles adjudicated incompetent to proceed in delinquency proceedings found, among other things, that the majority of individuals adjudicated incompetent had diagnoses of mental retardation and/or developmental disabilities, a finding quite different from cohorts of individuals found incompetent to stand trial in adult court where mental retardation typically is found in less than 10 percent of all cases (39). As juvenile competency (and potentially responsibility issues) (40) become more common in juvenile court, both policymakers and clinicians will need to address the issue of "fit" between legal standards and developmental issues; in addition, it will be important to develop standards for forensic assessment in this setting.

The assessment issues that arise under sexual predator statutes also raise questions of "fit" though in this context the overarching issue is whether the tools used by clinicians to address the central legal question (in this setting, future dangerousness) are appropriate to the task. Many of the tools developed for risk assessment in the last decade (the Sex Offender Risk Appraisal Guide, or SORAG (41); the Minnesota Sex Offender Screening Tool and Revised Screening Tool, or the MnSOST and MnSOST-R (42); and the Rapid Risk Assessment for Sexual Offense Recidivism, or RRASOR (43)) were developed for use in assessing individuals confined for sexual offending. The use of these instruments has been challenged on the ground that they do not enjoy broad scientific acceptance, one of the legal tests for determining whether certain types of evidence should be admitted as scientific evidence. In general, the courts have rejected such challenges (44).

While the courts appear for the most part willing to accept testimony regarding future risk based on the use of actuarial instruments, the *responsible* use of such instruments remains a major issue. In some circumstances, clinicians have not acknowledged the limitations of the instruments, leading to situations in which courts have characterized the instruments as able to "predict" future sexual offending in individual cases; this has the practical affect of inappropriately transforming a tool for assessing probabilities for future offending into something perceived as predictive for the defendant before the court (45). Because of judicial reliance on clinical expert testimony, it becomes incumbent upon the mental health professional to provide a realistic assessment of the tools he or she is using in offering an opinion about future risk, including clearly stating the limitations of the instrument in question.

Treatment and Detention Issues

The use of detention in juvenile cases and the growth of institutions housing individuals admitted under sexual predator statutes also raise important issues for the future. Two issues in particular will dominate discussion. The first is ameliorating the often inhumane conditions in such facilities, particularly those for juveniles; the second is how and under what conditions deinstitutionalization of these facilities will occur.

Juvenile detention facilities today raise stark questions regarding unsafe and inhumane conditions. Between 1985 and 1995, the average daily population in publicly operated juvenile detention facilities in the United States increased by 72 percent, with 6 of 10 youths placed in juvenile detention confined to an overcrowded institution (46). The use of detention (and problems associated with it) is nothing new; it has been used since the middle of the 19th century and in fact inhumane conditions in juvenile detention facilities contributed to the emergence of the rehabilitative juvenile court at the end of the 19th century (47). However, recent investigations by the United States Department of Justice and others suggests that conditions in many detention facilities continue to be brutal, with neglect of basic health and mental health care not uncommon. For example, one account described youth in one juvenile facility as regularly appearing at the infirmary "with black eyes, broken noses or jaws or perforated eardrums from beatings by the poorly paid, poorly trained guards or from fights with other boys... Meals are so meager that many boys lose weight. Clothing is so scarce that boys fight over shirts and shoes... Up to a fourth of the inmates are mentally ill or retarded, but a psychiatrist visits only one day a week... Emotionally disturbed boys who cannot follow guards' orders are locked in isolation cells for weeks at a time or have their sentences arbitrarily extended (48)." The result has been a resurgence of interest in litigation strategies designed to improve conditions (49).

There also have been many questions raised about the appropriateness of treatment provided individuals confined under sexual predator statutes (50,51). These questions, which include basic issues regarding the technologies available to treat and reduce risk among individuals committed as sexual predators, have acquired enhanced importance because of what appears to be the comparative indifference of the United States Supreme Court to legal questions regarding treatment raised by such statutes (52). A number of factors (the lack of standardized approaches to treatment, the fact that an individual must demonstrate that he is no longer a risk to third parties, the difficulty in securing community treatment settings for this population) make it difficult to discharge individuals quickly from the institutions that have been created since enactment of the most recent sexually violent predator statutes.

This suggests that a major challenge for the future, in the context of both juvenile detention facilities and facilities for individuals committed under sexual predator statutes, will be the deinstitutionalization of such institutions. Models exist for the creation of community-based systems for juveniles (53,54). There has also been discussion of the principles that might underlie transitional programs for individuals institutionalized under sexual offender statutes (55). However, as the experience with downsizing and eventually closing state psychiatric hospitals illustrates, it is difficult to wean a system from reliance on institutional care. This suggests that there will be no quick solution to the increased use of institutional care in some settings that occurred because of more conservative social policies. However, the search for alternatives, particularly in the areas of juvenile justice and sexual offender statutes, will be one of the critical issues that defines the forensic clinical and policy agenda in the next decade.

THE NEED TO BETTER UNDERSTAND THE USE OF COERCION AND MANDATES IN COMMUNITY TREATMENT

Coercion is perhaps the prototypical mental health law issue. While the assessment of capacity and risk lie at the heart of forensic practice, the use of coercion long has raised significant ethical, legal and clinical issues. Civil commitment is one of the only noncriminal areas of law where liberty may be taken without the person's consent; as such, it defined mental health law in its infancy, when mental health law emerged from constitutionally based civil rights law, and three decades later it continues to be a subject of intense controversy (56).

Coercion historically has been an issue of concern because of the use of institutional care. What is different today, and what will create the parameters for discussion of coercion by policymakers, practitioners, and researchers in the future is the use of coercion in the community. Coercion is no less important when used in the community than when used in the context of institutional care; however, the manner in which we think about coercion today, and will do so in the future, differs in important respects from the manner in which the issue was considered when applied to institutional settings.

The first difference has to do with the perspective by which certain interventions are viewed as coercive. Early discussions of coercion assumed that the "amount" of coercion contained in a particular intervention was tied to the legal countours of the intervention. For example, it was assumed that an involuntary civil commitment admission necessarily was more coercive than an admission that met voluntary admission standards. However, the manner in which coercion is defined changed with the introduction into mental health law research of the concepts of procedural justice and perceived coercion. Each of these concepts focuses on the perceptions of the individual subject to the intervention or legal process in question. For example, procedural justice attempts to gauge the subjective perspective of individuals involved in the process of case disposition; the theory is that the more the individual perceives the process as fair, the more likely it is that the process will facilitate the success of subsequent treatment (57). "Perceived coercion," developed as part of the research conducted by the MacArthur Foundation Network on Mental Health and the Law, examines the degree to which an individual subject to legal intervention perceives that he or she retains some degree of choice and control over the decisions that are part of the intervention (58). This represents a fundamental shift in the paradigm by which we understand "coercion." While *in general* more individuals perceive involuntary civil commitment as coercive than non-coercive, some individuals admitted as voluntary patients perceive admissions as quite coercive (59). The fact that we know this was made possible only by asking those subject to the interventions in question to describe their perceptions. Because of this research, it is no longer enough to assume that some types of legally sanctioned interventions are necessarily more coercive than others.

The second difference has to do with broadening our perspective on the circumstances in which coercion (and other types of leverage) is used in the community. Outpatient civil commitment has received the most attention as an example of the use of community-based coercion. In large part, this is because, like involuntary commitment in general, it is a sharply divisive issue in which ideological perspectives regarding the use of coercion have driven much of the debate (60). Yet as a seminal article by Monahan and his colleagues suggest, coercion and leverage are used in many other settings in the community (61). For example, coercion or the threat of sanction may be used in an effort to cause an individual with a mental illness to adhere to treatment as a condition of retaining housing. Similarly, a representative payee or other individual charged with controlling the use of money by a person with mental illness may impose conditions on the use of those resources that include following a treatment regimen. The courts may impose treatment conditions in exchange for placing an individual on probation rather than using incarceration. In addition, there are strategies that may be used to enable a person to exercise prospective control over their treatment, in anticipation of becoming incapacitated and thereby potentially reducing the use of coercion: A primary example is the use of an advance directive, a document permitted in many states by statute that enables a person to state in advance what types or conditions of treatment he or she desires if incapacitation results in the future (62).

While coercion and leverage may be used in many different settings, at present we know little about its use. Some of these issues have been explored, at least preliminarily. For example there has been research into the implementation of outpatient civil commitment statutes in North Carolina and New York (63,64). Mental health courts are increasingly the subject of research as well (65,66). In addition, journals are beginning to devote special issues to the topic of mandated community care, providing an opportunity for research into the use of mandates in a number of community settings to be considered together (67).

At the same time, our understanding of the use of coercion in community care is at an embryonic stage. The importance of the issue for practitioners and policy makers cannot be overstated. Many of the innovations in treatment in the last two decades have depended on expanding individual choice in defining the parameters of treatment (68). Yet our continued reliance on coercion, in a variety of settings and in activities (housing, control of money) that would seem essential to the exercise of choice, may be read as circumscribing unduly the continued expansion of individual choice. This is why it is essential to understand far better than we do the circumstances in which coercion is used, whether and to what degree certain interventions are perceived as coercive by those subject to them, and the ethical and legal questions that continue to swirl around the use of coercion in mental health and substance abuse treatment.

SUMMARY

There have been great strides in our knowledge regarding critical forensic issues such as capacity and risk assessment. In addition, the location of forensic assessment and treatment have changed and are much more likely to occur in the community. As a result, issues that formerly were considered primarily "forensic" issues now lie at the heart of much mental health practice. Practitioners who do not specialize in forensics have had to learn about forensic practice, because issues such as risk are no longer confined to forensic settings.

At the same time, it is useful to step back periodically and examine the types of issues that may define the forensic agenda (and by extension, much of the agenda in mental health policy and practice) in the future. This article suggests that four issues will dominate the agenda, including efforts to better integrate risk and treatment; the impact on system planning from the emergence of special jurisdiction courts such as mental health courts and drug courts; the need to address the continuing impact of conservative social policies particularly in the areas of juvenile justice and sexual predator statutes; and the need to understand the use of coercion in community settings that go far beyond civil commitment issues.

These issues affect practitioners, policy makers, and researchers. Many of these issues are not new. For example, the continuing struggle regarding the proper balance to draw between individual choice and the use of coercive strategies is a struggle that has gone on for decades. However, with the emergence of the consumer/survivor movement, the development of notions of procedural justice and perceived coercion, and the sweep toward more punitive social policies, the debate today may be more urgent and important than it has ever been.

Other issues here are of more recent vintage, for example, the efforts of courts to maintain a therapeutic stance in the face of broad social change that depends heavily on punishment. The assertion of this role has many implications for the role of the courts and of the lawyers representing individuals in such courts. It may also have implications for the mental health practitioner as well, as he or she may become engaged in treatment planning in which courts and lawyers assert a primary role.

Still others of these issues focus on the continuing effort to conform clinical and research knowledge with legal standards. The emerging debate regarding the appropriateness of utilizing adult competency standards to adjudicate juvenile competency illustrates the continuing difficulty of assuring that legal principles and knowledge about human development are congruent.

In all of this, forensic practitioners and policy makers can play a leading role, because of their knowledge of legal process and of the substantive issues (risk, capacity) that continue to be central in today's environment. What is different today is that those interested in forensics can exert influence in an arena that goes far beyond that available three decades ago: Far from being a backwater in the state-operated mental health system, forensics dominates much of the contemporary mental health practice, policy and research agenda.

ACKNOWLEDGMENTS

The author wishes to thank Joel Dvoskin, Ph.D., for his useful comments on earlier drafts of this article.

REFERENCES

1. Steadman H: Insanity acquittals in New York State, 1965-1978. American Journal of Psychiatry 137:321–326, 1980.
2. Monahan J: Predicting violent behavior: An assessment of clinical techniques. London, Sage, 1981.
3. Ennis BJ, Litwack TR: Psychology and the presumption of expertise: Flipping coins in the courtroom. California Law Review 62:671–693, 1974.
4. Bluestone H, Melella, J: A study of criminal defendants referred for competency to stand trial in New York City. Bulletin of The American Academy of Psychiatry and Law 7:166–178, 1979.
5. Petrila, J, Selle, J, Rouse, RC, et al: The pretrial examination process in Missouri: A descriptive study. Bulletin of The American Academy of Psychiatry and Law 9: 60–85, 1981.
6. Jackson v: Indiana, 406 U.S. 715, 1972.
7. Melton G, Petrila J, Poythress N, et al: Psychological Evaluations for the Courts: A Handbook for Mental Health Professionals and Lawyers, 2nd ed. New York, Guilford Press, 1997.
8. Monahan J, Steadman HJ, Silver E, et al: Rethinking Risk Assessment: The MacArthur Study of Mental Disorder and Violence. London, Oxford University Press, 2001.
9. Poythress NG, Nicholson R, Otto RK, et al: MacCAT-CA: The MacArthur Competence Assessment Tool—Criminal Adjudication (Professional Manual). Odessa, FL: Psychological Assessment Resources, 1999.
10. Rogers R, Ustad KL, Sewell KW, et al: Dimensions of incompetency: A factor analytic study of the Georgia court competency test. Behavioral Sciences and the Law 14:323–330, 1996.
11. Webster CD, Douglas KS, Eaves D, et al: HCR-20: Assessing Risk for Violence, Version 2. Burnaby, BC, Simon Fraser University, 1997.
12. Steadman HJ, Silver E, Monahan J, et al: A classification tree approach to the development of actuarial violence risk assessment tools. Law and Human Behavior 24:83–100, 2000.
13. Quinsey VL, Harris GT, Rice ME, et al: Violent offenders: Appraising and Managing risk. Washington DC, American Psychological Association, 1998.
14. Rodgers R: Clinical Assessment of Malingering and Deception, 2nd ed. New York, Guilford Press, 1997.
15. Hare RD: Manual for the Hare Psychopathy Checklist-Revised. Toronto ON, Multi-Health Systems, 1991.

16. Otto RK, Heilbrun K: The practice of forensic psychology: A look toward the future in light of the past. American Psychologist 57:5–18, 2002.
17. Dvoskin JA, Steadman HJ: Using intensive case management to reduce violence by mentally ill persons in the community. Hospital and Community Psychiatry 47:679–684, 1994.
18. Dvoskin JA, Heilbrun K: Risk assessment and release decision-making: Toward resolving the great debate. The Journal of the American Academy of Psychiatry and the Law 29:6–10, 2001.
19. Hodgins S (ed): Violence Among the Mentally Ill: Effective Treatment and Management Strategies. Boston, Kluwer Academic, 2000.
20. Borum R, Otto R: Advances in forensic assessment and treatment. Law and Human Behavior 24:1–7, 2000.
21. Hare R, Clar D, Grann M, et al: Psychopathy and the predictive validity of the PCL-R: An international perspective. Behavioral Sciences and the Law 18:623–645, 2000.
22. Dvoskin J: Knowledge is not power—knowledge is obligation. Journal of the American Academy of Psychiatry and the Law 30:533–540, 2002.
23. Hart S, Cox D, Hare R: Manual for the Psychopathy Checklist: Screening Version (PCL:SV). Toronto, Multi-Health Systems, 1995.
24. Skeem JL, Monahan J, Mulvey EP: Psychopathy, treatment involvement, and subsequent violence among civil psychiatric patients. Law and Human Behavior 26:577–603, 2002.
25. US Department of Justice. Mental Health and Treatment of Inmates and Probationers. Washington DC, Bureau of Justice Statistics, United States Department of Justice, 1999.
26. Dreyfuss RC: The sixth Abraham L. Pomerantz lecture: Forums of the future: The role of specialized courts in resolving business disputes. Brooklyn Law Review 61:1–16, 1995).
27. Petrila J: An introduction to special jurisdiction courts. International Journal of Law and Psychiatry 26:3–12, 2003.
28. Hora PF, Schma WG, Rosenthal JT: Therapeutic jurisprudence and the drug treatment court movement: Revolutionizing the criminal justice system's response to drug abuse and crime in America. Notre Dame Law Review 74:439–537, 1999.
29. Goldkamp JS: The drug court response: Issues and implications for justice change. Albany Law Review 63:923–961, 2000.
30. Maxwell S: Sanction threats in court-ordered programs: Examining their effects on offenders mandated into drug treatment. Crime and Delinquency 46:542–563, 2000.
31. Griffin PA, Steadman HJ, Petrila J: The use of criminal charges and sanctions in mental health courts. Psychiatric Services 53:1285–1289, 2002.
32. Glover R, Petrila J: Can the state mental health agency survive health care reform? Hospital and Community Psychiatry 45:911–913,1994.
33. Geraghyt TF, Drizin SA: Foreword—The debate over the future of juvenile courts: Can we reach consensus? Journal of Criminal Law and Criminology 88:1–13, 1997.
34. Bilchik S: Challenging the myths: 1999 national report series. Juvenile Justice Bulletin. Office of Justice Programs. Office of Juvenile Justice and Delinquency Prevention. Washington DC, United States Department of Justice, 2000.
35. In re Gault, 367 US 1, 1967.
36. Kansas v: Hendricks, 521 US 346, 1997.
37. Redding RE, Frost LE: Adjudicative competence in the modern juvenile court. Virginia Journal of Social Policy and the Law 9:353–409, 2001.

38. Grisso T: The competence of adolescents as trial defendants. Psychology, Public Policy, and Law 3:3–27, 1997.
39. McGaha AC, Otto RK, McClaren MD, et al: Juveniles adjudicated incompetent to proceed: A descriptive study of Florida's competence restoration program. Journal of the American Academy of Psychiatry and Law 29:472–482, 2001.
40. Taylor WC: Golden v State: Should the insanity defense exist in juvenile court? Arkansas Law Review, 54:703–725, 2001.
41. Quinsey VL, Harris GT, Rice ME, et al: Violent offenders: Appraising and managing risk. Washignton, DC, American Psychological Association, 1998.
42. Huot S, The referral process, in The Sexual Predator: Law, Policy, Evaluation, and Treatment. Edited by Schlank A, Cohen F, Kingston NY, Civic Research Institute, 1999.
43. Hanson RK. What do w eknow about sex offender risk assessment? Psychology, Public Policy, and Law 4:50–72, 1998.
44. Washington v. Strauss, 20 P. 3d 1022, 2001.
45. Petrila J, Otto RK. Admissibility of expert testimony in sexually violent predator proceedings. in The Sexual Predator: Legal Issues, Clinical Issues, Special Populations, vol. 2. Edited by Schlank A, Kingston NY, Civic Research Institute, 2001.
46. Wilson JJ. OJJDP Fact Sheet, November 2000, No. 18. Office of Justice Programs. Office of Juvenile Justice and Delinquency Prevention. Washington, DC, United States Department of Justice.
47. Macallair D. Emerging from darkness: Reinventing San Francisco's juvenile justice system. Stanford Law and Policy Review 7:31–39, 1995–1996.
48. Butterfield A. Hard time: A special report: Profits at a juvenile prison come with a chilling cost. New York Times July 15, 1998, Section A, p. 1.
49. Dale MJ. Lawsuits and public policy: The role of litigation in correcting conditions in juvenile detention centers. University of San Francisco Law Review 32:675–733, 1998.
50. Comment: Jimmy Ryce involuntary civil commitment for sexually violent predators' treatment and care act: Replacing criminal justice with civil commitment. Florida State University Law Review 26:487:516, 1999.
51. Walker JC, Freedom is to confinement as twilight is to dusk: The unfortunate logic of sexual predator statutes. University of Missouri Law Review 67:993–1017, 2002.
52. Kanas v. Crane, 534 US 407, 2002.
53. Research Preview: Reintegrating juvenile offenders into the community: OJJDP's intensive community-based aftercare demonstration program. Office of Justice Programs. National Institute of Justice. Washington, DC, United States Department of Justice, December, 1998.
54. Henggler SW, Borduin CM, Schoenwald SK, et al: Multisystemic treatment of antisocial behavior in children and adolescents. New York, Guilford, 1998.
55. Schlank A, Bidelman P: Transition—Challenges for the offender and the community, in The Sexual Predator: Legal Issues, Clinical Issues, Special Populations. Edited by Schlank A, Kingston NY, Civic Research Institute, 2001.
56. Petrila J. From constitution to contracts: Mental disability law at the turn of the century, The Evolution of Mental Health Law. Edited by Frost L, Bonnie, R, Washington DC: American Psychological Association, 2001.
57. Tyler TR. The psychological consequences of judicial processes: Implications for civil commitment hearings. Southern Methodist Law Review 46:433–445, 1992.
58. Gardner W, Hoge SK, Bennett N, et al: Two scales for measuring patients' perceptions of coercion during mental hospital admission. Behavioral Sciences and the Law 11:307–321, 1993.

59. Lidz C, Hoge S, Gardner W, et al: Perceived coercion in mental hospital admissions: Pressures and process. Archives of General Psychiatry 52:1034–1039, 1995.
60. Ridgely MS, Borum R, Petrila J: The effectiveness of involuntary outpatient treatment: Empirical evidence and the experience of eight states. Santa Monica CA, RAND Institute for Civil Justice, 2001.
61. Monahan J, Bonnie R, Appelbaum P, et al: Mandated community treatment: Beyond outpatient commitment. Psychiatric Services 52:1198–1205, 2001.
62. Swanson J, Swartz M, Hannon M, et al: Psychiatric advance directives: A survey of persons with schizophrenia, family members, and treatment providers. International Journal of Forensic Mental Health 2:73–86, 2003.
63. Swartz MS, Swanson JW, Hiday VA, et al: A randomized controlled trial of outpatient commitment in North Carolina. Psychiatric Services 52:325–329, 2001.
64. Steadman HJ, Gounis K, Dennis D, et al: Assessing the New York City involuntary outpatient commitment pilot program. Psychiatric Services 52:330–336, 2001.
65. Trupin E, Richards H. Seattle's mental health courts: Early indicators of effectiveness. International Journal of Law and Psychiatry 26:33–53, 2003.
66. Mcgaha A, Boothroyd, RA, Poythress NG, et al: Lessons from the Broward county mental health court evaluation. Evaluation and Program Planning 25:125–135, 2002.
67. Petrila J, Monahan J. An introduction to the special issue on mandated community treatment. Behavioral Sciences and the Law in press.
68. Anthony W. Psychiatric Rehabilitation, 2nd ed. Boston MA, Boston University Center for Psychiatric Rehabilitation, 2001.

Name Index